Inderbir Singh's Textbook of
HUMAN OSTEOLOGY
With Atlas of Muscle Attachments

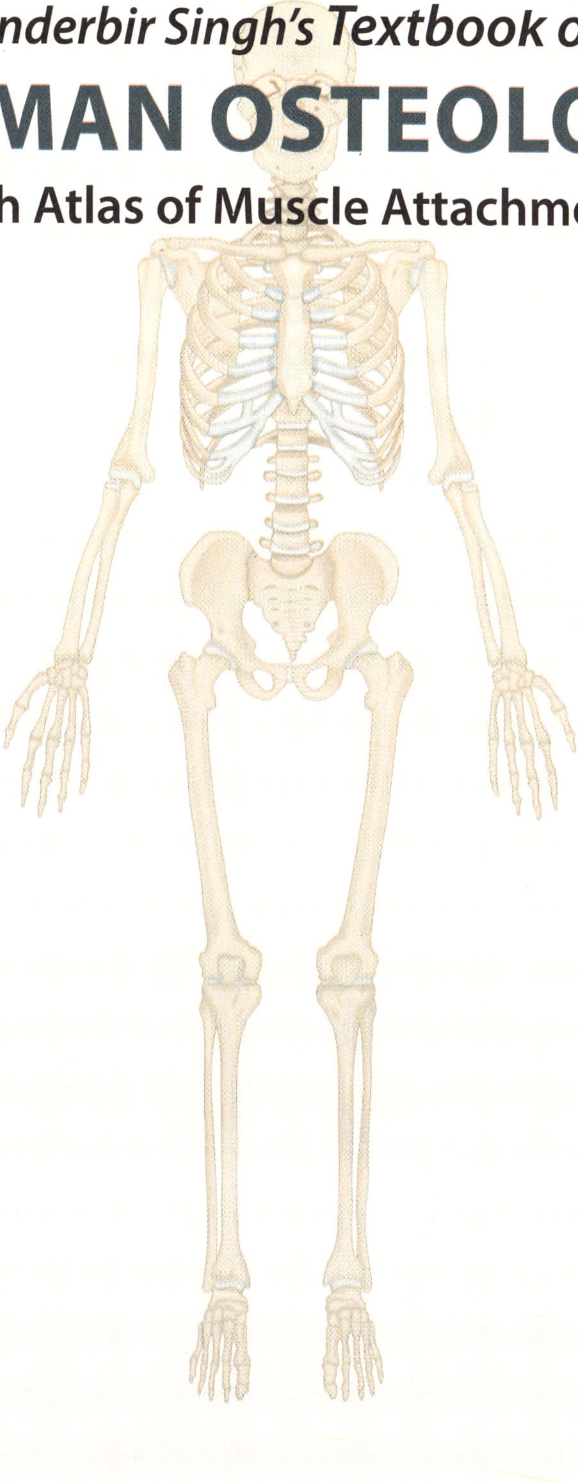

Inderbir Singh's Textbook of
HUMAN OSTEOLOGY
With Atlas of Muscle Attachments

As per the Competency-based Medical Education Curriculum (NMC)

Fifth Edition

Revised and Edited by

Brig (Dr) Sushil Kumar MBBS MS
Commandant, MH Mathura
Ex-Professor and Head
Department of Anatomy
Armed Forces Medical College
Pune, Maharashtra, India

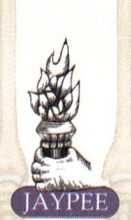

JAYPEE BROTHERS MEDICAL PUBLISHERS
The Health Sciences Publisher
New Delhi | London

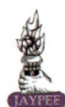

Jaypee Brothers Medical Publishers (P) Ltd

Headquarter

Jaypee Brothers Medical Publishers (P) Ltd
EMCA House, 23/23-B
Ansari Road, Daryaganj
New Delhi - 110 002, India
Landline: +91-11-23272143,+91-11-23272703,
+91-11-23282021,+91-11-23245672
Email: jaypee@jaypeebrothers.com

Corporate Office

Jaypee Brothers Medical Publishers (P) Ltd
4838/24, Ansari Road, Daryaganj
New Delhi 110 002, India
Phone: +91-11-43574357
Fax: +91-11-43574314
Email: jaypee@jaypeebrothers.com

Overseas Office

J.P. Medical Ltd
83 Victoria Street, London
SW1H 0HW (UK)
Phone: +44 20 3170 8910
Fax: +44 (0)20 3008 6180
Email: info@jpmedpub.com

Website: www.jaypeebrothers.com
Website: www.jaypeedigital.com

© 2023, Jaypee Brothers Medical Publishers

The views and opinions expressed in this book are solely those of the original contributor(s)/author(s) and do not necessarily represent those of editor(s) and publishers of the book.

All rights reserved. No part of this publication may be reproduced, stored or transmitted in any form or by any means, electronic, mechanical, photocopying, recording or otherwise, without the prior permission in writing of the publishers/editors.

All brand names and product names used in this book are trade names, service marks, trademarks or registered trademarks of their respective owners. The publisher is not associated with any product or vendor mentioned in this book.

Medical knowledge and practice change constantly. This book is designed to provide accurate, authoritative information about the subject matter in question. However, readers are advised to check the most current information available on procedures included and check information from the manufacturer of each product to be administered, to verify the recommended dose, formula, method and duration of administration, adverse effects and contraindications. It is the responsibility of the practitioner to take all appropriate safety precautions. Neither the publisher nor the author(s)/editor(s) assume any liability for any injury and/or damage to persons or property arising from or related to use of material in this book.

This book is sold on the understanding that the publisher is not engaged in providing professional medical services. If such advice or services are required, the services of a competent medical professional should be sought.

Every effort has been made where necessary to contact holders of copyright to obtain permission to reproduce copyright material. If any have been inadvertently overlooked, the publisher will be pleased to make the necessary arrangements at the first opportunity.

Inquiries for bulk sales may be solicited at: jaypee@jaypeebrothers.com

Inderbir Singh's Textbook of Human Osteology

First Edition: 1990;   Reprints: 1994, 1996, 1997, 2000

Second Edition: 2002;   Reprints: 2005, 2006

Third Edition: 2009;   Reprint: 2011

Fourth Edition: 2019

Fifth Edition: **2023**

ISBN 978-93-5465-177-9

Printed at Rajkamal Electric Press, Kundli, Haryana.

Dedicated to...

The all pervading presence of Almighty,
Benevolences of our revered Gurus,
Blessings of our respected teachers,
Care of our parents,
Affection of our understanding family members,
Best wishes of our inspiring friends,
and
Impetus of our adorable students
have made it possible to present this
humble offering.

Preface to the Fifth Edition

Study of osteology should be viewed in proper perspective. Osteology forms the base around which most of the anatomical facts are built. Thus, to comprehend regional anatomy, it is essential that the relevant bones are taught before or during gross anatomy lectures and/or dissection. The methodology to study the bones should be imbibed so as to act as a tool to take on bigger challenges.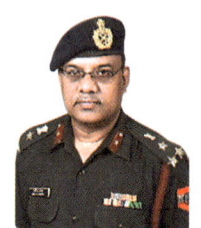

The casual approach to learn osteology to be addressed. In most medical colleges, osteology tutorials/demonstrations are covered by tutors or PG residents without much effort to generate interest in the students. The problem is further compounded by the inadequate number of bones provided in the class and the paucity of the diagrams drawn by the teacher. The student who has been exposed to this "small group teaching" finds it difficult to understand. Exasperation leads to procrastination and the base of anatomy gets a lower priority than what it deserves. To give structured text with diagrams and comprehensive tables takes care of most of the requirements of the students. This is precisely the aim of this book.

The *Textbook of Human Osteology* by Professor IB Singh was last published in 2009 (3rd edition) with subsequent reprint in 2011. This iconic and one of the best books in osteology was revived, thoroughly revised and edited book was republished in 2019 (4th edition) which was very well received by the students and faculty across the country.

The 5th edition of this book has been thoroughly revised and edited with an additional chapter on the Introduction to Osteology with added text at appropriate places and assigned competency number as given in the NMC directives. Thus, each bone and its sub-sections are shown with competency number and learning objectives. This is presented in a structured manner, amply supported with relevant diagrams and numerous tables for better understanding and easy recall. In addition, brief account of important clinical considerations with images provided at the end of the chapter will generate interest and instill a sense of purpose studying osteology. The questionnaire provided would be of great help for students to prepare for their viva-voce examinations.

I would like to place on record sincere thank to Dr Madhu Choudhary (Director–Educational Publishing) and their entire team, for their tireless efforts for the painstaking graphic artwork and text executed meticulously in bringing out this textbook to the utmost satisfying level.

I gratefully acknowledge Shri Jitendar P Vij (Group Chairman), Mr Ankit Vij (Managing Director), Mr MS Mani (Group President) and Ms Pooja Bhandari (Production Head) of M/s Jaypee Brothers Medical Publishers (P) Ltd, New Delhi, India, for reposing faith to revive and bringing out this standard textbook of osteology in its new avatar.

This *Textbook of Human Osteology* in its new avatar is a sincere tribute to Professor Inderbir Singh, legendary anatomist and medical teacher par excellence.

As teaching learning process is the continuous process the suggestions for the improvements for this book are more than welcome.

Happy Reading.......

Brig (Dr) Sushil Kumar

Preface to the First Edition

A sound knowledge of osteology continues to be fundamental to an understanding of the gross anatomy of the body. Traditionally, students in India have read osteology from large imported textbooks. However, in recent years, fewer and fewer students have had access to such texts. Further, with the changes in English usage in Western countries, our students are finding it increasingly difficult to follow these books. Most teachers of anatomy have felt the need for a complete, well-illustrated book on the subject. This book has been produced to fulfill this need.

This book has been written to meet the requirement of MBBS students. However, the matter should suffice for postgraduate students as well. For the benefit of the latter, sections on individual bones of the hands, the feet, and of the skull are included.

It is a pleasure to acknowledge the help in proofreading given by Dr (Mrs) Usha Dhall, and Dr SK Srivastava of the Department of Anatomy, Medical College, Rohtak, Haryana, India.

I shall welcome suggestions for improvement.

Inderbir Singh

Contents

1. **Introduction to Osteology** — 1
   - Anatomical Terminology — 1
   - General Features of Bones and Joints — 4
   - Cartilage (Gristle) — 6
   - Joints — 7
   - Fibrous Joints (Fixed/Synarthrosis) — 8
   - Cartilaginous Joints (Slightly Movable/Amphiarthroses) — 10
   - Synovial Joints (Freely Movable/Diarthroses) — 11

2. **Introduction to Skeleton** — 13
   - Preliminary Review of the Skull — 13
   - Vertebral Column — 14
   - Skeleton of the Thorax — 14
   - Skeleton of the Upper Limb — 15
   - Skeleton of the Lower Limb — 16

3. **Bones of Upper Limb** — 18
   - Clavicle (Collar Bone) — 18
   - Scapula (Shoulder Blade) — 23
   - Humerus (Arm Bone) — 30
   - Radius — 37
   - Ulna — 43
   - Skeleton of the Hand — 50
   - Movements at Major Upper Limb Joints — 65
   - **Atlas of Muscle Attachments: Upper Limb** — **69**

4. **Bones of Lower Limb** — 105
   - The Hip Bone — 105
   - The Femur — 116
   - The Patella (Knee Cap) — 124
   - The Tibia — 126
   - The Fibula — 135
   - The Skeleton of the Foot — 141
   - Movements at Major Lower Limb Joints — 160
   - **Atlas of Muscle Attachments: Lower Limb** — **163**

5. **Sternum and Ribs** — 207
   - The Sternum — 207
   - Typical Ribs — 213
   - Atypical Ribs — 216
   - Costal Cartilages (Hyaline Cartilage) — 223
   - **Atlas of Muscle Attachments: Thorax and Abdomen** — **225**

- **6. Vertebral Column** — **234**
  - Typical Vertebra — 234
  - Atypical Cervical Vertebrae — 243
  - Atypical Thoracic Vertebrae — 249
  - Lumbar Vertebrae — 252
  - Atypical Lumbar Vertebra — 252
  - Sacrum — 255
  - Coccyx — 258
  - Bony Pelvis — 261

7. **Bones of Head and Neck** — **268**
   - The Skull — 268
   - Skull from Above (Norma Verticalis) — 276
   - Skull from the Front (Norma Frontalis) — 277
   - Bony Orbit — 281
   - Skull from Behind (Norma Occipitalis) — 284
   - Skull from Lateral Side (Norma Lateralis) — 284
   - Skull from Below (Norma Basalis) — 293
   - Cranial Fossae — 300
   - Nasal Cavity — 311
   - Fetal Skull — 316

8. **Individual Bones of Skull** — **322**
   - Mandible — 322
   - Maxilla — 329
   - Zygomatic Bone — 333
   - Frontal Bone — 334
   - Parietal Bone — 337
   - Occipital Bone — 340
   - Temporal Bone — 342
   - Sphenoid Bone — 348
   - Palatine Bone — 351
   - Ethmoid Bone — 353
   - Lacrimal Bone — 354
   - Nasal Bone — 355
   - The Vomer — 355
   - Inferior Nasal Concha — 356
   - Hyoid Bone — 356

   Atlas of Muscle Attachments: Head and Neck — **360**

Index — 373

Competency Table

Number	COMPETENCY The student should be able to	Core (Y/N)	Chapter Number	Page Number
AN 1.1	Demonstrate normal anatomical position, various planes, relation, comparison, laterality and movement in our body	Y	1	1
AN 1.2	Describe composition of bone and bone marrow	Y	1	4
AN 2.1	Describe parts, blood and nerve supply of a long bone	Y	1	4
AN 2.2	Enumerate laws of ossification	N	1	6
AN 2.3	Enumerate special features of a sesamoid bone	N	1	6
AN 2.4	Describe various types of cartilage with its structure and distribution in body	Y	1	6
AN 2.5	Describe various joints with subtypes and examples	Y	1	7
AN 2.6	Explain the concept of nerve supply of joints and Hilton's law	Y	1	12
AN 8.1	Identify the given bone, its side, important features and keep it in anatomical position	Y	3	18
AN 8.2	Identify and describe joints formed by the given bone	Y	3	18
AN 8.3	Enumerate peculiarities of clavicle	Y	3	18
AN 8.4	Demonstrate important muscle attachment on the given bone	Y	3	18
AN 8.5	Identify and name various bones in articulated hand, specify the parts of metacarpals and phalanges and enumerate the peculiarities of pisiform	Y	3	50, 53, 56
AN 8.6	Describe scaphoid fracture and explain the anatomical basis of avascular necrosis	N	3	51
AN 13.4	Describe sternoclavicular joint, acromioclavicular joint, carpometacarpal joints and metacarpophalangeal joint	N	3 5	22, 60, 65, 208
AN 14.1	Identify the given bone, its side, important features and keep it in anatomical position	Y	4	105
AN 14.2	Identify and describe joints formed by the given bone	Y	4	105
AN 14.3	Describe the importance of ossification of lower end of femur and upper end of tibia	Y	4	120
AN 14.4	Identify and name various bones in the articulated foot with individual muscle attachment	N	4	105
AN 20.1	Describe and demonstrate the type, articular surfaces, capsule, synovial membrane, ligaments, relations, movements and muscles involved, blood and nerve supply of tibiofibular and ankle joint	Y	4	132
AN 20.2	Describe the subtalar and transverse tarsal joints	N	4	145, 147
AN 21.1	Identify and describe the salient features of sternum, typical rib, 1st rib and typical thoracic vertebra	Y	5 6	207, 213, 216, 234
AN 21.2	Identify and describe the features of 2nd, 11th and 12th ribs, 1st, 11th and 12th thoracic vertebrae	N	6	249
AN 21.8	Describe and demonstrate type, articular surfaces and movements of manubriosternal, costovertebral, costotransverse and xiphisternal joints	Y	5	211, 216

Competency Table

Number	COMPETENCY The student should be able to	Core (Y/N)	Chapter Number	Page Number
AN 21.10	Describe costochondral and interchondral joints	N	5	216
AN 21.11	Mention boundaries and contents of the superior, anterior, middle and posterior mediastinum	Y	5	208
AN 26.1	Demonstrate anatomical position of skull, identify and locate individual skull bones in skull	Y	7	268
AN 26.2	Describe the features of norma frontalis, verticalis, occipitalis, lateralis and basalis	Y	7	268
AN 26.3	Describe cranial cavity, its subdivisions, foramina and structures passing through them	Y	7	272
AN 26.4	Describe morphological features of mandible	Y	8	322
AN 26.5	Describe features of typical and atypical cervical vertebrae (atlas and axis)	Y	6	243
AN 26.6	Explain the concept of bones that ossify in membrane	N	6	248
AN 26.7	Describe the features of the 7th cervical vertebra	N	6	247
AN 30.1	Describe the cranial fossae and identify related structures	Y	7	300
AN 30.2	Describe and identify major foramina with structures passing through them	Y	7	305
AN 43.1	Describe and demonstrate the movements with muscles producing the movements of atlantooccipital joint and atlantoaxial joint	Y	6	246
AN 50.1	Describe the curvatures of the vertebral column	Y	6	241
AN 50.2	Describe and demonstrate the type, articular ends, ligaments and movements of intervertebral joints, sacroiliac joints and pubic symphysis	Y	6	241, 257
AN 51.1	Describe and identify the cross-section at the level of T8, T10 and L1 (transpyloric plane)	Y	6	242
AN 53.2	Demonstrate the anatomical position of bony pelvis and show boundaries of pelvic inlet, pelvic cavity, pelvic outlet	Y	6	260
AN 53.3	Define true pelvis and false pelvis and demonstrate sex determination in male and female bony pelvis	Y	6	262
AN 53.4	Explain and demonstrate clinical importance of bones of abdominopelvic region (sacralization of lumbar vertebra, lumbarization of 1st sacral vertebra, types of bony pelvis and coccyx)	N	6	252, 265

CHAPTER 1: Introduction to Osteology

AN1.1 Demonstrate normal anatomical position, various planes, relation, comparison, laterality and movements in our body.

ANATOMICAL TERMINOLOGY

Body Positions (Fig 1.1)

Anatomical position: Person is standing erect, with the arms by the sides of trunk and the palms facing forward. The lower limbs are joined together with the toes pointing forward. The face is directed forwards and the eyes look straight to the horizon.

Supine position: Body in recumbent position; lying down with the face directed upwards.

Prone position: Body in recumbent position; lying down with the face directed downwards.

Lithotomy position: Body in supine position with buttocks at the edge of the examination table. The hips and knees are flexed and thighs are wide apart. It is used in vaginal deliveries and perineal surgeries.

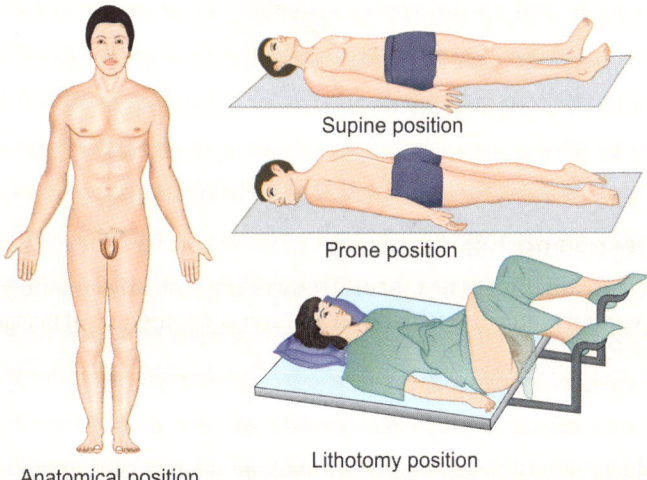

Fig. 1.1: Anatomical positions.

Anatomical Planes of Reference (Fig. 1.2)

Sagittal plane: This imaginary vertical plane (*after sagittal suture of skull*) passes longitudinally through the body; divides it into right and left equal halves.

Coronal plane (*frontal plane: after coronal suture of skull*): Vertical plane that intersects sagittal plane at right angle; separates the body into anterior and posterior parts.

Horizontal plane: This plane at right angle to both sagittal and coronal planes separates body into upper and lower parts.

Transverse plane: It passes at right angle to the longitudinal axis of a structure. Thus, a transverse section through an artery is not necessarily horizontal. A transverse section through the hand is horizontal, whereas a transverse section through the foot is coronal.

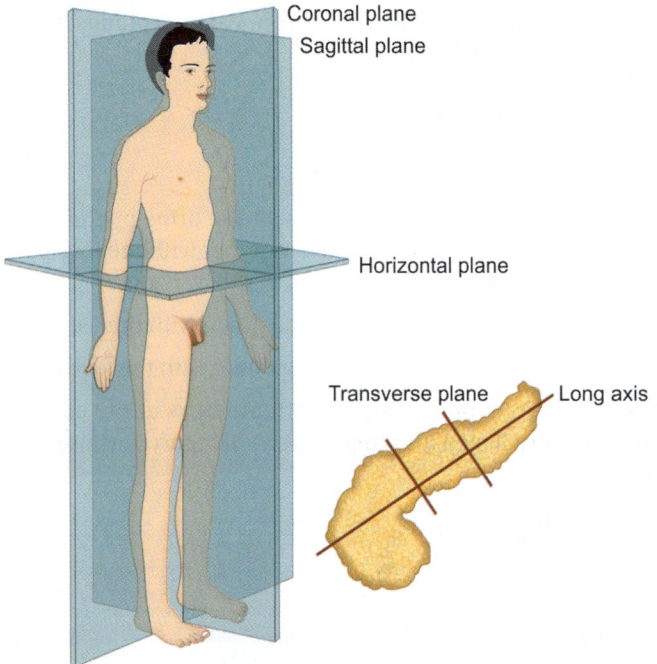

Fig. 1.2: Planes of reference.

Movements (Figs. 1.3 and 1.4)

Flexion: It is the approximation of flexor surfaces whereby the angle of the joint is reduced. It takes place in the sagittal plane. It is usually an anterior movement; but occasionally posterior, e.g., flexion at knee joint.

Extension: To extend is to stretch out or to straighten (*opposite of flexion*). Here the angle at the joint is increased. It usually takes place in a posterior direction.

Lateral flexion: Movement of the trunk in a coronal plane; may be right or left lateral flexion.

Adduction: Movement towards the median plane (*central axis*).

Abduction: It is the movement away from the median plane (*central axis*).

Circumduction: Movements of flexion, abduction, extension and adduction in a sequence.

Rotation: Movement of a part of the body around its long axis. In *medial rotation* the anterior surface of the part faces medially (internal rotation). In *lateral rotation* anterior surface of the part faces laterally (external rotation).

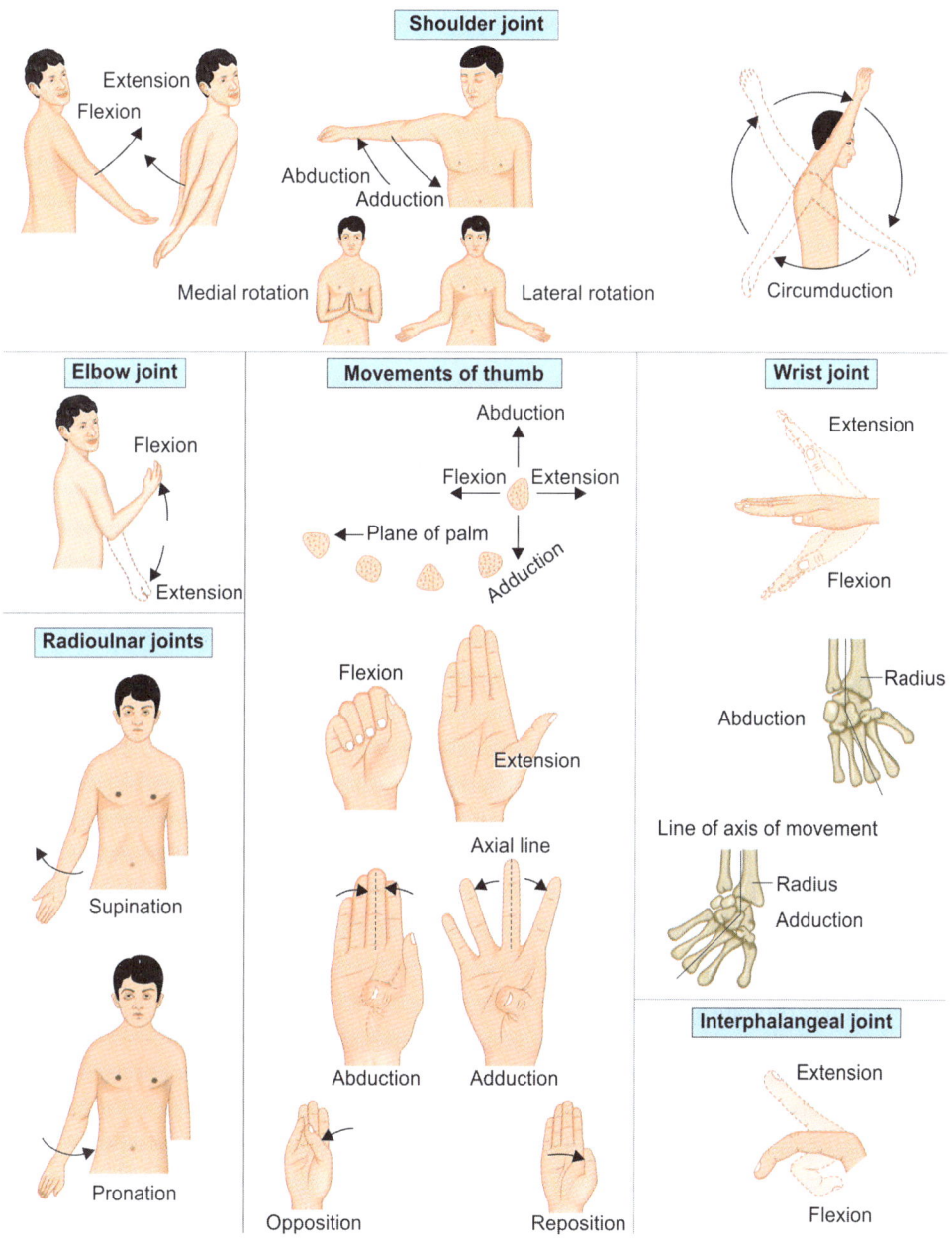

Fig. 1.3: Movements.

Supination: It is the lateral rotation of forearm from the pronated position, so that the palm faces anteriorly.

Pronation: It is the medial rotation of forearm resulting in the palm to face posteriorly.

Inversion: In this movement medial border of foot is raised and the sole faces inwards.

Eversion: Opposite to inversion where lateral border of foot is raised and sole faces outwards.

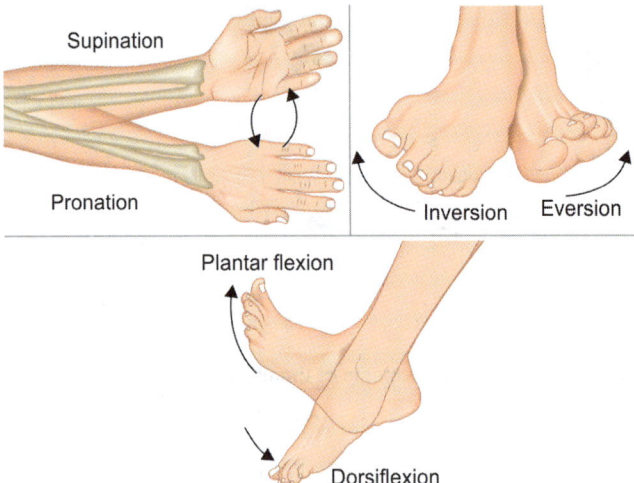

Fig. 1.4: Special movements.

GENERAL FEATURES OF BONES AND JOINTS

AN 1.2 Describe composition of bone and bone marrow.

AN 2.1 Describe parts, blood and nerve supply of a long bone.

The bone (*osseous tissue*) is a rigid form of connective tissue consisting of cells and specialized connective tissue covering called the periosteum. Three cell types (*osteoblasts, osteocytes and osteoclasts*) are noted. **Osteoblasts** are associated with bone formation; found in relation to bone surface where osseous matrix is being deposited. **Osteocytes** (*bone cells*) are trapped osteoblasts within bone matrix. **Osteoclasts** (*multinucleated giant cells*) are involved in bone resorption.

Bone matrix comprises organic and inorganic components. **Organic portion** (35% of weight of bone) is mainly composed of *osteocollagenous fibers* (difficult to see in H&E preparation). It makes bone tough and resilient that can afford resistance to tensile forces. **Inorganic portion** (65% of weight of bone) is composed of minerals mainly as crystals of calcium phosphate and partly calcium carbonate and other salts. It makes bone hard and rigid that can afford resistance to compressive forces. The bone matrix is arranged characteristically in lamellae. These result from concentrically deposited matrix. The fibres in any lamella are parallel to each other and take a spiral loop.

Periosteum (fibrous sheath) envelops bone except articular surfaces. It consists of two layers. The outer layer is composed of dense fibrous tissue, containing network of blood vessels. The inner layer contains spindle shaped connective tissue cells (*osteoprogenitor cells*) which on stimulation become activated as seen in fracture.

Endosteum (delicate layer lining marrow cavities) consists of condensed reticular tissue with both osteogenic and hemopoietic potencies.

Parts of a Long Bone (Fig. 1.6)

At birth, both ends of a long bone are cartilaginous. The part of bone between cartilaginous ends is *diaphysis*. There is a casing of compact bone, enclosing a medullary cavity. Before ossification is completed, the following parts are seen:

a. **Epiphysis** is bone end that ossifies from the secondary center. They are of following types: ***Pressure epiphysis*** is articular and takes part in weight transmission (head of humerus, condyles of femur). ***Traction epiphysis*** is non-articular and does not take part in weight transmission. It develops at the sites of attachments of certain tendons (trochanters of femur, tubercles of humerus). ***Atavistic epiphysis*** is phylogenetically separate bone (independent) but during evolution has fused with other bone (coracoid process of scapula). ***Aberrant epiphysis*** is not always present (epiphysis at head of 1st metacarpal) (**Fig. 1.5**).

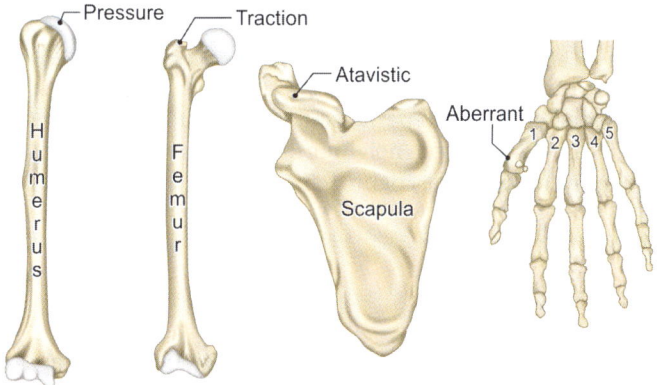

Fig. 1.5: Types of epiphyses.

b. **Diaphysis** is the elongated shaft that develops from one primary center of ossification.
c. **Metaphysis** is the epiphyseal end of diaphysis; zone of active growth. Before epiphyseal fusion, it is richly supplied by blood vessels through end arteries.
d. **Epiphyseal plate of cartilage** separates epiphysis from metaphysis. Proliferation of cells here are responsible for lengthwise growth of bone. After epiphyseal fusion, bone no longer grows in length. The epiphyseal fusion is earlier in females compared to males.

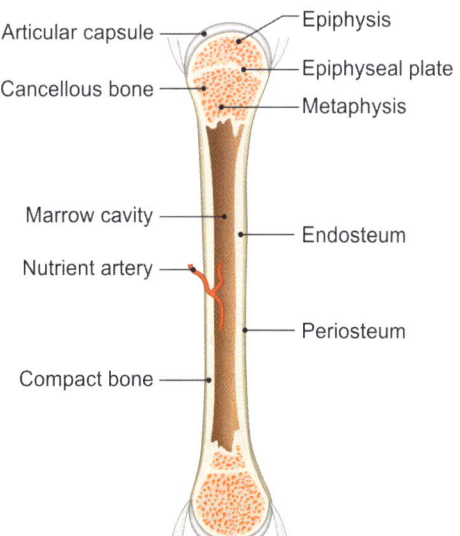

Fig. 1.6: Parts of long bone.

Blood Supply of a Long Bone

It is supplied by many sources that include:

Nutrient artery is the main artery of shaft (*medullary artery*) that enters bone through nutrient foramen and runs obliquely through the cortex. After entering, it divides into ascending and descending branches in medullary cavity. Each branch further subdivides into many small parallel channels that terminate in adult metaphysis. It supplies medullary cavity, inner two third of cortex and metaphysis.

Periosteal twigs enter shaft at many points. These run in small longitudinal (*Haversian*) canals and supply outer 1/3rd of the cortex.

Twigs from articular arteries are derived from epiphyseal and metaphyseal arteries:
- *Epiphyseal arteries* are derived from periarticular vascular arcade (*circulus vasculosus*).
- *Metaphyseal arteries* are derived from neighboring arteries which pass directly to metaphysis and reinforce metaphyseal branches of nutrient artery.

Laws of Ossification

AN 2.2 Enumerate laws of ossification.

Laws of ossification are as under:
- Bone develops from one primary center (*prenatal*) and many secondary centers (*postnatal*) of ossification (exception being clavicle which develops from two primary centers)
- Secondary center for growing end appears first and fuses last (except fibula).

Sesamoid Bones (*Arabic: seed like*)

AN 2.3 Enumerate special features of sesamoid bones.

These are nodules of bones that develop in certain tendons. Special features include:
- Periosteum is absent, hence no regeneration
- Free surface is covered with articular cartilage
- Postnatal development (*appear after birth*).

Functional aspects:
a) Minimize friction
b) Alter direction of pull of muscle
c) Resist pressure
d) Maintain local circulation.

Examples: Patella (*largest sesamoid bone*), pisiform, fabella, etc.

CARTILAGE (GRISTLE)

AN 2.4 Describe various types of cartilage with its structure and distribution in body.

It is a connective tissue where a solid ground substance (more resilient than bone) forms the matrix. It is composed of cells (*chondrocytes*) and fibers (*collagen or yellow elastic*) embedded in a firm gel-like matrix rich in mucopolysaccharides.

Features (Fig. 1.7)
- No blood vessels or lymphatics; nutrition diffuses through matrix
- No nerves thus insensitive to pain

- ❖ Surrounded by perichondrium; similar to periosteum
- ❖ When calcified, chondrocytes die; cartilage is replaced by bone.
1. **Hyaline cartilage:** It is white and resilient (potential bone). All bones (*except clavicle and certain skull bones*) are performed in hyaline cartilage. It persists in adult life at articular ends of bones as articular cartilage, sternal ends of ribs as costal cartilage and cartilages of nose, trachea, bronchi and larynx.
2. **Fibrocartilage:** It has same structure as fibrous tissue with addition of cartilage ground substance. Whenever fibrous tissue is subjected to great pressure, it is replaced by fibrocartilage that is tough, strong and resilient. It appears white and opaque due to abundance of dense collagen fibers. Example: intervertebral discs, articular discs (*menisci of knee joint*), etc.
3. **Elastic cartilage:** Here, the cartilage cells are numerous and the solid ground work is pervaded by yellow elastic fibers, making it more pliable. It maintains the shape of the structure while allowing considerable flexibility. It is found in external ear, small cartilages guarding entrance of the larynx.

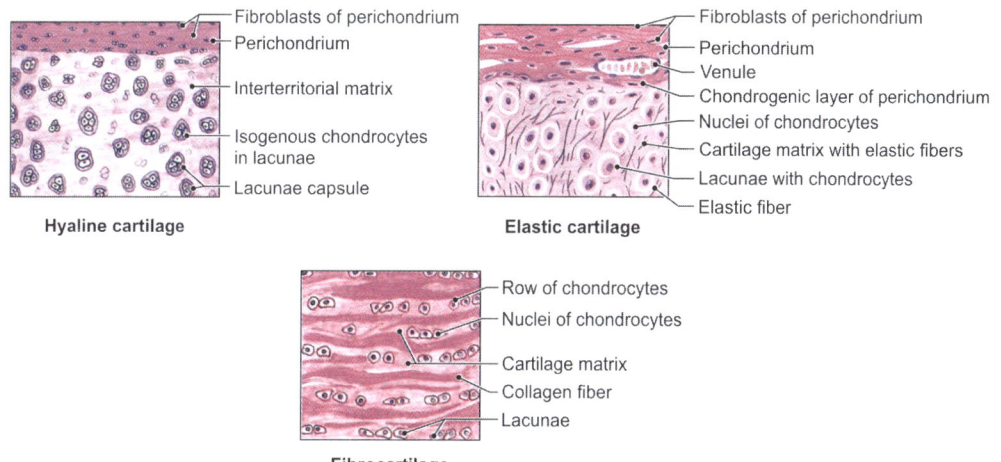

Fig. 1.7: The cartilages.

JOINTS

AN 2.5 Describe various joints with subtypes and examples.

A joint (*articulation*) said to exist whenever two or more bones or cartilages meet. Thus a joint is a junction between bones or cartilages. These permit movements while the immovable joints are meant for growth (permit molding during childbirth).

Classification of Joints

Structural	Functional	Regional
On the basis of intervening tissue	On the basis of movements permitted	On the basis of location
Fibrous	Synarthroses (immovable), e.g., Fibrous joints	Skull type (immovable)

Structural	Functional	Regional
Cartilaginous	Amphiarthroses (slightly movable), e.g., Cartilaginous joints	Vertebral type (slightly movable)
Synovial	Diarthroses (freely movable), e.g., Synovial joints	Limb type (freely movable)

Classification of Joints and Subtypes

Fibrous Fixed (Synarthroses)	Cartilaginous Slightly movable (Amphiarthroses)	Synovial Freely movable (Diarthroses)
Types	Types	Types

1. Sutures
  a. Plane
  b. Squamous
  c. Limbous
  d. Serrate
  e. Dentate
	Primary cartilaginous joints (Synchondroses)
	
	Secondary cartilaginous joints (Syndesmoses)
		a. Plane
		b. Hinge
		c. Pivot
		d. Condylar
		e. Ellipsoid
		f. Saddle

2. Gomphosis		
3. Syndesmosis		
4. Schindylesis		

FIBROUS JOINTS (FIXED/SYNARTHROSIS)

They are generally limited to skull. They are of following varieties:
1. **Sutures:** Skull bones are lined outside by pericranium and inside by endocranium (*outer layer of dura mater*). These membranes pass across from one bone to other and unite them. Some fibrous tissue intervenes that passes from one side to the other; continues with pericranium called *sutural ligament*. Part of this ligament that lies near bone ends is cellular and contains osteogenic cells. In young subjects, these cells lay down new bone and help skull to grow. Sutures start disappearing (*by bone fusion*) around 30 years of age. Fusion starts on inner surface and gradually extends to outer surface (**Fig. 1.8**).
Functions:
   - Provide slight perinatal flexibility in some locations
   - Essential structural mechanism for sutural bone growth
   - Provide rigidity and geometry in the upper neurocranium, nasofacial and palatine skeleton
      a. *Plane suture:* In this there is simple apposition of contiguous surfaces which are usually rough and reciprocally irregular. Example: Intermaxillary, interpalatine, palatomaxillary sutures.
      b. *Squamous suture:* Adjacent bone surfaces are reciprocally bevelled. Example: Anterior squamous, anterior temporal and parietal sutures.
      c. *Limbus suture:* Adjacent bone surfaces are reciprocally bevelled and mutually ridged or serrated. Example: Posterior squamous suture, posterior temporal and parietal sutures.

d. ***Serrate suture:*** Edges are like serrations of a saw. Example: Sagittal and corona sutures.
e. ***Dentate suture***: Edges have small tooth projections; often widen towards their ends to provide even more effective interlocking. Example: Lambdoid suture.

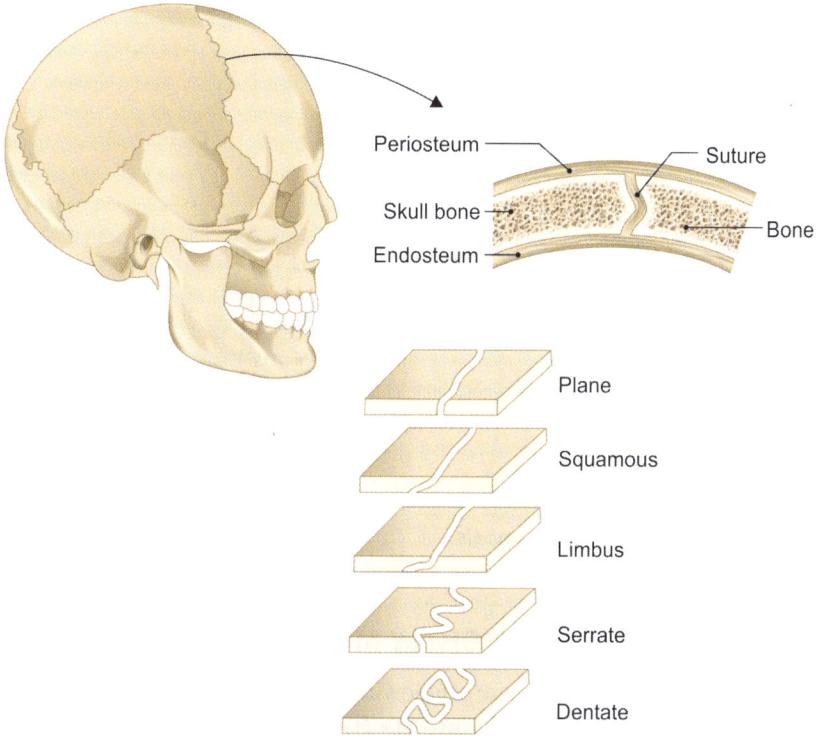

Fig. 1.8: Sutures.

2. **Schindylesis (Fig. 1.9):** This is wedge and groove type of joint. Ex: Rostrum of sphenoid and ala of vomer.
3. **Gomphosis (Peg and socket joint) (Fig. 1.9):** The cavity in the jaw and root of teeth are connected by some fibrous tissue; collagen of periodontium connects dental cement (alveolar bone). Example: Joint between tooth and jaw (alveolar socket).
4. **Syndesmosis (Fig. 1.9):** Here bony surfaces are bound together by an interosseous ligament, slender fibrous cord or an aponeurotic membrane. This usually allows slight but occasionally more extensive movement between them. The ligament is mainly made up of collagen fibers but may contain elastic fibers.
Examples include: Inferior tibiofibular joint, dorsal part of sacroiliac junction, interosseous membrane and oblique cord of forearm and interosseous membrane and anterior and posterior tibiofibular ligaments of leg, etc. Syndesmoses also include pterygospinous, stylohyoid, interspinous and intertransverse joints with ligamentum flava and ligamentum nuchae.

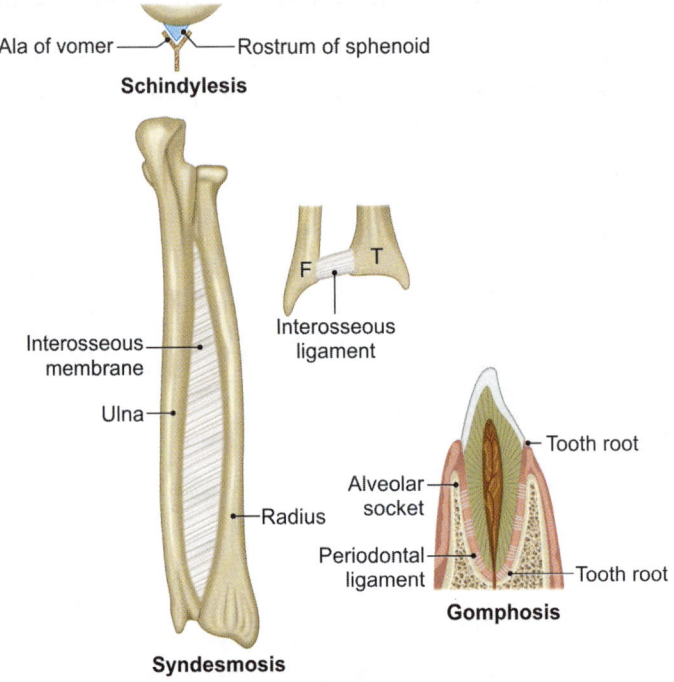

Fig. 1.9: Schindylesis, gomphosis and syndesmosis.

CARTILAGINOUS JOINTS (SLIGHTLY MOVABLE/AMPHIARTHROSES)

The bones are united by cartilage. They are of following types:

1. **Primary cartilaginous joint (*Synchondrosis/Hyaline cartilage joint*) (Fig. 1.10)**
   The bones are united by a plate of hyaline cartilage (two ossifying ends are closely bonded by a specialized hyaline growth cartilage). The joint is immovable but strong. It is temporary because cartilage plate is replaced by bone later (*synostosis*). Functionally synchondrosis is primarily a growth mechanism although they also contribute to slightly more flexible skeleton in youth (*resist: forces, compression, tension shear or torsion*).
   Example: Joints between diaphysis and epiphysis, neurocentral synchondrosis, first costochondral joint

2. **Secondary cartilaginous joint (*Symphysis/Fibrocartilaginous joint*) (Fig. 1.10)**
   The bone ends forming such joints are covered with a thin layer of hyaline cartilage; united by an intervening layer of fibrocartilage. The ligaments join the bones; but capsule is absent. These joints are permanent; persist throughout life. They are typically seen in midline. They permit

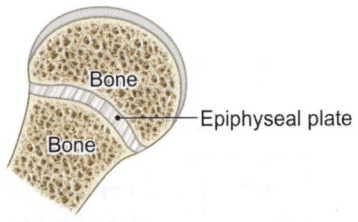

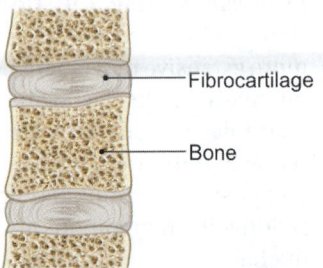

Fig. 10: Cartilaginous joints.

limited movements due to compressible pad of fibrocartilage, thickness of which is directly proportional to the range of movements. These joints represent an intermediate stage in the evolution of synovial joints. Example: joints between bodies of vertebrae, pubic symphysis, etc.

SYNOVIAL JOINTS (FREELY MOVABLE/DIARTHROSES)

These are most evolved and most mobile joints in the body. The bony ends are not directly connected by any tissue and have smooth articular surfaces covered with hyaline or articular cartilages (**Fig. 1.11**). The bones are held together by articular (*fibrous*) capsule made up of fibrous tissue enclosing the articular surfaces in a joint cavity. Inside of the capsule is lined by the synovial membrane that is absent over articular surfaces. The joint cavity is filled with synovial fluid (*lubricating and nutritive functions*). The capsule is richly innervated; sensitive to stretches imposed by movements. The capsule is reinforced by ligaments. *True ligaments* represent thickening of fibrous capsule (intracapsular or extracapsular). *Accessory ligaments* are placed away from the capsule.

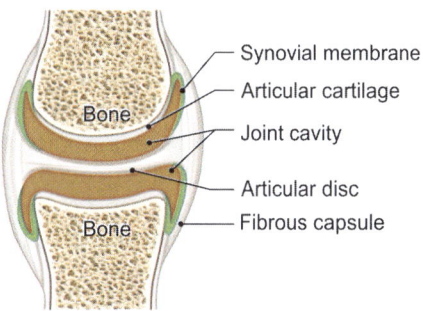

Fig. 1.11: Synovial joint.

Morphological Classification of Synovial Joints (Fig. 1.12)

Plane (Gliding)	Uniaxial	Biaxial	Polyaxial (Multiaxial)
Plane	• Hinge • Pivot	• Condylar • Ellipsoid • Saddle (*Sellar*)	Ball and socket

1. **Plane (*Gliding*) joints:** These are formed by flat articular surfaces; permit gliding movements (*translation*) in various directions. There is no axis in these joints. Example: Intercarpal joints, joints between articular processes of vertebrae.
2. **Hinge (*Ginglymus*) joints:** These are uniaxial (*transverse axis*); generally pulley shaped. The articular surfaces are moulded so as to largely restrict to and fro movements in one plane. The movements are around a transverse axis. These joints are typically provided with strong collateral ligaments. Example: Elbow joint (*humeroulnar part*), interphalangeal joints, etc.
3. **Pivot (*Trochoid*) joints:** These are uniaxial (*longitudinal axis*). The joint comprises a central bony pivot surrounded by an osteoligamentous ring. The movement is rotation around a longitudinal axis, passing through the center of pivot. Either pivot may rotate with in the ring (*superior and inferior radioulnar joints*) or ring may rotate around the pivot (*median atlantoaxial joint*).
4. **Condylar joints:** The articular surfaces include condyle shaped articular surface (male surface) fitting into reciprocally concave female surface sometimes inappropriately called condyles. They are generally uniaxial; principal movements occurring largely in one plane, but in addition, limited rotation is possible about a second axis - orthogonal (set at 90°) to the principal axis. Movements occur mainly around a transverse axis; rotation can occur around the vertical axis. Example: Knee joint, temporomandibular joint, etc.
5. **Ellipsoid joints:** These are biaxial; formed by oval convex male surface fitting into an elliptical female concavity. The primary movements are possible in two axes set at right

angle (*flexion/extension and adduction/abduction*). The combination of these foregoing movements produces circumduction. Example: Wrist joint (radiocarpal joint), atlanto-occipital joint, etc.

6. **Saddle (*Sellar*) joints:** These are biaxial; for functional purposes considered as polyaxial joint. The articular surfaces are reciprocally concavo-convex. The principal movements occur in two planes set at right angles but because of their articular geometry, these are accompanied by rotation. Such "*conjunct rotation*" cannot occur independently. Example: 1st carpometacarpal joint (thumb joint), calcaneocuboid joint, etc.

7. **Ball and socket (*Spheroidal*) joints:** These are multiaxial; formed by globular head fitting into a cup-shaped socket. The movements take place independently around three axes. Their surfaces, though resembling parts of spheres are not strictly spherical but slightly ovoid. Thus, in most positions, congruence is not perfect but occurs only in one position at the end of the movement under consideration. The movements of flexion and extension, adduction and abduction, medial and lateral rotations and circumduction occur quite freely. Example: Shoulder joint, hip joint, etc.

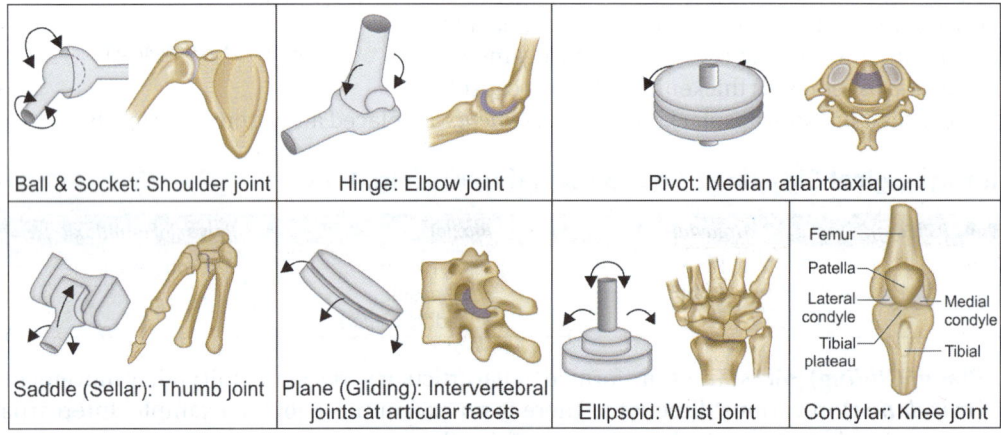

Fig. 1.12: Types of synovial joints.

Nerve Supply of Joints and Hilton's Law

AN 2.6 Explain the concept of nerve supply of joints and Hilton's law.

Nerve supply of joints: The articular capsule and joint ligaments have rich nerve supply; thus pain sensitive. The synovial membrane has poor nerve supply. The articular cartilage is non-nervous; insensitive to pain. The articular nerves contain sensory and autonomic fibers. Some sensory fibers are proprioceptive; sensitive to position and movement. They are concerned with reflex control of posture and locomotion. Other sensory fibers are sensitive to pain. The autonomic fibers are vasomotor (*vasosensory*).

Hilton's law: It states that a motor nerve to the muscle acting on a joint tends to give a branch to that joint and another branch to the skin covering the joint. This concept was elucidated by Gardner, accordingly, each nerve innervates a specific region of the capsule and that the part of the capsule rendered taut by a given muscle is innervated by the nerve supplying its antagonists. Thus, the pattern of innervation is concerned with the maintenance of an efficient stability at the joint.

2 CHAPTER

Introduction to Skeleton

INTRODUCTION

The human skeleton is divided into:
- *Axial skeleton:* It is made up of bones of the head, neck, and trunk.
- *Appendicular skeleton:* It is consisting of the bones of the limbs.

PRELIMINARY REVIEW OF THE SKULL

The skeleton of the head is the skull. The skull contains a large *cranial cavity* which contains the brain. Just below the forehead the skull shows two large depressions called the orbits, in which the eyes are lodged. In the region of the nose and mouth there are apertures that lead to the interior of the skull (**Figs. 2.1 and 2.2**).

The skull is made up of many bones; firmly joined together. In the forehead region the *frontal bone* is seen. At the back of the head (*occiput*) there is the *occipital bone*. The top of the skull and parts of its side walls are formed mainly by the right and left *parietal bones*. The region of the head just above the ears is the *temple*, and the bone here is the *temporal bone*.

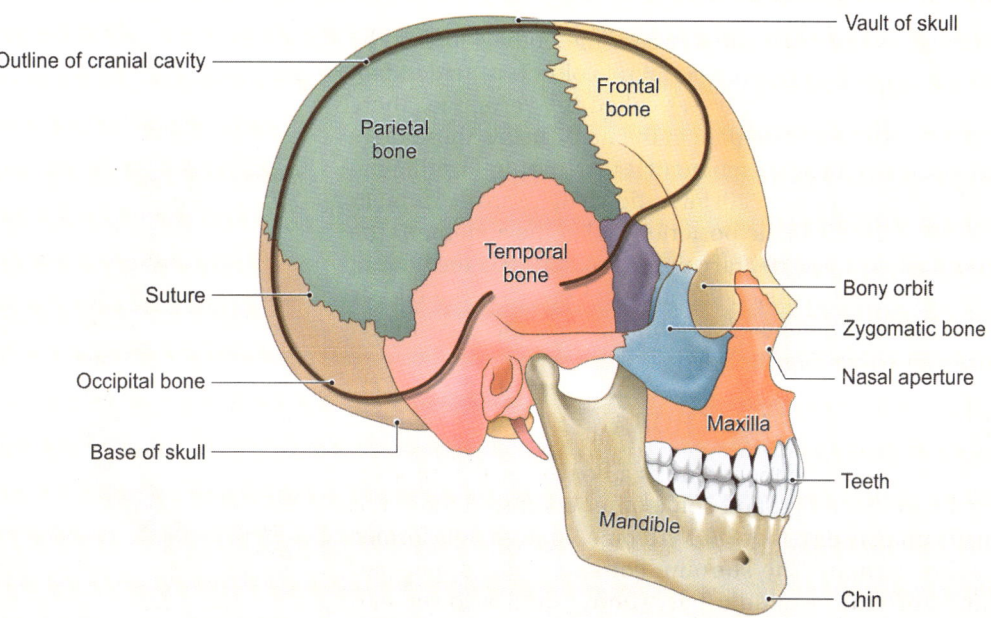

Fig. 2.1: Skull from the right side.

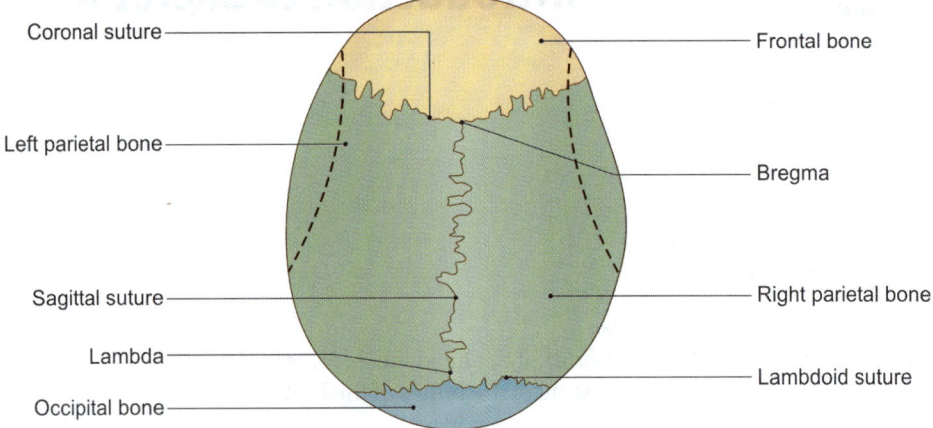

Fig. 2.2: Skull from above.

The bone forming the upper jaw bearing the upper teeth is the maxilla. The prominence of the cheek is formed by the zygomatic bone. In the floor of the cranial cavity an unpaired sphenoid bone is placed. The bone of the lower jaw is the mandible which is separated from the rest of the skull. In addition, there are several smaller bones that will be identified during the study of the skull in detail.

VERTEBRAL COLUMN

Below the skull, the central axis of the body is formed by the vertebral column. The vertebral column is made up of many irregular-shaped bones called the vertebrae. There are seven cervical vertebrae in the neck. Below these there are twelve thoracic vertebrae that take part in forming the skeleton of the thorax. Still lower down there are five lumbar vertebrae that lie in the posterior wall of the abdomen. The lowest part of the vertebral column is made up of the sacrum (consisting of five fused sacral vertebrae) and the coccyx (four fused rudimentary vertebrae). Thus, there are thirty-three vertebrae (**Fig. 2.3**).

SKELETON OF THE THORAX

The skeleton of the thorax forms a bony cage that protects the heart, the lungs, and some other organs. Behind, it is made up of twelve thoracic vertebrae. In front, it is formed by the sternum. The sternum consists of an upper part (manubrium), a middle part (body), and a lower part (xiphoid process). The side walls of the thorax are formed by twelve ribs on either side.

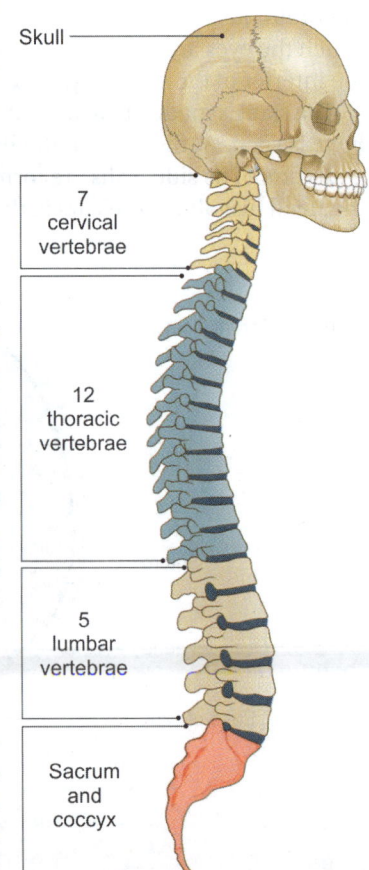

Fig. 2.3: Skull and vertebral column (right lateral view).

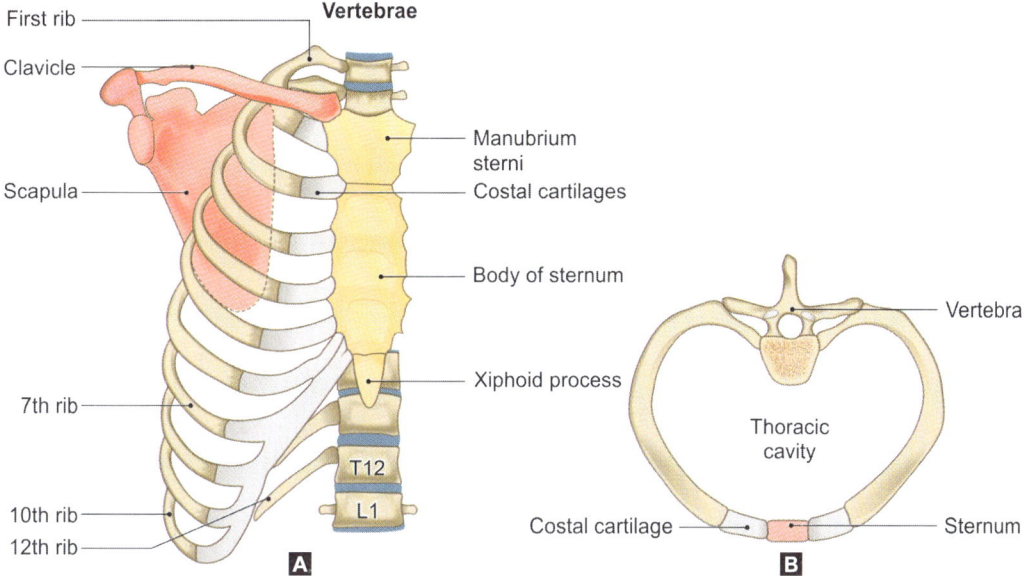

Figs. 2.4A and B: (A) Skeleton of the thorax from the front. Bones of the shoulder girdle are also shown; (B) Section across thorax.

Each rib is a long curved bone that is attached posteriorly to the vertebral column. It curves round the sides of the thorax. Its anterior end through the *costal cartilage* is attached to the sternum **(Figs. 2.4A and B)**. This arrangement is present in the upper seven ribs; called *vertebrosternal ribs* (true ribs). The 8th, 9th, and 10th costal cartilages do not reach the sternum; attached to 7th costal cartilage. These are called *vertebrochondral ribs* (false ribs). The *anterior ends of the 11th and 12th ribs are* free, called the *floating ribs.*

SKELETON OF THE UPPER LIMB

Skeleton of the upper limb consists of the bones of:
* Pectoral girdle *(*shoulder girdle)
* Free limb.

The pectoral girdle consists of the *clavicle* (collar bone) and the *scapula* (shoulder blade). The clavicle is placed in front of the upper part of the thorax. Medially, it is attached to the manubrium sterni, and laterally to the scapula. The scapula is a triangular-shaped bone placed behind the upper part of the thorax.

The bone of the arm is the *humerus.* There are two bones in the forearm. The bone placed laterally (toward thumb) is the *radius;* and the bone placed medially (toward little finger) is the *ulna.* The humerus, radius, and ulna are long bones. They have a cylindrical middle part (*shaft*) and expanded upper and lower *ends.*

In the wrist, there are eight small, roughly cuboidal, *carpal bones.* The skeleton of the palm is made up of five *metacarpals.* The skeleton of the fingers (digits) is made up of the *phalanges.* There are three phalanges (*proximal, middle, and distal*) in each digit *except* the thumb that has only two phalanges (proximal and distal) **(Fig. 2.5)**.

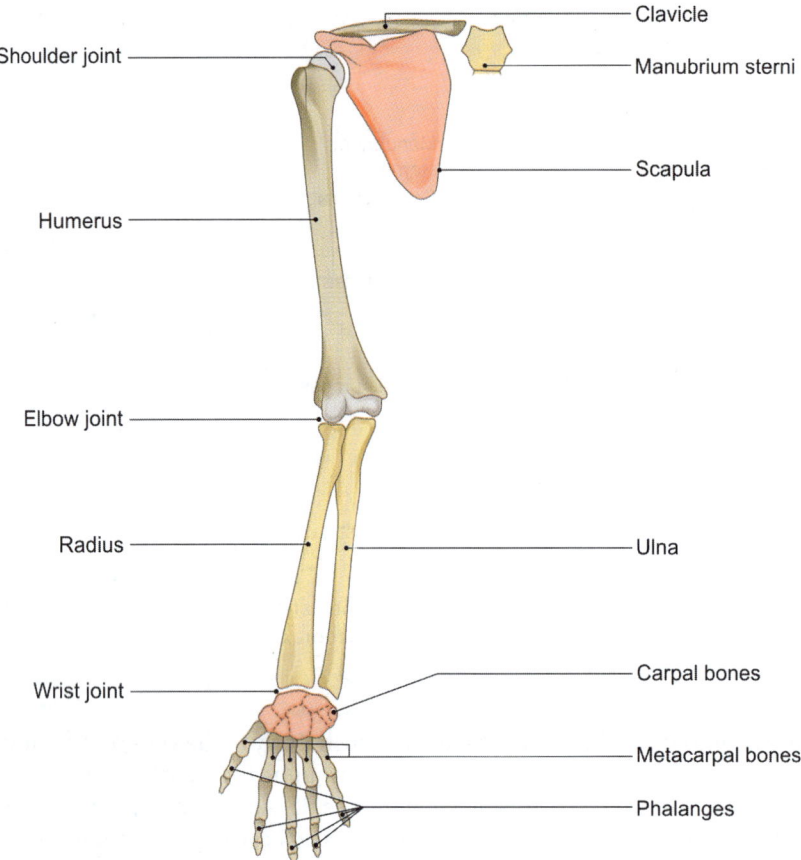

Fig. 2.5: Skeleton of the right upper limb (manubrium sterni for orientation).

The upper end of the humerus is joined with the scapula at the shoulder joint and its lower end is joined with the upper ends of the radius and ulna to form the elbow joint. The wrist joint is formed by the union of the lower ends of the radius and ulna with the carpals (scaphoid and lunate). The upper and lower ends of the radius and ulna are united to form superior and inferior radioulnar joints. There are many small joints in the hand. These include:
- *Intercarpal joints* between carpals themselves
- *Carpometacarpal joints* between carpals and metacarpals
- *Metacarpophalangeal joints* between each metacarpal and proximal phalanx
- *Interphalangeal joints* between the phalanges themselves.

SKELETON OF THE LOWER LIMB

Skeleton of the lower limb consists of the bones of:
- Pelvic girdle
- Free limb.

The pelvic girdle is made up of both *hip bones*. Each hip bone is made up of three fused parts. The upper expanded part is the *ilium*. The *pubis* lies in the front. The lower part is the *ischium*.

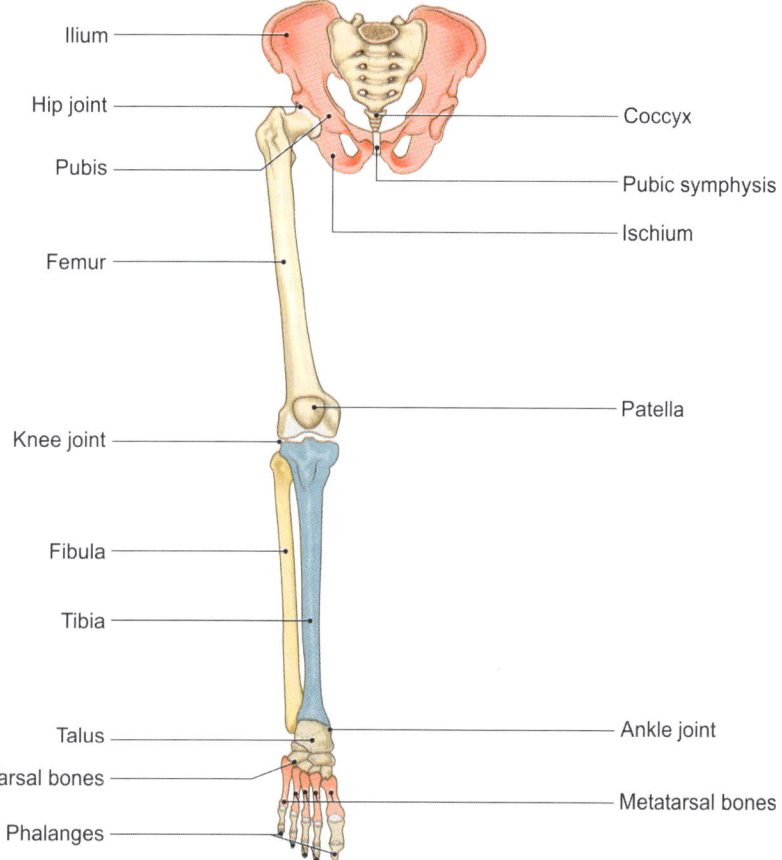

Fig. 2.6: Skeleton of the pelvis and right lower limb.

Anteriorly, the two pubic bones meet in the midline to form *pubic symphysis.* Posteriorly, the sacrum is wedged in between the two hip bones. The hip bones and sacrum (with coccyx) form the *bony pelvis* (**Fig. 2.6**).

The bone of the thigh is the *femur.* There are two bones in the leg—the medial bone (toward great toe) is the *tibia,* while the outer bone is the *fibula.* The femur, tibia and fibula are long bones; present cylindrical shafts with expanded upper and lower ends. In the foot there are seven roughly cuboidal *tarsal bones.* The *calcaneus* is the largest tarsal bone, which forms the heel. Next in size is the *talus.* In the anterior part of the foot there are five *metatarsals.* Each digit (toe) has three *phalanges,* proximal, middle, and distal. However, the great toe has only two phalanges proximal and distal.

The upper end of the femur fits into a deep socket in the hip bone (*acetabulum*) to form the *hip joint.* The lower end of the femur joins the tibia to form the *knee joint.* A small bone called the *patella* (sesamoid bone) is placed in front of the knee. The tibia and fibula are joined to each other at their upper and lower ends to form the superior and inferior *tibiofibular joints.* The lower ends of the tibia and fibula with the talus form the *ankle joint.* Within the foot there are *intertarsal, tarsometatarsal, metatarsophalangeal* and *interphalangeal joints* on a similar pattern as seen in the hand.

Bones of Upper Limb

CHAPTER 3

AN 8.1 Identify the given bone, its side, important features and keep it in anatomical position.
AN 8.2 Identify and describe joints formed by the given bone.
AN 8.4 Demonstrate important muscle attachment on the given bone.

CLAVICLE (COLLAR BONE)

The clavicle (*modified long bone*) presents shaft, and two ends. The medial end is quadrilateral; distinguished from the flattened lateral end. The shaft shows a gentle S-shaped curve (convex forward in medial two-third; concave forward in lateral one-third). The inferior aspect of the shaft presents a shallow groove **(Figs. 3.1 and 3.2)**.

Side Determination

- *Medial:* Quadrilateral sternal end.
- *Anterior*: Convexity of medial two-third of the shaft.
- *Inferior*: Groove for subclavius, conoid tubercle, and trapezoid line.

Anatomical Position

Placed horizontally in the body.

AN 8.3 Enumerate peculiarities of clavicle.

Peculiarities of Clavicle

- First bone to start ossifying in the body
- Only long bone that ossifies in membrane (greater part)
- Only long bone which has two primary centers of ossification
- Only long bone placed horizontally
- Only long bone that lacks medullary cavity
- Subcutaneous throughout its extent
- Occasionally pierced by middle supraclavicular nerve.

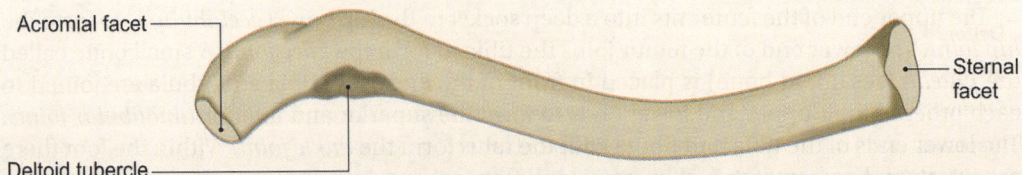

Fig. 3.1: Right clavicle from above.

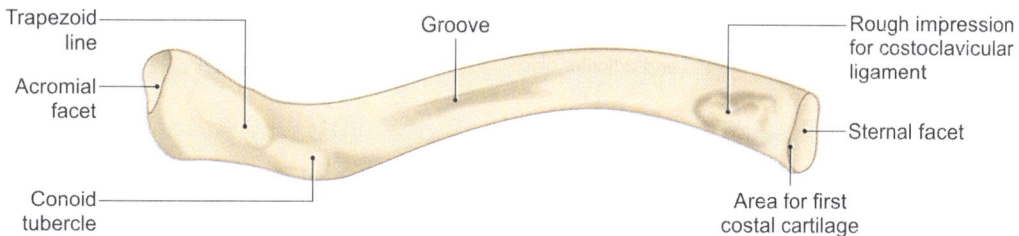

Fig. 3.2: Right clavicle from below.

Functions

- Supports shoulder laterally and backward so that the arm can swing clearly away from the trunk.
- Transmits the weight/force from the upper limb to the sternum
- Clavicular movements at sternoclavicular joint permits overhead abduction.

General Features

Shaft: The shaft is divided into the lateral one-third (flattened) and the cylindrical medial two-thirds. *Lateral one-third* of the shaft has superior and inferior surfaces; separated by anterior and posterior borders. The anterior border is concave and shows a small *deltoid tubercle*. The inferior surface shows a prominent thickening near the posterior border—the *conoid tubercle*. Lateral to the tubercle, a rough ridge runs obliquely up to the lateral end of the bone called the *trapezoid line*.

Medial two-thirds of the shaft presents four surfaces (anterior, posterior, superior, and inferior) which merge with each other.

Ends: *Lateral (acromial end)* has a smooth facet which articulates with the acromion of the scapula to form the acromioclavicular joint.

Medial (sternal end) articulates with the manubrium sterni and the first costal cartilage. The articular area is smooth; extends for a short distance on to the inferior surface of the bone. The sternal end forms a prominent bulge which extends above the upper border of the manubrium sterni (**Fig. 3.3**).

Movements: Clavicle moves round an axis of the costoclavicular ligament. Thus, the two ends of the bone move in opposite directions.

Attachments on the Clavicle (Figs. 3.4 and 3.5)

Muscles

Muscle	Attachment
Pectoralis major *(clavicular head)*	Anterior surface of the medial half of shaft *(origin)*
Deltoid	Anterior border of lateral one-third of shaft *(origin)*
Sternocleidomastoid *(clavicular head)*	Medial part of the upper surface *(origin)*
Sternohyoid	Lower part of posterior surface near sternal end *(origin)*
Trapezius	Posterior border of lateral one-third of shaft *(insertion)*
Subclavius	Groove on the inferior surface of shaft *(insertion)*

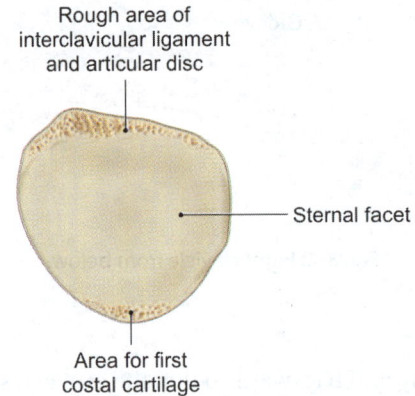

Fig. 3.3: Medial end of clavicle: Medial aspect.

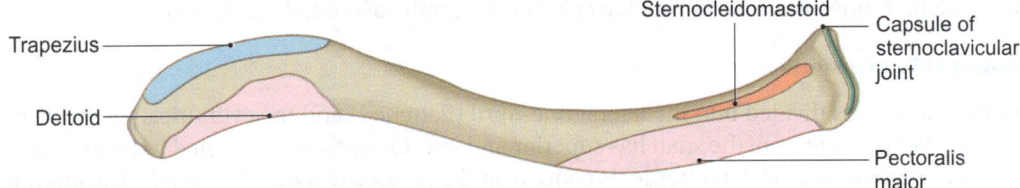

Fig. 3.4: Right clavicle: Attachments from above.

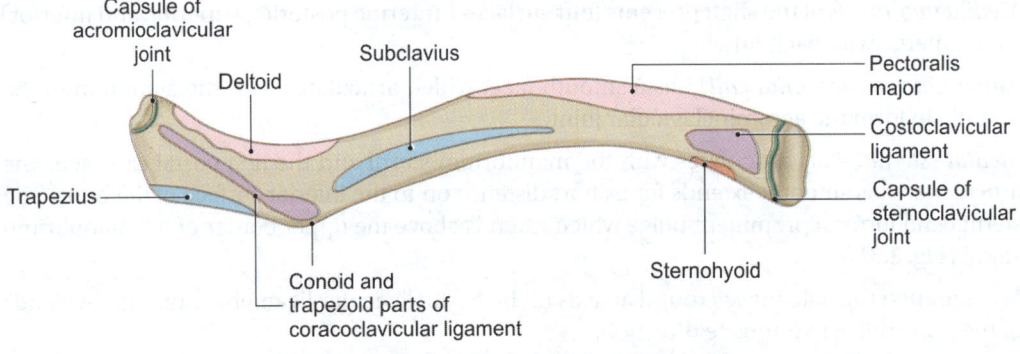

Fig. 3.5: Right clavicle: Attachments from below.

Other Attachments

Structure	Attachment
Clavipectoral fascia	Edges of the groove for subclavius
Interclavicular ligament and articular disc of sternoclavicular joint	Rough area above articular surface for manubrium sterni
Costoclavicular ligament	Medial end of clavicle
Conoid part of coracoclavicular ligament	Conoid tubercle
Trapezoid part of coracoclavicular ligament	Trapezoid line
Articular capsules of acromioclavicular and sternoclavicular joints	Margins of articular areas for these joints

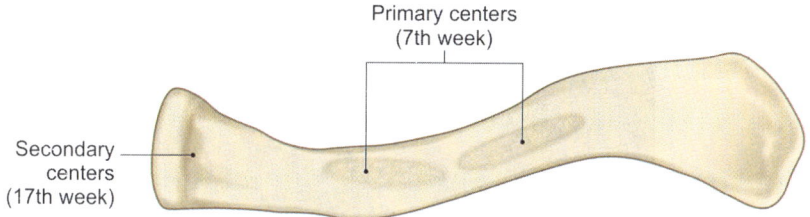

Fig. 3.6: Clavicle: Ossification.

Ligaments Attached at Medial End
- Capsule of sternoclavicular joint
- Articular disc of sternoclavicular joint
- Anterior and posterior sternoclavicular ligaments
- Costoclavicular ligament
- Interclavicular ligament.

Ossification
- Clavicle is the first bone to start ossifying. Two primary centers appear in the shaft during 6th week of fetal life; soon fuse with each other.
- Sternal end ossifies from one secondary center that appears between 15 years and 20 years of age; fuses with shaft by 25 years of age. Additional center may appear in the acromion (**Fig. 3.6**).
- Greater part of clavicle develops in membrane (*intramembranous ossification*). Sternal and acromial ends are preformed in cartilage.
- Medial (sternal) end is the growing end of the bone.

Sexual Differences

Feature	Male	Female
Acromial end	Slightly above the sternal end	Slightly below the sternal end
Muscular impressions	More pronounced	Less pronounced
Mid-shaft circumference	33 mm (average)	25 mm (average)
Curvature	More sinuously curved	Less curved
Length	Longer	Shorter
Thickness	Thicker	Thinner

Clinical Anatomy
- *Fractures of clavicle:* Clavicle is one of the *most frequently fractured bones*; common in children. Indirect forces due to a fall on the outstretched hand cause most fractures. It may be due to a direct blow to the shoulder.
- *Fractures of middle third* are most common fractures. The medial fragment is displaced upward by the pull of sternocleidomastoid while the lateral fragment is displaced downward by the weight of the shoulder (gravity). In young children, clavicle fracture presents a *greenstick pattern* (**Fig. 3.7**).

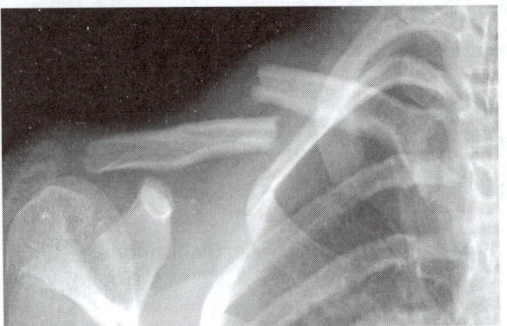

Fig. 3.7: Fracture clavicle.

- ***Weight transmission from upper limb:*** Clavicle is a connection between appendicular and axial skeleton. Coracoclavicular ligament transmits weight from the upper limb onto the clavicle which passes it onto the sternum.
- ***Craniocleido-dysostosis:*** There is faulty ossification of the membranous bones. This rare abnormality is associated with congenital absence of one or both clavicles. The patient can bring both shoulders close to each other in front of chest **(Fig. 3.8)**.

Measurement of Upper Limb

Following bony landmarks are used:
- Tip of acromion process to medial epicondyle of humerus.
- From medial epicondyle of humerus to styloid process of ulna.

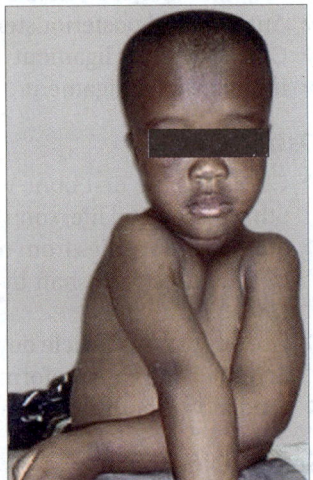

Fig. 3.8: *Craniocleido-dysostosis.*

AN 13.4 Describe acromioclavicular joint.

Acromioclavicular Joint

Acromioclavicular joint (*synovial: plane variety*) allows gliding and rotatory movements of the scapula. It is reinforced by the conoid and trapezoid ligaments (*parts of coracoclavicular ligament*).

Dislocation of acromioclavicular joint results from a fall on the shoulder or on the outstretched arm. The shoulder is separated from the clavicle when the joint dislocates with rupture of coracoclavicular ligament. It is repaired by fixing clavicle to coracoid process and repairing coracoclavicular ligament.

> **QUESTIONNAIRE**
> - Classify the bone. How does it differ from other long bones?
> - Side determination and anatomical position.
> - Enumerate the peculiarities of the clavicle.
> - What are the joints associated with clavicle and their types?

- Mark the attachments of:

Ligaments	Muscles
Costoclavicular	On medial one-third of shaft
Coracoclavicular (conoid and trapezoid parts)	On lateral one-third of shaft
Interclavicular	On subclavius groove
Clavipectoral fascia	

- Comment on its ossification. Which is the growing end?
- Which is the most vulnerable part of the clavicle? Why?
- What is the function of the coracoclavicular ligament?

SCAPULA (SHOULDER BLADE)

The scapula is a large triangular (*flat*) bone. It is placed on the posterolateral side of the chest wall. It extends from the second to the seventh ribs.

Side Determination

- *Lateral*: Glenoid cavity
- *Inferior*: Inferior angle
- *Dorsal*: Spinous process.

Anatomical Position

- Glenoid cavity is directed anterolaterally
- Costal surface is directed medially and forward.

The greater part of the scapula (flat triangular plate) is the *body*. The upper part of the body is broad (*base of triangle*) and the inferior end (*apex*) is pointed. The body presents anterior (costal) and posterior (dorsal) surfaces. The anterior surface is smooth. The upper part of the posterior surface has a large projection called the spine or spinous process. At its lateral angle, scapula presents large shallow depression called the *glenoid cavity* which articulates with the head of the humerus **(Figs. 3.9 to 3.11)**. The body presents:

- *Three angles*: (a) Superior, (b) inferior, and (c) lateral.
- *Three borders*: (a) Medial, (b) lateral, and (c) superior.

Three processes arise from the body:
- Spinous process
- Acromion process
- Coracoid process.

Lateral border runs from the glenoid cavity to the inferior angle.
Medial border extends from the superior angle to the inferior angle.
Superior border passes laterally from the superior angle; separated from the glenoid cavity (*lateral angle*) by the root of coracoid process. The *suprascapular notch* is seen at the lateral end of the superior border.

The concave *costal surface* lies against the posterolateral part of the chest wall. The spine divides *dorsal surface* into *supraspinous* and *infraspinous fossae*. Both fossae communicate through the *spinoglenoid notch*.

The bone adjoining the lateral border is thickened to form a longitudinal bar of bone. The dorsal aspect of the scapula adjoining lateral border is rough for muscular attachments.

CHAPTER 3 ✦ Bones of Upper Limb

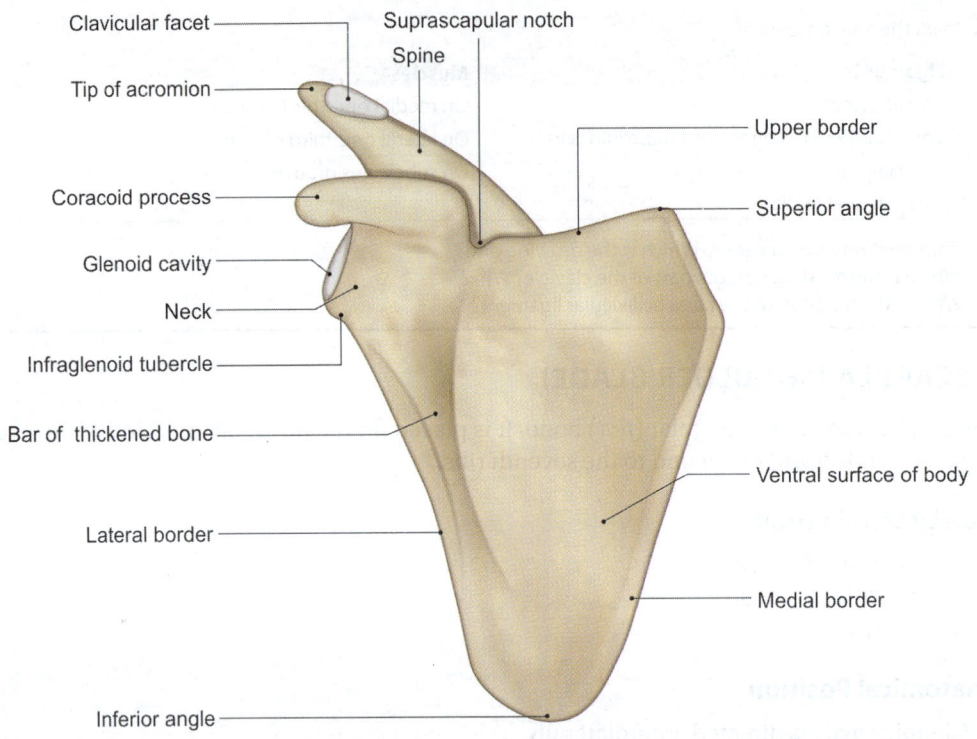

Fig. 3.9: Right scapula: From the front.

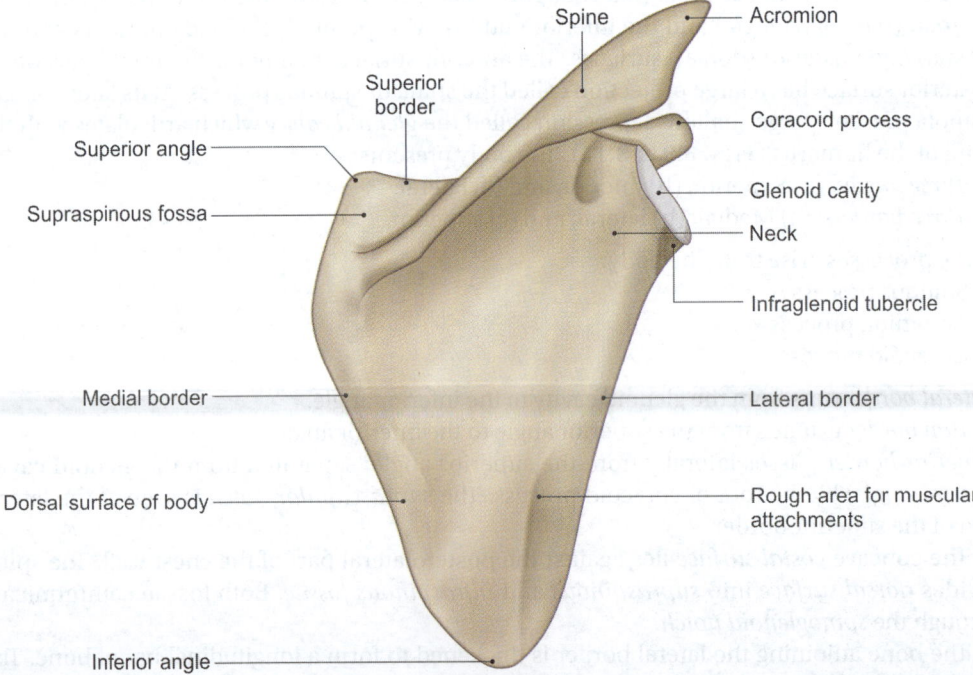

Fig. 3.10: Right scapula: From behind.

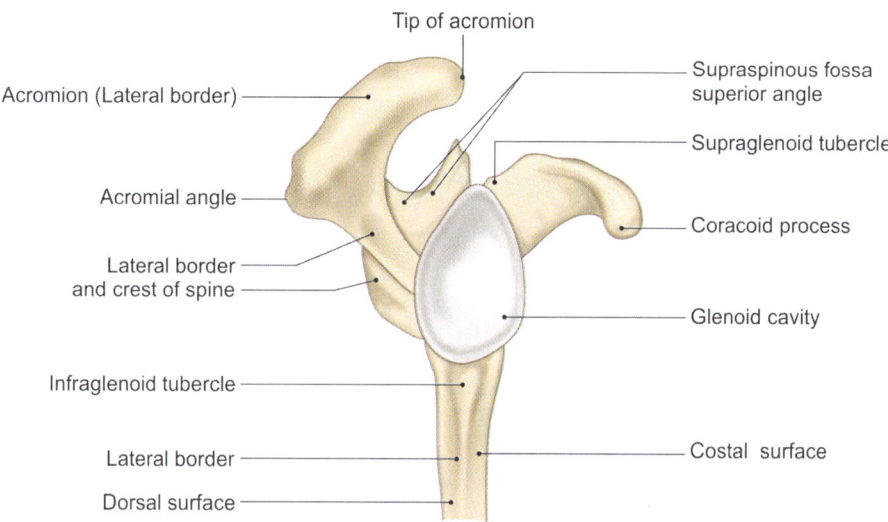

Fig. 3.11: Upper part of right scapula: From the lateral side.

The pear-shaped *glenoid cavity* (*head of scapula*) forms the shoulder joint with the head of the humerus. Just below the cavity the lateral border shows a rough raised area called the *infraglenoid tubercle*. Immediately above the glenoid cavity *supraglenoid tubercle* is noted. Immediately beyond glenoid cavity there is a constriction which constitutes the *neck*.

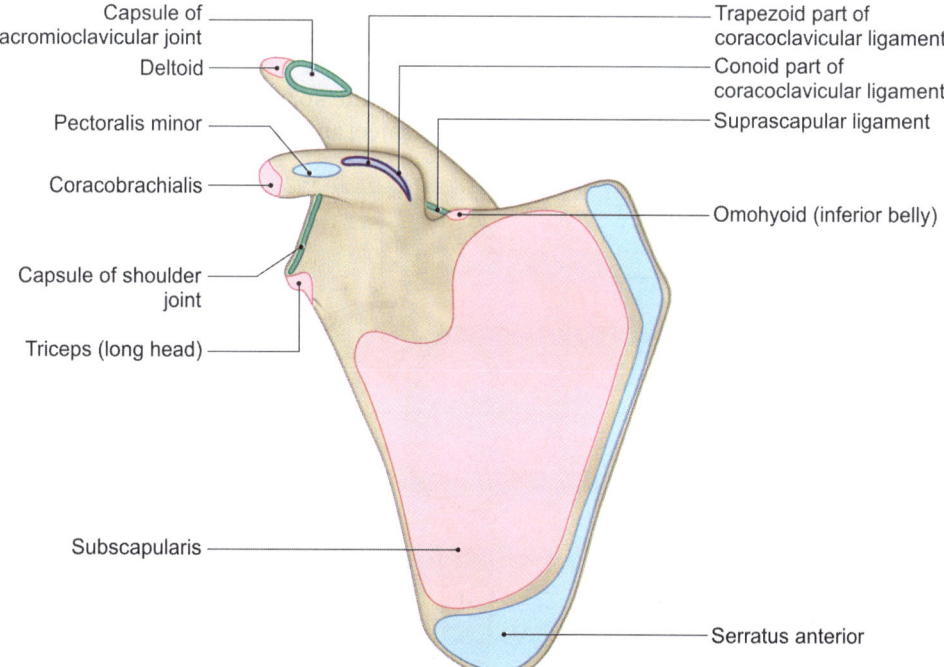

Fig. 3.12: Right scapula: Attachments seen from the front.

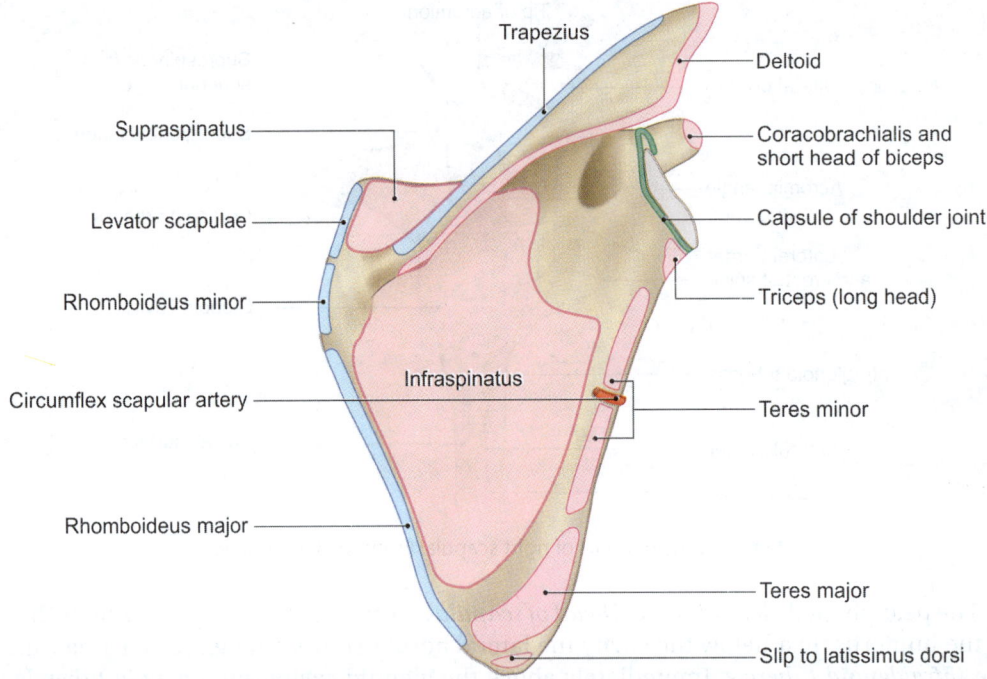

Fig. 3.13: Right scapula: Attachments from behind.

Spinous process is triangular shaped. Its anterior border is attached to the dorsal surface of the body. Its posterior border is free and forms the *crest of spine*. The medial end of the spine forms the *root of spine*. The lateral border of the spine is free and forms the medial boundary of the *spinoglenoid notch*.

Acromion process continues with the lateral end of the spine; forms a projection that is directed forward. It has lateral and medial borders that meet anteriorly at the tip of the acromion.

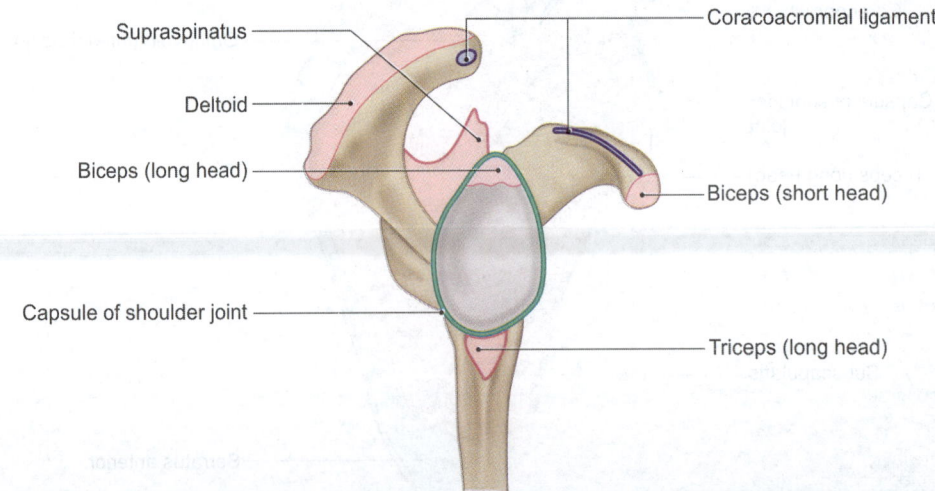

Fig. 3.14: Right scapula: Attachments seen from lateral side.

The lateral border meets the crest of the spine at a sharp angle—the *acromial angle*. The medial border shows a small oval facet for articulation with the lateral end of the clavicle. Acromion presents upper and lower surfaces.

Coracoid process is shaped like a bent finger. The root of the process is attached to the body of the scapula just above the glenoid cavity. The lower part of the root is marked by the supraglenoid tubercle. The tip of the coracoid process is directed forward. (*note*: costal surface of the body of scapula faces anteromedially; glenoid cavity faces forward and laterally).

Attachments

Muscles (Figs. 3.12 to 3.14)

Muscle	Attachment
Deltoid	Lower border of the crest of spine; lateral margin, tip and upper surface of acromion (*origin*)
Trapezius	Upper border of the crest of spine and medial border of acromion (*insertion*)
Biceps brachii (short head)	Tip of coracoid process (*origin*)
Biceps brachii (long head)	Supraglenoid tubercle (*origin*)
Coracobrachialis	Medial part of the tip of coracoid process (*origin*)
Long head of triceps	Infraglenoid tubercle (*origin*)
Pectoralis minor	Superior aspect of coracoid process (*insertion*)
Inferior belly of omohyoid	Upper border near suprascapular notch (*origin*)
Subscapularis	Costal surface, except for a small part near neck (*origin*)
Serratus anterior	Costal surface along medial border: *First digitation* extends from superior angle to root of spine, *next 2–3 digitations* into a narrow line along the medial border, *lower 4–5 digitations* into triangular area over inferior angle (*insertion*)
Supraspinatus	Medial two-thirds of supraspinous fossa, including upper surface of spine (*origin*)
Infraspinatus	Greater part of infraspinous fossa, except near lateral border and neck (*origin*)
Teres minor	Upper two-thirds on the lateral border; dorsal surface (*origin*)
Teres major	Lower one-third along the dorsal aspect of lateral border up to inferior angle (*origin*)
Levator scapulae	Dorsal aspect of medial border, extending from superior angle to root of spine (*origin*)
Rhomboideus minor	Dorsal aspect of medial border, opposite root of spine (*origin*)
Rhomboideus major	Dorsal aspect of medial border, from root of spine to inferior angle (*origin*)
Latissimus dorsi	Dorsal surface of inferior angle (*origin*)

Ligaments

Ligament	Attachment
Capsule of shoulder joint and glenoid labrum	Margins of glenoid cavity; in upper part, capsular attachment extends above supraglenoid tubercle (origin of long head of biceps brachii is intracapsular)
Capsule of acromioclavicular joint	Margins of the facet for the clavicle
Coracoacromial ligament	Anteromedial end to lateral border of coracoid process; lateral end to medial aspect of the tip of acromion in front of clavicular facet
Coracoclavicular ligament	Coracoid process: *Trapezoid part* on superior aspect and *conoid part* near the root
Suprascapular ligament	Suprascapular notch; converts it into a foramen—transmits suprascapular nerve; suprascapular vessels pass above the ligament

Ossification

Scapula has eight centers of ossification.
- A center appears in the body during 8th week of fetal life; spine ossifies by extension from this center.
- Greater part of coracoid process ossifies from a center that appears during first year. At puberty second center appears at the root of coracoid process—*subcoracoid center*. Extension of ossification from this center forms upper part of glenoid cavity.
- At puberty two centers appear in acromion and one each in the lower part of glenoid cavity, inferior angle and medial border.
- Subcoracoid center fuses with the body by 15th year. Other centers fuse with the body by 20th year **(Figs. 3.15A and B)**.

Clinical Anatomy

- ***Inferior angle of scapula as bony landmark:*** Inferior angle of scapula corresponds to spine of T-7 vertebra.
- ***Triangle of auscultation:*** It is bounded by trapezius, latissimus dorsi, and medial border of scapula. Rhomboid major forms its floor. This triangle is used for auscultating breath sounds as this area is least covered with muscles.
- ***Winging of scapula:*** Serratus anterior keeps medial border of scapula closely applied to chest wall. Injury to long thoracic nerve (Bell's) causes paralysis of serratus anterior. When the patient is asked to push against resistance medial border of scapula on the affected side stands out called the *winged scapula* **(Fig. 3.16)**.
- ***Pulsating scapula:*** There exists rich arterial anastomosis around the scapula. When the circulation in axillary/brachial artery is affected (coarctation of aorta or blockade in main vessels) this necessitates opening up the collaterals. It leads to dilatation and tortuosity of the collaterals makes the scapula pulsatile.

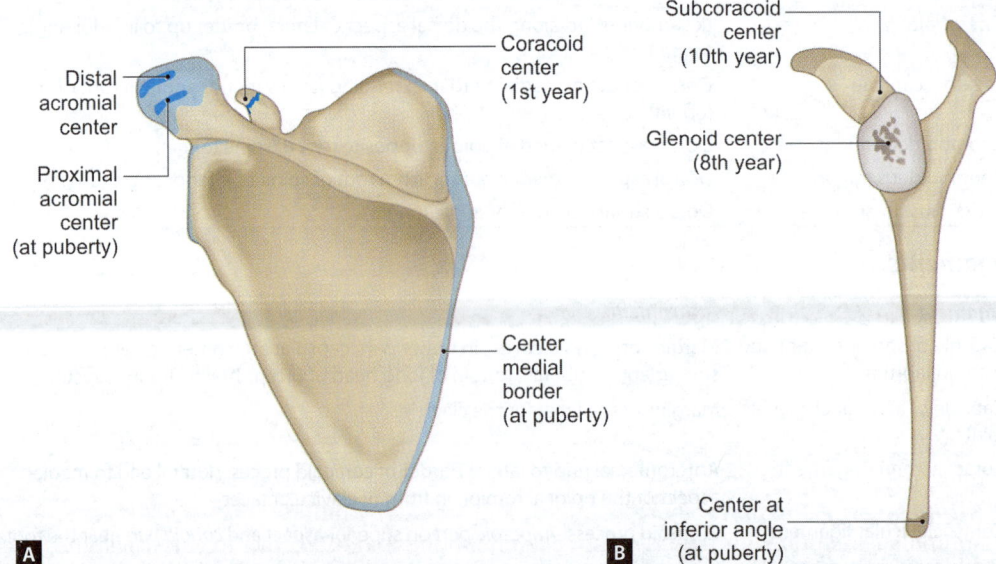

Figs. 3.15A and B: Ossification of scapula: (A) Dorsal aspect; (B) Lateral aspect.

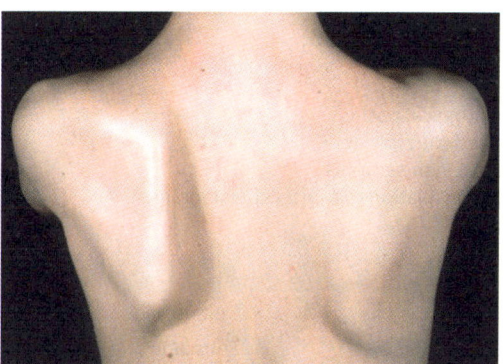

Fig. 3.16: Left winged scapula.

- **Scaphoid scapula:** Developmental anomaly where the medial border of the scapula is concave.
- **Painful arc syndrome (supraspinatus syndrome):** It is characterized by thickening of supraspinatus tendon with pain during 60–120° abduction. There is impingement of supraspinatus tendon against coracoacromial arch. Important causes include tear of supraspinatus tendon and calcified deposit in the supraspinatus tendon.
- **Frozen shoulder:** It is due to tendinitis involving rotator cuff. All shoulder movements are restricted due to adhesions.
- **Shoulder arthrodesis:** Surgical fixation (joint fusion) is arthrodesis. Optimal position of shoulder arthrodesis is 45° abduction and 20° flexion in front of coronal plane (palm of hand touching back of neck) **(Fig. 3.17)**.
- **Sprengel's deformity:** In this congenital deformity scapula remains elevated **(Fig. 3.18)**. This failure of scapular descent is due to failure of migration from cervical to thoracic region. Such individual may have other skeletal anomalies (abnormal vertebrae or hypoplasia of pectoral muscles).
- **Klippel–Feil syndrome:** There is bilateral failure of scapulae descent. The associated anomalies include failure of fusion of occipital bone and the defect in cervical spine. This results in webbing of neck and limited neck movements.

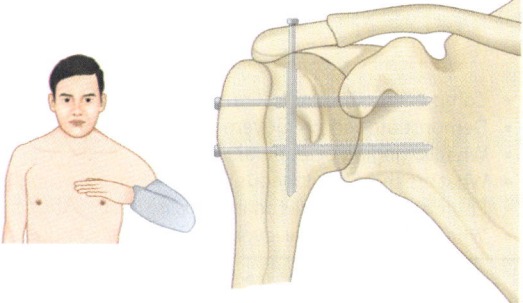

Fig. 3.17: Arthrodesis of shoulder joint.

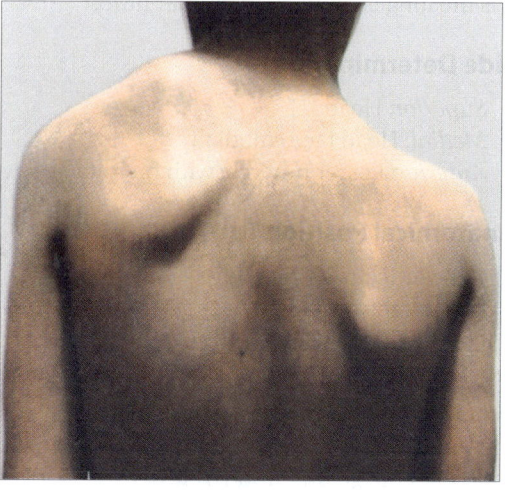

Fig. 3.18: Sprengel's deformity.

CHAPTER 3 ✦ Bones of Upper Limb

QUESTIONNAIRE

- Classify the bone.
- Side determination and anatomical position.
- What are the joints associated with this bone?
- How many angles are present in the scapula?
- Name the structures passing in relation to suprascapular foramen.
- Mark the attachments of:

Ligaments	Muscles
Capsule of shoulder joint	Deltoid and trapezius
Transverse scapular	Subscapularis
Coracoclavicular	Teres major and minor
Coracohumeral	Supraspinatus and infraspinatus
Coracoacromial arch	Serratus anterior
	Latissimus dorsi
	Biceps and triceps (long heads)

- Comment on the ossification of this bone.
- Demonstrate various movements of the scapula.
- What is winging of scapula?
- What are the subcutaneous palpable parts of scapula?
- Enumerate the arteries anastomosing around the scapula.
- What are the vertebral levels in relation to scapula?

HUMERUS (ARM BONE)

It is the longest bone of the upper limb.

Side Determination

- ❖ *Superior*: Head
- ❖ *Medial*: Head faces medially
- ❖ *Anterior*: Lesser tubercle with bicipital groove on its lateral side.

Anatomical Position

Placed vertically in the body.

The humerus (*long bone*) presents cylindrical *shaft*, and enlarged *upper and lower ends*. The upper end bears a large rounded head. The anterior aspect of the upper end shows a vertical groove called the *intertubercular sulcus* (**Figs. 3.19A and B**).

Upper end: The rounded and articular *head* is directed medially, backward and upward. It forms the shoulder joint with the glenoid cavity of the scapula. The upper end shows two prominences called (a) *the greater* and (b) *lesser tubercles* (tuberosities); separated by the *intertubercular sulcus* (bicipital groove).

- ❖ *Lesser tubercle* lies on the anterior aspect medial to the sulcus.
- ❖ *Greater tubercle* is on the lateral aspect of the upper end; shows three impressions for muscles attachments.

CHAPTER 3 ✦ Bones of Upper Limb

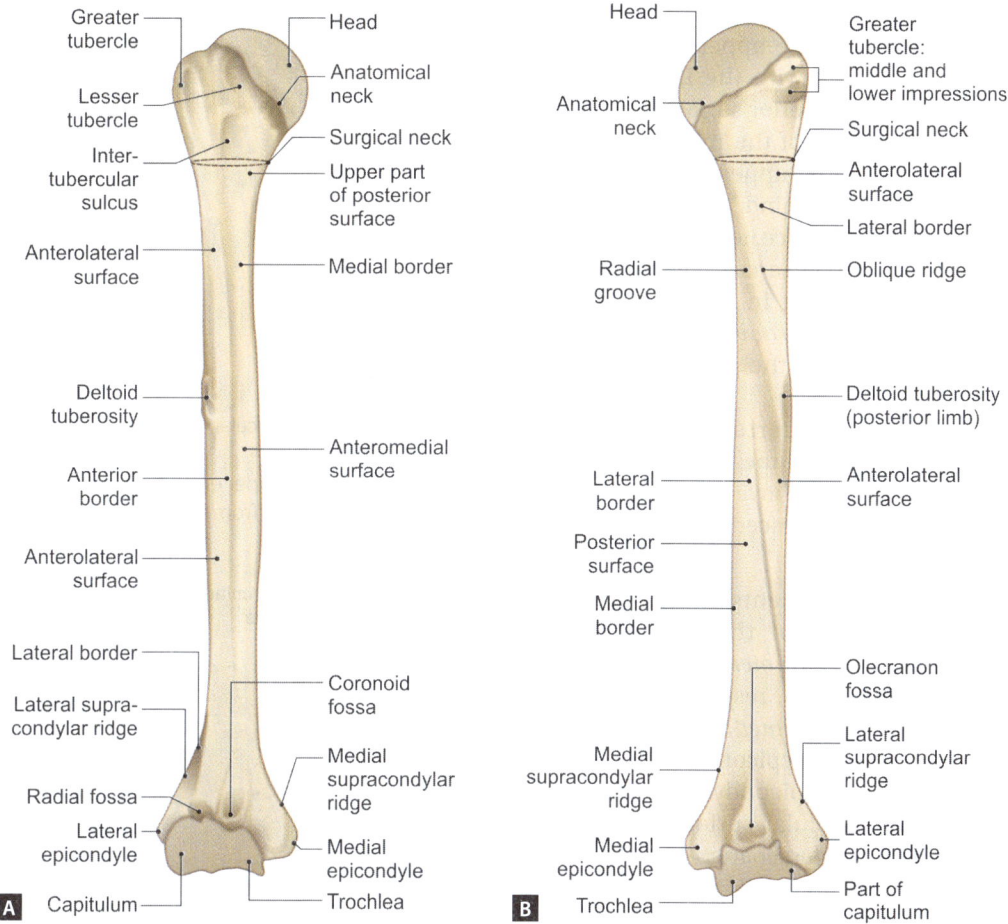

Figs. 3.19A and B: (A) Right humerus from the front; (B) Right humerus from behind.

Upper end shows two distinct *necks*:
a) *Anatomical neck* at the junction of the head with the upper end.
b) *Surgical neck* at the junction of the upper end with the shaft.

Shaft

The *shaft* has three borders: (a) anterior, (b) medial, and (c) lateral. When traced upward the *anterior border* continues with the anterior margin of the greater tubercle (*lateral lip of intertubercular sulcus*). The *medial border* can be traced to the lower end of the lesser tubercle and to its sharp lateral margin (*medial lip of intertubercular sulcus*). The lower part of the *lateral border* can be seen from the front, but its upper part runs upward on the posterior aspect of the bone.

Three borders divide shaft into three surfaces:
a) *Anterolateral surface*: Between anterior and lateral borders.
b) *Anteromedial surface*: Between anterior and medial borders.
c) *Posterior surface*: Between medial and lateral borders.

Because of the convergence of the anterior and medial borders in the upper part, the anteromedial surface continues with the intertubercular sulcus and part of the posterior surface seen from the front. Similarly, because of the medial inclination of the lateral border in its upper part of the anterolateral surface seen from behind.

Anterolateral surface near the middle of the surface has a V-shaped rough area called the *deltoid tuberosity*. Posteriorly the shaft in its upper part is crossed by shallow *radial groove* which runs downward and laterally across the posterior and anterolateral surfaces.

Radial groove interrupts the lateral border of the shaft. The part of the border below the groove is indistinct; the part above the groove is also not well marked, but can be traced to the posterior part of the greater tuberosity.

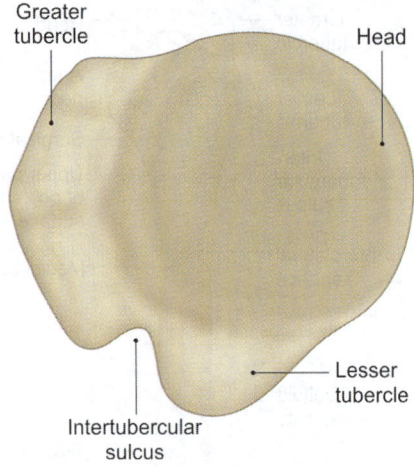

Fig. 3.20: Upper end of right humerus from above.

Lower end: It presents the *condyles*. The lowest parts of the medial and lateral borders form *medial* and *lateral supracondylar ridges,* respectively. Their lower ends end in *medial* and *lateral epicondyles* (medial epicondyle is larger). Between the two epicondyles, the lower end presents articular surface; divisible into medial and lateral parts.

Rounded lateral part is the *capitulum*; articulates with the head of the radius.

Pulley-shaped medial part is the *trochlea*; articulates with the upper end (*trochlear notch*) of the ulna. The medial margin of the trochlea projects downwards much below the level of the capitulum.

The anterior aspect of the lower end above capitulum and trochlea shows two depressions. The depression above the capitulum is the *radial fossa* and above the trochlea is the *coronoid fossa*. Parts of the head of the radius and the coronoid process of the ulna lie in these fossae in fully flexed elbow. Depression above the trochlea on the posterior aspect of the lower end is the *olecranon fossa* that lodges the olecranon process of the ulna in fully extended elbow **(Figs. 3.20 and 3.21)**.

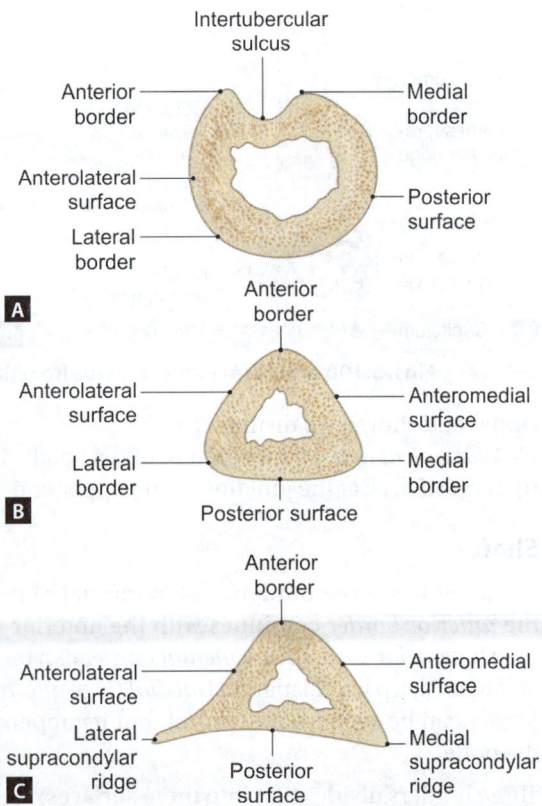

Figs. 3.21A to C: Transverse section (TS) through shaft of humerus (viewed from below). (A) Near upper end; (B) At its middle; (C) Near lower end.

Humerus: Attachments (Figs. 3.22 to 3.24)

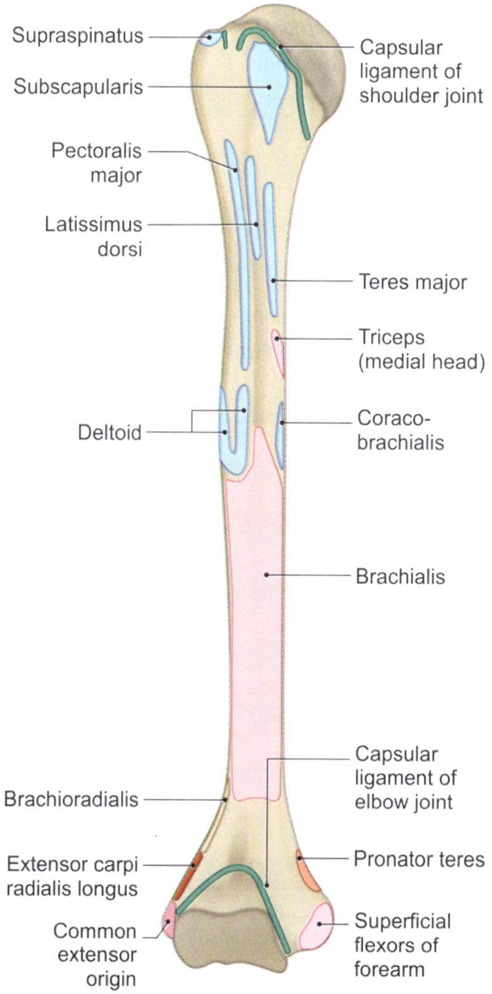

Fig. 3.22: Right humerus: Attachments seen from the front.

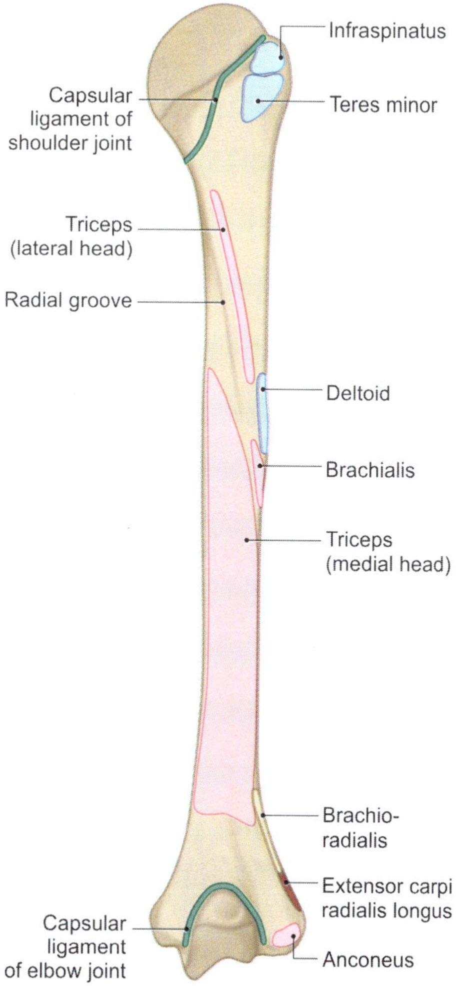

Fig. 3.23: Right humerus: Attachments seen from behind.

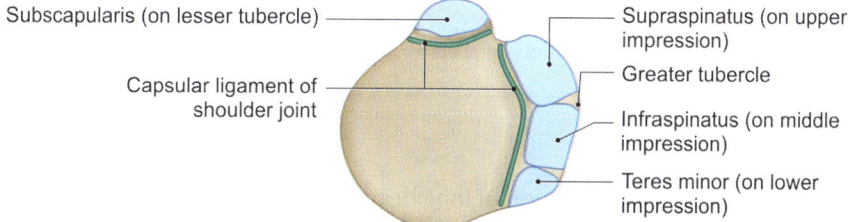

Fig. 3.24: Upper end of right humerus: Attachments seen from above.

Muscles

Muscle	Attachment
Supraspinatus	Upper impression on the greater tubercle (*insertion*)
Infraspinatus	Middle impression on the greater tubercle (*insertion*)
Teres minor	Lower impression on the greater tubercle (*insertion*)
Subscapularis	Lesser tubercle (*insertion*)
Pectoralis major	Lateral lip of intertubercular sulcus (*insertion*)
Latissimus dorsi	Floor of intertubercular sulcus (*insertion*)
Teres major	Medial lip of intertubercular sulcus (*insertion*)
Deltoid	Deltoid tuberosity (*insertion*)
Coracobrachialis	Rough area on the middle of medial border (*insertion*)
Brachialis	Lower halves of anteromedial and anterolateral surfaces of shaft; area extends onto posterior aspect (*origin*)
Pronator teres (*humeral head*)	Anteromedial surface, near lower end of medial supracondylar ridge (*origin*)
Brachioradialis	Upper two-thirds of lateral supracondylar ridge (*origin*)
Extensor carpi radialis longus	Lower one-third of lateral supracondylar ridge (*origin*)
Forearm: Superficial flexors	Anterior aspect of medial epicondyle (*origin*)
Forearm: Common extensor	Anterior aspect of lateral condyle (*origin*)
Triceps (*lateral head*)	Oblique ridge on the upper part of posterior surface, above radial groove (*origin*)
Triceps (*medial head*)	Posterior surface below radial groove; extends on to anterior aspect of shaft (*origin*)
Anconeus	Posterior surface of lateral epicondyle (*origin*)

Other Attachments

Structure	Attachment
Capsular ligament of shoulder joint	Anatomical neck *except* on medial side where attachment dips down one centimeter; attachment interrupted at intertubercular sulcus for tendon of long head of biceps that leaves joint cavity
Capsular ligament of elbow joint	• Attachment include radial and coronoid fossae, (*anteriorly*) and olecranon fossa (*posteriorly*) (*fossae within joint cavity*) • Medially, attachment passes between medial epicondyle and trochlea • On lateral side passes between lateral epicondyle and capitulum
Medial and lateral intermuscular septa	Medial and lateral supracondylar ridges
Ulnar and radial collateral ligaments	Medial and lateral epicondyles

Humerus: Relations

❖ **Intertubercular sulcus** lodges tendon of long head of biceps brachii with ascending branch of anterior circumflex humeral artery.

- *Surgical neck* is related to axillary nerve and anterior and posterior circumflex humeral vessels.
- *Radial groove* lodges radial nerve and the profunda brachii vessels.
- *Medial epicondyle* posteriorly is crossed by ulnar nerve.

Ossification

One primary center appears in the shaft during 8th fetal week. The greater part of the bone is formed from this center.

Secondary centers appear for:
- Head in first year
- Greater tubercle in second year
- Lesser tubercle in fifth year

These fuse with each other in the sixth year to form a single epiphysis for the upper end which fuses with the shaft about 18–20 years.

At the lower end a center appears in:
- Capitulum during first year
- Medial part of the trochlea in ninth or 10th year
- Lateral epicondyle around 12th year.

These fuse to form a single epiphysis which fuses with the shaft around 15 years.

A separate center appears in the medial epicondyle around fifth year; fuses with the shaft about 20th year **(Fig. 3.25)**.

Clinical Anatomy

- *Palpation of the ulnar nerve*: It can be palpated behind the medial epicondyle in a semiflexed elbow.
- *Fracture of surgical neck of humerus*: Axillary nerve winds around surgical neck of humerus. It may get damaged in fracture of surgical neck. There will be loss of contour of affected shoulder, abduction from 16–90° and sensation over lower half of deltoid.

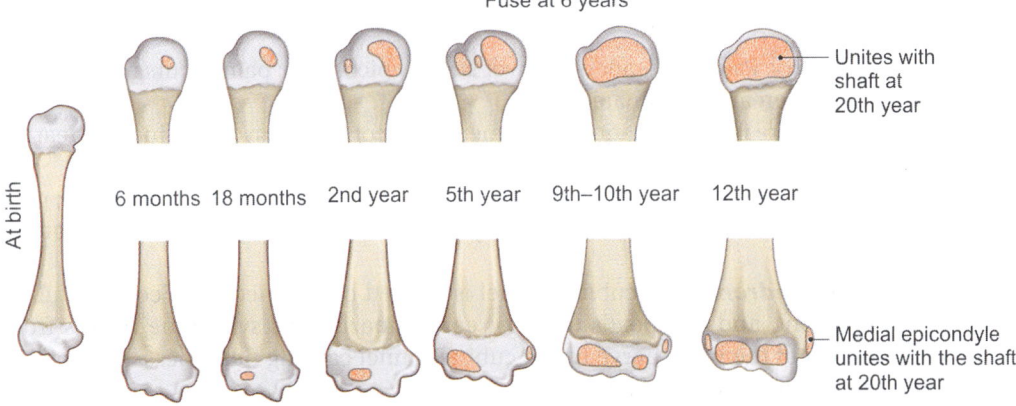

Fig. 3.25: Humerus: Ossification.

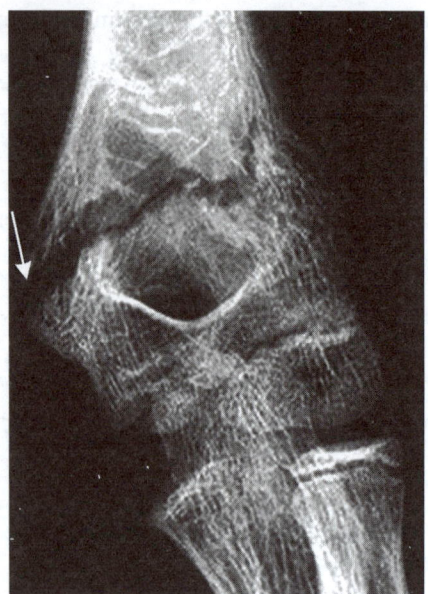

Fig. 3.26: Supracondylar fracture of humerus.

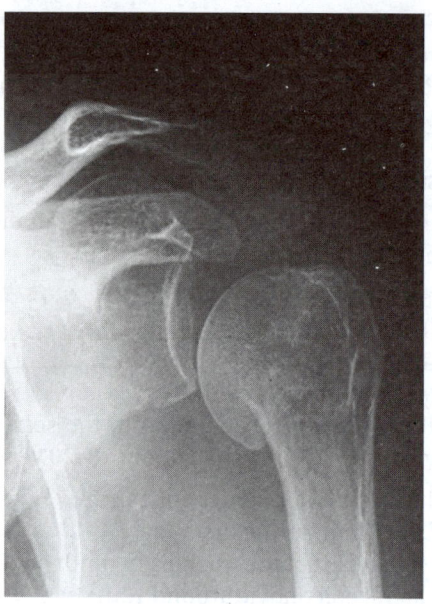

Fig. 3.27: Dislocation of shoulder joint.

- ❖ **Supracondylar fracture of humerus (Fig. 3.26):** This (*common in children and adolescents*) occurs due to fall on the outstretched hand. At times it may involve brachial artery resulting in *Volkmann's ischemic contracture*. Radial and median nerves may be involved from the displaced fracture fragment.
- ❖ **Dislocation (subluxation) of shoulder joint (Fig. 3.27):** It occurs usually in the anteroinferior direction (*no support by rotator cuff*). It may damage axillary nerve and posterior humeral circumflex vessels.
- ❖ **Tennis elbow:** This most common cause of elbow pain is due to inflammation of tissues surrounding humeral lateral epicondyle. Causes include spasm of radial collateral ligament and tearing of common extensor origin **(Fig. 3.28)**.
    - ▪ *Mechanism:* Repeated violent extension of wrist with forearm pronated (backhand stroke in lawn tennis).
    - ▪ *Clinical features:* Pain and tenderness over lateral epicondyle; pain occurs on extension of elbow when forearm is pronated.
- ❖ **Golfer's elbow:** There is inflammation at the medial epicondyle. The causes include tearing of ulnar collateral ligament or tearing of common flexor origin.
    - ▪ *Clinical features:* Pain and tenderness over anterior aspect of medial epicondyle; pain aggravates by stretching flexor tendons by forcible extension of wrist while patient flexes it.
- ❖ **Cubital tunnel syndrome:** The cubital tunnel is formed by the medial epicondyle, ulnar collateral ligament, and two heads of flexor carpi ulnaris. This syndrome results from the compression of the ulnar nerve in the cubital tunnel causing numbness and tingling sensations in the ring and little fingers.

CHAPTER 3 ✦ Bones of Upper Limb

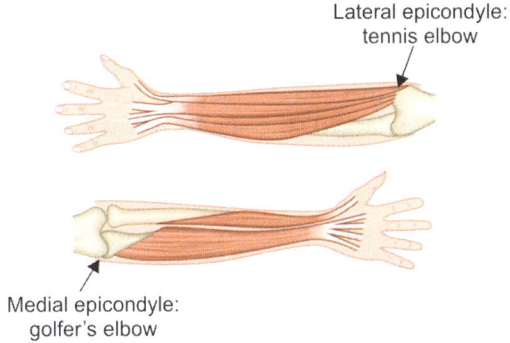

Fig. 3.28: Tennis elbow and golfer's elbow.

QUESTIONNAIRE

- Side determination and anatomical position.
- Name the joints associated with it and their types.
- What are the three necks of the humerus?
- Mark the nerves closely related to this bone.
- Mark the attachments of:

Ligaments	Muscles
Capsule of shoulder joint	Shoulder cuff muscles
Transverse humeral	On intertubercular sulcus
Glenohumeral	Deltoid
Coracohumeral	Brachialis and coracobrachialis
Capsule of elbow joint	Triceps (medial and lateral heads)
Radial collateral ligament of elbow joint	Common flexors origin
Ulnar collateral ligament of elbow joint	Common extensors origin

- Demonstrate the movements of the shoulder joint.
- Demonstrate the movements at elbow joint.
- Mark the epiphyseal lines at the upper and lower ends.
- What is supracondylar spur?
- What is ligament of Struthers'?
- What do you understand by Volkmann's ischemic contracture?

RADIUS

It is the lateral bone of the forearm (long bone); homologous with tibia of lower limb.

Side Determination

- ❖ *Superior*: Head of radius.
- ❖ *Medial*: Sharp interosseous border.
- ❖ *Anterior*: Concavity at the lower end.

38 CHAPTER 3 ✦ Bones of Upper Limb

Anatomical Position

Placed vertically in the body.

The radius presents a shaft and two ends (upper and lower). The upper end bears a disc-shaped head. The lower end is enlarged. The shaft is convex laterally with a sharp medial (*interosseous*) border. The posterior aspect of the lower end is marked by many ridges and grooves **(Figs. 3.29 to 3.33)**.

Upper end: It consists of head, neck and tuberosity. The *head* is disc-shaped. Its upper surface is concave and articulates with the capitulum of humerus. The circumference of the head is smooth and articular. Medially it articulates with the ulnar notch; remaining part is enclosed by the annular ligament. This joint is the superior radioulnar joint (*pivot joint*) **(Fig. 3.30)**.

The constricted region just below the head is the *neck*. Just below the medial part of the neck there is *radial tuberosity*. The tuberosity is rough posteriorly; smooth anteriorly.

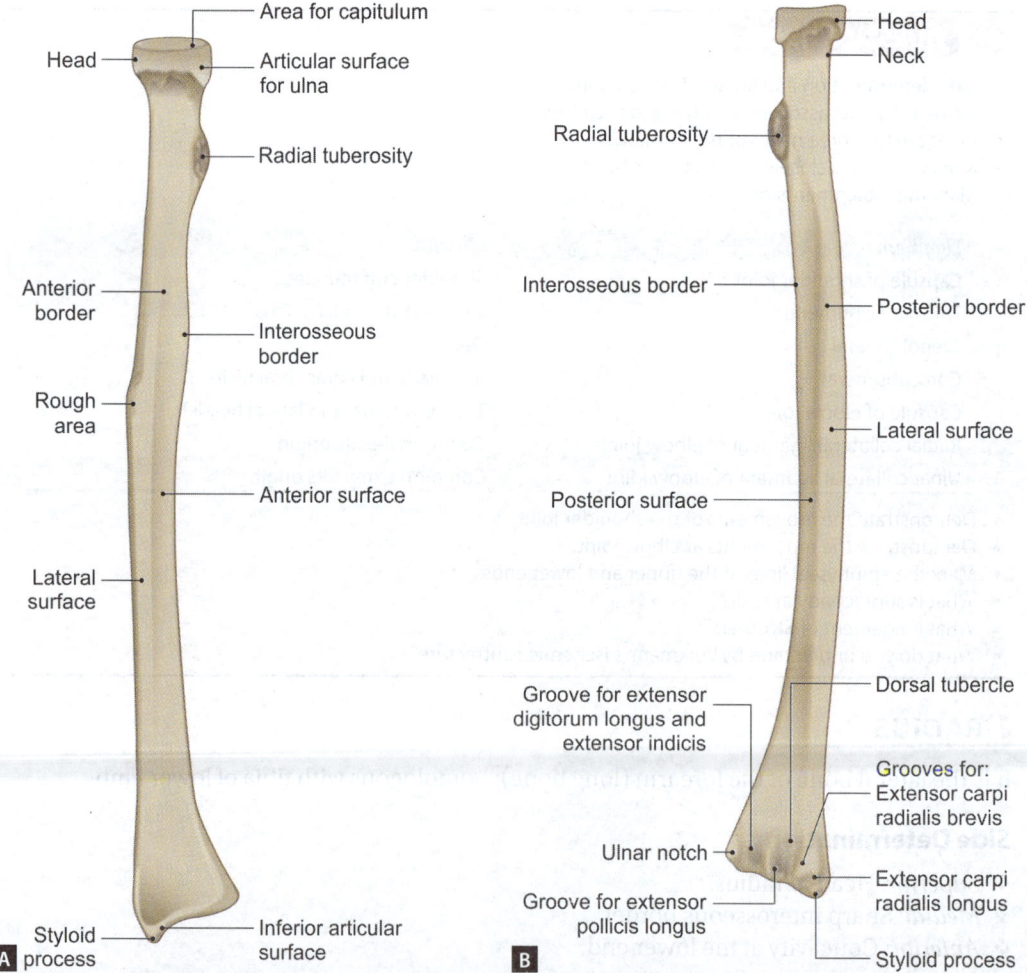

Figs. 3.29A and B: (A) Right radius seen from the front; (B) Right radius seen from behind.

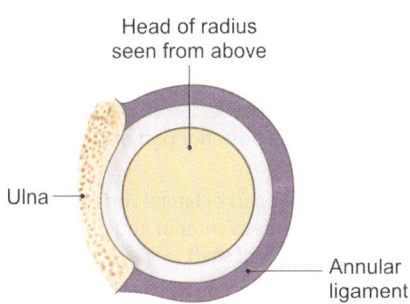

Fig. 3.30: Relationship of head of radius to the ulna and annular ligament.

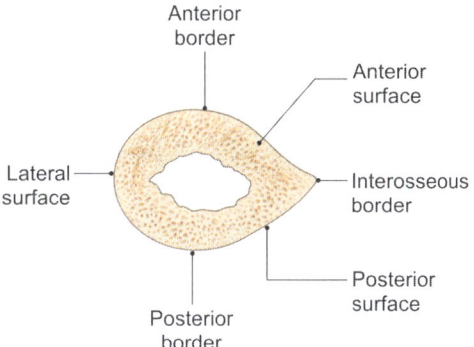

Fig. 3.31: Transverse section (TS) middle of shaft to show its borders and surfaces.

Shaft: The shaft presents **(Fig. 3.31)**:
- Three borders—(a) anterior, (b) posterior, and (c) interosseous.
- Three surfaces—(a) anterior, (b) posterior, and (c) lateral.

1. *Anterior border* begins at the radial tuberosity and runs downward and laterally across the anterior aspect of the shaft. This part of the border is the *anterior oblique line*. It then runs downward and forms the lateral boundary of the smooth anterior aspect of the lower part of the shaft.
2. *Posterior border:* Upper part of this border runs downward and laterally from the posterior part of radial tuberosity. The lower part of posterior border runs downward along the middle of the posterior aspect of the shaft to the lower end.
3. *Interosseous* (sharp and medial) *border* extends just below the radial tuberosity to the lower end of the shaft. Near the lower end this border forms the posterior margin of a small triangular area.

Shaft presents three surfaces:
a) *Anterior surface*: Between interosseous and anterior borders.
b) *Posterior surface*: Between interosseous and posterior borders.
c) *Lateral surface*: Between anterior and posterior borders.

In the upper part, the *lateral surface* expands into a wide triangular area. The lateral surface shows a rough area near the middle part of the shaft.

Lower end: It presents anterior, lateral, and posterior surfaces that continue with the corresponding surfaces of the shaft. In addition, it presents medial and inferior surfaces. The lateral surface is prolonged downward as the *styloid process*. The medial aspect of the lower end shows an articular area called the *ulnar notch*. It articulates with the lower end of ulna (*head*) to form the inferior radioulnar joint (*pivot joint*). Just above the notch there is a triangular area. The posterior aspect of the lower end is marked by a number of vertical grooves separated by ridges. The most prominent ridge is the *dorsal tubercle* (midway between medial and lateral aspects of lower end). Immediately medial to the tubercle there is a narrow oblique groove, and still medially there is a wide shallow groove. The area lateral to the dorsal tubercle shows two grooves separated by a ridge. The inferior surface of the lower end is articular. It forms the wrist joint. It is subdivided into a medial quadrangular area that articulates with the lunate and a lateral triangular area that articulates with the scaphoid **(Figs. 3.32A and B)**.

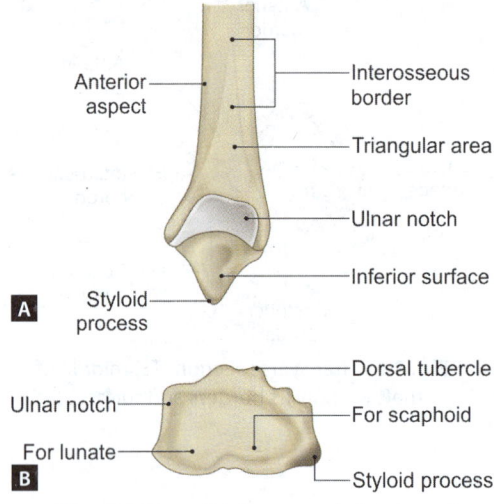

Figs. 3.32A and B: Lower end of right radius: (A) From medial side; (B) From below side.

Attachments on the Radius (Figs. 3.33A and B)

Muscles Insertion

Muscle	Insertion
Biceps brachii	Rough posterior part of radial tuberosity
Supinator	Upper part of lateral surface; extends to anterior and posterior aspects of shaft
Pronator teres	Rough area on the middle of lateral surface
Brachioradialis	Lowest part of lateral surface above styloid process
Pronator quadratus	Lower part of anterior surface and triangular area on the medial side of lower end

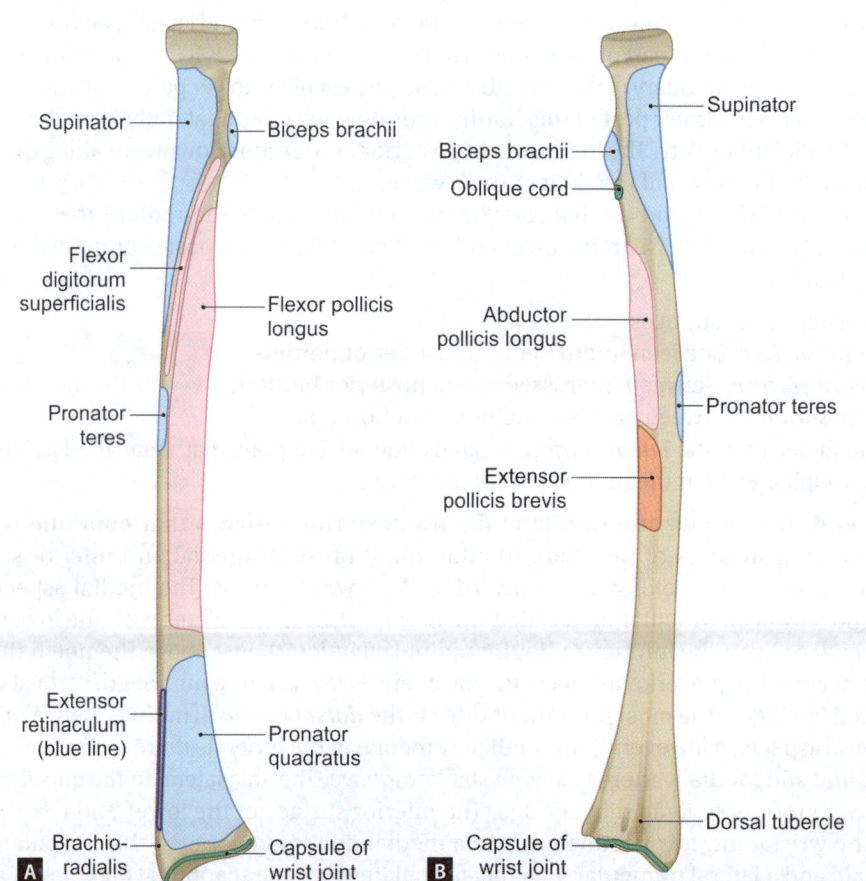

Figs. 3.33A and B: Right radius: (A) Attachments from the front; (B) Attachments from behind.

CHAPTER 3 ✦ Bones of Upper Limb

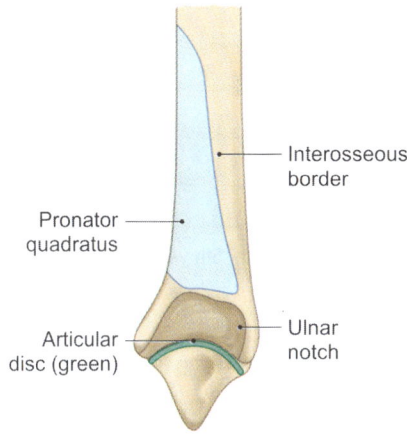

Fig. 3.34: Lower end of right radius: Attachments seen from medial side.

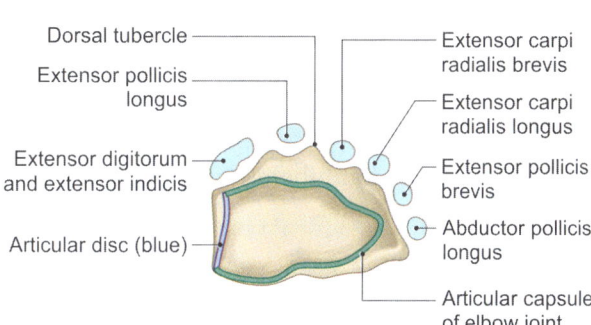

Fig. 3.35: Lower end of right radius from below: Related tendons.

Muscles Origin

Muscle	Origin
Flexor digitorum superficialis (*radial head*)	Upper part of anterior border (oblique line)
Flexor pollicis longus	Upper two-thirds of anterior surface
Abductor pollicis longus	Upper part of posterior surface
Extensor pollicis brevis	Small area on the posterior surface below the area for abductor pollicis longus

Other Attachments (Fig. 3.34)

Structure	Attachment
Articular capsule of wrist joint	Anterior and posterior margins of the lower end and styloid process
Articular disc of inferior radioulnar joint	Lower border of ulnar notch
Interosseous membrane	Lower three-fourths of interosseous border
Oblique cord	Just below radial tuberosity
Extensor retinaculum	Lower part of anterior border

Lower End of Radius: Tendons Related (Fig. 3.35)

Groove	Tendons related
Groove behind medial part of lower end	Extensor digitorum and extensor indicis
Oblique groove medial to dorsal tubercle	Extensor pollicis longus
Groove lateral to dorsal tubercle	Extensor carpi radialis longus and brevis

Lateral aspect of the lower end of the radius is crossed by the tendon of abductor pollicis longus and extensor pollicis brevis.

Ossification (Fig. 3.36)

- A primary center appears in the shaft during 8th week of fetal life.
- A secondary center appears in the lower end in first year; joins shaft around 18 years.
- A secondary center appears in the head during fourth or fifth year; fuses with shaft around 16th year.
- Occasionally radial tuberosity may ossify from a separate center.

Clinical Anatomy

- **Subluxation of radial head (pulled elbow):** This is common in young children.
    - *Mechanism of injury:* Annular ligament is funnel-shaped in adults; tubular in children. When the child is suddenly lifted or pulled up by forearm (forearm is pronated), the head of radius slips out of the annular ligament called subluxation (incomplete dislocation).
    - *Clinical features:* Inability to use the limb from a fall or jerk, child complains of pain and restricted supination and the child keeps elbow fixed/supported in slight flexion and pronation.
  Subluxation is reduced by firm supination of elbow while pushing radius in proximal direction.
- **Colles' fracture:** It is due to a fall on the outstretched hand. Deformity caused by dorsal displacement of distal radius segment is the *dinner fork deformity* (**Fig. 3.37**).
- **Smith–Petersen fracture:** It is reverse Colles' fracture. Here, distal one-fourth of radius is fractured when a person falls on hyperflexed wrist. Distal fragment is displaced downward and forward (**Fig. 3.38**).
- **Weight transmission:** During fall, the palm hits the ground and the force of impact is received by the hand. At wrist joint, major contribution is by the radius. Thus, the impact is transmitted

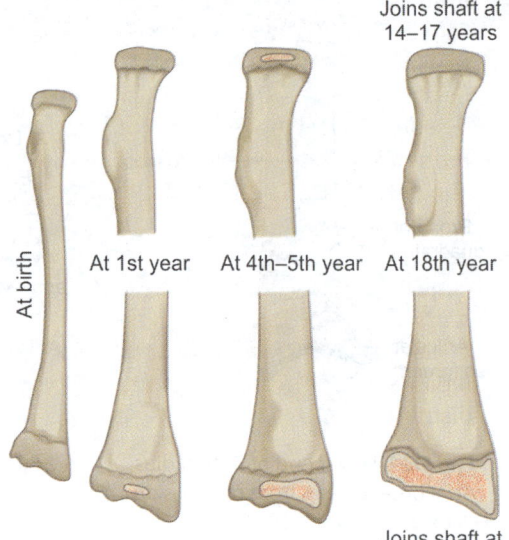

Fig. 3.36: Radius: Ossification.

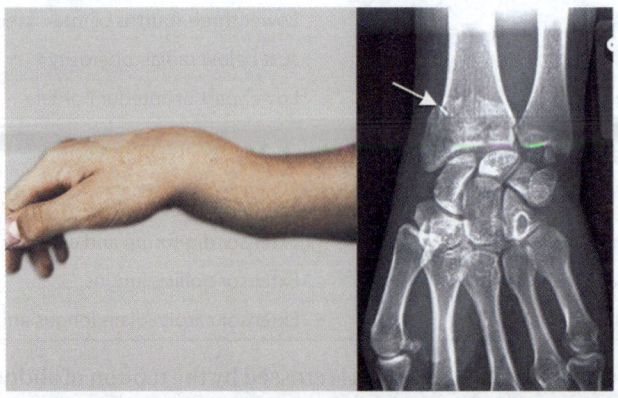

Fig. 3.37: Colles' fracture with dinner fork deformity.

from the palm to the forearm along the radius. At elbow joint, ulna has a major contribution than radius. Therefore, line of force transmission passes from the radius onto the ulna via the interosseous membrane (*fibers in interosseous membrane directed downward from radius to ulna*). The ulna transmits force to humerus. From the head of humerus, force is received by glenoid cavity; majority carried to coracoid process. The coracoclavicular ligament (*conoid and trapezoid parts*) transmits the impact onto the lateral end of clavicle. From the medial end of the clavicle it passes to the sternum. From sternum, force is distributed along the ribs to the vertebral column.

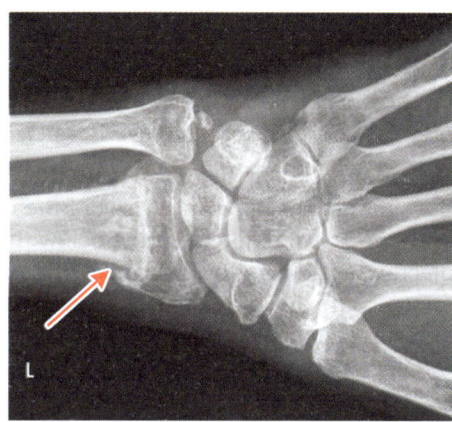

Fig. 3.38: Smith-Peterson fracture.

QUESTIONNAIRE

- Side determination and anatomical position.
- What are the joints associated with this bone and their types?
- Mark the attachments of:

Ligaments	Muscles
Capsule of elbow joint	Biceps brachii
Radial collateral ligament of elbow joint	Supinator
Annular ligament	Flexor pollicis longus
Quadrate ligament	Flexor digitorum superficialis
Interosseous membrane	Pronator quadratus
Articular disc of inferior radioulnar joint	Brachioradialis
Ulnar collateral ligament of elbow joint	Of posterior compartment of forearm

- Mark the attachments of capsule of elbow joint, annular, and quadrate ligaments.
- Identify the dorsal tubercle. Enumerate the tendons in relation to it.
- Comment on its ossification. Which is the growing end?
- How and where the radial head is palpated?
- Demonstrate the movements at superior and inferior radioulnar joints.
- Demonstrate the movements at wrist joint. Enumerate the muscles causing them.
- What is tennis elbow?
- What is pulled elbow? Why it is common in young children?
- What is Colles' fracture and dinner fork deformity?

ULNA

It is the medial bone of the forearm (long bone); homologous with the fibula of the lower limb.

Side Determination

- ❖ *Superior*: Hook like olecranon process.
- ❖ *Lateral*: Sharp interosseous border.
- ❖ *Anterior*: Trochlear notch.

Anatomical Position

Placed vertically in the body.

The ulna presents a *shaft* and two *ends*. The upper end is large and irregular, the lower end presents head. The upper end anteriorly presents *trochlear notch* (**Figs. 3.39A and B**).

Upper end: It consists of two processes. The *olecranon process* is the upward continuation of the shaft; forms uppermost part of the ulna. The *coronoid process* projects forward from the anterior aspect of the ulna just below the olecranon process. The *trochlear notch* is between olecranon and coronoid processes. It articulates with the trochlea of the humerus; forms elbow joint. The trochlear notch is divided into medial and lateral areas corresponding to the medial and lateral flanges of the trochlea.

Olecranon process presents anterior, superior, posterior, medial and lateral surfaces.

The upper surface of coronoid process forms the lower part of the trochlear notch. In addition it has anterior, medial and lateral surfaces. The anterior surface is triangular. Its lower part shows a rough projection called the ulnar tuberosity. The upper part of the lateral surface of the coronoid process shows the radial notch (concave articular facet); articulates with the head of the radius to form superior radioulnar joint (*pivot joint*). There is a depression just below the radial notch. The posterior border of this depression is formed by a ridge called the *supinator crest* (**Figs. 3.40 and 3.41**).

Lower end: It consists of a disc-like *head* and *styloid process*. The head has a circular inferior surface. This surface is separated from the cavity of the wrist joint by an articular disc. The

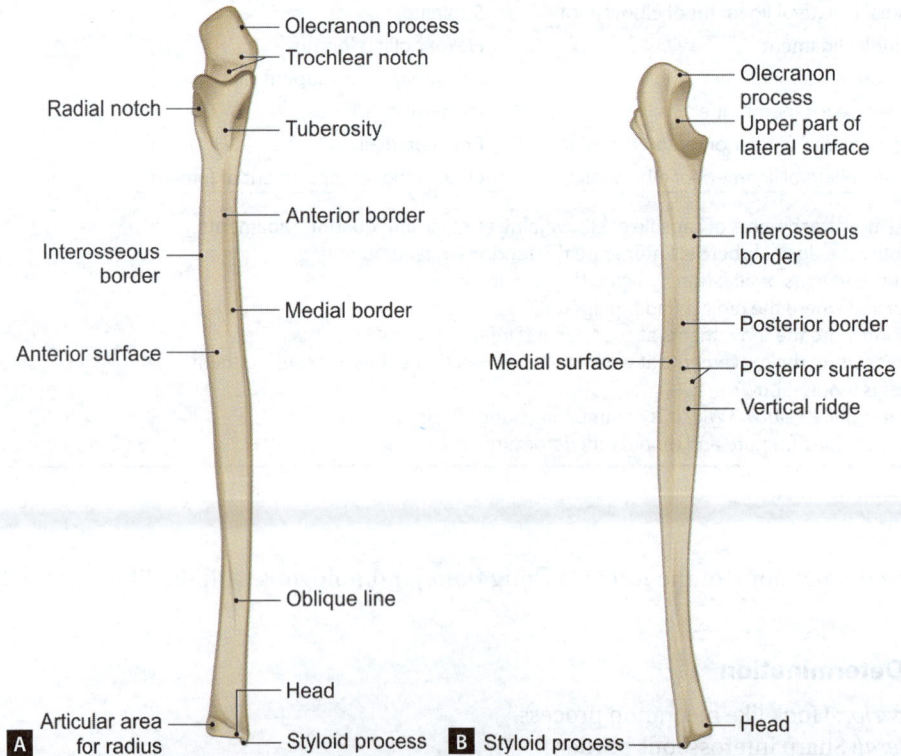

Figs. 3.39A and B: (A) Right ulna from the front; (B) Right ulna from behind.

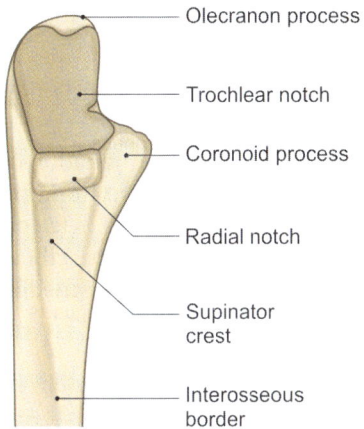

Fig. 3.40: Upper part of right ulna from lateral side.

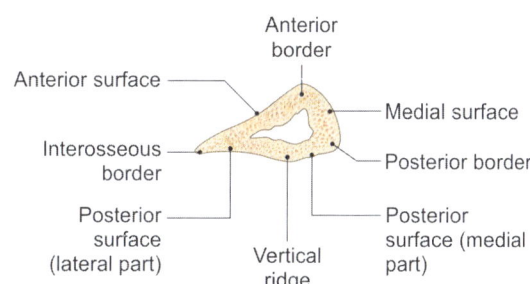

Fig. 3.41: Transverse section (TS) middle of the shaft of ulna: Surfaces and borders.

head has another convex articular surface on its lateral side. It articulates with the ulnar notch of the radius to form the inferior radioulnar joint (*pivot joint*). The styloid process (downward projection) lies on the posteromedial aspect of the head. Between the styloid process and the head, the posterior aspect is marked by a vertical groove. The tip of the styloid process of the ulna is at a higher level than that of the radius.

Shaft: The shaft has anterior, posterior and sharp lateral (*interosseous*) borders and anterior, posterior, and medial surfaces.

Upper part of *interosseous border* continues with the supinator crest.

Anterior border begins at ulnar tuberosity. Near its lower end it curves backward to end in front of the styloid process.

Posterior border begins at the apex of the triangular area on the posterior aspect of the olecranon process and ends at the styloid process.

Anterior surface (between interosseous and anterior borders) in its lower part shows oblique ridge that runs downward and medially from the interosseous border.

Medial surface lies between the anterior and posterior borders.

Posterior surface (between interosseous and posterior borders) is marked by two lines that divide it into three areas.
a. Upper line (runs obliquely downwards and medially) starts at posterior end of the radial notch and terminates by joining the posterior border
b. Part of the posterior surface above the line is triangular
c. Part below the oblique line is subdivided into medial and lateral parts by a vertical ridge.

Ulna: Attachments (Figs. 3.42 to 3.44)

Muscles Insertion

Muscle	Insertion
Brachialis	Anterior surface of coronoid process and ulnar tuberosity
Triceps	Posterior part of superior surface of olecranon process
Anconeus	Lateral aspect of olecranon process and upper one-fourth of posterior surface of shaft

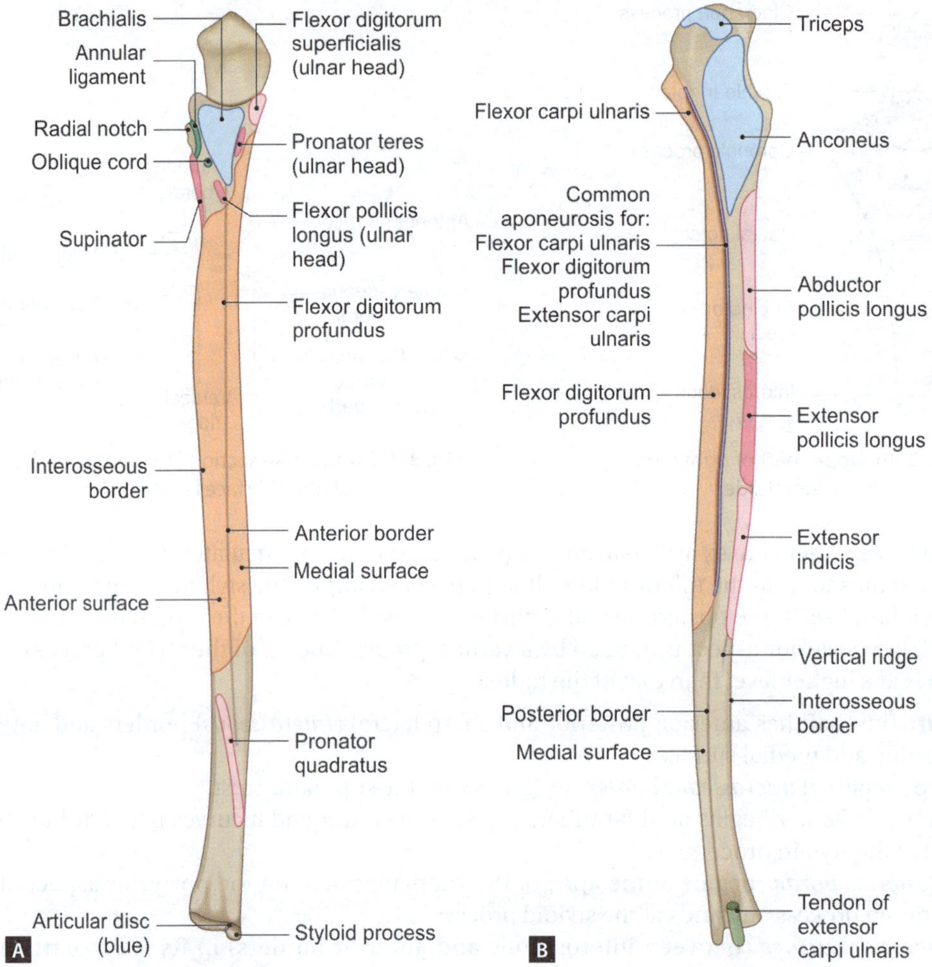

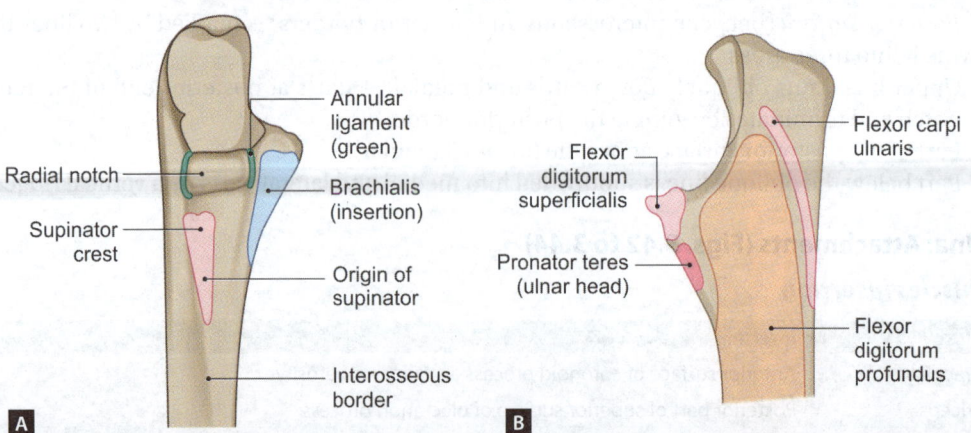

Figs. 3.42A and B: Right ulna: (A) Attachments from front; (B) Attachments from behind.

Figs. 3.43A and B: Upper end of right ulna: (A) Attachments from lateral side; (B) Attachments from medial side.

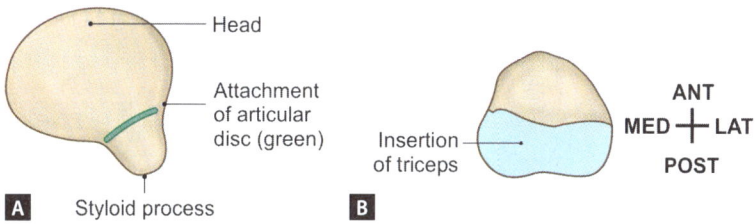

Figs. 3.44A and B: (A) Lower end of right ulna from below; (B) Olecranon process from above.

Muscles Origin

Muscle	Origin
Flexor digitorum profundus	• Upper three-fourths of anterior and medial surfaces; extends to medial surfaces of coronoid and olecranon processes • Also from posterior border through common aponeurosis of flexor carpi ulnaris and extensor carpi ulnaris
Supinator	Supinator crest and triangular area in front of it
Flexor pollicis longus	Lateral border of coronoid process
Flexor digitorum superficialis (*ulnar head*)	Tubercle at the upper end of medial margin of coronoid process
Pronator teres (*ulnar head*)	Medial margin of coronoid process
Pronator quadratus	Oblique ridge on the lower part of anterior surface of the shaft
Flexor carpi ulnaris (*ulnar head*)	Medial side of olecranon process and upper two-thirds of posterior border through aponeurosis common to it, extensor carpi ulnaris and flexor digitorum profundus
Extensor carpi ulnaris (*ulnar head*)	Posterior border by aponeurosis common to it, flexor carpi ulnaris and flexor digitorum profundus; posterior surface of ulna is divided into medial and lateral parts by vertical ridge, lateral part lies between vertical ridge and interosseous border; this part of posterior surface is divided into four parts: a) *Uppermost part*: Abductor pollicis longus b) *Next part*: Extensor pollicis longus c) *Third part*: Extensor indicis d) *Lowest part* is devoid of attachments

Other Attachments

Structure	Attachment
Interosseous membrane	Interosseous border
Oblique cord	Lateral side of the tuberosity
Capsular ligament of elbow joint	Margins of trochlear notch (coronoid and olecranon processes)
Annular ligament	Anterior and posterior borders of radial notch
Ulnar collateral ligament	Styloid process
Articular disc of inferior radioulnar joint	Rough area lateral to styloid process

Tendon of *extensor carpi ulnaris* lies in a groove on the posterior aspect of the lower end of the ulna.

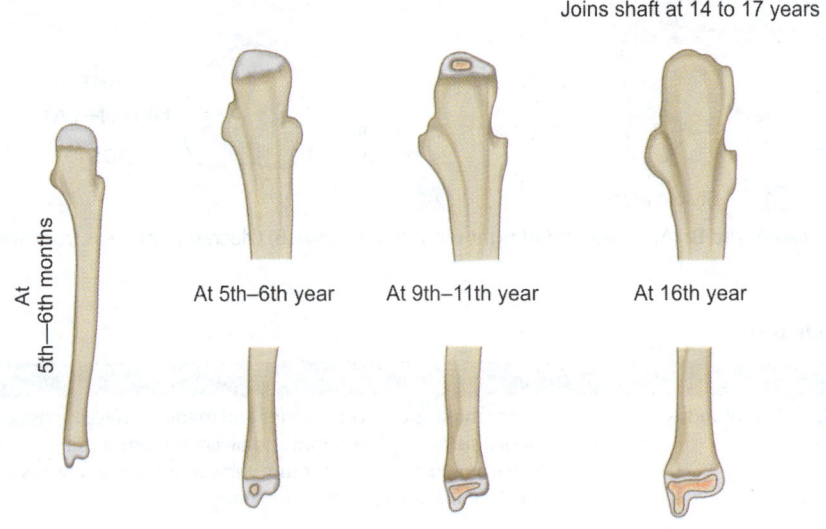

Fig. 3.45: Ulna: Ossification.

Ossification (Fig. 3.45)

- One primary center appears in the shaft in 8th fetal week; forms greater part of ulna.
- One center for lower end appears around fifth to sixth year; joins shaft by 18th year.
- Greater part of olecranon ossifies by extension from primary center. Proximal part of olecranon process ossifies from two centers that appear about 10th year; joins shaft around 15th year.

Clinical Anatomy

- ***Equilateral triangle at elbow:*** Two epicondyles of humerus and tip of olecranon process lie in the same line in the extended elbow. In flexed elbow, these three points form an equilateral triangle. In dislocation of the elbow joint this relationship is altered (**Fig. 3.46**).

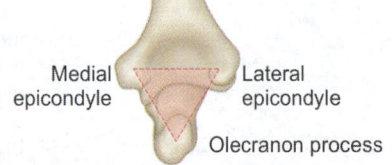

Fig. 3.46: Equilateral triangle at elbow.

- ***Dislocation of the elbow:*** It is produced by a fall on the outstretched hand with the elbow slightly flexed. The olecranon shifts posteriorly and the elbow is fixed in slight flexion.
- ***Student's elbow (Miner's elbow):*** There is inflammation of subcutaneous olecranon bursa which causes a round, fluctuating and painful swelling over olecranon process. It is due to repeated friction, or infection from abrasions of skin covering olecranon process (**Fig. 3.47**).
- ***Cubitus valgus:*** There is increase in carrying angle at elbow (also seen in Turner's syndrome).
- ***Carrying angle:*** It is formed by the long axis of the arm and forearm; opens laterally when the elbow is extended. The medial edge of the trochlea projects more inferiorly than its lateral edge and the forearm deviates (5-15°) laterally (**Fig. 3.48**). It is more in women than in men. The angle disappears when the forearm is flexed or pronated.

CHAPTER 3 ✦ Bones of Upper Limb

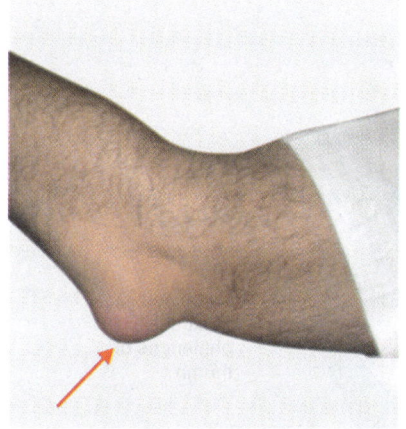

Fig. 3.47: Student's elbow.

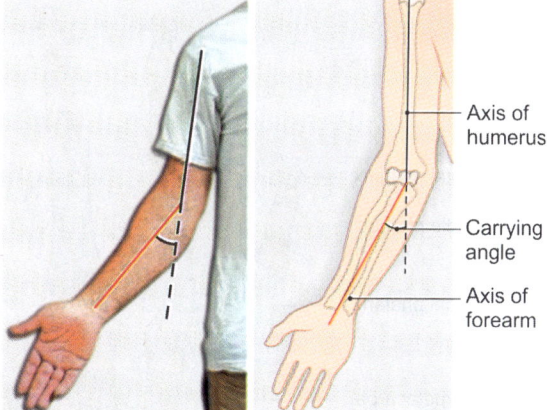

Fig. 3.48: Carrying angle.

❖ **Fracture of olecranon and coronoid processes:**
- Olecranon fracture is caused by a fall on the point of the elbow
- Coronoid process fracture (uncommon); accompanies dislocation of the elbow.

QUESTIONNAIRE

- Side determination and anatomical position.
- What are the joints associated with it and their types?
- Mark the attachments of:

Ligaments	Muscles
Capsule of elbow joint	Triceps brachii and anconeus
Ulnar collateral ligament of elbow joint	Supinator
Annular ligament	Brachialis
Quadrate ligament	Flexor digitorum superficialis
Interosseous membrane	Flexor digitorum profundus
Articular disc of inferior radioulnar joint	Pronator quadratus
Ulnar collateral ligament of elbow joint	Of posterior compartment of forearm

- What are the processes of ulna?
- Which tendon forms the groove on the posterior aspect of the head of ulna?
- Comment in its ossification. Which is the growing end of this bone?
- What are the subcutaneous palpable parts of ulna?
- Does ulna move during supination? If so, which muscles bring this about?
- Demonstrate the movements at radioulnar joints. What is their axis? Name the muscles responsible for these movements.
- Comment on the functional aspect of interosseous membrane.
- What is student's elbow?

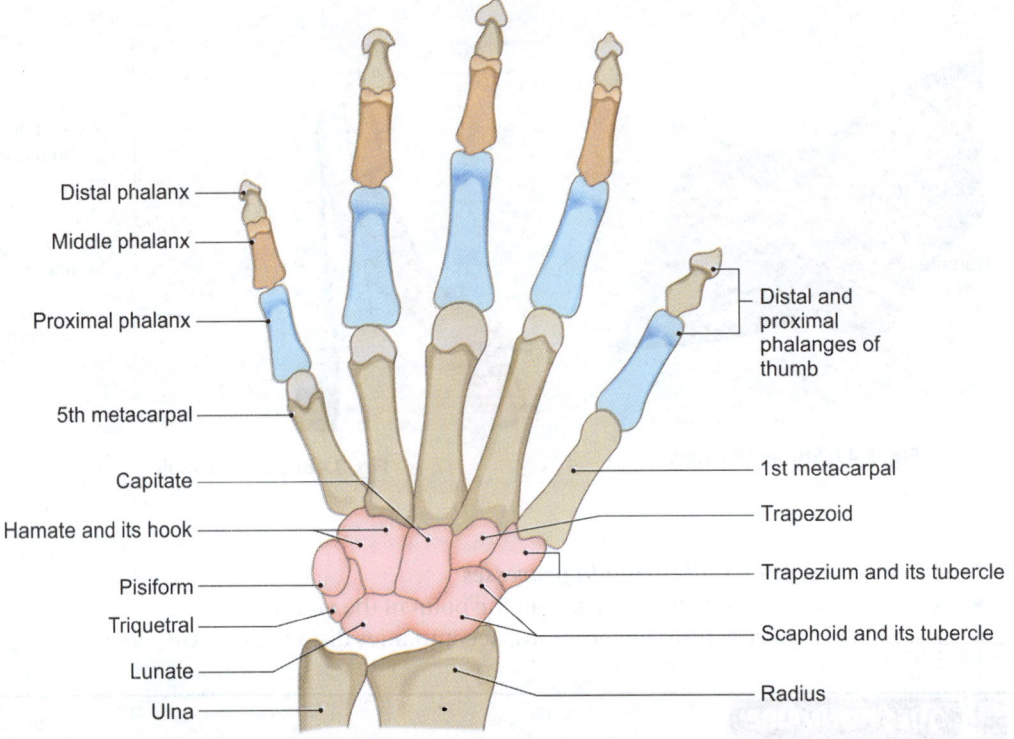

Fig. 3.49: Skeleton of the hand: Palmar aspect.

SKELETON OF THE HAND

AN 8.5 Identify and name various bones in articulated hand.

Skeleton of the hand consists of the bones of the:
- **Wrist:** Skeleton of the wrist consists of eight (*roughly cuboidal*) carpal bones.
- **Palm:** Skeleton of the palm is made up of five metacarpals (*miniature long bones*).
- **Digits:** Skeleton of the fingers is made up of the phalanges. There are three phalanges (proximal, middle, and distal) in each digit except the thumb which has two phalanges (proximal and distal) **(Figs. 3.49 and 3.50)**.

Carpal Bones

The carpal bones are arranged in proximal and distal rows.
- Proximal row is made up (*from lateral to medial side*) of:
  a. Scaphoid   b. Lunate   c. Triquetral   d. Pisiform
- Distal row is made up (*from lateral to medial side*) of:
  a. Trapezium   b. Trapezoid   c. Capitate   d. Hamate

Carpals of the proximal row (*except pisiform*) take part in forming the wrist joint. Distal carpals articulate with the metacarpals. Each carpal bone articulates with neighboring carpal bones to form *intercarpal joints*.

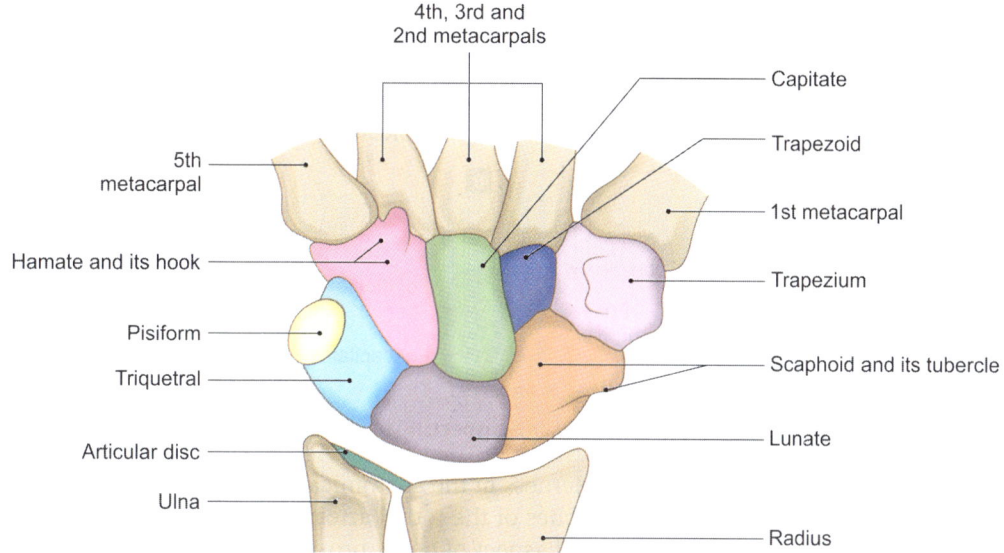

Fig. 3.50: Right carpus from the front.

Scaphoid

It is a boat-shaped bone. The proximal part of the bone shows a large, convex, articular surface for the radius. Distally and laterally the palmar surface of the bone shows a projection called the *tubercle* **(Figs. 3.51A to C)**.

Side Determination

- Proximal side bears large convex facet for radius; tubercle is placed distally.
- Palmar aspect bears tubercle (on distal and lateral part); dorsal surface is narrower than palmar surface.
- Medial and lateral aspects can be distinguished by the tubercle which lies laterally; medial aspect bears a flat semilunar facet for lunate, and concave facet for capitate.

Articulations

- Medial surface articulates with:
  - Lunate (proximally)
  - Capitate (distally).
- Distal surface articulates with:
  - Trapezium (laterally)
  - Trapezoid (medially).

Fracture of Scaphoid and Avascular Necrosis (Fig. 3.52)

AN 8.6 **Describe scaphoid fracture and explain the anatomical basis of avascular necrosis.**

Scaphoid is the most commonly fractured (*70-80% of all carpal fractures*) carpal bone. Generally it occurs after a fall on the outstretched hand causing fracture through the waist of scaphoid

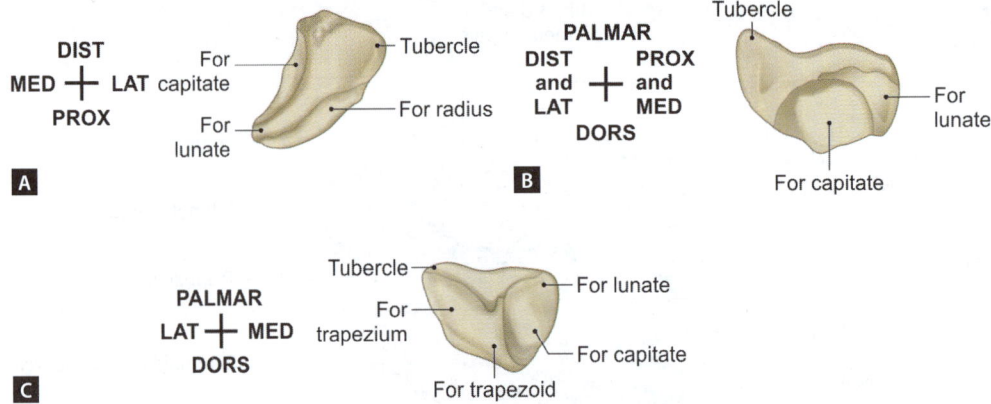

Figs. 3.51A to C: Right scaphoid: (A) Palmar aspect; (B) Medial aspect; (C) Distal aspect.

(about 65% cases). It presents with tenderness in the anatomical snuffbox. The blood supply to scaphoid comes from different branches of the radial artery. Major blood supply to the scaphoid enters distal pole on the dorsal aspect of bone; proximal pole has relatively poor blood supply. Fractures through the waist of scaphoid may disrupt blood supply to proximal pole leading to avascular necrosis.

Lunate (Figs. 3.53A and B)

The lunate bone is lunar crescent shaped.

Side Determination

- Palmar surface is larger than dorsal surface (both surfaces nonarticular and rough).
- Proximal aspect bears a convex facet (for radius); distal aspect has a concave facet (for capitate).
- Medial surface bears a square facet (for triquetral); lateral surface presents a semilunar facet (for scaphoid).

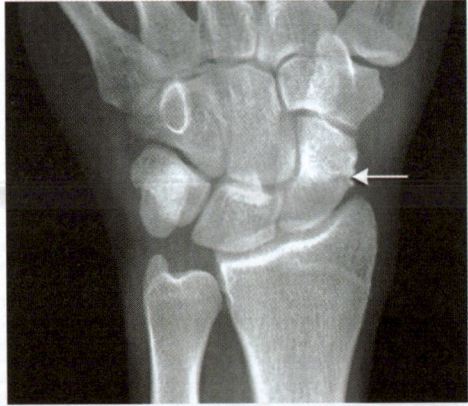

Fig. 3.52: Scaphoid fracture.

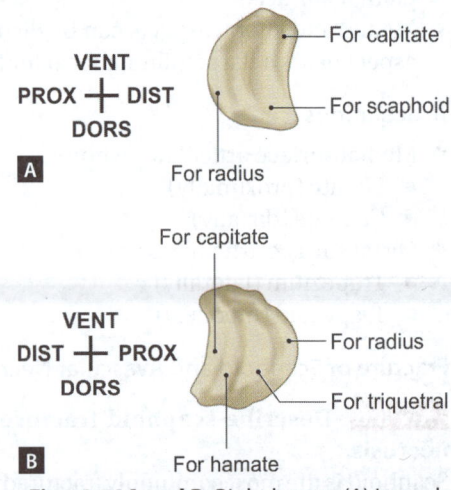

Figs. 3.53A and B: Right lunate: (A) Lateral aspect; (B) Medial aspect.

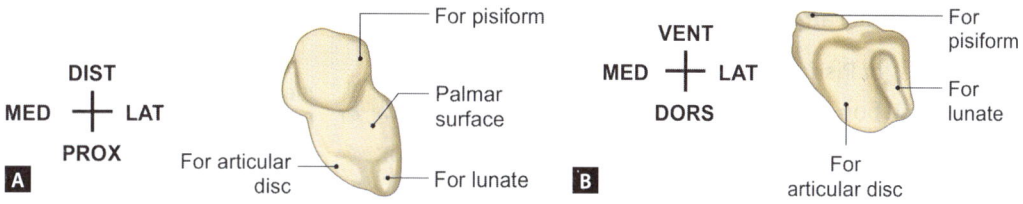

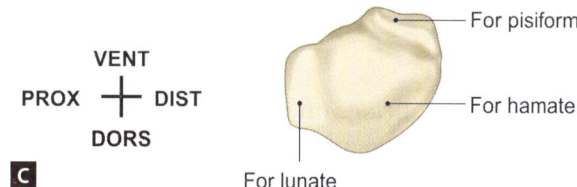

Figs. 3.54A to C: Right triquetral: (A) Palmar aspect; (B) Proximal aspect; (C) Lateral aspect.

Proximally, the lunate has a convex articular facet that takes part in forming the wrist joint.

Lunate Articulates with
- *Scaphoid*: Laterally
- *Triquetral*: Medially
- *Capitate*: Distally.

Triquetral (Figs. 3.54A to C)

It is small roughly cuboidal-shaped bone. It presents palmar, dorsal, proximal, distal, medial, and lateral surfaces.

Side Determination
- Palmar aspect bears oval facet (for pisiform); dorsal aspect is nonarticular.
- Distal aspect can be distinguished: Facet for pisiform is on the distal part of the palmar surface.
- Medial surface bears a convex facet (for wrist joint); lateral surface has a concavo-convex facet (for hamate).

Articulations
- Distal part of palmar surface articulates with pisiform.
- Medial surface is in contact with articular disc of inferior radioulnar joint.
- Lateral surface articulates with hamate.
- Proximal surface articulates with lunate.

Pisiform (Fig. 3.55)

The pisiform bone is pea-shaped. Its dorsal aspect bears a single facet for articulation with the triquetral bone.

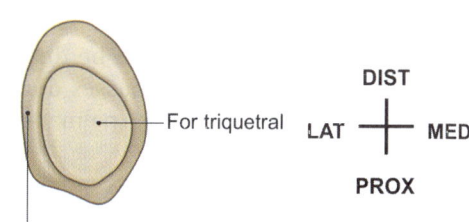

Fig. 3.55: Right pisiform: Dorsal aspect.

AN 8.5 Enumerate the peculiarities of pisiform.

Peculiarities of Pisiform

- Sesamoid bone
- Develops in the tendon of flexor carpi ulnaris
- Smallest carpal bone
- Does not take part in the formation of wrist joint in any position
- Last carpal bone to develop (12th year)
- Lacks periosteum.

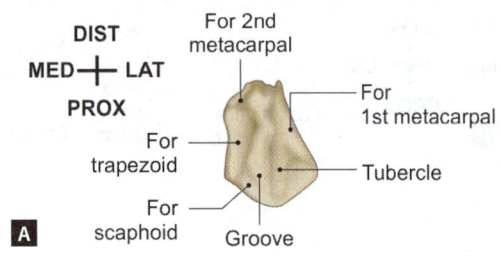

Trapezium (Figs. 3.56A to C)

This bone has a thick prominent *ridge* on its palmar aspect called the *tubercle*.

Side Determination

- Palmar surface bears the tubercle.
- Medial and lateral aspects can be distinguished by examining the palmar surface: Presence of deep groove on the medial side of the tubercle.
- Distal surface bears concavo-convex facet (for first metacarpal); proximal surface has small concave facet (for scaphoid).

Trapezium Articulates with

- *Scaphoid*: Proximally and medially.
- *First metacarpal*: Distally and laterally.
- *Trapezoid*: Medially.
- *Base of second metacarpal*: Distally and medially.

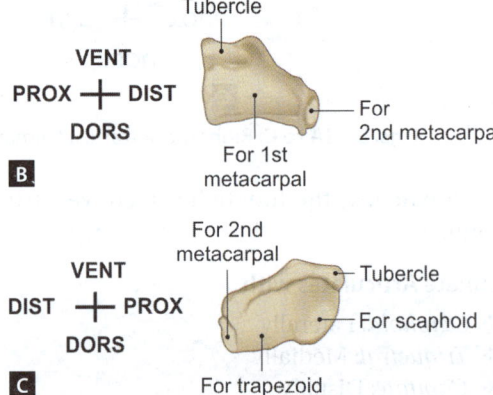

Figs. 3.56A to C: Right trapezium: (A) Palmar aspect; (B) Distal and lateral aspect; (C) Proximal and medial aspect.

Trapezoid (Figs. 3.57A and B)

The trapezoid is small and irregular; shape resembles that of a shoe.

Side Determination

- Palmar surface is much smaller than the dorsal aspect.
- Distal aspect bears concavo-convex facet for base of second metacarpal.
- Medial and lateral sides can be distinguished: rough, nonarticular strip passes dorsally from lateral (and distal) part of the palmar surface.

Trapezoid Articulates with

- *Base of second metacarpal*: Distally.
- *Trapezium*: Laterally.
- *Capitate*: Medially.
- *Scaphoid*: Proximally.

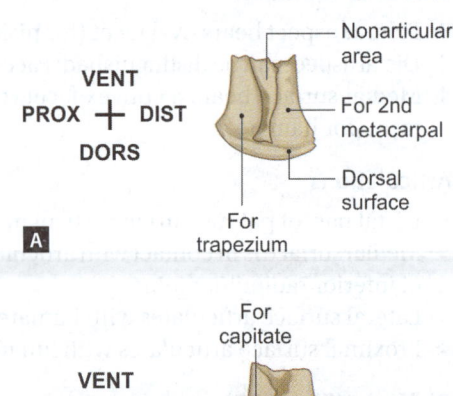

Figs. 3.57A and B: Right trapezoid: (A) Lateral aspect; (B) Medial aspect.

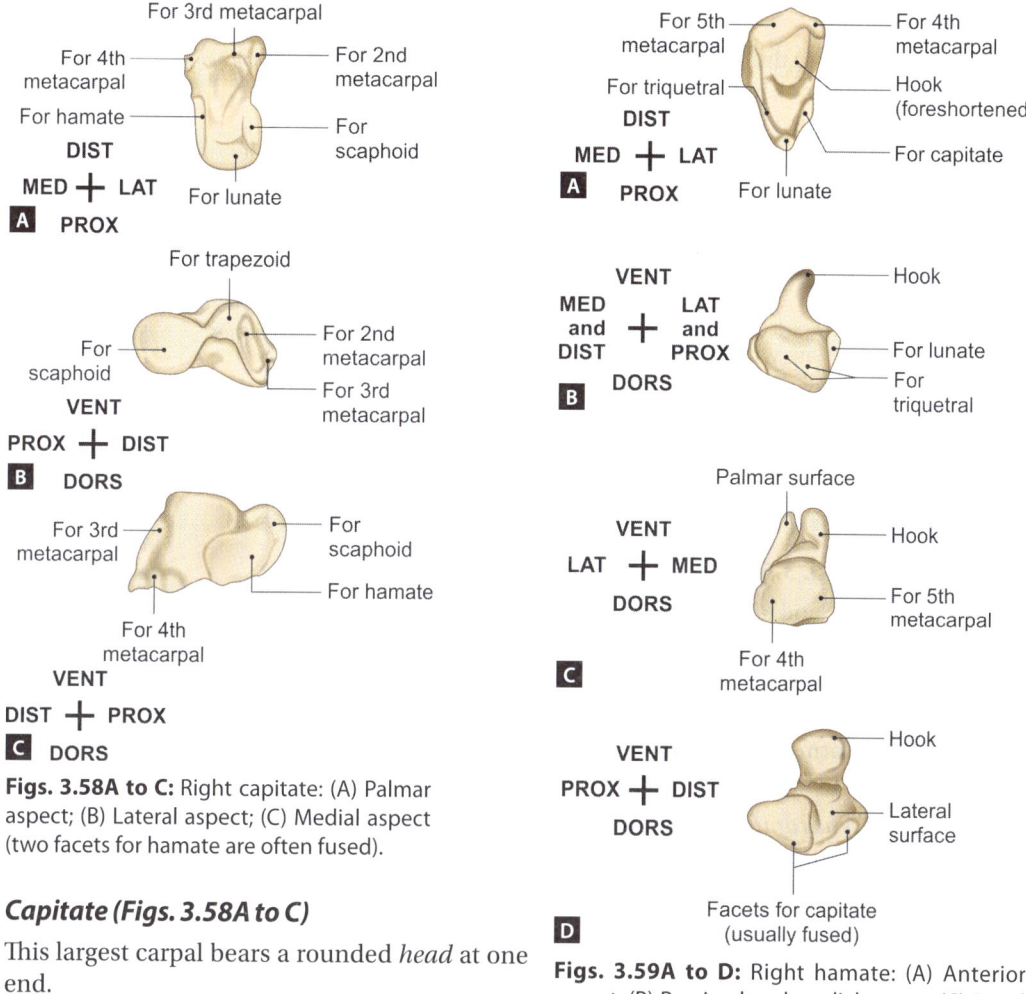

Figs. 3.58A to C: Right capitate: (A) Palmar aspect; (B) Lateral aspect; (C) Medial aspect (two facets for hamate are often fused).

Figs. 3.59A to D: Right hamate: (A) Anterior aspect; (B) Proximal and medial aspect; (C) Distal aspect; (D) Lateral aspect.

Capitate (Figs. 3.58A to C)

This largest carpal bears a rounded *head* at one end.

Side Determination

* Rounded head is proximal; distal surface is triangular.
* Dorsal surface is larger than the palmar surface (both are rough).
* Medial aspect bears a large facet for the hamate; lateral surface presents a smaller facet for the trapezoid.

Articulations

* *Proximally*: Lunate (*head fits into a socket formed by lunate and scaphoid*).
* *Distally*: Mainly with third metacarpal; also with second and fourth metacarpals.
* *Lateral aspect*: Scaphoid (proximally) and trapezoid (distally).
* *Medially*: Hamate.

Hamate (Figs. 3.59A to D)

The hamate presents prominent hook-like process attached to the distal and medial part of its palmar aspect.

Side Determination
- Hook is attached to the palmar surface.
- Concavity of the hook is directed laterally.
- Hook is attached near the distal end of the palmar aspect.

Viewed from palmar aspect: Hamate is triangular shaped (apex directed proximally).

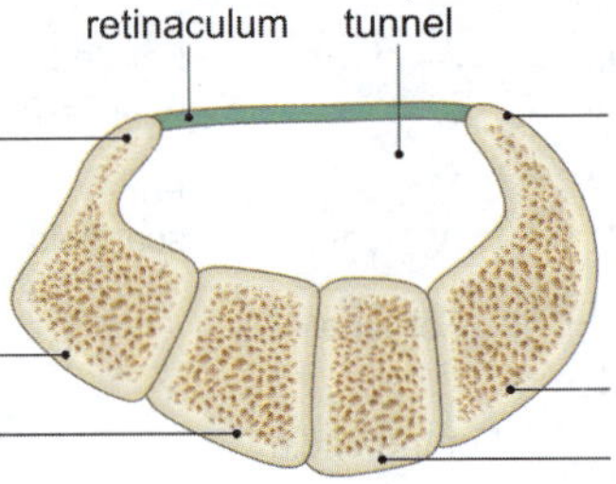

Articulations
- Apex may articulate with lunate.
- Distally articulates with fourth and fifth metacarpals.
- Medially and proximally articulates with triquetral.
- Laterally with capitate.
- Distal aspect has a facet; divided into two parts by a ridge, for articulation with fourth and fifth metacarpals.

Fig. 3.60: Schematic section across the distal row of carpal bones.

Carpal Tunnel (Fig. 3.60)

The dorsal, medial, and lateral surfaces of the carpals form one convex surface while the palmar surface is deeply concave. This concavity is converted into the carpal tunnel by the *flexor retinaculum* (modified deep fascia).

Attachments of flexor retinaculum:
- *Medially*: Pisiform and hook of hamate
- *Laterally*: Tubercle of scaphoid and crest of trapezium.

Carpal tunnel syndrome: Most common site of injury to the median nerve is the carpal tunnel (*most common entrapment neuropathy*). Median nerve passes through the carpal tunnel with long flexor tendons. Anything that increases pressure within tunnel will compress median nerve. Carpal tunnel may be narrowed by:
a) Arthritic changes in wrist joint.
b) Anterior dislocation of lunate.
c) Soft tissue thickening (myxedema and acromegaly).
d) Edema and obesity including pregnancy.

Surgically, it is treated by partial or complete division of the flexor retinaculum.

AN 8.5 Specify the parts of metacarpals and phalanges.

Metacarpals (Figs. 3.61 and 3.62)

The metacarpals and phalanges are miniature long bones. Each bone consists of a shaft and two ends (proximal base and distal head).

The hand has five metacarpal bones. They are numbered from lateral to medial side (bone related to thumb is the first metacarpal; to the little finger is the fifth). A metacarpal (*miniature long bone*) presents a shaft and proximal and distal ends.

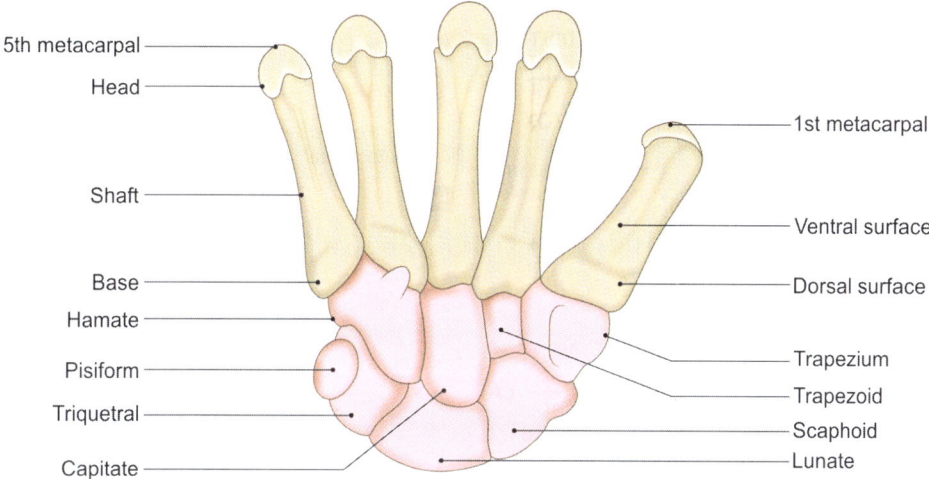

Fig. 3.61: Carpals and metacarpals of the right hand: Seen from the front.

Distal end (rounded head) bears convex articular surface that articulates with the proximal phalanx of the corresponding digit.

Shaft (triangular in cross-section) has medial, lateral, and dorsal surfaces. The bases (proximal ends) articulate with the distal row of carpals.

Bases of second and third, third and fourth, and fourth and fifth metacarpals also articulate with each other. The bases of metacarpals have certain characteristics to distinguish them from each other.

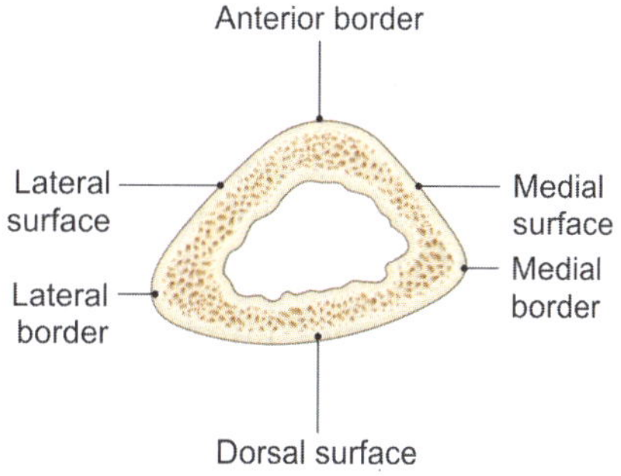

Fig. 3.62: Transverse section (TS) across the shaft of a metacarpal.

Individual Metacarpals

First metacarpal: Its *base* has a saddle-shaped articular surface on its proximal aspect for articulation with the trapezium. The medial and lateral sides of the base are nonarticular. It is shorter and thicker compared to other metacarpals. The first metacarpal is widely separated from the other metacarpals; much more mobile. It has been rotated through 90° so that its palmar surface faces medially (*not forward*), and the dorsal surface faces laterally (*not backward*). The palmar surface of the shaft is subdivided by a ridge into larger lateral part and smaller medial part **(Figs. 3.63A to C)**.

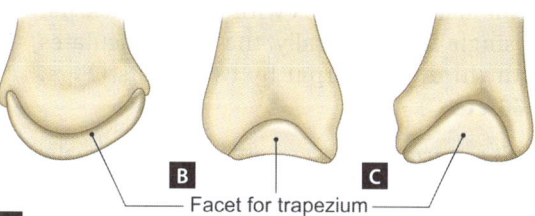

Figs. 3.63A to C: Base of right first metacarpal: (A) Anterior aspect; (B) Lateral aspect; (C) Medial aspect.

Second metacarpal: It has a grooved base which articulates with the trapezoid.

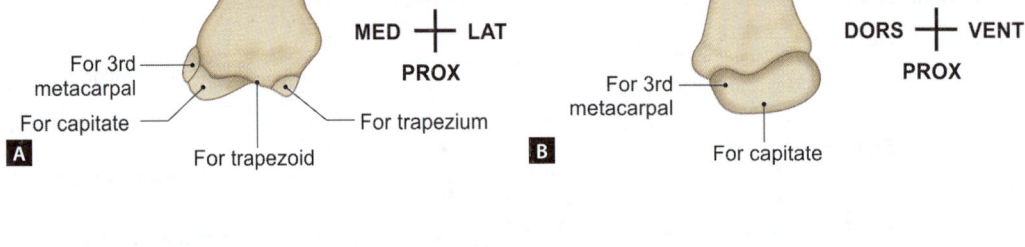

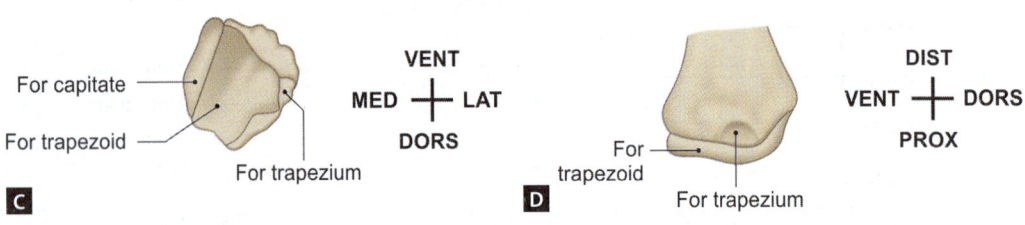

Figs. 3.64A to D: Base of right second metacarpal: (A) Anterior aspect; (B) Inferior aspect; (C) Medial aspect; (D) Lateral aspect.

The groove is medially bounded by a ridge which articulates with the capitate. The base also articulates laterally with trapezium and with the base of third metacarpal medially **(Figs. 3.64A to D)**.

Third metacarpal: It presents *styloid process* which is attached to the lateral and dorsal part of the base. The proximal aspect of the base articulates with the capitate. The base also articulates laterally with second metacarpal and medially with fourth metacarpal **(Figs. 3.65A to C)**.

Fourth metacarpal: Its *base* articulates proximally with the hamate. The medial side of the base articulates with fifth metacarpal by single facet. Laterally, the base articulates with third metacarpal by two facets **(Figs. 3.66A to C)**.

Fifth metacarpal: Its *base* articulates proximally with the hamate. Its lateral side articulates with fourth metacarpal; medial side is nonarticular **(Figs. 3.67A to C)**.

The fourth and fifth metacarpals can be distinguished from each other by their medial and lateral sides of bases. The fifth metacarpal

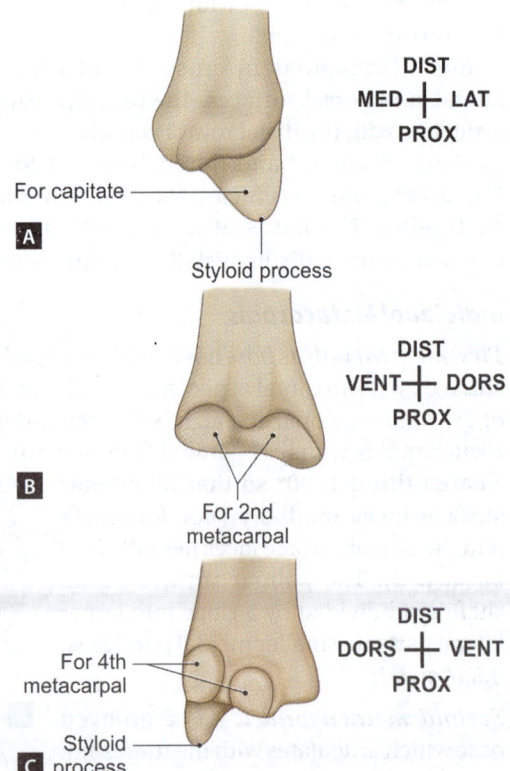

Figs. 3.65A to C: Base of right third metacarpal: (A) Anterior aspect; (B) Lateral aspect; (C) Medial aspect.

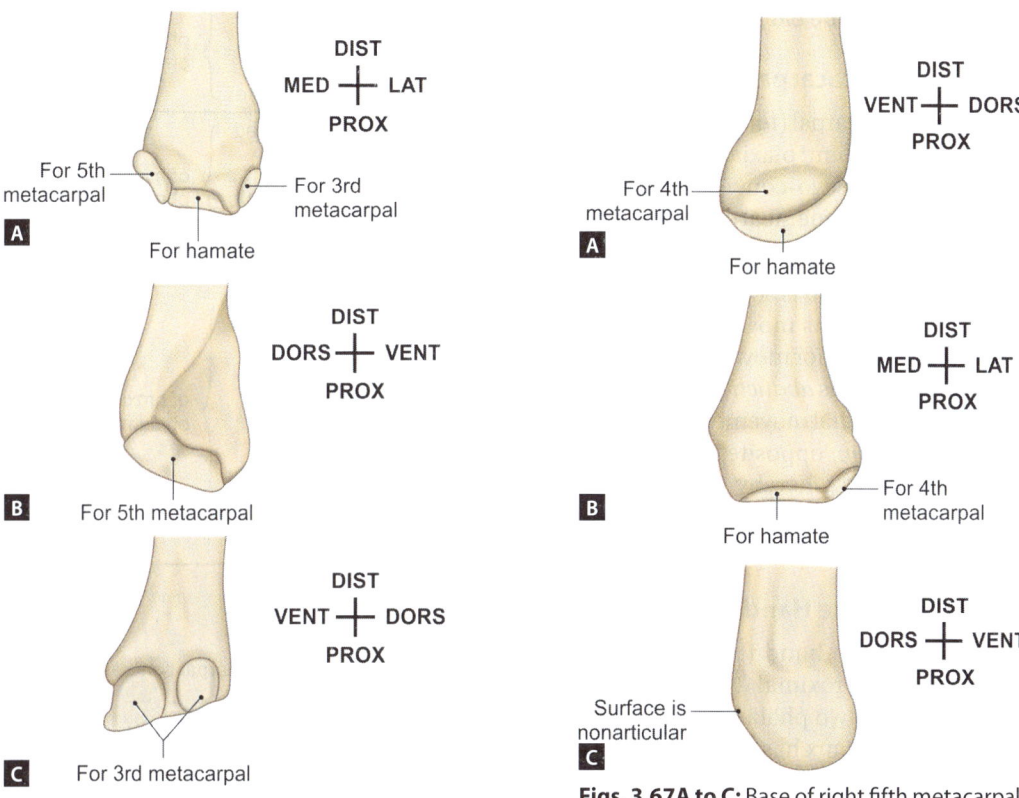

Figs. 3.66A to C: Base of right fourth metacarpal: (A) Anterior aspect; (B) Medial aspect; (C) Lateral aspect.

Figs. 3.67A to C: Base of right fifth metacarpal: (A) Lateral aspect; (B) Anterior aspect; (C) Medial aspect.

has a facet only on one (lateral) side, while fourth metacarpal has facets on both lateral and medial sides of its base.

Side Determination of Metacarpals

Proximal and distal ends: Head of the bone is distal.

Palmar and dorsal aspects: Shaft is concave on the palmar aspect; convex dorsally.

Side to which a metacarpal belongs can be determined by distinguishing between the medial and lateral sides of the bone.

- *First metacarpal*: Palmar surface of the shaft is divided into larger lateral and smaller medial parts.
- *Second metacarpal*: Ridge on the base is medial to the groove.
- *Third metacarpal*: Styloid process is attached to the lateral part of the base.
- *Fourth metacarpal*: Two facets on the lateral side of the base; only one on the medial side.
- *Fifth metacarpal*: Medial side of the base is nonarticular; lateral side has a facet for fourth metacarpal.

AN 13.4 Describe carpometacarpal joint.

First Carpometacarpal Joint

First carpometacarpal (*thumb joint*) joint is a synovial (*saddle variety*) joint; biaxial in nature. It is formed by reciprocally concavo-convex surfaces of trapezium and base of first metacarpal bone. The ligaments reinforce the capsule.

Movements: Thumb is set at an angle to the plane of the palm. Hence, its movements are different from other fingers. Anterior movement of thumb as a whole (away from palm) is *abduction*; opposite movement is *adduction*. A medial movement of thumb in the plane of palm is *flexion*; opposite is *extension*. Opposition is the movement whereby palmar aspect of thumb touches palmar aspect of another finger of same hand; opposite movement is *reposition*.

Phalanges of the Hand

Each digit of the hand (except thumb) has three phalanges: (a) proximal, (b) middle and (c) distal. The thumb has two phalanges: (a) proximal and (b) distal. Each phalanx has distal end (head), proximal end (base), and a shaft.

The base of each proximal phalanx is concave for articulation with the rounded head of the corresponding metacarpal. The head is pulley shaped. The base of the middle phalanx bears two small concave facets (separated by a ridge) to fit the two convexities on the head of the proximal phalanx. Its distal end is pulley shaped like that of the proximal phalanx. The proximal end of the distal phalanx is similar to that of the middle phalanx. Its distal end is nonarticular and irregular shaped **(Fig. 3.68)**.

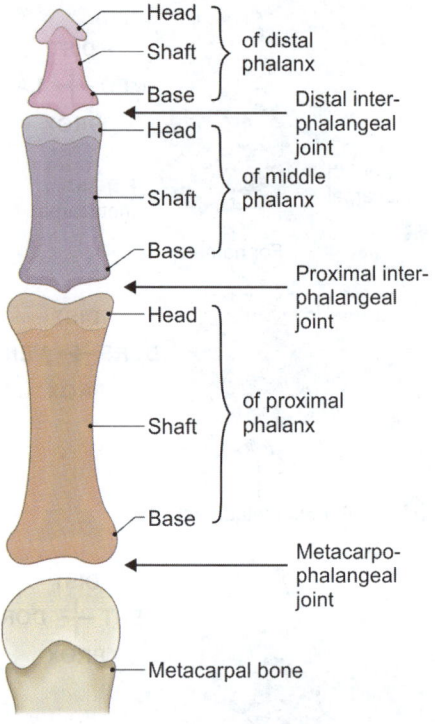

Fig. 3.68: Phalanges of a typical digit of the hand.

Attachments on the Skeleton of Hand (Fig. 3.69)

Many muscles are attached to the bones of the hand. These include intrinsic muscles of the hand and muscles in the forearm, but their tendons are inserted into bones of the hand.

Muscles of the Anterior Compartment of Forearm

Muscle	Insertion
Flexor carpi radialis	Palmar surface of the bases of second and third metacarpals
Flexor carpi ulnaris	Proximal part of pisiform
Flexor digitorum superficialis	Both sides of middle phalanges of all digits *except* thumb
Flexor digitorum profundus	Bases of distal phalanges of all digits *except* thumb
Flexor pollicis longus	Palmar surface of the base of distal phalanx of thumb

CHAPTER 3 ✦ Bones of Upper Limb

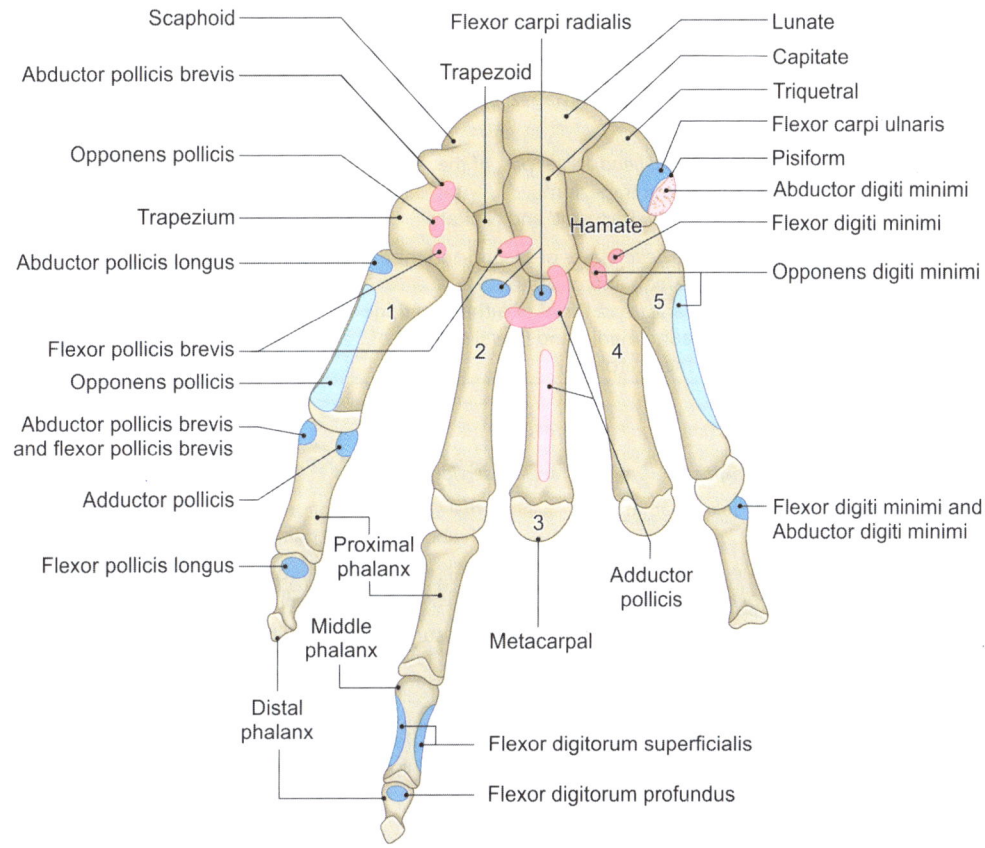

Fig. 3.69: Skeleton of the right hand: Attachments on the palmar aspect.

Muscles of the Posterior Compartment of Forearm

Muscle	Insertion
Extensor carpi ulnaris	Base of fifth metacarpal: Medial side
Extensor carpi radialis brevis	Bases of second and third metacarpals: Dorsal aspect
Extensor carpi radialis longus	Base of second metacarpal: Dorsal aspect
Abductor pollicis longus	Lateral side of base of first metacarpal
Extensor pollicis brevis	Base of proximal phalanx of thumb: Dorsal aspect
Extensor pollicis longus	Base of the distal phalanx of thumb
Extensor digitorum	Bases of middle and distal phalanges of all digits *except* thumb

Thenar Muscles

Muscle	Origin	Insertion
Abductor pollicis brevis	Tubercle of scaphoid and proximal part of tubercle of trapezium	Lateral side of the base of proximal phalanx of thumb

Contd...

Contd...

Muscle	Origin	Insertion
Opponens pollicis	Middle of tubercle of trapezium	Lateral part of palmar surface of the shaft of first metacarpal
Flexor pollicis brevis (*two heads*)	• *Superficial head*: Distal part of the tubercle of trapezium • *Deep head*: Trapezoid and capitate	Lateral side of the base of proximal phalanx of thumb
Adductor pollicis (*two heads*)	• *Oblique head*: Bases of second and third metacarpals and capitate • *Transverse head*: Distal two-thirds of ridge separating medial and lateral surfaces of third metacarpal	Medial side of the base of proximal phalanx of thumb

Hypothenar Muscles

Muscle	Origin	Insertion
Flexor digiti minimi	Hook of hamate	Medial side of base of proximal phalanx of little finger (with abductor digiti minimi)
Abductor digiti minimi	Medial and distal part of pisiform	Medial side of base of proximal phalanx of little finger (with flexor digiti minimi)
Opponens digiti minimi	Hook of hamate	Medial surface of fifth metacarpal

Attachments of Interossei (Figs. 3.70 and 3.71)

There are four palmar and four dorsal interossei. Each palmar interosseous muscle arises from one metacarpal; and each dorsal interosseous muscle from adjacent sides of two metacarpals.

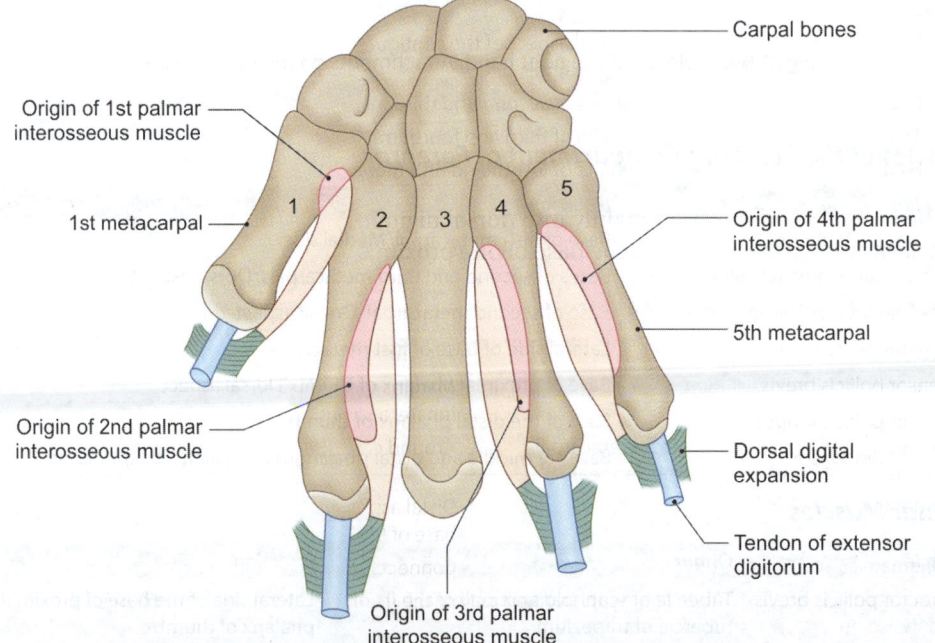

Fig. 3.70: Attachments of palmar interossei (note: insertions into dorsal digital expansions).

CHAPTER 3 ✦ Bones of Upper Limb

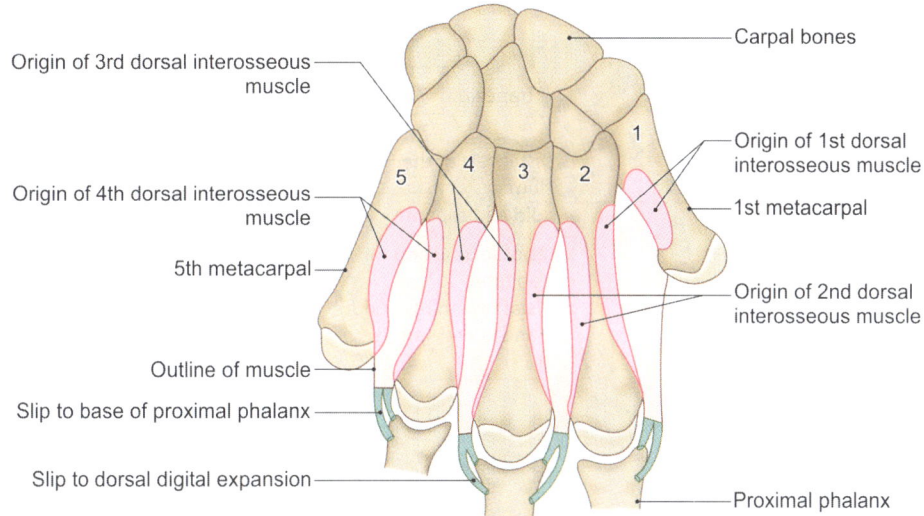

Fig. 3.71: Attachments of dorsal interossei (note: insertions into dorsal digital expansions).

Palmar interossei		
1	First palmar interosseous	Medial side of the base of first metacarpal
2	Second palmar interosseous	Medial surface of the palmar aspect of the shaft of second metacarpal
3	Third palmar interosseous	Lateral surface of the palmar aspect of the shaft of fourth metacarpal
4	Fourth palmar interosseous	Lateral surface of the palmar aspect of the shaft of fifth metacarpal
Dorsal interossei		
1	First dorsal interosseous	Dorsal aspect of the contiguous sides of the shafts of the first and second metacarpals
2	Second dorsal interosseous	Shafts of second and third metacarpals: Contiguous sides
3	Third dorsal interosseous	Shafts of third and fourth metacarpals: Contiguous sides
4	Fourth dorsal interosseous	Shafts of fourth and fifth metacarpals: Contiguous sides

All the interossei are inserted mainly into dorsal digital expansions. Each dorsal interosseous muscle also gains insertion into the base of one proximal phalanx.

Other Attachments (Fig. 3.72)

Structure	Attachment
Capsular ligament of wrist joint	Margins of the articular surface formed by scaphoid, lunate, and triquetral bones
Capsules of joints (intercarpal, carpometacarpal, metacarpophalangeal, and interphalangeal)	Around corresponding articular surfaces
Pisometacarpal ligament	Distal aspect of pisiform and anterior aspect of the base of fifth metacarpal
Pisohamate ligament	Connects pisiform to hook of hamate
Pisometacarpal and pisohamate ligaments transmit pull of the flexor carpi ulnaris to the fifth metacarpal and hamate	

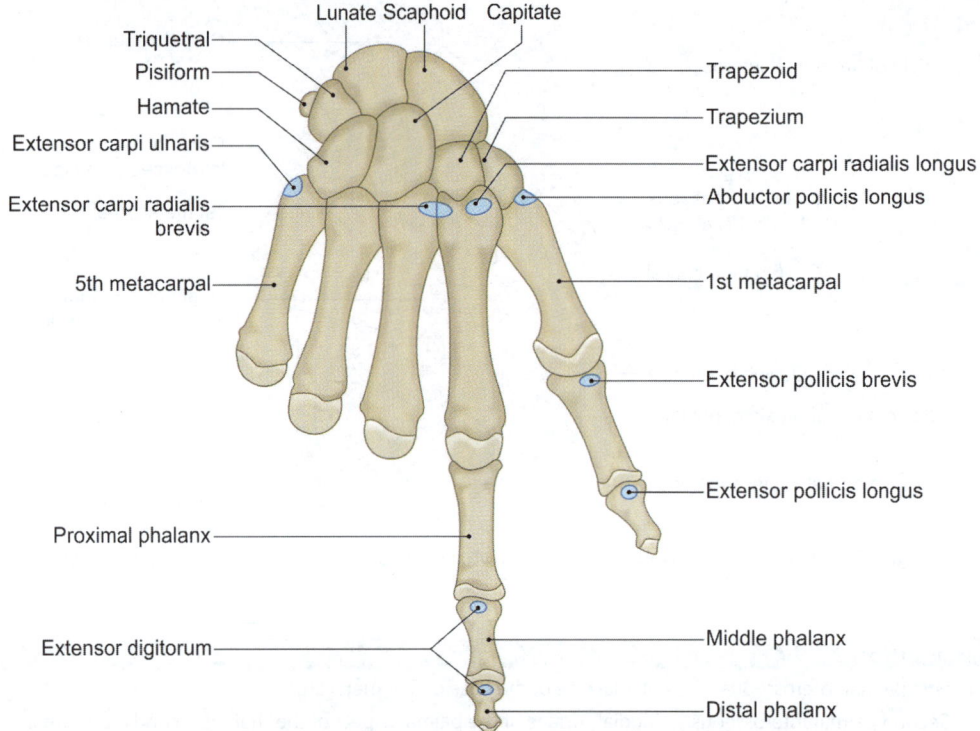

Fig. 3.72: Skeleton of the right hand: Attachments on the dorsal aspect.

Structure	Attachment
Flexor retinaculum	Medially: Pisiform and hook of hamate laterally: tubercle of scaphoid and crest of trapezium
Extensor retinaculum (medially)	Triquetral and pisiform
Fibrous flexor sheaths	Palmar aspect of each phalanx lateral margins

Dorsal aspects of the phalanges are covered by the dorsal digital expansions.

Ossification

Each carpal bone is ossified from one center that appears as follows:

Capite	2nd month	Scaphoid	4th–5th year
Hamate	3rd month	Trapezium	4th–5th year
Triquetral	3rd year	Trapezoid	4th–5th year
Lunate	4th year	Pisiform	About 10th-12th years

- *Each metacarpal* has a primary center for the shaft; appears in 9th week of intrauterine life.
- *First metacarpal* has a secondary center for the base; appears in second or third year, and unites with the shaft at about 16 years.
- *Other metacarpals* have secondary centers in the heads (*not in base*): appear at about 2 years of age and unite with the shaft between 16 years and 18 years.
- *Each phalanx* has a primary center for the shaft and a secondary center for its proximal end.

Primary Center Appears

- First in the distal phalanges (8th week)
- Next in the proximal phalanges (10th week)
- Last in the middle phalanges (12th fetal week).

Secondary Centers Appear

- First in the proximal phalanges (second year)
- Later in the middle and distal phalanges (third or fourth year). They unite with the shafts between 16–18 years.

AN 13.4 Describe metacarpophalangeal joint.

Metacarpophalangeal Joint

The MP joints are synovial joints (*condylar variety*) which are biaxial in nature. The movements permitted are flexion and extension and abduction and adduction.

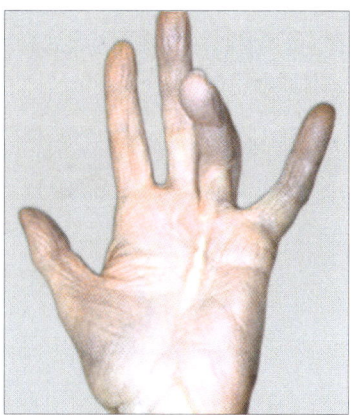

Fig. 3.73: Dupuytren's contracture.

Clinical Anatomy

Fracture of the hamate: It may injure the ulnar nerve and artery because they are near the hook of the hamate.

Dupuytren's ischemic contracture: It is the progressive thickening, shortening, and fibrosis of the palmar aponeurosis. It causes a flexion deformity of fingers where the fingers are flexed, especially the third and fourth fingers (**Fig. 3.73**).

Mallet finger (hammer or baseball finger): It shows permanent flexion of the distal phalanx due to an avulsion of the lateral bands of the extensor tendon to the distal phalanx (**Fig. 3.74**).

QUESTIONNAIRE

- Identification of carpal bones.
- Scaphoid: Why avascular necrosis of scaphoid is common?
- Lunate: What are the muscles attached to it?
- Pisiform: Type of bone and ossification.
- Hamate: Which nerve is related to hook of hamate?
- Trapezium: What is attached to its groove?
- What are the attachments of the flexor retinaculum?
- Enumerate the structures passing superficial and deep to flexor retinaculum?
- Comment on the ossification of the carpal bones.
- Classify the joints in the hand:
  - Radiocarpal joint
  - First carpometacarpal joint
  - Carpometacarpal joints of fingers
  - Interphalangeal joints.

MOVEMENTS AT MAJOR UPPER LIMB JOINTS

Shoulder Joint (Fig. 3.75)

Type	Axis	Movements
Ball and socket	Multiaxial	Flexion and extension, Abduction and adduction, Medial and lateral rotations and Circumduction

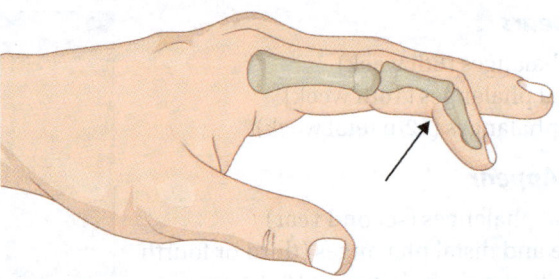
Fig. 3.74: Mallet finger.

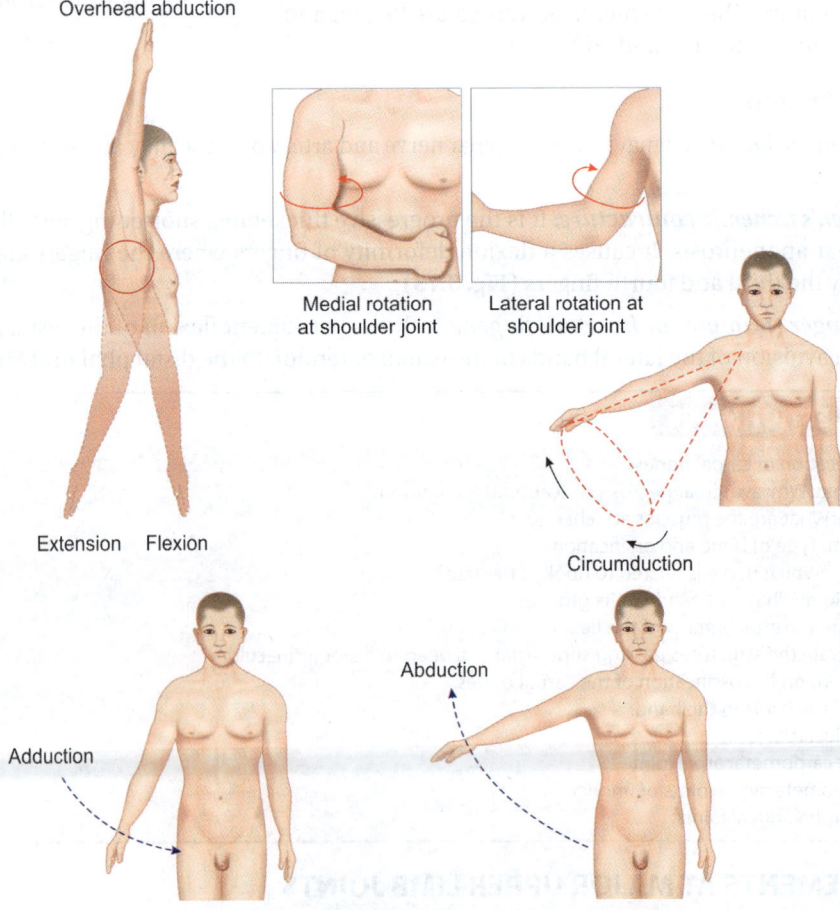
Fig. 3.75: Shoulder joint.

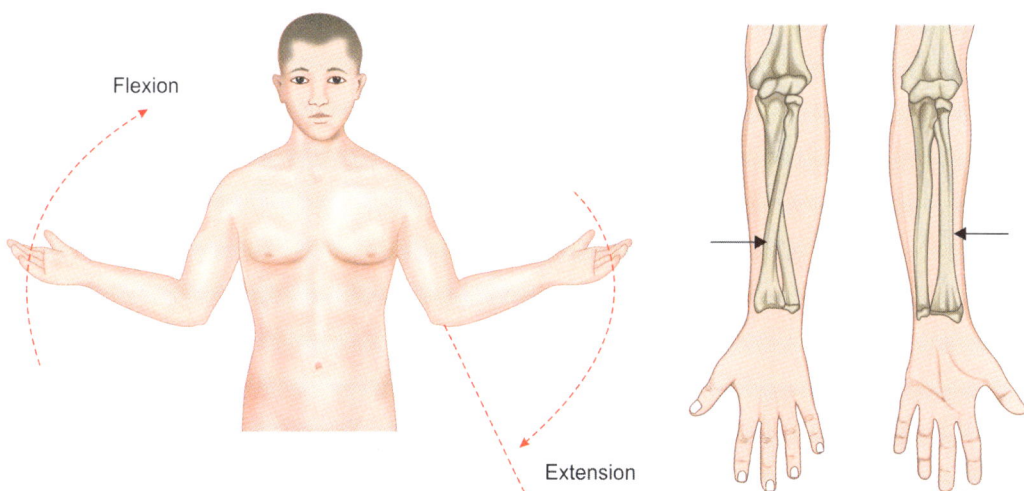

Fig. 3.76: Movements at elbow joint.

Fig. 3.77: Movements at radioulnar joints (Pronation and Supination).

Elbow Joint (Fig. 3.76)

Type	Axis	Movements
Hinge	Uniaxial	Flexion and extension

Superior and Inferior Radioulnar Joints (Fig. 3.77)

Type	Axis	Movements
Pivot	Uniaxial	Supination and pronation

Wrist Joint (Figs. 3.78A to D)

Type	Axis	Movements
Ellipsoid	Biaxial	Flexion and extension, Abduction and adduction, circumduction

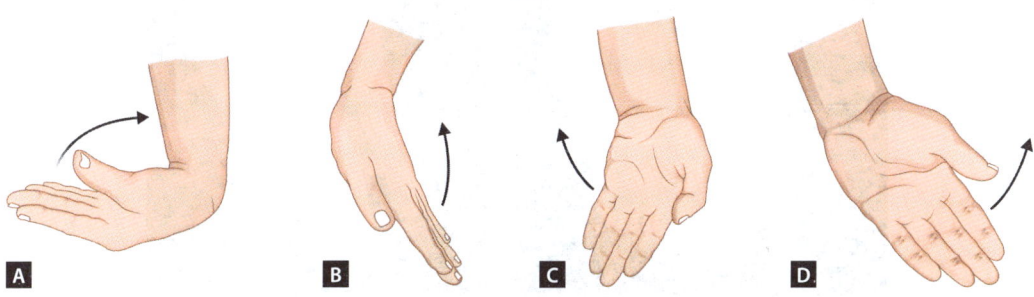

Figs. 3.78A to D: Movements at wrist joint: (A) Flexion; (B) Extension; (C) Adduction; (D) Abduction.

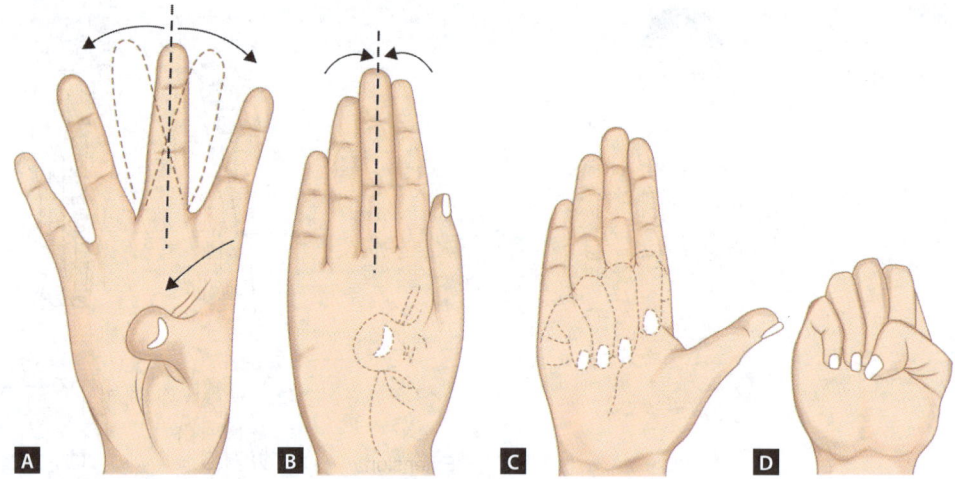

Figs. 3.79A to D: Movements at metacarpophalangeal joints: (A) Abduction; (B) Adduction; (C) Extension; (D) Flexion.

Metacarpophalangeal Joints (Figs. 3.79A to D)

Type	Axis	Movements
Condylar	Biaxial	Flexion and extension Abduction and adduction

Interphalangeal Joints (Figs. 3.80A and B)

Type	Axis	Movements
Hinge	Uniaxial	Flexion and extension

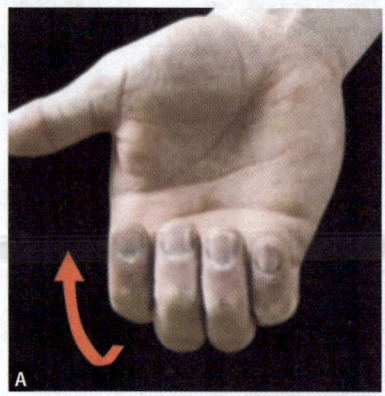 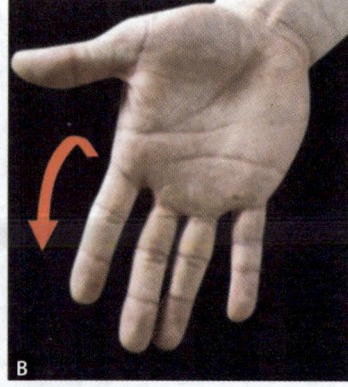

Figs. 3.80A and B: Movements at interphalangeal (IP) joint: (A) Flexion at IP joint; (B) Extension at IP joint.

ATLAS OF MUSCLE ATTACHMENTS: UPPER LIMB

Plate 1
Pectoralis Major

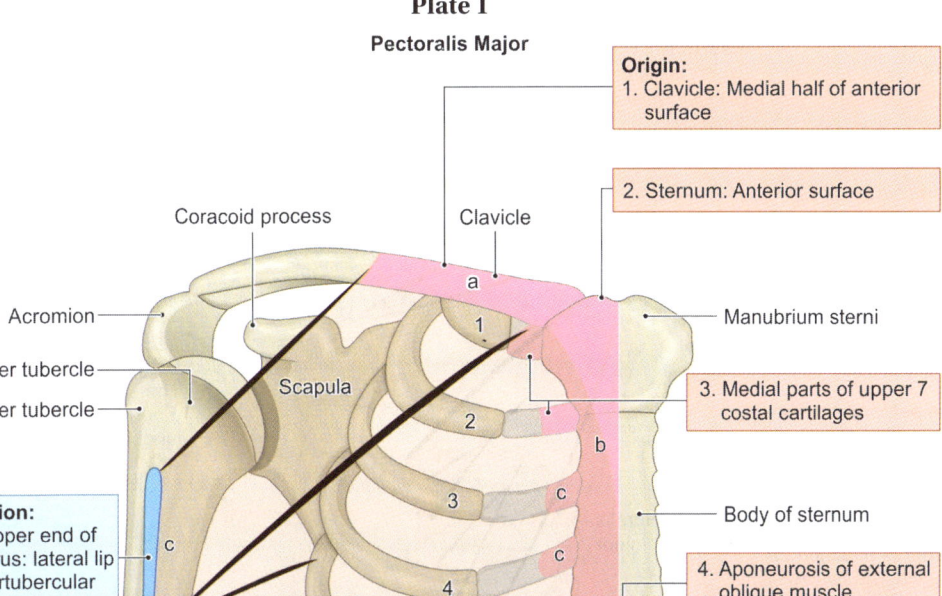

Origin:
1. Clavicle: Medial half of anterior surface
2. Sternum: Anterior surface
3. Medial parts of upper 7 costal cartilages
4. Aponeurosis of external oblique muscle

Insertion:
Into upper end of humerus: lateral lip of intertubercular sulcus

Nerve supply:
Lateral and medial pectoral nerves (C5, 6, 7, 8, T1)

Actions:
Adductor and medial rotator of arm.
The clavicular fibers (acting with the anterior fibers of the deltoid) can flex the arm.
The sternocostal fibers can extend the flexed arm against resistance (helped by latissimus dorsi and teres major). The muscle can also cause forward movement of the extended arm as in giving a blow. When the arm is fixed the muscle can raise the thorax.

Notes:
1. The tendon of the muscle is bilaminar. The anterior lamina receives the clavicular and upper sternocostal fibers. The posterior lamina receives the fibers from the lower costal cartilage and from the aponeurosis of the external oblique.
2. The muscle forms the anterior fold of the axilla. It is related to the mammary gland. Deep to it there are the pectoralis minor and the clavipectoral fascia. The lateral part of the muscle lies over the biceps brachii and the coracobrachialis.

Atlas of Muscle Attachments: Upper Limb

Plate 2

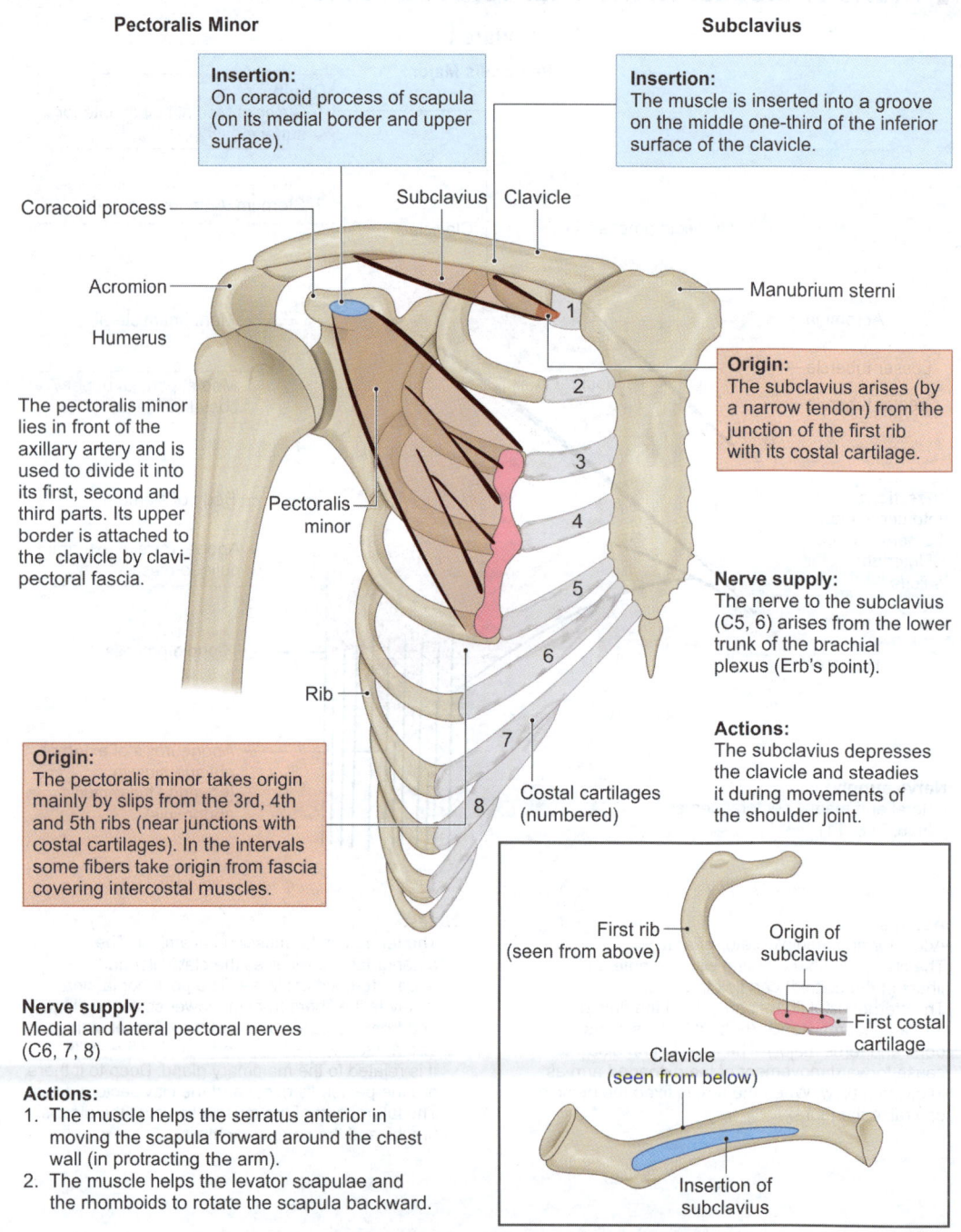

Pectoralis Minor

Insertion:
On coracoid process of scapula (on its medial border and upper surface).

The pectoralis minor lies in front of the axillary artery and is used to divide it into its first, second and third parts. Its upper border is attached to the clavicle by clavipectoral fascia.

Origin:
The pectoralis minor takes origin mainly by slips from the 3rd, 4th and 5th ribs (near junctions with costal cartilages). In the intervals some fibers take origin from fascia covering intercostal muscles.

Nerve supply:
Medial and lateral pectoral nerves (C6, 7, 8).

Actions:
1. The muscle helps the serratus anterior in moving the scapula forward around the chest wall (in protracting the arm).
2. The muscle helps the levator scapulae and the rhomboids to rotate the scapula backward.

Subclavius

Insertion:
The muscle is inserted into a groove on the middle one-third of the inferior surface of the clavicle.

Origin:
The subclavius arises (by a narrow tendon) from the junction of the first rib with its costal cartilage.

Nerve supply:
The nerve to the subclavius (C5, 6) arises from the lower trunk of the brachial plexus (Erb's point).

Actions:
The subclavius depresses the clavicle and steadies it during movements of the shoulder joint.

Atlas of Muscle Attachments: Upper Limb

Plate 3
Serratus Anterior

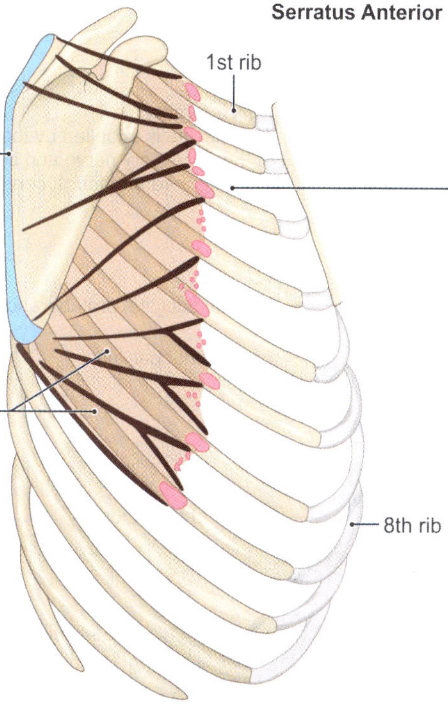

Origin:
The serratus anterior takes origin by several digitations from the outer surfaces of the upper eight (or nine) ribs, and from fascia covering intercostal muscle.

Insertion:
The entire muscle is inserted into the costal surface of the scapula along its medial border. The first digitation is inserted from the angle to the root of the spine (a). The next two or three digitations are inserted lower down on the medial border (b). The lower four or five digitations are inserted into a large triangular area (c) over the inferior angle.

Nerve supply:
The nerve to the serratus anterior is a branch of the brachial plexus and arises from the roots C5, 6, 7.

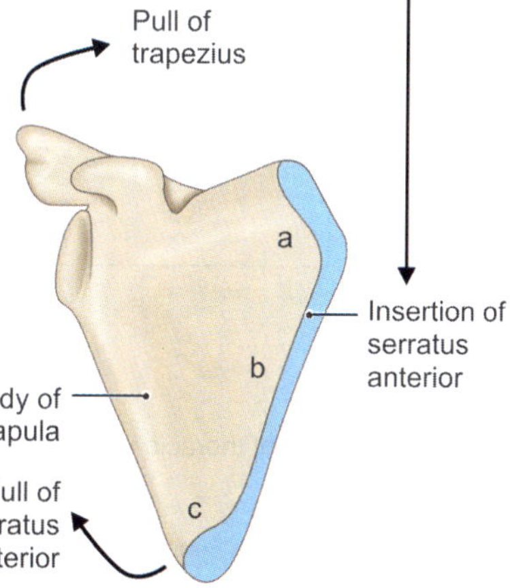

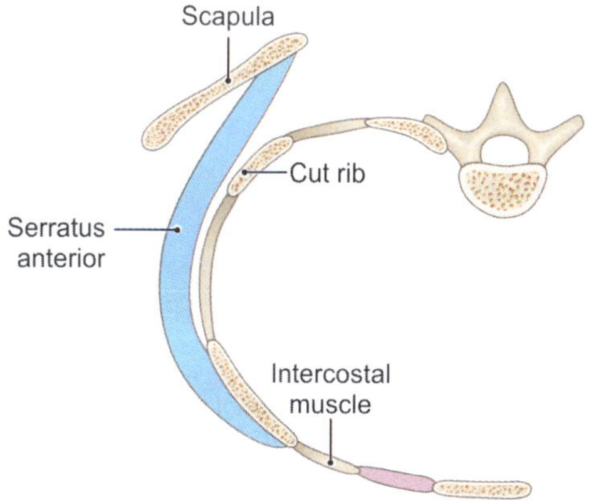

Actions:
1. Helped by the pectoralis minor the muscle pulls the scapula forwards around the chest wall to protract the upper limb (as in pushing or giving a blow).
2. The fibers inserted into the inferior angle of the scapula pull it forward and rotate the scapula so that the glenoid cavity is turned upward. In this action the serratus anterior acts along with the trapezius, which contributes to the rotation by pulling acromion upward and backward.

Atlas of Muscle Attachments: Upper Limb

Plate 4
Trapezius

Origin:
The muscles has a long linear origin from the following structures:
1. Medial one-third of superior nuchal line.
2. External occipital protuberance.
3. Ligamentum nuchae.
4. Spine of 7th cervical vertebra.
5. Spines of all thoracic vertebrae and intervening supraspinous ligaments.

Nerve supply:
The muscle is supplied by the spinal part of the accessory nerve and by branches from the third and fourth cervical nerves.

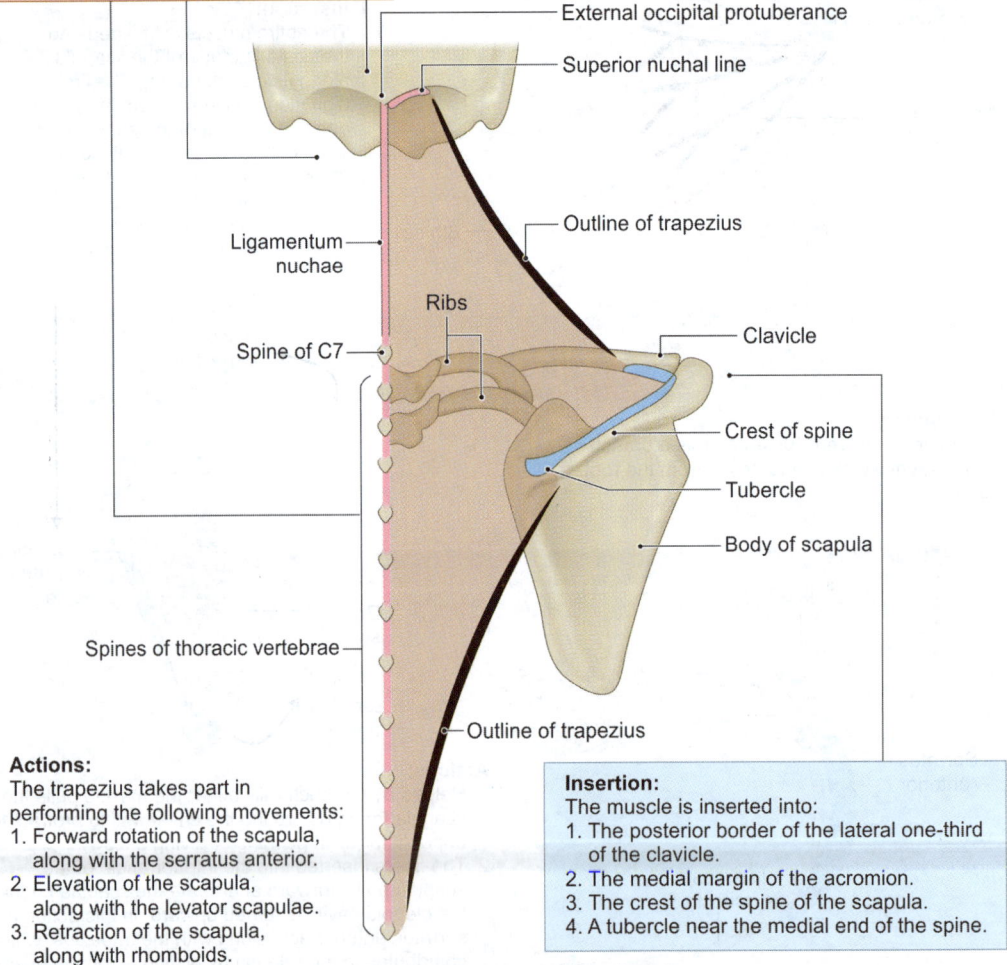

- External occipital protuberance
- Superior nuchal line
- Outline of trapezius
- Ligamentum nuchae
- Ribs
- Clavicle
- Spine of C7
- Crest of spine
- Tubercle
- Body of scapula
- Spines of thoracic vertebrae
- Outline of trapezius

Actions:
The trapezius takes part in performing the following movements:
1. Forward rotation of the scapula, along with the serratus anterior.
2. Elevation of the scapula, along with the levator scapulae.
3. Retraction of the scapula, along with rhomboids.
4. The muscles of the two sides acting together draw the head backward. Each muscle acting alone draws the head backward and laterally to its own side.

Insertion:
The muscle is inserted into:
1. The posterior border of the lateral one-third of the clavicle.
2. The medial margin of the acromion.
3. The crest of the spine of the scapula.
4. A tubercle near the medial end of the spine.

Atlas of Muscle Attachments: Upper Limb

Plate 5
Latissimus Dorsi

Nerve supply:
The muscle is supplied by the thoracodorsal nerve (C6, C7, C8).

Insertion:
The muscle ends in a tendon which is inserted into the anterior aspect of the upper end of the humerus, in the floor of the intertubercular sulcus.

Origin:
The latissimus dorsi has a long origin from the following:
1. The spines of the lower six thoracic vertebrae and the intervening supraspinous ligaments.
2. The lumbar fascia (and thus indirectly form the lumbar) and sacral spines.
3. The iliac crest.

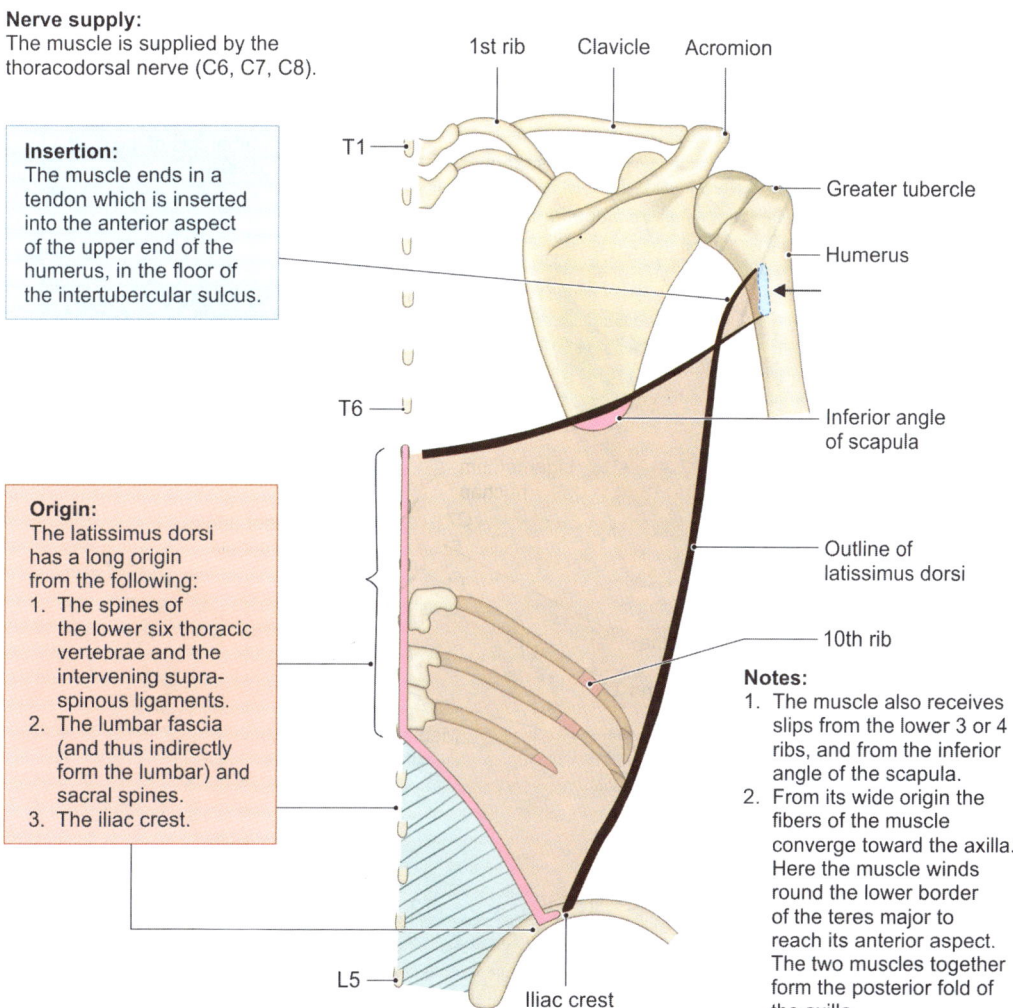

Notes:
1. The muscle also receives slips from the lower 3 or 4 ribs, and from the inferior angle of the scapula.
2. From its wide origin the fibers of the muscle converge toward the axilla. Here the muscle winds round the lower border of the teres major to reach its anterior aspect. The two muscles together form the posterior fold of the axilla.

Actions:
1. Adduction of the arm.
2. Medial rotation of the arm (because the tendon passes anterior to the axis of rotation).
3. Extension of the arm (especially when the flexed arm is extended against resistance).
4. It can depress the raised arm against resistance (along with the pectoralis major).
5. It can elevate the trunk if the arm is raised and fixed (as in exercising on parallel bars) (again along with the pectoralis major).

Plate 6
Levator Scapulae

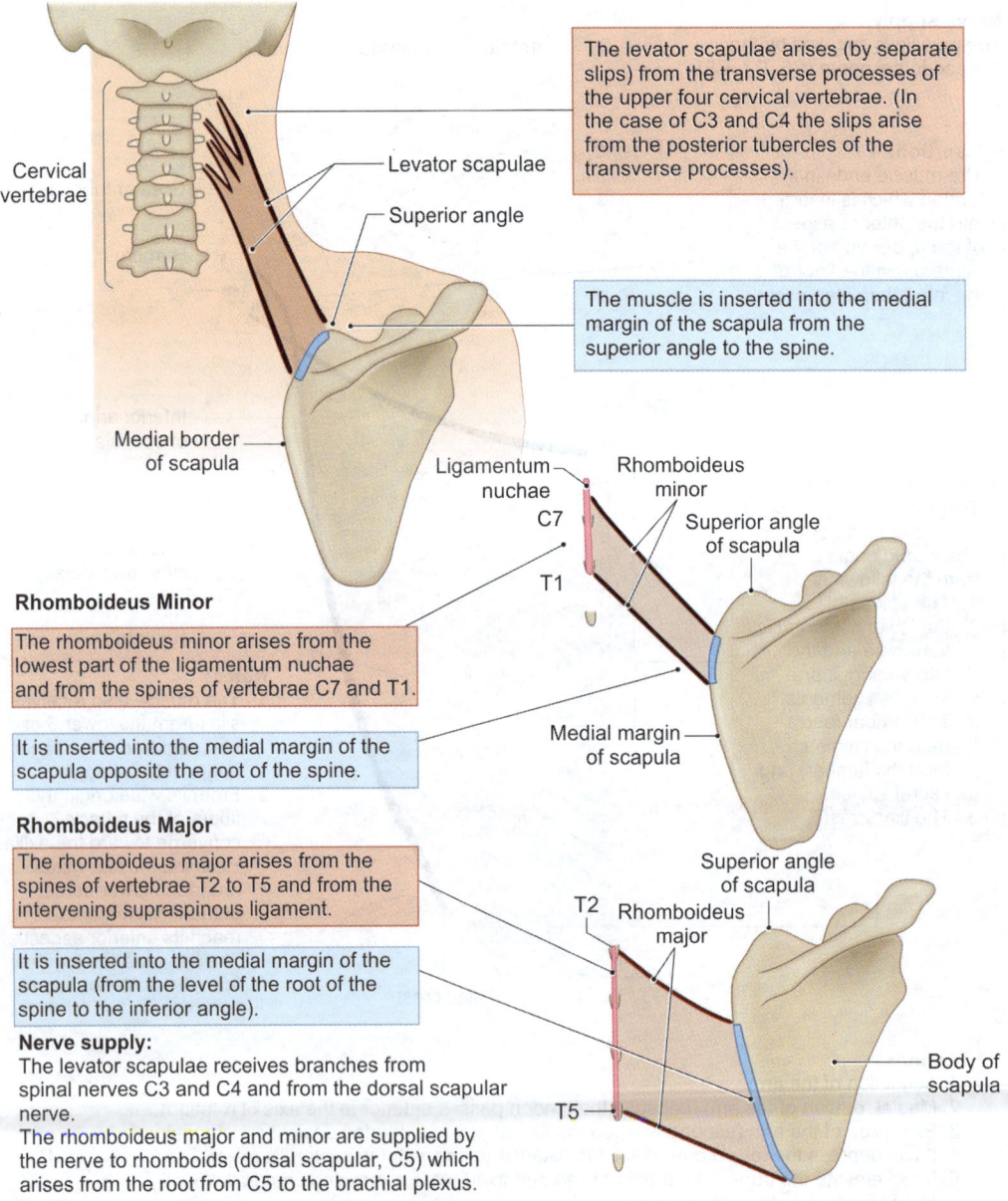

The levator scapulae arises (by separate slips) from the transverse processes of the upper four cervical vertebrae. (In the case of C3 and C4 the slips arise from the posterior tubercles of the transverse processes).

The muscle is inserted into the medial margin of the scapula from the superior angle to the spine.

Rhomboideus Minor

The rhomboideus minor arises from the lowest part of the ligamentum nuchae and from the spines of vertebrae C7 and T1.

It is inserted into the medial margin of the scapula opposite the root of the spine.

Rhomboideus Major

The rhomboideus major arises from the spines of vertebrae T2 to T5 and from the intervening supraspinous ligament.

It is inserted into the medial margin of the scapula (from the level of the root of the spine to the inferior angle).

Nerve supply:
The levator scapulae receives branches from spinal nerves C3 and C4 and from the dorsal scapular nerve.
The rhomboideus major and minor are supplied by the nerve to rhomboids (dorsal scapular, C5) which arises from the root from C5 to the brachial plexus.

Actions:
The levator scapulae elevates the scapula, while the rhomboids retract it. Acting together they steady the scapula during movements of the upper limb. They also produce backward rotation of the scapula.

Atlas of Muscle Attachments: Upper Limb

Plate 7
Deltoid

Origin:
The deltoid has one continuous origin from the following:
1. The upper surface and anterior border of the lateral one-third of the clavicle.
2. The lateral margin and upper surface of the acromion.
3. The lower lip of the crest of the spine of the scapula.

Insertion:
The muscle is inserted into the V-shaped deltoid tuberosity on the lateral aspect of the shaft of the humerus.

Nerve supply:
Axillary nerve (C5, C6).

Actions:
1. The acromial part of the muscle produces abduction of the arm at the shoulder joint.
2. The anterior fibers cause flexion and medial rotation of the humerus.
3. The posterior fibers cause extension and lateral rotation.

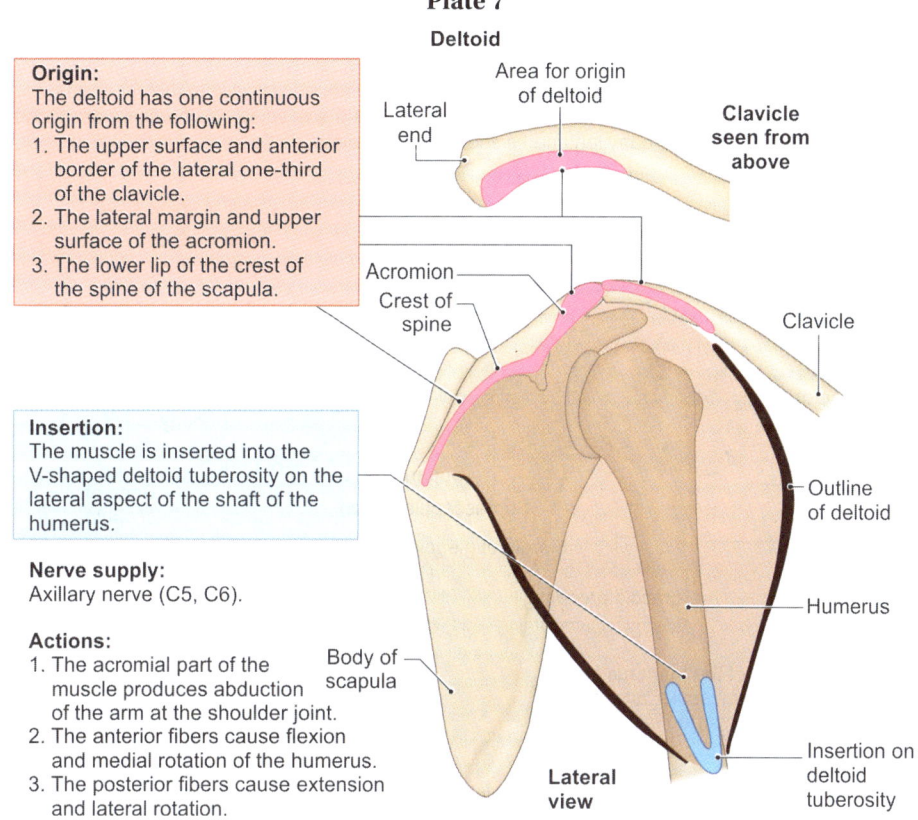

Mechanism of Abduction of the Arm

Abduction of the arm is a complex movement and the deltoid is one of the most important muscles for it. This is, therefore, an appropriate place for us to examine the contribution of various muscles to this movement. Abduction of the arm takes place partly at the shoulder joint, and partly by rotation of the scapula. The first few degrees of abduction at the shoulder joint are produced by the supraspinatus, the deltoid being able to act efficiently only after this has been done. The pull of the acromial fibers of the deltoid can be resolved into a lateral pull (which causes abduction) and an upward pull because of which the head of the humerus is in danger of getting stuck under the coracoacromial arch. This upward pull is neutralized by the downward pull of the subscapularis, the infraspinatus and the teres minor. These muscles are said to form a couple with the deltoid and supraspinatus to ensure smooth movement. The movement is also assisted by the anterior and posterior fibers of the deltoid; they contract to prevent side away. Abduction of the arm at the shoulder joint is limited to about 90 degrees. Further abduction is produced by forward rotation of the scapula produced by the serratus anterior and the trapezius acting together. However, the components of the movement at the shoulder joint, and by rotation of the scapula, take place simultaneously. Abduction of the arm is thus seen to be a complicated movement involving several muscles that act synergistically. In overhead abduction of the arm the greater tuberosity of the humerus slides under the acromion. This sliding is greatly facilitated by the presence of a large subacromial bursa in this situation.

Atlas of Muscle Attachments: Upper Limb

Plate 8

Supraspinatus

This muscle covers the posterior aspect of the scapula above the spine, and passes to the uppermost part of the humerus. The attachments of this muscle are best visualized when the scapula and humerus are viewed from above. It is good to first identify the bony landmarks seen in such a view.

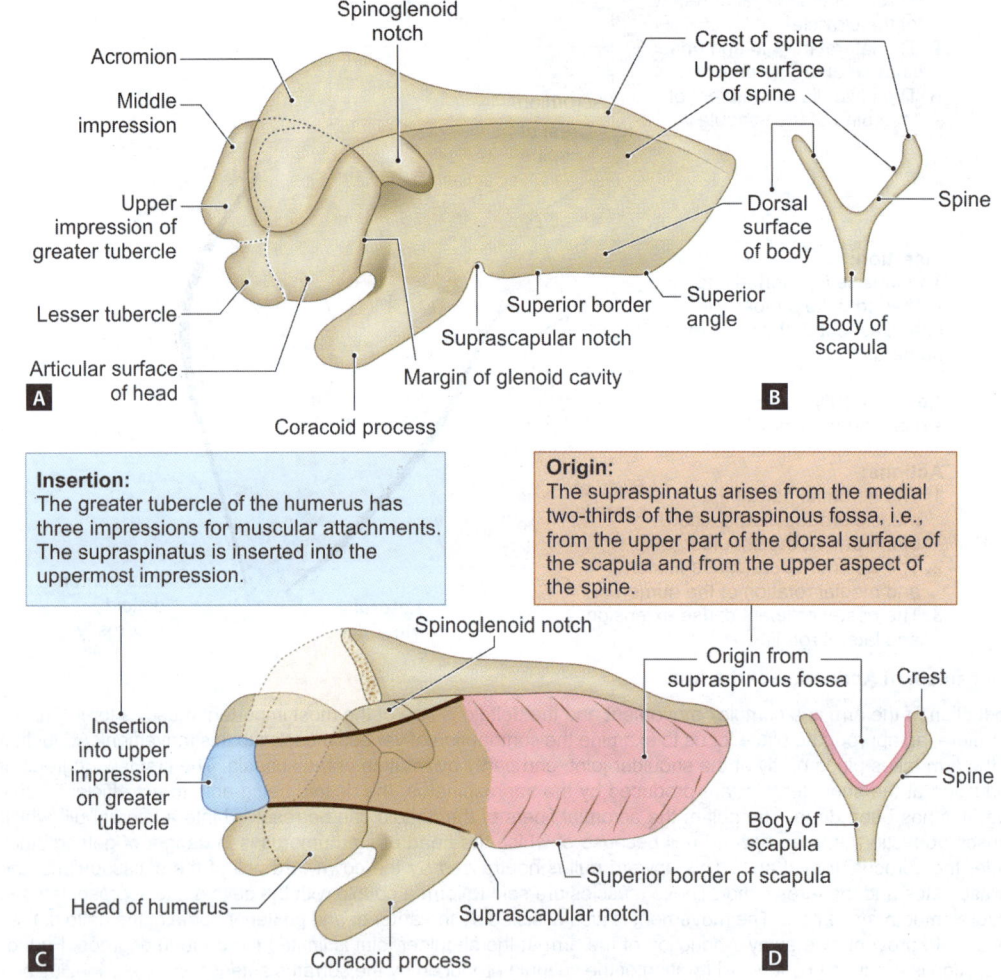

Insertion:
The greater tubercle of the humerus has three impressions for muscular attachments. The supraspinatus is inserted into the uppermost impression.

Origin:
The supraspinatus arises from the medial two-thirds of the supraspinous fossa, i.e., from the upper part of the dorsal surface of the scapula and from the upper aspect of the spine.

Nerve supply: By suprascapular nerve.
Actions:
1. Supraspinatus, acting along with other muscles, around the shoulder joint, stabilizes it.
2. It is an abductor of the arm. It is generally said to be muscle that initiates abduction, the deltoid being able to act only after a few degrees of abduction have taken place (as described under deltoid).

Note:
1. The muscle passes under cover of the coracoacromial arch to reach its insertion.
2. Strain of this muscle can result in pain over the scapula. This usually occurs when acts like writing or typing (involving slight abduction of the arm) are performed over long periods.

Atlas of Muscle Attachments: Upper Limb

Plate 9

Infraspinatus

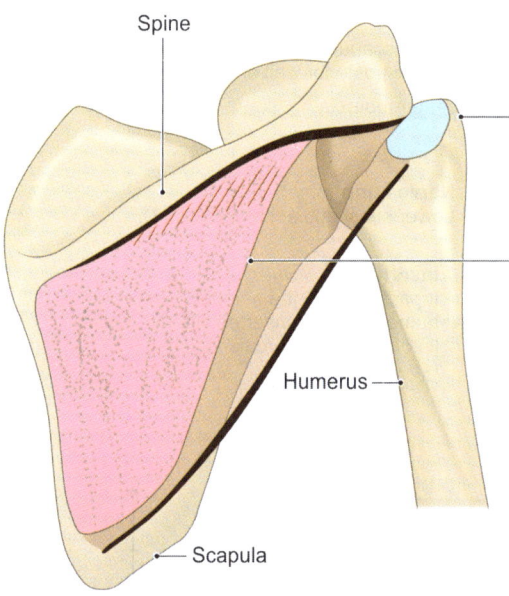

Insertion:
The greater tubercle of the humerus has three impressions, upper, middle and inferior. The infraspinatus is inserted into the middle impression.

Origin:
The infraspinatus arises from the posterior aspect of the scapula. The area of origin includes the medial two-thirds of the infraspinous fossa, and the inferior aspect of the spine.

Nerve supply:
Suprascapular nerve

Actions:
(common to infraspinatus and teres minor)
1. These muscle are adductors and lateral rotators of the humerus.
2. They stabilize the shoulder joint and strengthen the posterior part of its capsule.
3. During abduction of the arm (by the deltoid and the supraspinatus) their downward pull prevents the head of the humerus from getting stuck under the coracoacromial arch. This allows abduction to take place smoothly (The subscapularis has a similar role).

Teres Minor

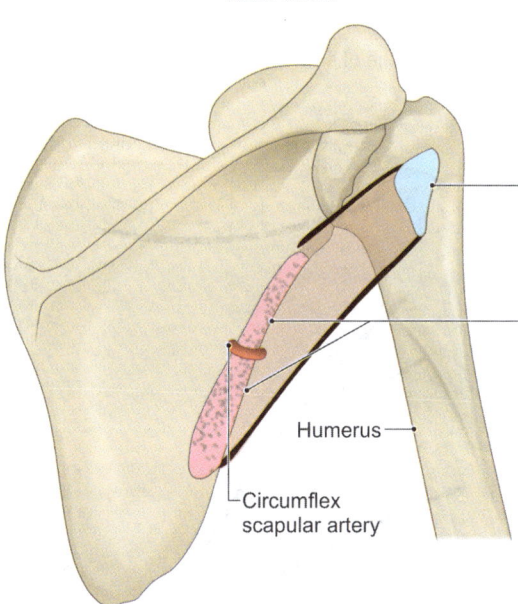

Insertion:
The teres minor is inserted into the lowest impression on the greater tubercle of the humerus.

Origin:
The teres minor arises from the dorsal surface of the scapula along the upper two-thirds of the lateral border. The area of origin is interrupted by the circumflex scapular artery.

Nerve supply:
Axillary nerve.

Plate 10

Teres Major

Note: The subscapularis and the teres major form the posterior wall of the axilla.

Greater tubercle

Nerve supply: Lower subscapular nerves (C6, 7).

Insertion: It passes on to the anterior aspect of the humerus and is inserted into the medial lip of the intertubercular sulcus (see lower figure).

Scapula (infraspinous fossa)

Origin: From dorsal surface of scapula (inferior angle and lower one-third of lateral border).

Actions: Both the teres major and the subscapularis are adductors and medial rotators of the arm. In addition the teres major can extend the arm. During abduction of the arm (by the deltoid and supraspinatus) these two muscles pull the head of the humerus downward and thus prevent it from getting stuck under the coracoacromial arch. Along with other muscles surrounding the shoulder joint these muscles strengthen the capsule and stabilize the joint.

Subscapularis

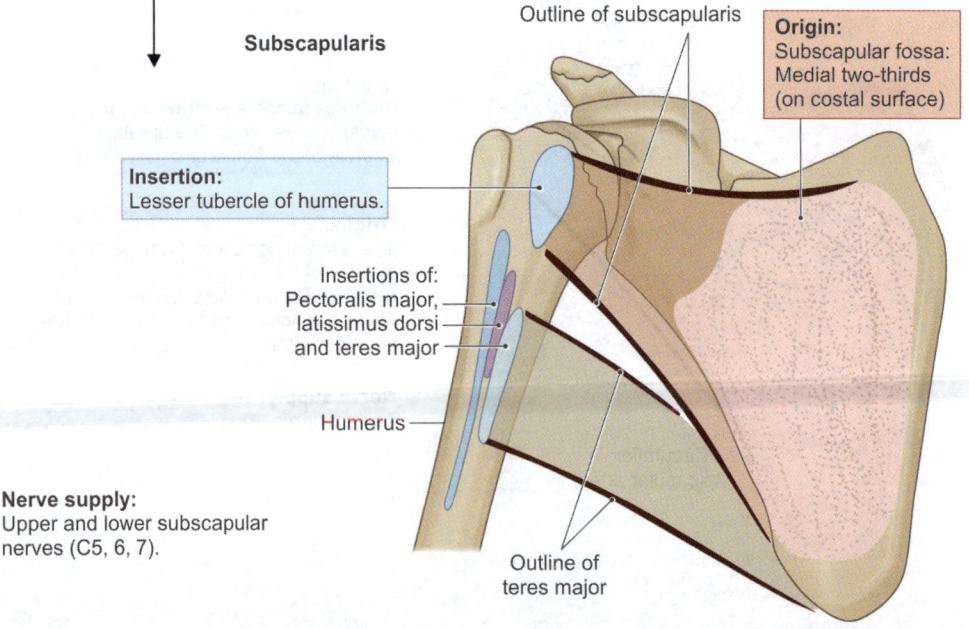

Outline of subscapularis

Origin: Subscapular fossa: Medial two-thirds (on costal surface)

Insertion: Lesser tubercle of humerus.

Insertions of:
Pectoralis major,
latissimus dorsi
and teres major

Humerus

Nerve supply: Upper and lower subscapular nerves (C5, 6, 7).

Outline of teres major

Atlas of Muscle Attachments: Upper Limb

Plate 11
Biceps Brachii

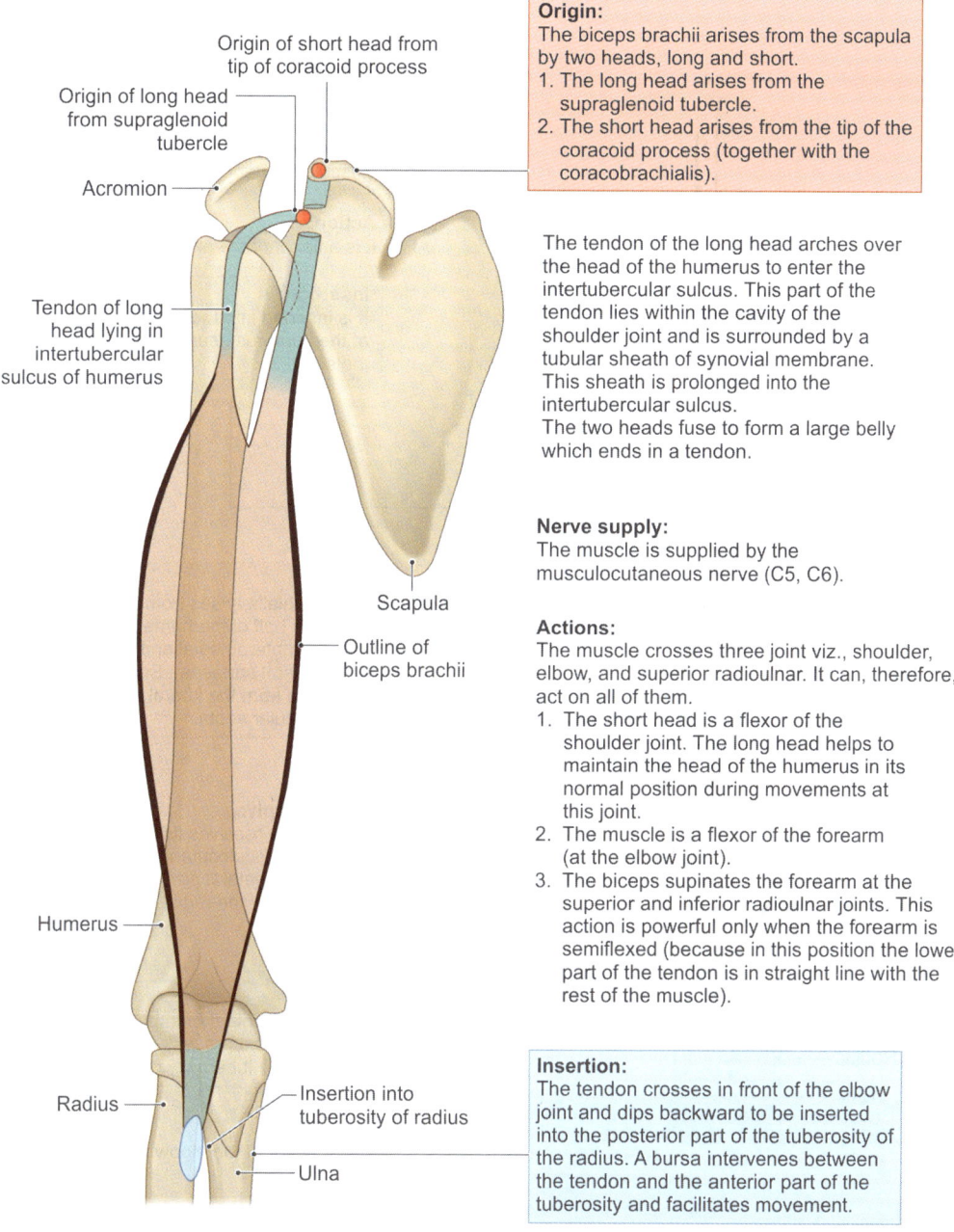

Origin:
The biceps brachii arises from the scapula by two heads, long and short.
1. The long head arises from the supraglenoid tubercle.
2. The short head arises from the tip of the coracoid process (together with the coracobrachialis).

The tendon of the long head arches over the head of the humerus to enter the intertubercular sulcus. This part of the tendon lies within the cavity of the shoulder joint and is surrounded by a tubular sheath of synovial membrane. This sheath is prolonged into the intertubercular sulcus.
The two heads fuse to form a large belly which ends in a tendon.

Nerve supply:
The muscle is supplied by the musculocutaneous nerve (C5, C6).

Actions:
The muscle crosses three joint viz., shoulder, elbow, and superior radioulnar. It can, therefore, act on all of them.
1. The short head is a flexor of the shoulder joint. The long head helps to maintain the head of the humerus in its normal position during movements at this joint.
2. The muscle is a flexor of the forearm (at the elbow joint).
3. The biceps supinates the forearm at the superior and inferior radioulnar joints. This action is powerful only when the forearm is semiflexed (because in this position the lowest part of the tendon is in straight line with the rest of the muscle).

Insertion:
The tendon crosses in front of the elbow joint and dips backward to be inserted into the posterior part of the tuberosity of the radius. A bursa intervenes between the tendon and the anterior part of the tuberosity and facilitates movement.

Atlas of Muscle Attachments: Upper Limb

Plate 12

Coracobrachialis

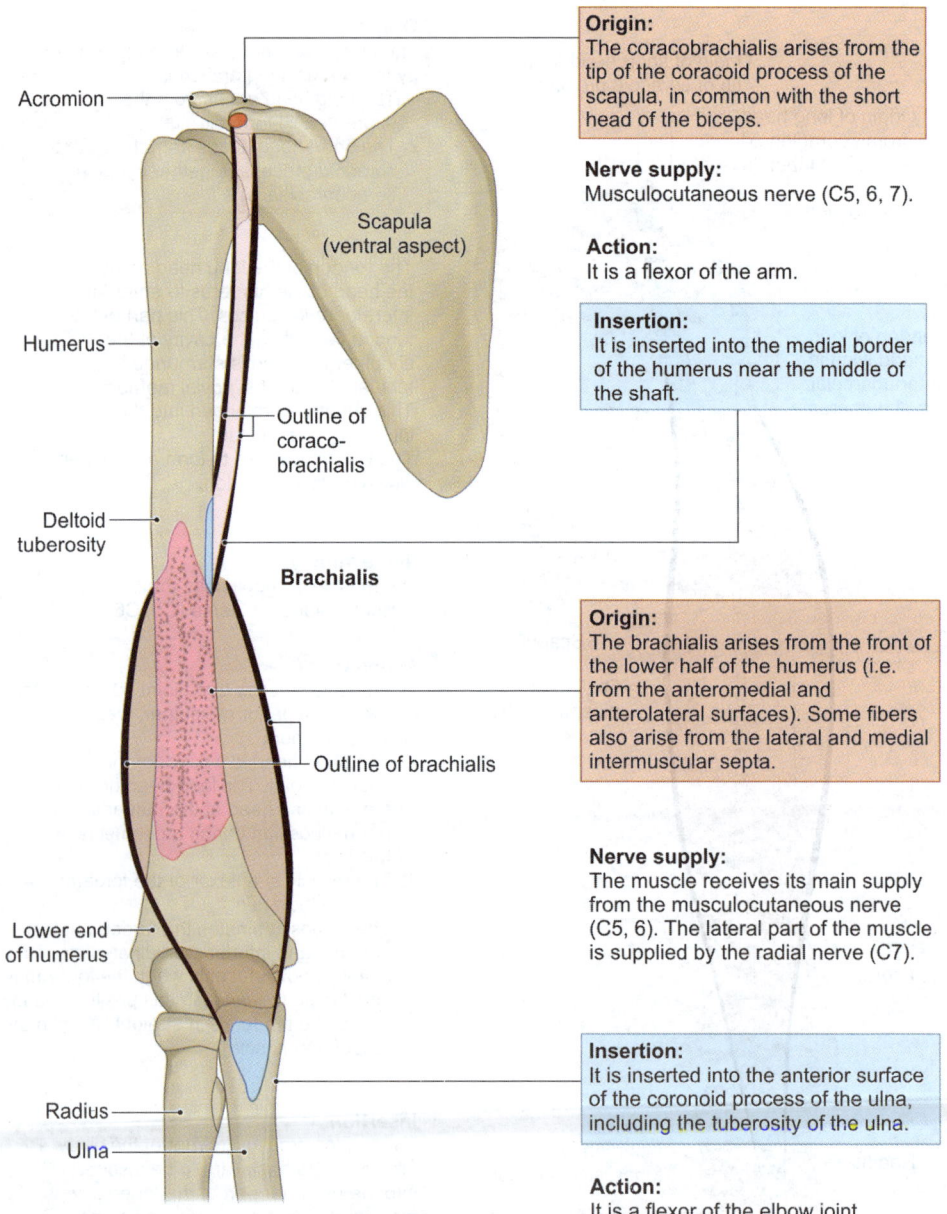

Origin:
The coracobrachialis arises from the tip of the coracoid process of the scapula, in common with the short head of the biceps.

Nerve supply:
Musculocutaneous nerve (C5, 6, 7).

Action:
It is a flexor of the arm.

Insertion:
It is inserted into the medial border of the humerus near the middle of the shaft.

Brachialis

Origin:
The brachialis arises from the front of the lower half of the humerus (i.e. from the anteromedial and anterolateral surfaces). Some fibers also arise from the lateral and medial intermuscular septa.

Nerve supply:
The muscle receives its main supply from the musculocutaneous nerve (C5, 6). The lateral part of the muscle is supplied by the radial nerve (C7).

Insertion:
It is inserted into the anterior surface of the coronoid process of the ulna, including the tuberosity of the ulna.

Action:
It is a flexor of the elbow joint.

Atlas of Muscle Attachments: Upper Limb

Plate 13
Triceps

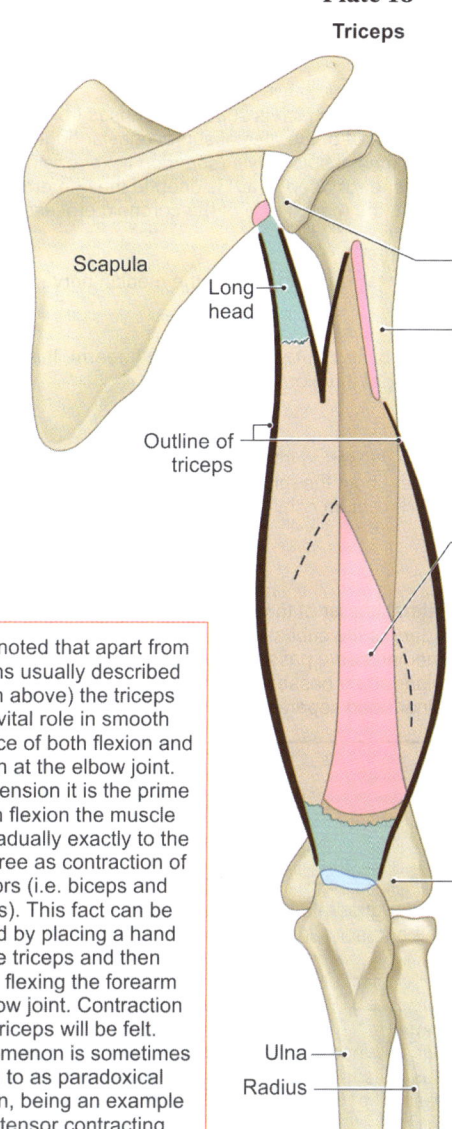

Origin:
As indicated by its name the muscle has three heads of origin.

1. The long head arises from the infraglenoid tubercle of the scapula.

2. The lateral head arises from a ridge on the posterior aspect of the humerus. The ridge corresponds to the upper part of the lateral border of the bone. The upper end of the ridge reaches the greater tubercle; the lower end lies near the deltoid tuberosity.

3. The medial head arises from the posterior surface of the humerus below the radial groove; and also from the medial and lateral intermuscular septa.

Insertion:
The muscle is inserted into the posterior part of the superior surface of the olecranon process of the ulna.

Nerve supply:
Radial nerve.

Actions:
The triceps extends the forearm at the elbow joint. The long head helps in bringing back the abducted or extended arm to the side of the body. It supports the lower part of the capsule of the shoulder joint when the arm is abducted.

It may be noted that apart from the actions usually described (as given above) the triceps plays a vital role in smooth performance of both flexion and extension at the elbow joint. During extension it is the prime mover. In flexion the muscle relaxes gradually exactly to the same degree as contraction of the flexors (i.e. biceps and brachialis). This fact can be confirmed by placing a hand over the triceps and then gradually flexing the forearm at the elbow joint. Contraction of the triceps will be felt. The phenomenon is sometimes referred to as paradoxical contraction, being an example of an extensor contracting during flexion.

Plate 14

Pronator Teres

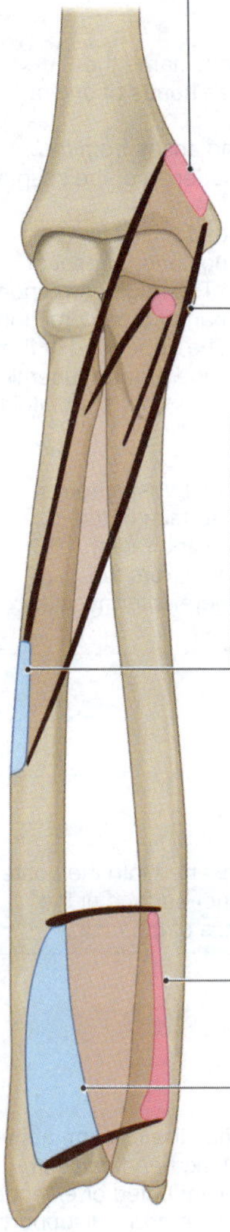

Origin:
The pronator teres has two heads of origin.
The humeral head (which is superficial) arises from:
1. The lowest part of the medial supracondylar ridge, and
2. From the medial epicondyle (common flexor origin).
The ulnar head (or deep head) is deep to the humeral head. It arises from the medial side of the coronoid process.

Nerve supply:
The pronator teres is supplied by the median nerve (C6, 7).

Actions:
As indicated by its name it pronates the forearm. It is also a weak flexor of the elbow.

Insertion:
The muscle is inserted into the lateral surface of the shaft of the radius at about the middle of the bone. The insertion is at the site of maximum convexity of the shaft of the radius.

Notes:
1. The lateral border of the pronator teres forms the medial boundary of the cubital fossa.
2. The median nerve passes between the humeral and ulnar heads.
3. The ulnar artery passes deep to the ulnar head. In other words, the ulnar head separates the ulnar artery from the median nerve.

Pronator Quadratus

Origin:
The pronator quadratus arises from an oblique ridge on the lower part of the anterior surface of the ulna. The area of origin widens inferiorly.

Insertion:
The muscle is inserted into the anterior surface of the shaft of the radius in its lower one-fourth. The insertion extends on to the medial aspect of the radius: on the triangular area above the ulnar notch.

Nerve supply:
The pronator quadratus is supplied by the median nerve through its anterior interosseous branch (C8, T1).

Actions:
It is the chief pronator of the forearm. It prevents separation of the radius and ulna.

Atlas of Muscle Attachments: Upper Limb

Plate 15
Flexor Carpi Radialis

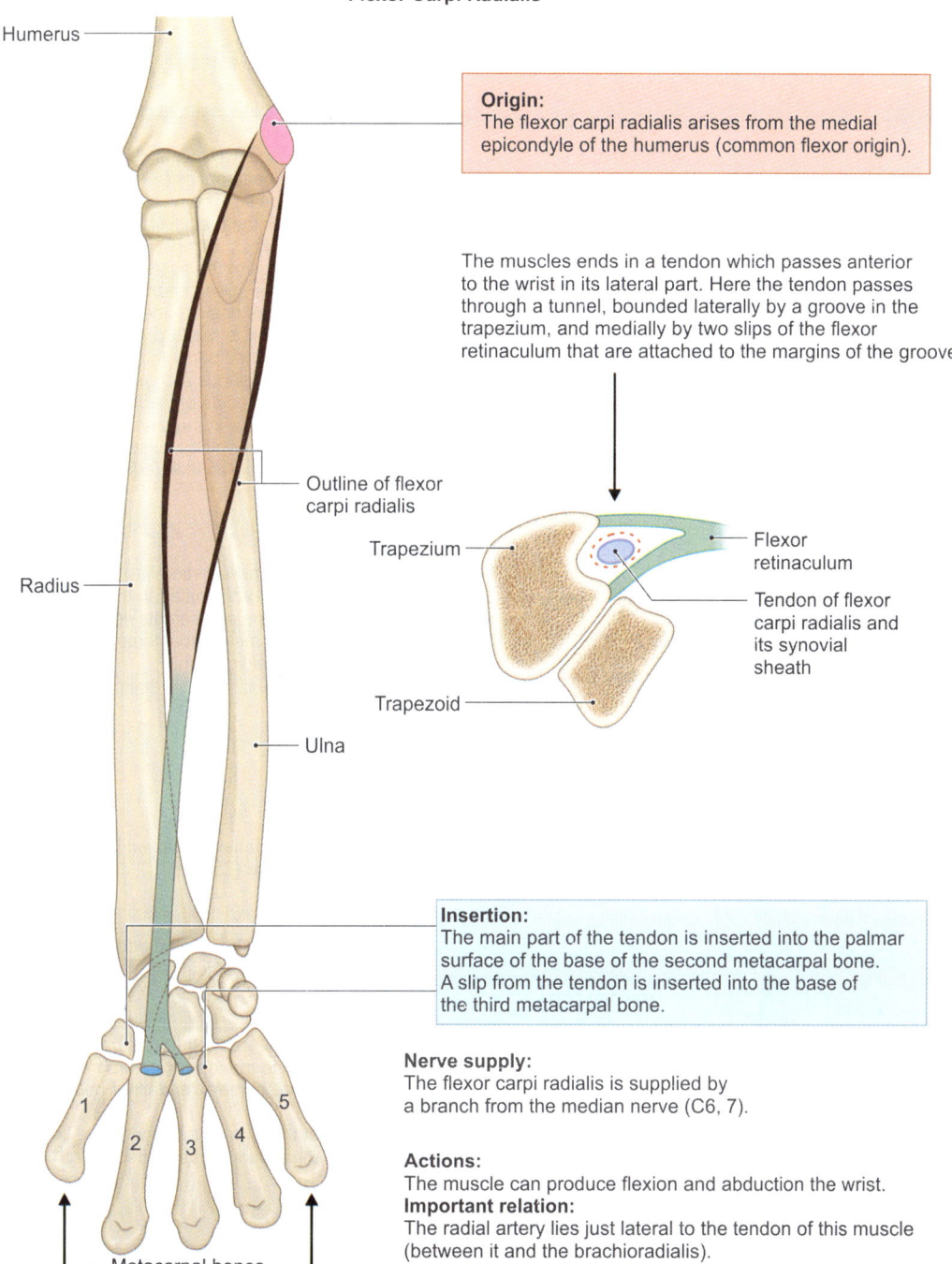

Origin:
The flexor carpi radialis arises from the medial epicondyle of the humerus (common flexor origin).

The muscles ends in a tendon which passes anterior to the wrist in its lateral part. Here the tendon passes through a tunnel, bounded laterally by a groove in the trapezium, and medially by two slips of the flexor retinaculum that are attached to the margins of the groove.

Insertion:
The main part of the tendon is inserted into the palmar surface of the base of the second metacarpal bone. A slip from the tendon is inserted into the base of the third metacarpal bone.

Nerve supply:
The flexor carpi radialis is supplied by a branch from the median nerve (C6, 7).

Actions:
The muscle can produce flexion and abduction the wrist.
Important relation:
The radial artery lies just lateral to the tendon of this muscle (between it and the brachioradialis).

Plate 16
Flexor Carpi Ulnaris

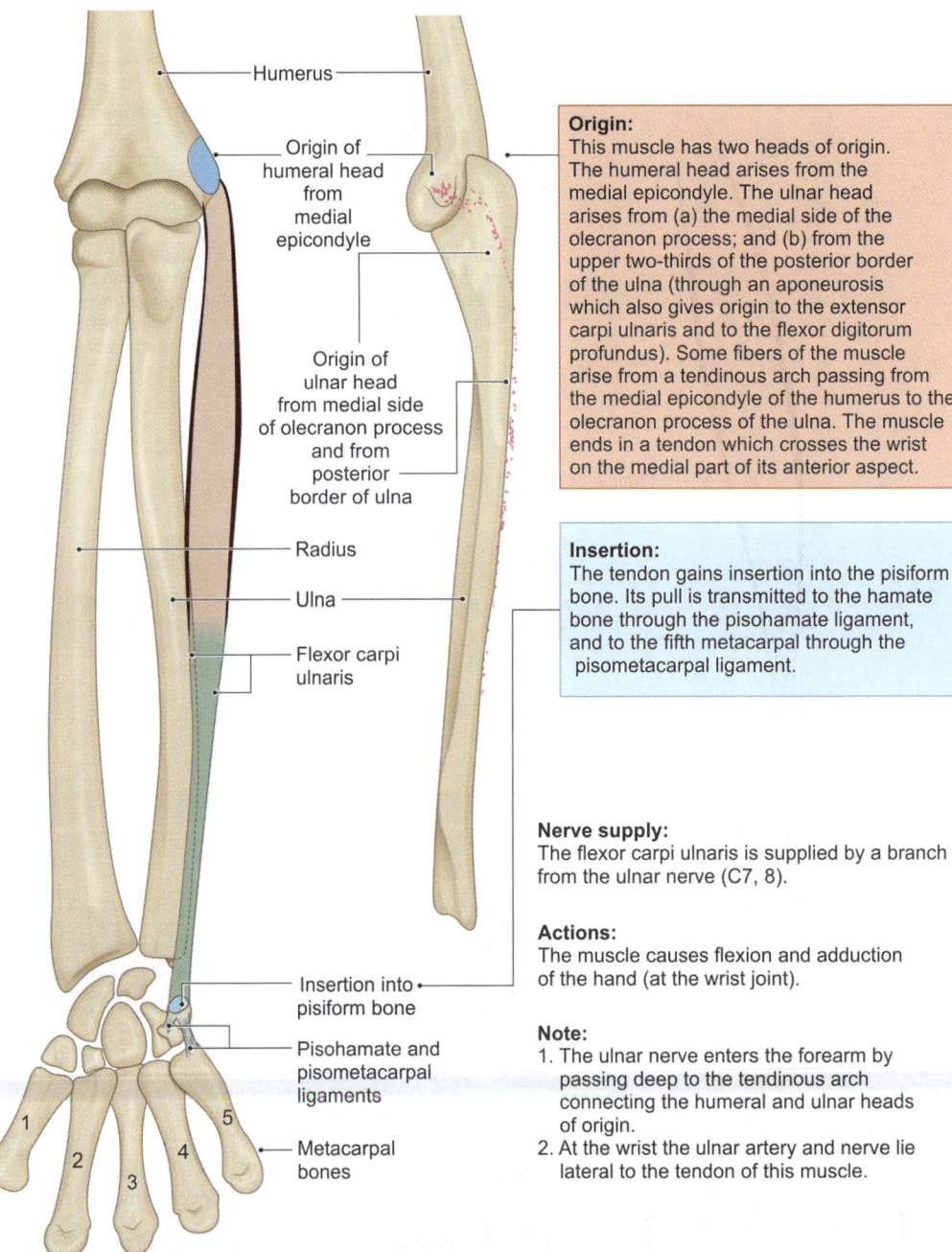

Origin:
This muscle has two heads of origin. The humeral head arises from the medial epicondyle. The ulnar head arises from (a) the medial side of the olecranon process; and (b) from the upper two-thirds of the posterior border of the ulna (through an aponeurosis which also gives origin to the extensor carpi ulnaris and to the flexor digitorum profundus). Some fibers of the muscle arise from a tendinous arch passing from the medial epicondyle of the humerus to the olecranon process of the ulna. The muscle ends in a tendon which crosses the wrist on the medial part of its anterior aspect.

Insertion:
The tendon gains insertion into the pisiform bone. Its pull is transmitted to the hamate bone through the pisohamate ligament, and to the fifth metacarpal through the pisometacarpal ligament.

Nerve supply:
The flexor carpi ulnaris is supplied by a branch from the ulnar nerve (C7, 8).

Actions:
The muscle causes flexion and adduction of the hand (at the wrist joint).

Note:
1. The ulnar nerve enters the forearm by passing deep to the tendinous arch connecting the humeral and ulnar heads of origin.
2. At the wrist the ulnar artery and nerve lie lateral to the tendon of this muscle.

Atlas of Muscle Attachments: Upper Limb

Plate 17
Flexor Digitorum Superficialis

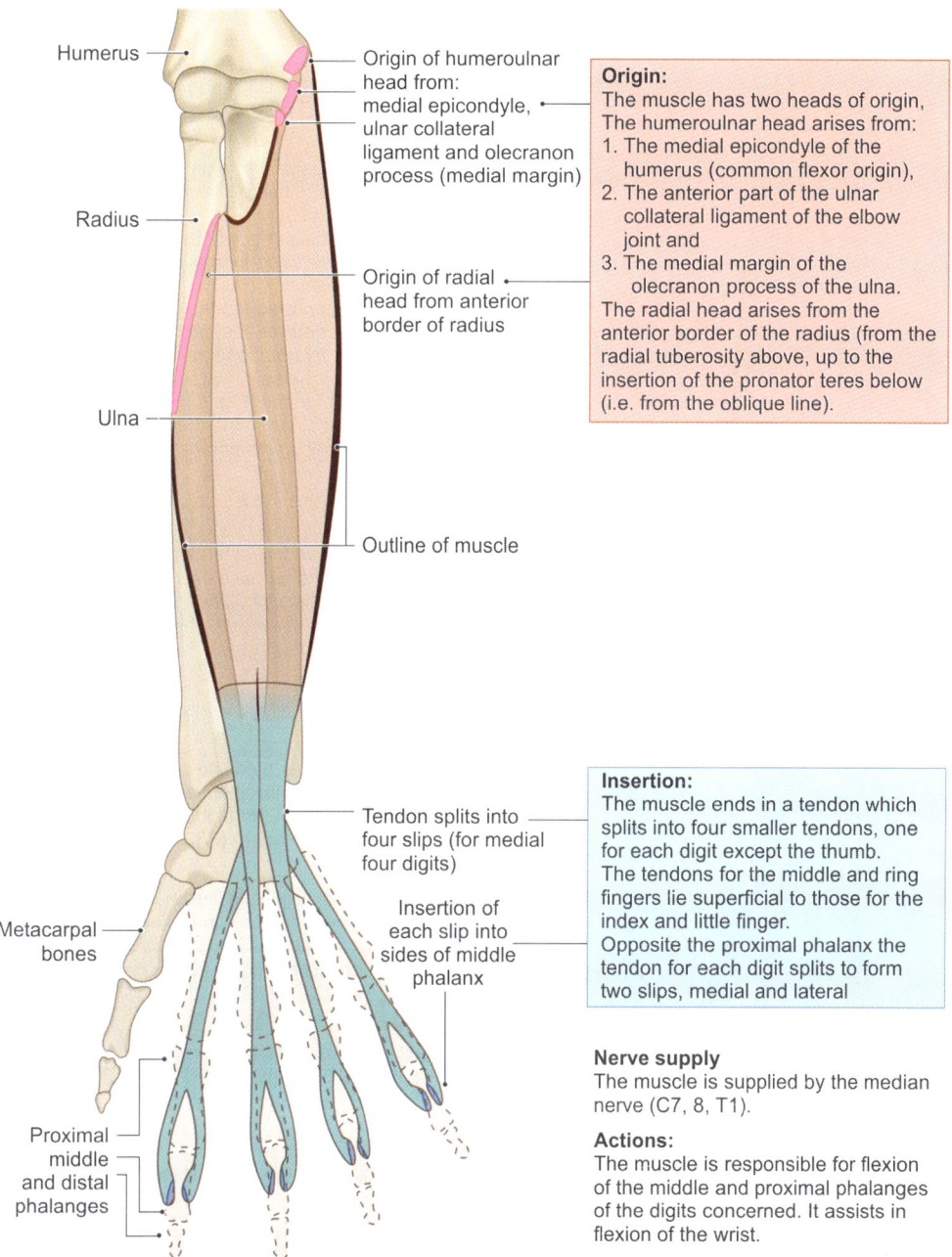

Origin:
The muscle has two heads of origin,
The humeroulnar head arises from:
1. The medial epicondyle of the humerus (common flexor origin),
2. The anterior part of the ulnar collateral ligament of the elbow joint and
3. The medial margin of the olecranon process of the ulna.
The radial head arises from the anterior border of the radius (from the radial tuberosity above, up to the insertion of the pronator teres below (i.e. from the oblique line).

Insertion:
The muscle ends in a tendon which splits into four smaller tendons, one for each digit except the thumb. The tendons for the middle and ring fingers lie superficial to those for the index and little finger.
Opposite the proximal phalanx the tendon for each digit splits to form two slips, medial and lateral

Nerve supply
The muscle is supplied by the median nerve (C7, 8, T1).

Actions:
The muscle is responsible for flexion of the middle and proximal phalanges of the digits concerned. It assists in flexion of the wrist.

Atlas of Muscle Attachments: Upper Limb

Plate 18
Flexor Digitorum Profundus

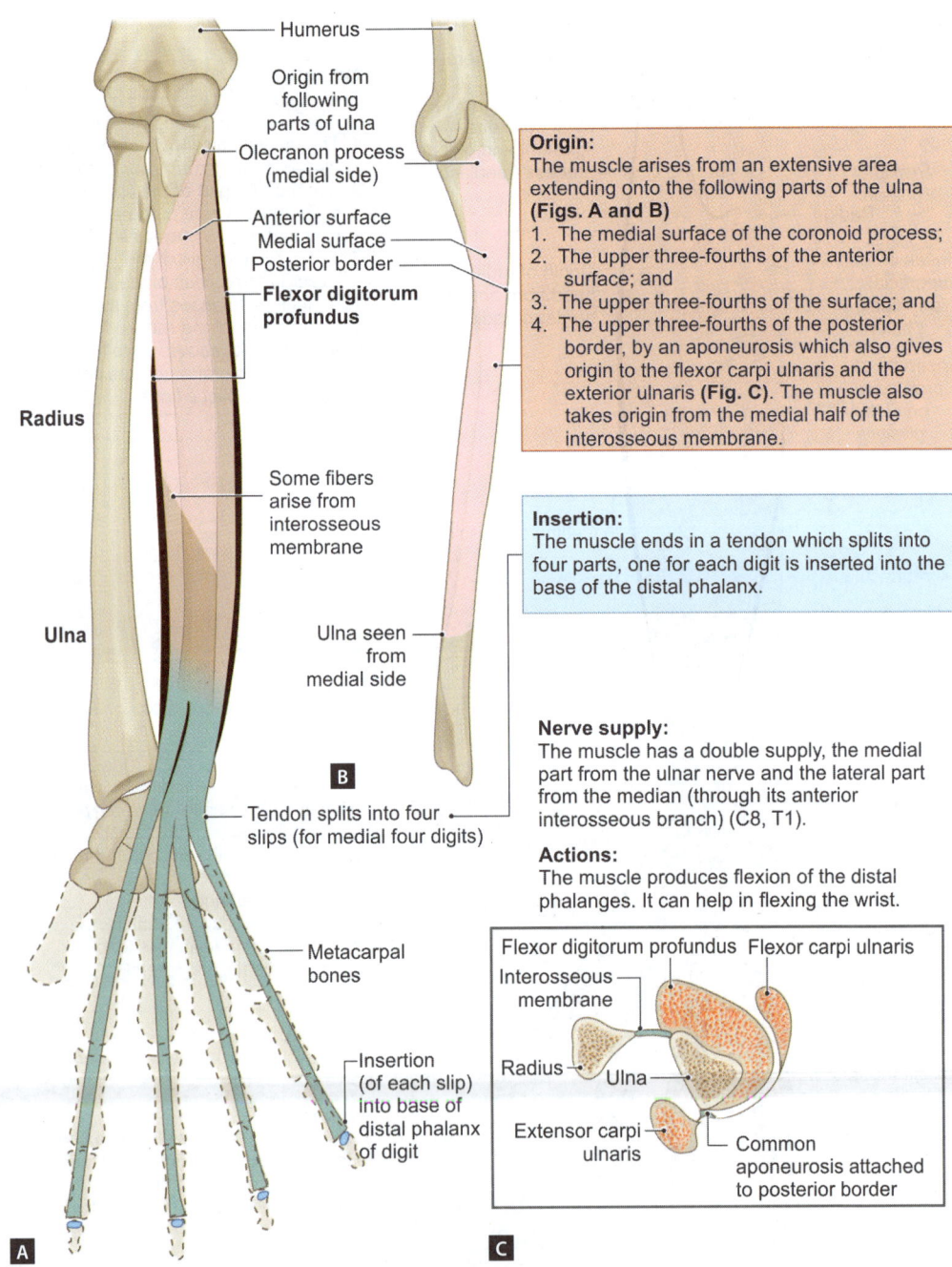

Origin:
The muscle arises from an extensive area extending onto the following parts of the ulna (**Figs. A and B**)
1. The medial surface of the coronoid process;
2. The upper three-fourths of the anterior surface; and
3. The upper three-fourths of the surface; and
4. The upper three-fourths of the posterior border, by an aponeurosis which also gives origin to the flexor carpi ulnaris and the exterior ulnaris (**Fig. C**). The muscle also takes origin from the medial half of the interosseous membrane.

Insertion:
The muscle ends in a tendon which splits into four parts, one for each digit is inserted into the base of the distal phalanx.

Nerve supply:
The muscle has a double supply, the medial part from the ulnar nerve and the lateral part from the median (through its anterior interosseous branch) (C8, T1).

Actions:
The muscle produces flexion of the distal phalanges. It can help in flexing the wrist.

Atlas of Muscle Attachments: Upper Limb

Plate 19

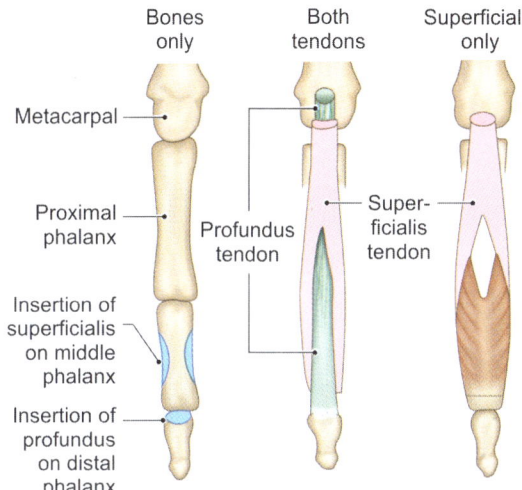

Additional Notes on Flexor Digitorum Superficialis and Profundus

1. Further details of arrangement in the digits (Fig. A):
Over the base of the proximal phalanx, the profundus tendon lies deep to that of the superficialis. Over the middle of the proximal phalanx, the superficialis tendon splits into two slips. The profundus tendon passes through the interval between these slips. Behind the profundus tendon the slips of the superficialis reunite and partially decussate. They form a groove over which the profundus tendon passes. Finally, the slips are inserted on the sides of the middle phalanx. The profundus tendon passes over the groove formed by the superficialis tendon to reach the base of the distal phalanx.

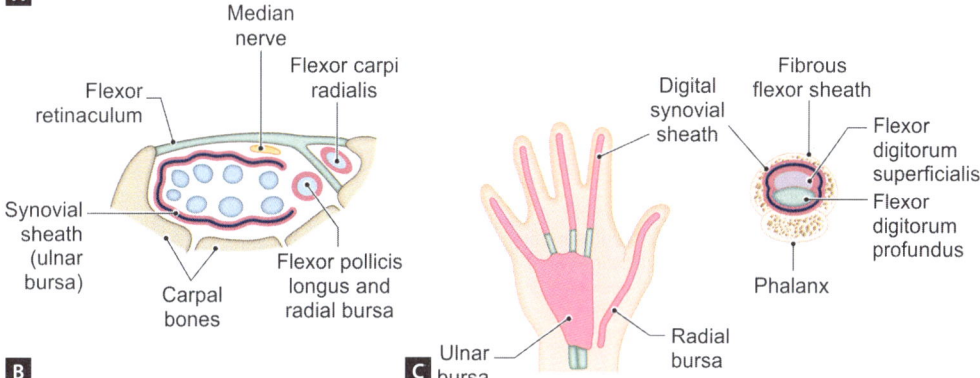

2. Fibrous flexor sheath:
During their course over the ventral aspect of the digits, the tendons of the flexor digitorum superficialis and profundus (for that digit) lie in a common canal; bounded posteriorly by the phalanges and anteriorly (and on the sides) by a fibrous membrane. This membrane is called the fibrous flexor sheath. It holds the tendons in place (**Fig. C**).

3. Synovial sheaths:
At the wrist, the four tendons of the flexor digitorum superficialis lie superficial to the four tendons of the profundus. All the eight tendons pass through the carpal tunnel which is bounded, in front by the flexor retinaculum; and behind by the carpal bones (**Fig. B**). Here the tendons are surrounded by a common synovial sheath (ulnar bursa). Proximally, the sheath extends into the forearm for about 2.5 cm proximal to the flexor retinaculum. Distally, it extends to the middle of the palm.

Over the digits, the tendons are surrounded by a common digital synovial sheath (**Fig. C**), which lines the inside of the fibrous flexor sheath. Each digital sheath extends from the level of the metacarpophalangeal joint (proximally) to the insertion of the profundus tendon (distally). The digital sheath of the little finger is continuous proximally with the ulnar bursa. The synovial sheath surrounding the flexor pollicis longus is called the radial bursa.

Plate 20

Flexor Pollicis Longus

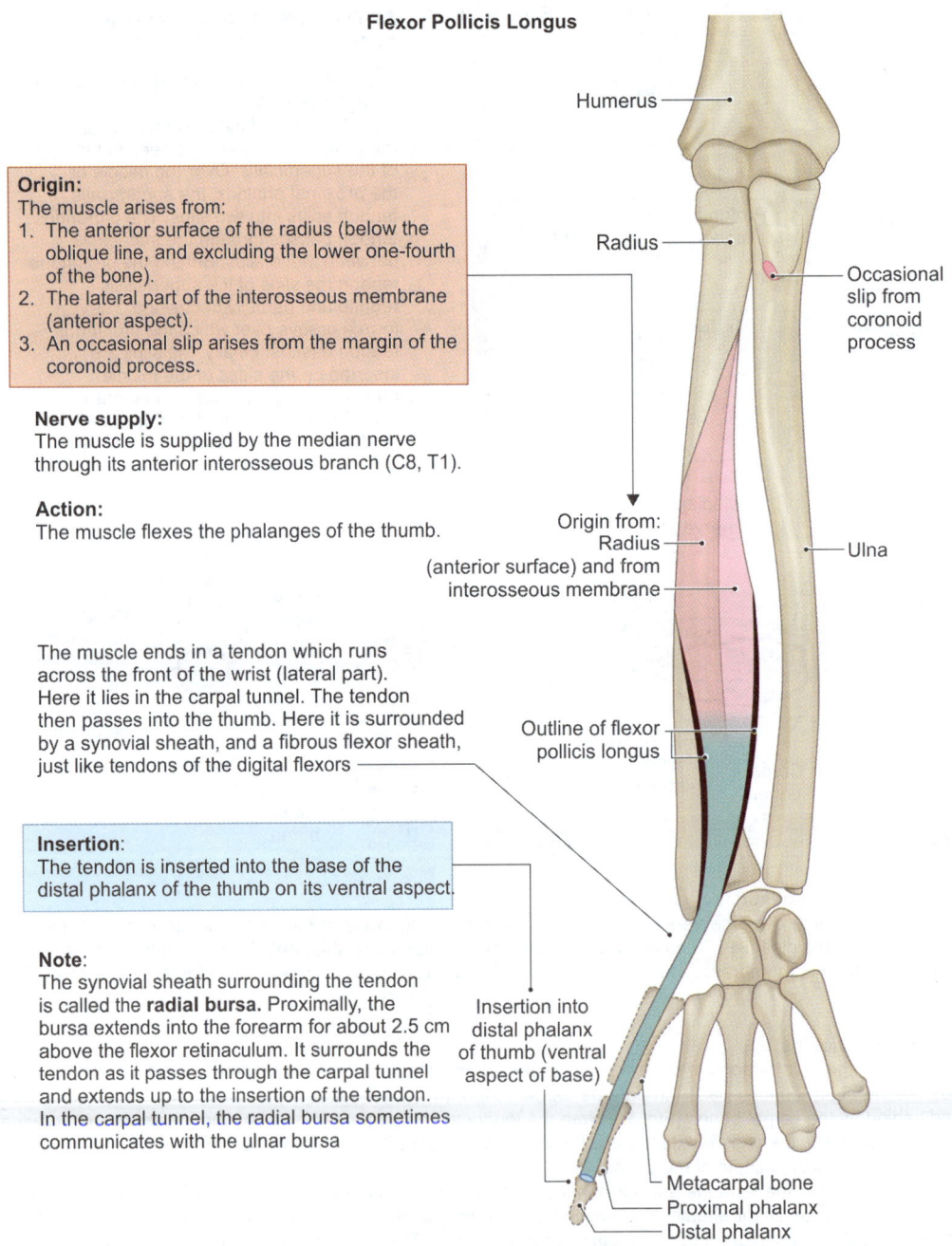

Origin:
The muscle arises from:
1. The anterior surface of the radius (below the oblique line, and excluding the lower one-fourth of the bone).
2. The lateral part of the interosseous membrane (anterior aspect).
3. An occasional slip arises from the margin of the coronoid process.

Nerve supply:
The muscle is supplied by the median nerve through its anterior interosseous branch (C8, T1).

Action:
The muscle flexes the phalanges of the thumb.

The muscle ends in a tendon which runs across the front of the wrist (lateral part). Here it lies in the carpal tunnel. The tendon then passes into the thumb. Here it is surrounded by a synovial sheath, and a fibrous flexor sheath, just like tendons of the digital flexors

Insertion:
The tendon is inserted into the base of the distal phalanx of the thumb on its ventral aspect.

Note:
The synovial sheath surrounding the tendon is called the **radial bursa**. Proximally, the bursa extends into the forearm for about 2.5 cm above the flexor retinaculum. It surrounds the tendon as it passes through the carpal tunnel and extends up to the insertion of the tendon. In the carpal tunnel, the radial bursa sometimes communicates with the ulnar bursa

Plate 21

Flexor Retinaculum

This strong band of fascia stretches across the ventral aspect of the carpal bones; between the retinaculum and the carpal bones is the *carpal tunnel*. It transmits the long flexor tendons (flexor digitorum superficialis and profundus and flexor pollicis longus) and the median nerve.

The flexor retinaculum is attached medially to the pisiform bone, and to the hook of the hamate bone. Laterally, it splits into a superficial and a deep layer. The superficial layer is attached to the tubercle of the scaphoid, and to the tubercle of the trapezium. The deep layer is attached to the trapezium posterior to the groove for the flexor carpi radialis.

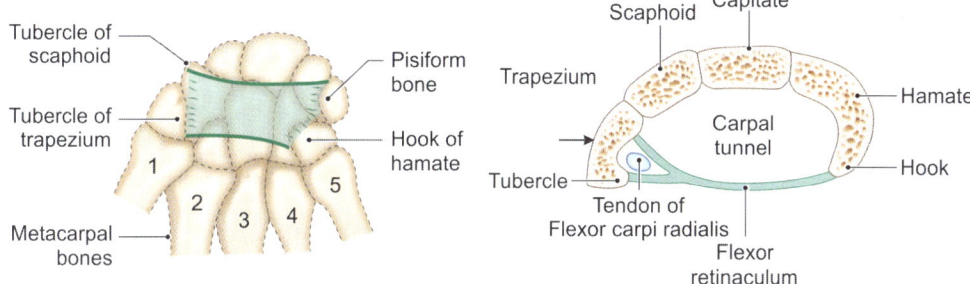

Lumbrical Muscles

These are four small muscles that take origin from the tendons of the flexor digitorum profundus. They are numbered from lateral to medial side.

Nerve supply: The first and second lumbricals receive branches from the median nerve (C8, T1) and the third and fourth from the deep branch of the ulnar (C8, T1).

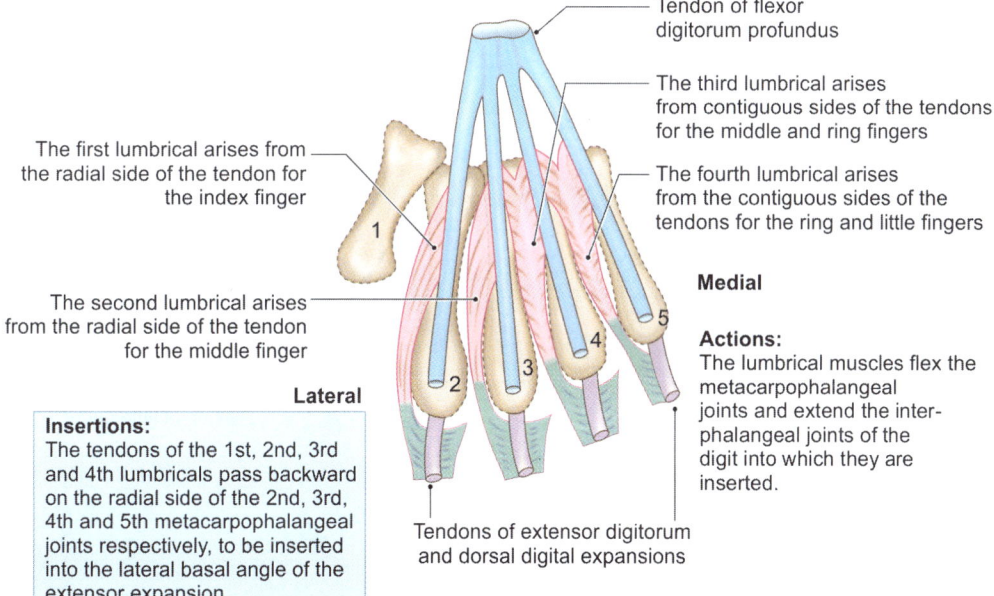

Insertions:
The tendons of the 1st, 2nd, 3rd and 4th lumbricals pass backward on the radial side of the 2nd, 3rd, 4th and 5th metacarpophalangeal joints respectively, to be inserted into the lateral basal angle of the extensor expansion.

Actions:
The lumbrical muscles flex the metacarpophalangeal joints and extend the interphalangeal joints of the digit into which they are inserted.

Atlas of Muscle Attachments: Upper Limb

Plate 22

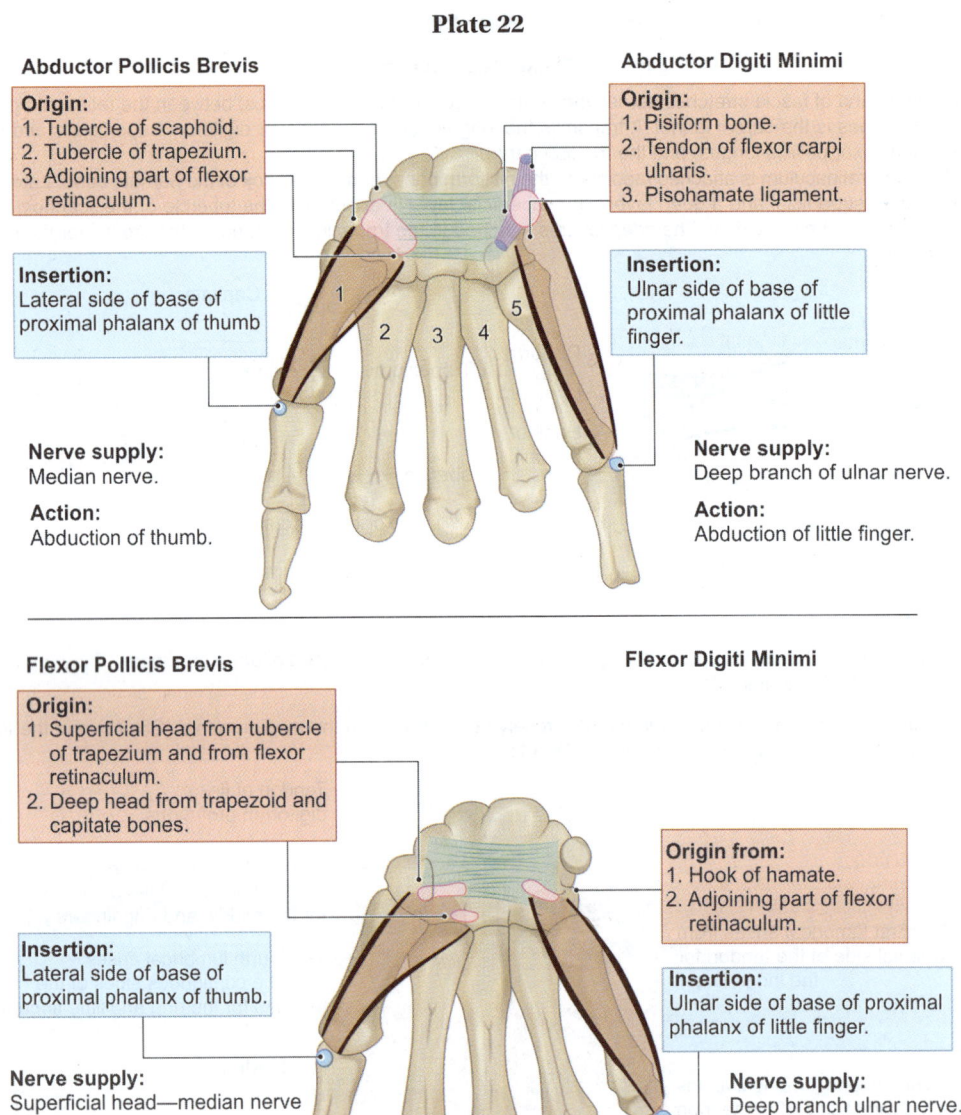

Abductor Pollicis Brevis

Origin:
1. Tubercle of scaphoid.
2. Tubercle of trapezium.
3. Adjoining part of flexor retinaculum.

Insertion:
Lateral side of base of proximal phalanx of thumb

Nerve supply:
Median nerve.

Action:
Abduction of thumb.

Abductor Digiti Minimi

Origin:
1. Pisiform bone.
2. Tendon of flexor carpi ulnaris.
3. Pisohamate ligament.

Insertion:
Ulnar side of base of proximal phalanx of little finger.

Nerve supply:
Deep branch of ulnar nerve.

Action:
Abduction of little finger.

Flexor Pollicis Brevis

Origin:
1. Superficial head from tubercle of trapezium and from flexor retinaculum.
2. Deep head from trapezoid and capitate bones.

Insertion:
Lateral side of base of proximal phalanx of thumb.

Nerve supply:
Superficial head—median nerve
Deep head—deep branch ulnar nerve.

Action:
Flexion of thumb.

Flexor Digiti Minimi

Origin from:
1. Hook of hamate.
2. Adjoining part of flexor retinaculum.

Insertion:
Ulnar side of base of proximal phalanx of little finger.

Nerve supply:
Deep branch ulnar nerve.

Action:
Flexion of little finger.

Atlas of Muscle Attachments: Upper Limb

Plate 23

Opponens Pollicis

Origin from:
1. Tubercle of trapezium
2. Adjoining part of flexor retinaculum.

Insertion into:
Lateral half of palmar surface of first metacarpal bone.

Nerve supply:
Median nerve.

Action:
Opposition of thumb.

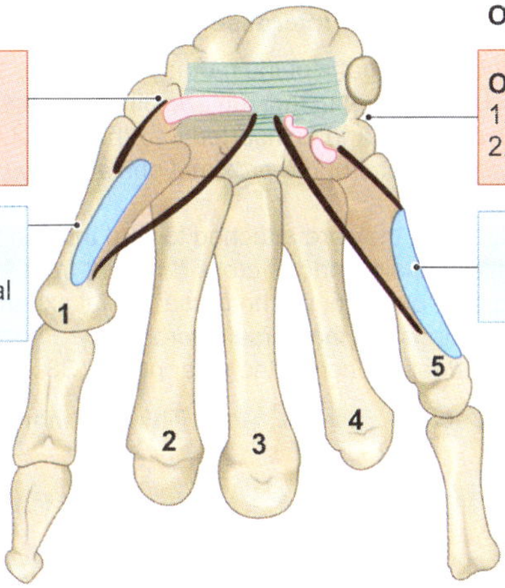

Opponens Digiti Minimi

Origin from:
1. Hook of hamate
2. Adjoining part of flexor retinaculum.

Insertion into:
Medial surface of fifth metacarpal bone.

Nerve supply:
Deep branch ulnar nerve.

Action:
1. Making palm hollow
2. Little finger touches tip of thumb.

Addcutor Pollicis

Origin of oblique head from:
1. Capitate bone
2. Base of 2nd and 3rd metacarpal bones.

Origin of transverse head from:
Shaft of third metacarpal bone.

Insertion:
Proximal phalanx of thumb (medial side of base).

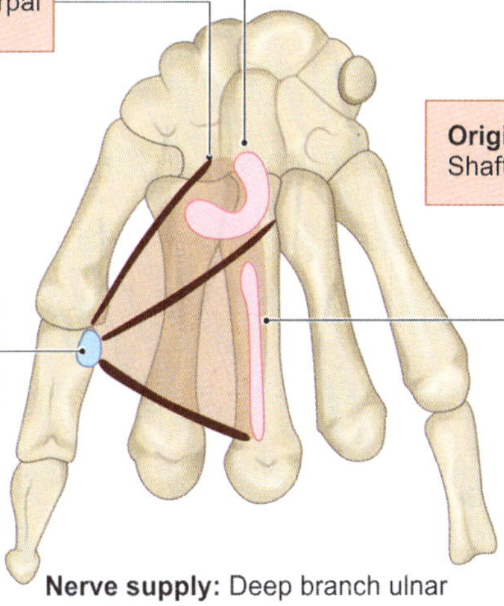

Nerve supply: Deep branch ulnar
Action: Adduction of thumb

Plate 24

Palmar Interossei

These are four small muscles placed between the shafts of the metacarpal bones. They are numbered from lateral to medial side. There is one muscle each from the 1st, 2nd, 4th and 5th digits, there being none for the 3rd digit.

Each muscle arises from one metacarpal bone and is inserted into the dorsal digital expansion of the same digit. It may have an additional insertion on the base of the proximal phalanx. The attachment of each muscle is shown below.

All palmar interossei adduct the digit to which they are attached toward the middle finger. In addition, they flex the digit at the metacarpophalangeal joint, as their tendons cross this joint from front to back. They extend the digit at the interphalangeal joints exerting their pull through the dorsal digital expansion. (Compare these actions with those of the lumbrical muscles and with those of the dorsal interossei).

All palmar interossei are supplied by the deep branch of the ulnar nerve (C8, T1).

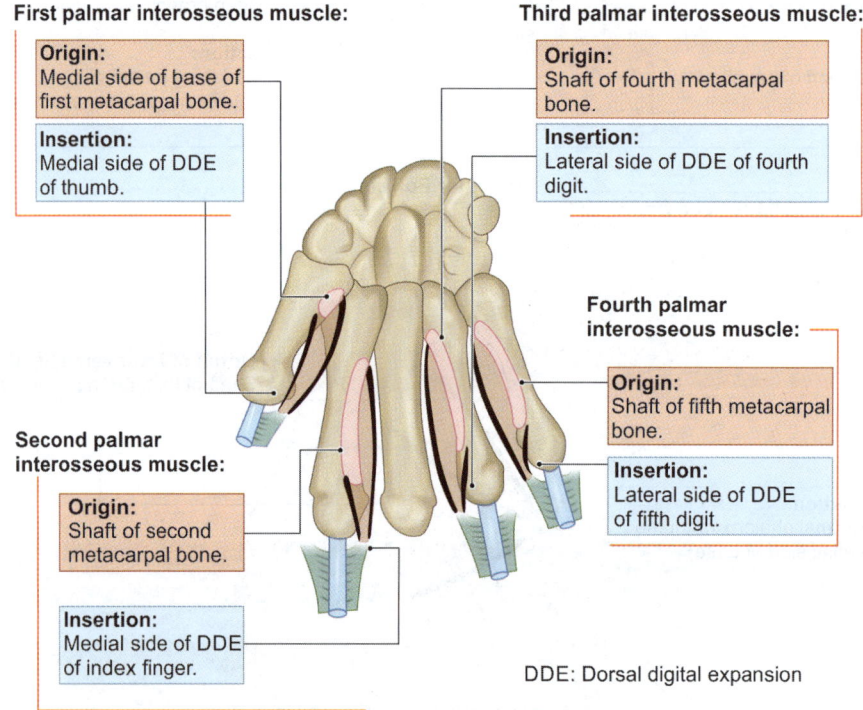

First palmar interosseous muscle:
Origin: Medial side of base of first metacarpal bone.
Insertion: Medial side of DDE of thumb.

Second palmar interosseous muscle:
Origin: Shaft of second metacarpal bone.
Insertion: Medial side of DDE of index finger.

Third palmar interosseous muscle:
Origin: Shaft of fourth metacarpal bone.
Insertion: Lateral side of DDE of fourth digit.

Fourth palmar interosseous muscle:
Origin: Shaft of fifth metacarpal bone.
Insertion: Lateral side of DDE of fifth digit.

DDE: Dorsal digital expansion

Atlas of Muscle Attachments: Upper Limb

Plate 25

Dorsal Interossei

Like the palmar interossei the dorsal interossei are four small muscles placed between the metacarpal bones, and numbered from the lateral to the medial side.

Each muscle arises from the contiguous sides of two metacarpal bones. For details of each muscle see below.

It is inserted (a) into a dorsal digital expansion, and (b) into side of the base of a proximal phalanx, see below. All dorsal interossei are abductors of the digits, i.e. they move the digits, away from the line of the middle finger.

In addition (like the palmar interossei), they flex the metacarpophalangeal joint and extend the interphalangeal joint.

All dorsal interossei are supplied by the deep branch of the ulnar nerve (C8, T1).

In the figure, the areas of origin of these muscles are shown as seen from the dorsal aspect. Note, however, that the areas pass right round the sides of the bones and can be seen from the front also.

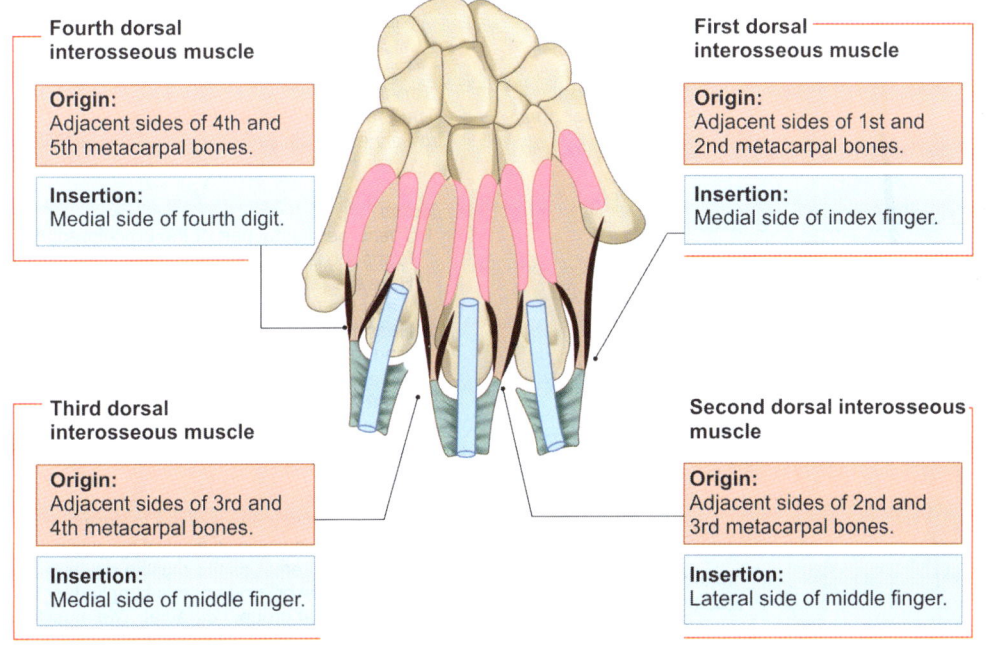

Fourth dorsal interosseous muscle

Origin:
Adjacent sides of 4th and 5th metacarpal bones.

Insertion:
Medial side of fourth digit.

First dorsal interosseous muscle

Origin:
Adjacent sides of 1st and 2nd metacarpal bones.

Insertion:
Medial side of index finger.

Third dorsal interosseous muscle

Origin:
Adjacent sides of 3rd and 4th metacarpal bones.

Insertion:
Medial side of middle finger.

Second dorsal interosseous muscle

Origin:
Adjacent sides of 2nd and 3rd metacarpal bones.

Insertion:
Lateral side of middle finger.

94 Atlas of Muscle Attachments: Upper Limb

Plate 26
Brachioradialis

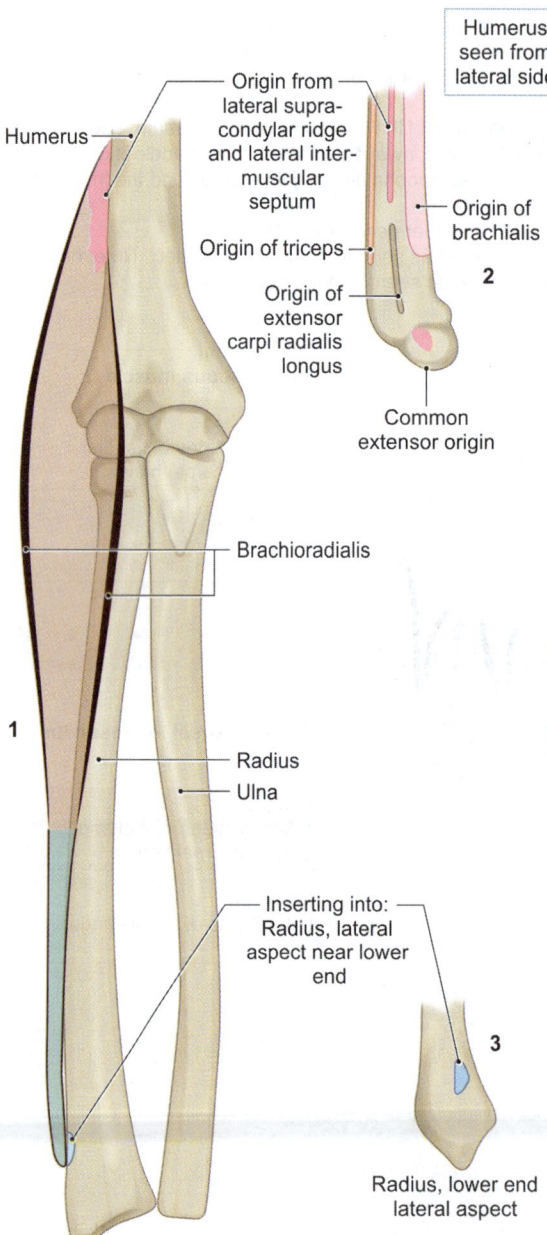

Origin:
This muscle arises from:
1. The upper two-thirds of the lateral supracondylar ridge of the humerus, and
2. The lateral intermuscular septum.

Insertion:
The muscle ends in a tendon which is inserted into the lateral side of the radius just above the styloid process.

Nerve supply:
The brachioradialis is supplied by the radial nerve (C5, 6, 7).

Notes:
1. The upper fleshy part of the brachioradialis forms the lateral boundary of the cubital fossa. Here the radial nerve is deep to it (between it and the brachialis).
2. Near its insertion its tendon is crossed by tendons of the abductor pollicis longus and the extensor pollicis brevis.
3. At the wrist, the radial artery is medial to the tendon (between it and the tendon of the flexor carpi radialis).

Actions:
1. The muscle is a flexor of the forearm (because it crosses in front of the elbow joint). This is of interest as the muscle belongs to the extensor group and is supplied by the nerve of that group, i.e. radial. The muscle acts best as a flexor when the forearm is in the midprone position.
2. It supinates the fully pronated forearm; and pronates the fully supinated forearm, to bring it to the midprone position (This action is controversial).

Atlas of Muscle Attachments: Upper Limb

Plate 27
Extensor Carpi Radialis Longus

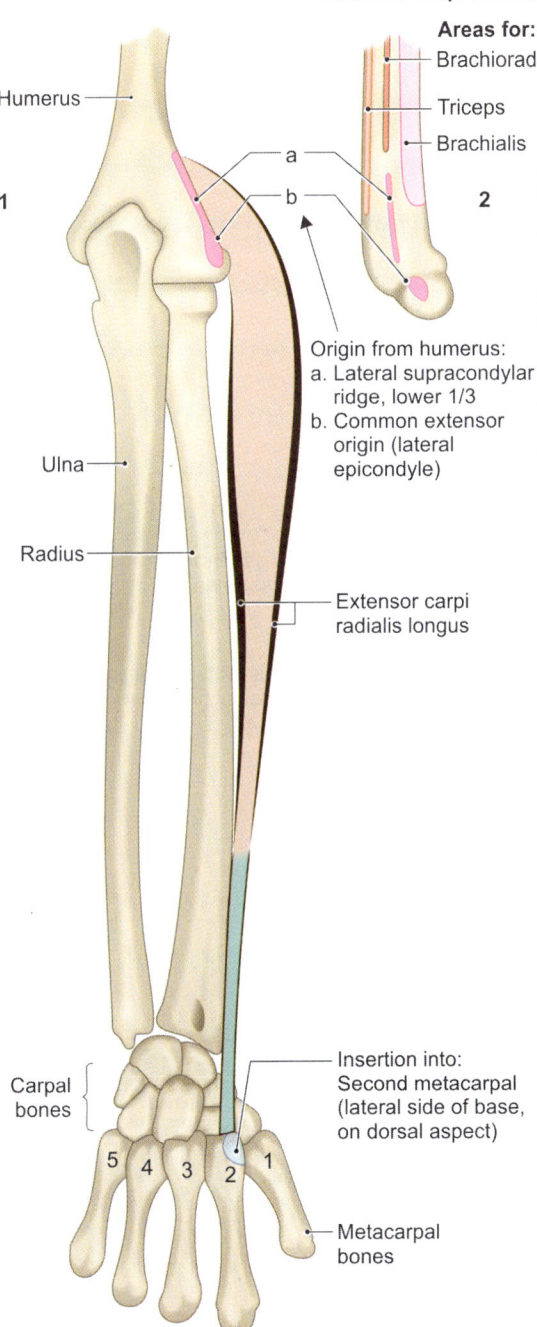

Areas for:
- Brachioradialis
- Triceps
- Brachialis

Origin from humerus:
a. Lateral supracondylar ridge, lower 1/3
b. Common extensor origin (lateral epicondyle)

Extensor carpi radialis longus

Insertion into: Second metacarpal (lateral side of base, on dorsal aspect)

Metacarpal bones

Carpal bones

Origin:
This muscle arises from:
1. The lower one-third of the lateral supracondylar ridge of the humerus.
2. Some fibers arise from the common extensor origin (i.e. lateral epicondyle).
3. Some fibers also arise from the lateral intermuscular septum (not shown).

Insertion:
The muscle ends in a tendon which is inserted into the lateral side of the base of the second metacarpal bone.

Nerve supply: Radial nerve (C6, C7)

Action:
These are common to the extensor carpi radialis longus and brevis.
1. These muscles produce extension of the wrist (along with extensor carpi ulnaris).
2. They abduct the wrist (along with the flexor carpi radialis).
3. They assist movements of the digits by fixing the wrist.

Notes:
(Common to extensor carpi radialis longus and brevis)
1. The extensor carpi radialis longus is superficial to the brevis.
2. The tendons of the two muscles run distally along the lateral side of the radius. They pass deep to the abductor pollicis longus and the extensor pollicis brevis muscles.
3. At the lower end of the radius, the tendons occupy a groove just behind the styloid process (and lateral to the dorsal tubercle). The longus tendon lies lateral to the brevis tendon. Here the two tendons pass deep to the extensor retinaculum. They are surrounded by a common synovial sheath.
4. A little above their insertion, the tendons are crossed by the tendon of the extensor pollicis longus.

Plate 28
Extensor Carpi Radialis Brevis

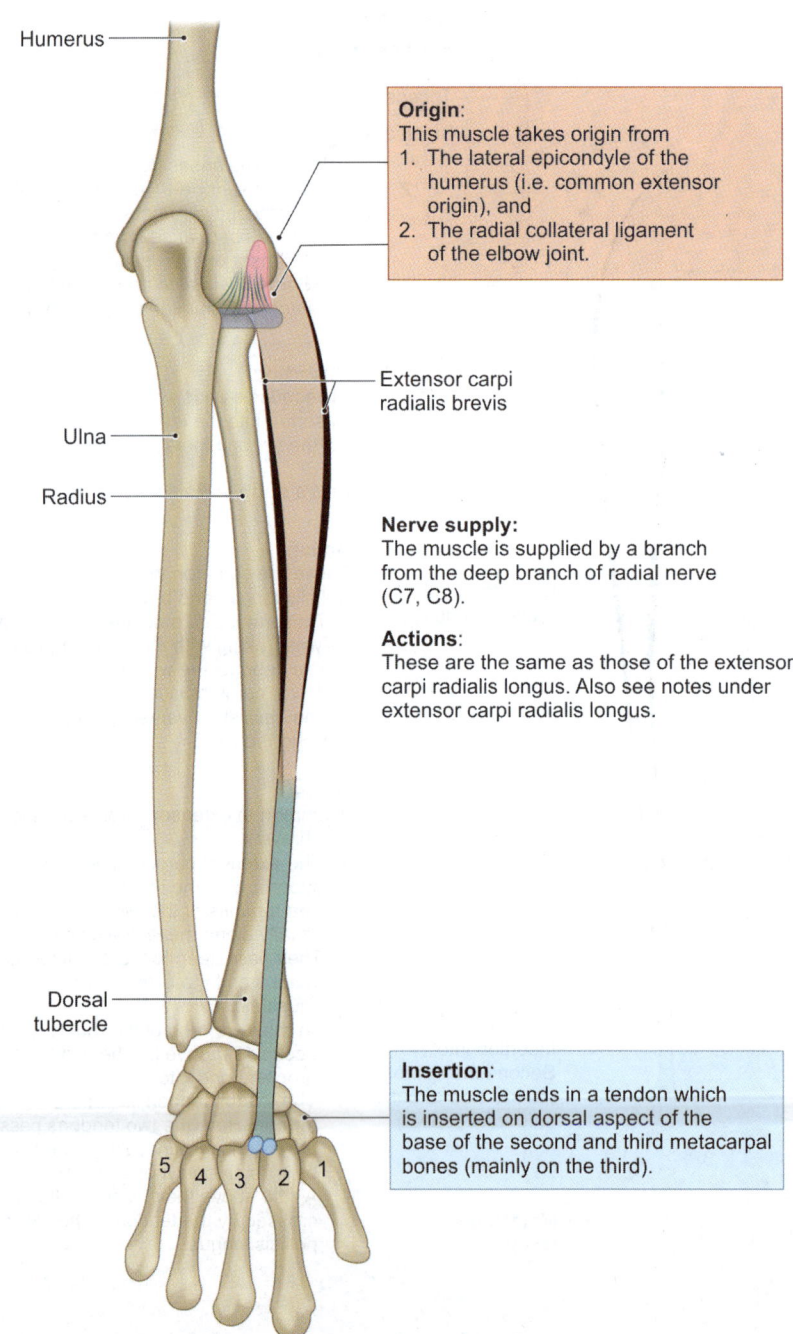

Origin:
This muscle takes origin from
1. The lateral epicondyle of the humerus (i.e. common extensor origin), and
2. The radial collateral ligament of the elbow joint.

Nerve supply:
The muscle is supplied by a branch from the deep branch of radial nerve (C7, C8).

Actions:
These are the same as those of the extensor carpi radialis longus. Also see notes under extensor carpi radialis longus.

Insertion:
The muscle ends in a tendon which is inserted on dorsal aspect of the base of the second and third metacarpal bones (mainly on the third).

Atlas of Muscle Attachments: Upper Limb

Plate 29
Extensor Digitorum

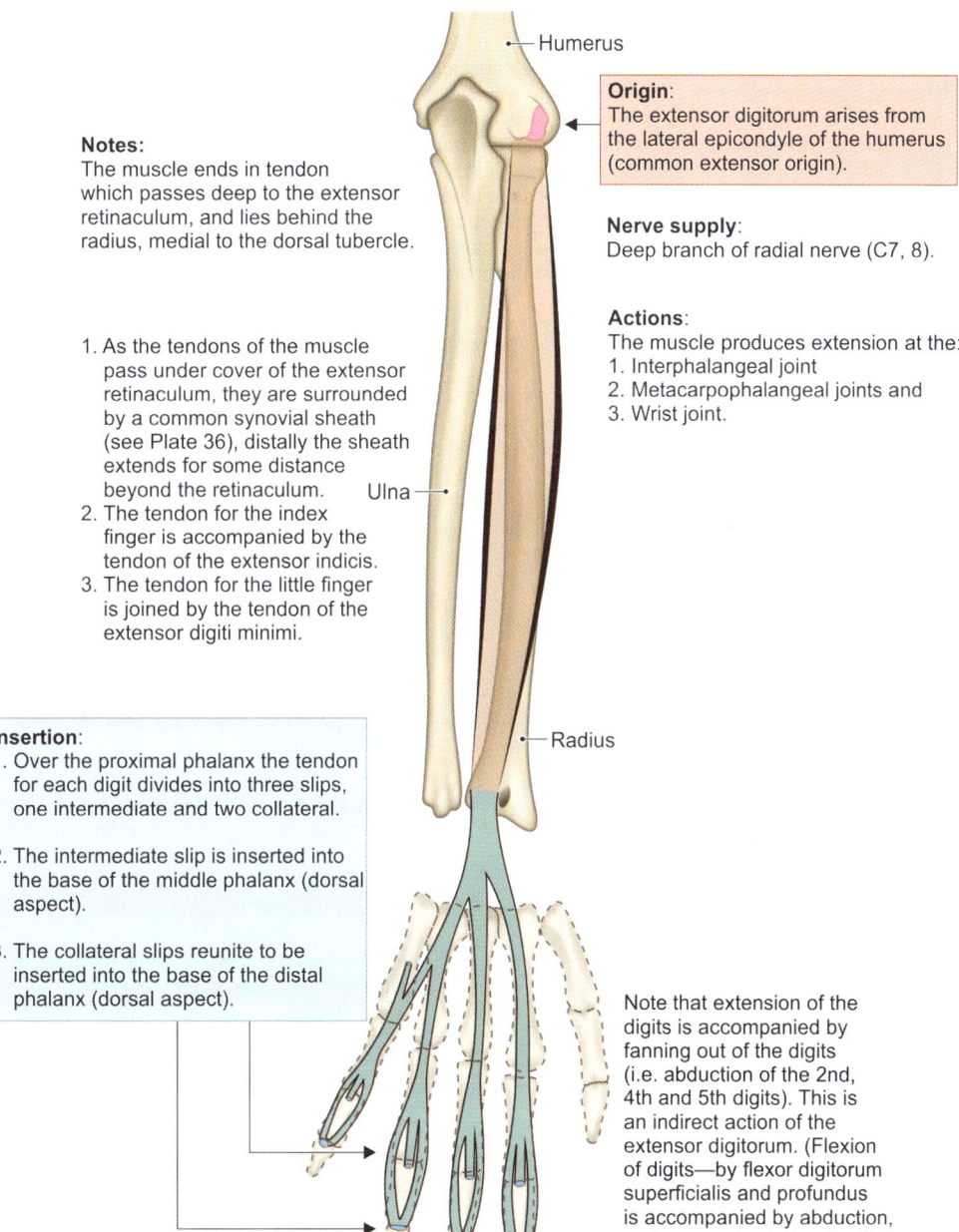

Origin:
The extensor digitorum arises from the lateral epicondyle of the humerus (common extensor origin).

Nerve supply:
Deep branch of radial nerve (C7, 8).

Actions:
The muscle produces extension at the:
1. Interphalangeal joint
2. Metacarpophalangeal joints and
3. Wrist joint.

Notes:
The muscle ends in tendon which passes deep to the extensor retinaculum, and lies behind the radius, medial to the dorsal tubercle.

1. As the tendons of the muscle pass under cover of the extensor retinaculum, they are surrounded by a common synovial sheath (see Plate 36), distally the sheath extends for some distance beyond the retinaculum.
2. The tendon for the index finger is accompanied by the tendon of the extensor indicis.
3. The tendon for the little finger is joined by the tendon of the extensor digiti minimi.

Insertion:
1. Over the proximal phalanx the tendon for each digit divides into three slips, one intermediate and two collateral.
2. The intermediate slip is inserted into the base of the middle phalanx (dorsal aspect).
3. The collateral slips reunite to be inserted into the base of the distal phalanx (dorsal aspect).

Note that extension of the digits is accompanied by fanning out of the digits (i.e. abduction of the 2nd, 4th and 5th digits). This is an indirect action of the extensor digitorum. (Flexion of digits—by flexor digitorum superficialis and profundus is accompanied by abduction, as happens in closing the fist).

Plate 30

Dorsal Digital Expansion

The dorsal digital expansion is an aponeurosis present on the dorsal aspect of the proximal phalanx, and the metacarpophalangeal joint. The expansion is triangular. It has an apex directed distally, and a broad base that lies dorsal to the metacarpophalangeal joint. The expansion may be regarded as an aponeurotic extension of the tendon of the extensor digitorum. This tendon joins the central part of the base of the expansion, and divides into its intermediate and collateral slips in the substance of the expansion. The expansion also gives attachment to the lumbrical and interosseous muscles of the digit. The lateral angle of the base gives attachment to one interosseous muscle alone. In addition to these muscles, the expansion for the index finger receives the tendon of the extensor indicis and that of the little finger receives the tendon of the extensor digiti minimi.

A similar expansion is also seen in relation to the tendon of the extensor pollicis longus as it crosses behind the metacarpophalangeal joint of the thumb. On its lateral side, it receives part of the tendon of the abductor pollicis brevis; and on the medial side, it receives the first palmar interosseous muscle, and part of the abductor pollicis brevis.

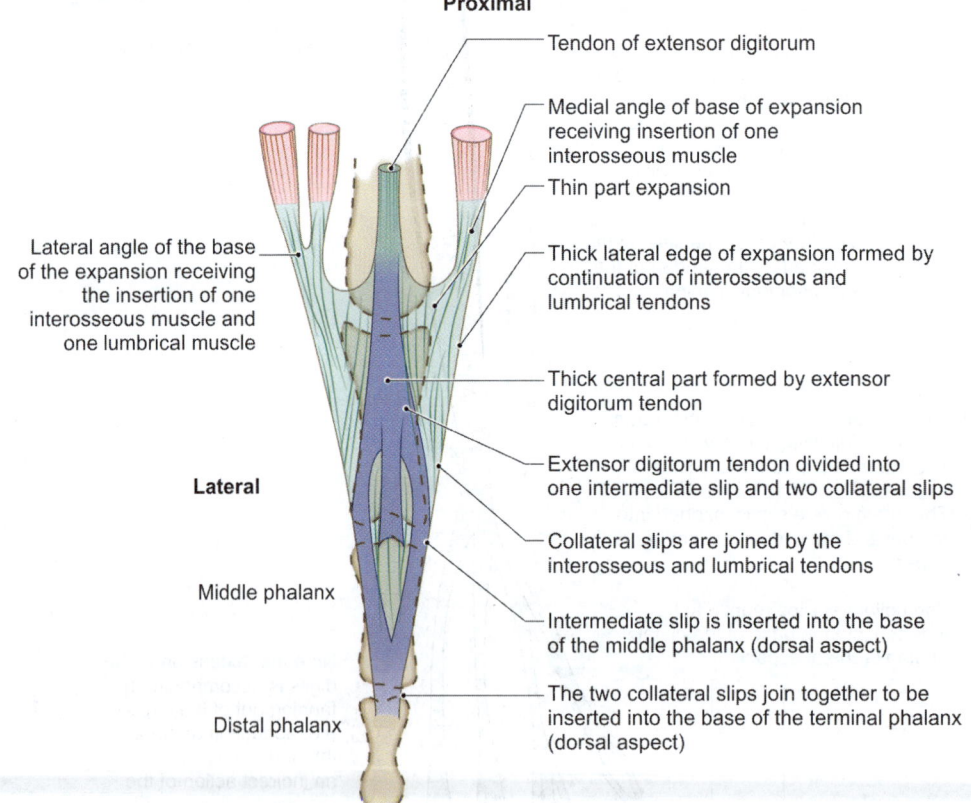

Plate 31
Extensor Digiti Minimi

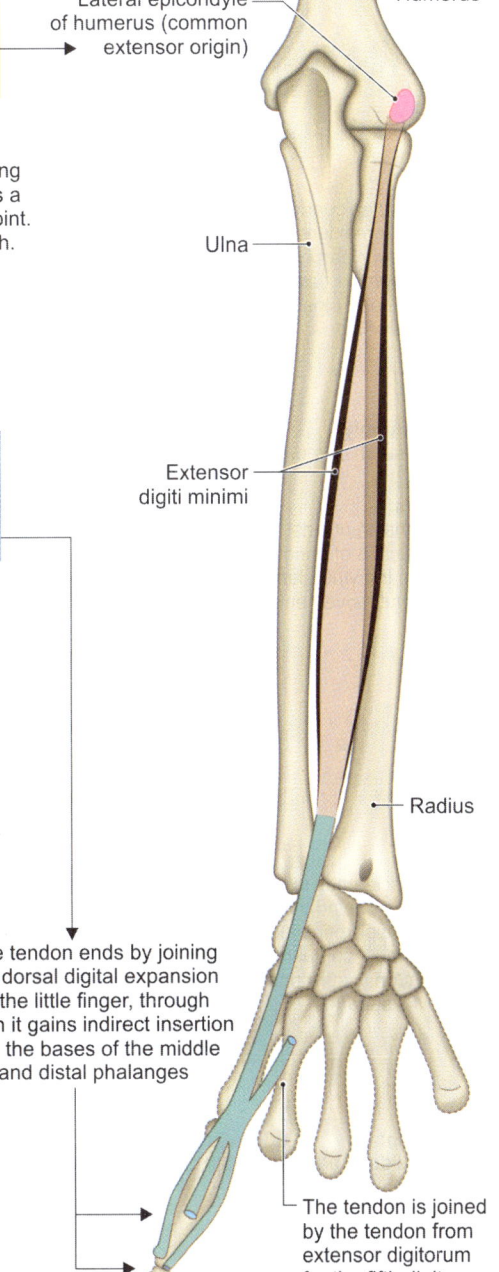

Origin:
The muscle arises from the lateral epicondyle of the humerus (common extensor origin).

The tendon runs across the back of the wrist passing deep to the extensor retinaculum where it occupies a separate compartment just behind the radioulnar joint. Here the tendon is surrounded by a synovial sheath.

Over the metacarpophalangeal joint, the tendon is joined by the tendon of the extensor digitorum for the fifth digit.

Insertion:
The tendon ends in the dorsal digital expansion through which it is inserted into the dorsal aspect of the base of the middle phalanx, and the base of the distal phalanx.

Nerve supply:
Deep branch of radial nerve.

Actions:
The muscle produces extension of the little finger at the interphalangeal and metacarpophalangeal joints. It can help in extending the wrist joint.

Lateral epicondyle of humerus (common extensor origin)

Humerus

Ulna

Extensor digiti minimi

Radius

The tendon ends by joining the dorsal digital expansion of the little finger, through which it gains indirect insertion into the bases of the middle and distal phalanges

The tendon is joined by the tendon from extensor digitorum for the fifth digit

Plate 32

Extensor Carpi Ulnaris

Origin:
1. Lateral epicondyle of the humerus (common extensor origin).
2. Posterior border of ulna (by an aponeurosis common to it, the flexor carpi ulnaris and the flexor digit profundus.

Nerve supply:
Deep branch of radial nerve.

Actions:
1. Extension of wrist
2. Abduction of hand
3. Fixes the wrist during forceful movements.

The muscle ends in a tendon that descends behind the wrist deep to the extensor retinaculum in the medial-most compartment. Here the tendon is surrounded by a synovial sheath.

Insertion:
Medial side of base of the 5th metatarsal bone.

Anconeus

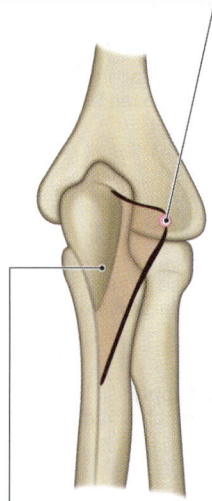

Origin:
The anconeus arises from a small area on the posterior aspect of the lateral epicondyle of the humerus (The area is medial to the common extensor origin).

Insertion:
The muscle fans out to be inserted (a) into the lateral aspect of the olecranon process of the ulna, and (b) into the upper one-fourth of its posterior surface.

Nerve supply:
The anconeus is supplied by a branch of the radial nerve (C7, C8, T1) which travels to it through the substance of the medial head of the triceps.

Actions:
The muscle is a weak extensor of the elbow. It moves the ulna laterally during pronation.

Atlas of Muscle Attachments: Upper Limb

Plate 33

Supinator

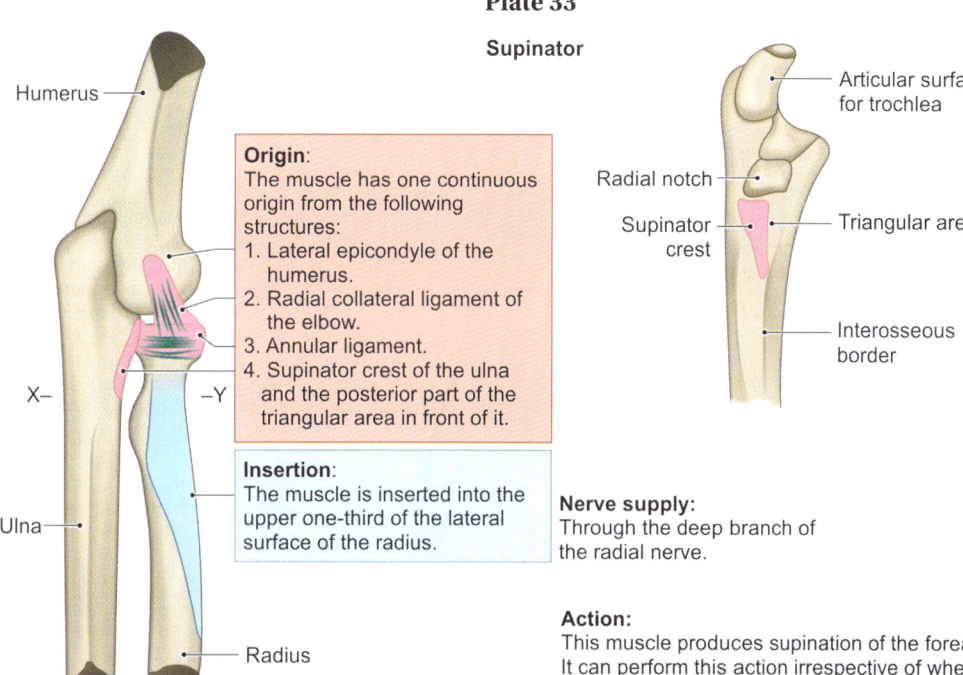

Origin:
The muscle has one continuous origin from the following structures:
1. Lateral epicondyle of the humerus.
2. Radial collateral ligament of the elbow.
3. Annular ligament.
4. Supinator crest of the ulna and the posterior part of the triangular area in front of it.

Insertion:
The muscle is inserted into the upper one-third of the lateral surface of the radius.

Nerve supply:
Through the deep branch of the radial nerve.

Action:
This muscle produces supination of the forearm. It can perform this action irrespective of whether the elbow is flexed or extended. In contrast, the biceps brachii (another powerful supinator) can produce this movement only when the elbow is semiflexed. The role of the brachioradialis in supination and pronation is controversial.

Notes:
1. Starting from their origin, the fibers of the supinator wind round the posterior, lateral and anterior aspects of the radius (in that order) to reach their insertion. The fibers thus have a spiral course (figure below) that enables them to rotate the radius with ease
2. The muscle has two layers, superficial and deep. The deep branch of radial nerve runs downward between these layers.

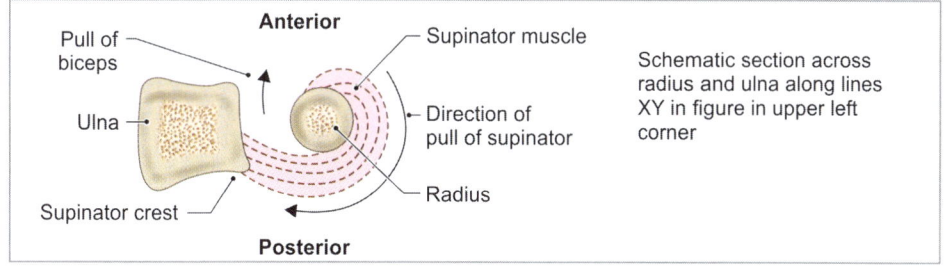

Schematic section across radius and ulna along lines XY in figure in upper left corner

Plate 34

Extensor Pollicis Longus

- Insertion of anconeus
- Insertion of supinator
- Ridge dividing posterior surface of ulna into medial and lateral parts

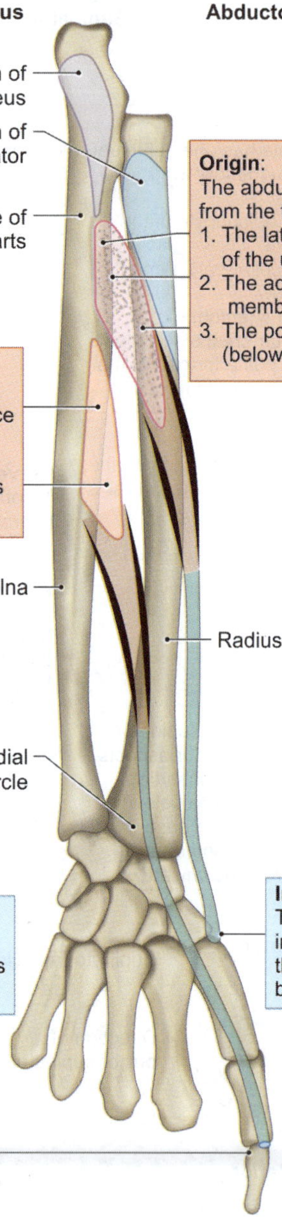

Origin:
The extensor pollicis longus arises from:
1. The lateral part of the posterior surface of the ulna (below the origin of the abductor pollicis longus), and from
2. The adjoining part of the interosseous membrane.

Ulna

Tendon lies medial to dorsal tubercle

Insertion:
It is inserted into the base of the distal phalanx of the thumb on its dorsal aspect.

Actions:
It extends the distal phalanx, the proximal phalanx and the metacarpal of the thumb. Further contraction of the muscle leads to abduction and lateral rotation of the thumb.

Nerve supply:
Deep branch of radial nerve (C7, 8).

Abductor Pollicis Longus

Origin:
The abductor pollicis longus arises from the following:
1. The lateral part of the posterior surface of the ulna (below insertion of anconeus).
2. The adjoining part of the interosseous membrane.
3. The posterior surface of the radius (below insertion of the supinator).

Nerve supply:
Deep branch of radial nerve (C7, 8).

Actions:
Abduction and extension of the thumb. These movements take place at the carpometacarpal joint of the thumb.

Radius

Insertion:
The abductor pollicis longus is inserted into the radial side of the base of the first metacarpal bone; and on the trapezium.

Plate 35

Extensor Indicis

Nerve supply:
Deep branch of radial nerve (C7, 8).

Actions:
The muscle extends the index finger and helps to extend the wrist.

Area for origin of abductor pollicis longus

Origin:
The extensor indicis arises from the posterior surface of the ulna below the origin of the extensor pollicis longus, and from the adjoining part of the interosseous membrane.

The muscle ends in a tendon which passes across the back of the wrist, deep to the extensor retinaculum. It shares the compartment and synovial sheath with the tendons of the extensor digitorum.

Insertion:
The tendon ends by joining the ulnar side of the extensor digitorum tendon for the index finger (through which it may be regarded as being inserted into the dorsal aspect of the middle and distal phalanges).

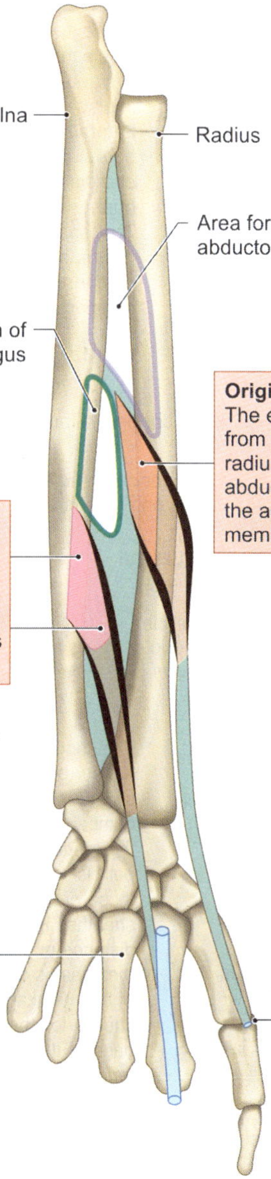

Extensor Pollicis Brevis

Ulna

Radius

Area for origin of abductor pollicis longus

Origin:
The extensor pollicis brevis arises from the posterior surface of the radius below the origin of the abductor pollicis longus, and from the adjoining part of the interosseous membrane.

Nerve supply:
Deep branch of radial nerve (C7, 8).

Actions:
The muscle extends the proximal phalanx and the metacarpal bone of the thumb.

Insertion:
The tendon is inserted into the dorsal surface of the base of the proximal phalanx of the thumb.

The tendon of the muscle is closely associated in its course with that of the abductor pollicis longus.

Plate 36

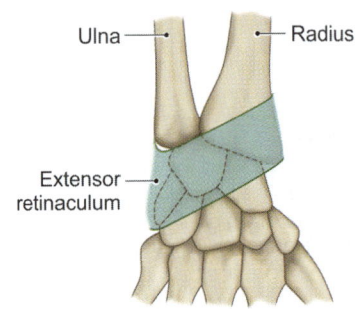

Extensor Retinaculum

The extensor retinaculum is a thickened band of deep fascia that runs across the back (and sides) of the wrist. It is about 2.5 cm in width. It holds the extensor tendons in place and facilitates their action by acting as a pulley. Laterally, the retinaculum is attached to the anterior border of the radius. From here the bers run medially and distally to be attached to the triquetral and pisiform bones.

The space between the deep surface of the retinaculum and the underlying bones is divided into six compartments. Note the tendons passing through each compartment.

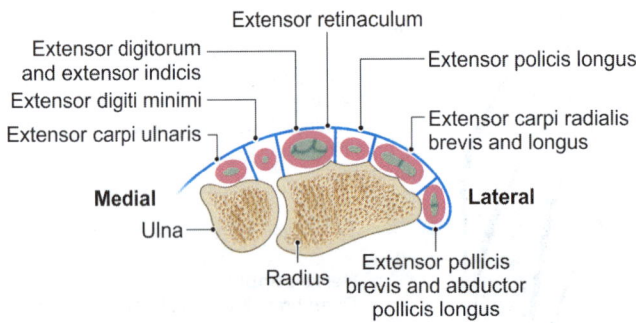

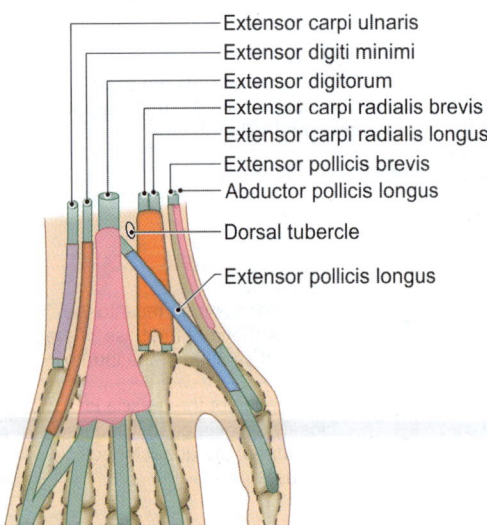

Synovial Sheaths

The tendons passing under the extensor retinaculum are surrounded by synovial sheaths. Normally, there are six sheaths—one for the tendons passing through each compartment under the extensor retinaculum. However, the tendons of the first compartment (i.e. the abductor pollicis longus and the extensor pollicis brevis), and those of the second compartment, may have individual sheaths. Proximally, the sheaths extend for a short distance proximal to the extensor retinaculum. Distally, the sheaths of tendons that gain insertion into the bases of the metacarpal bones extend up to the insertion. The sheath for the extensor pollicis brevis extends to the base of the first metacarpal bone. The sheaths for the tendons going to the digits, and that for the extensor pollicis longus, extend to the level of the middle of the metacarpus.

4 Bones of Lower Limb

CHAPTER

AN 14.1 Identify the given bone, its side, important features and keep it in anatomical position.

AN 14.2 Identify and describe joints formed by the given bone.

AN 14.4 Identify and name various bones in the articulated foot with individual muscle attachment.

THE HIP BONE

Introduction

The hip bone constitutes the pelvic girdle. Both hip bones with the sacrum and coccyx form the *bony pelvis* (**Figs. 4.1 to 4.3**).

Each hip bone consists of three parts: (a) ilium, (b) pubis, and (c) ischium. These parts meet at the *acetabulum* (deep cavity on its lateral aspect). The acetabulum forms the hip joint with the head of the femur. Below and medial to the acetabulum, the hip bone shows a large oval or triangular gap called the *obturator foramen*.

Ilium consists of a large expanded upper part above and behind the acetabulum. It forms the side wall of the greater pelvis. Its upper border is called the *iliac crest*. The posterior part of the ilium shows a large rough articular area on its medial side for articulation with the sacrum.

Pubis lies in relation to the upper and medial part of the obturator foramen. The two pubic bones meet anteriorly in the middle line to form the *pubic symphysis*.

Ischium forms the lowest part of the hip bone; lies below and behind the acetabulum and the obturator foramen.

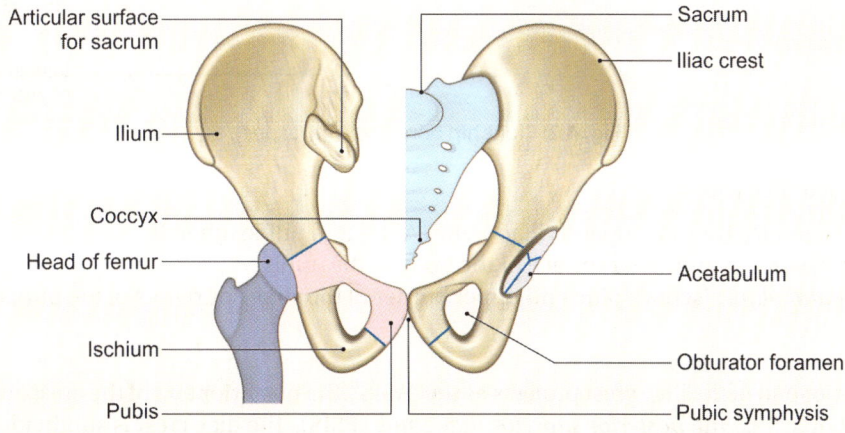

Fig. 4.1: Pelvis viewed from the front; sacrum shown in left half and femur on right side.

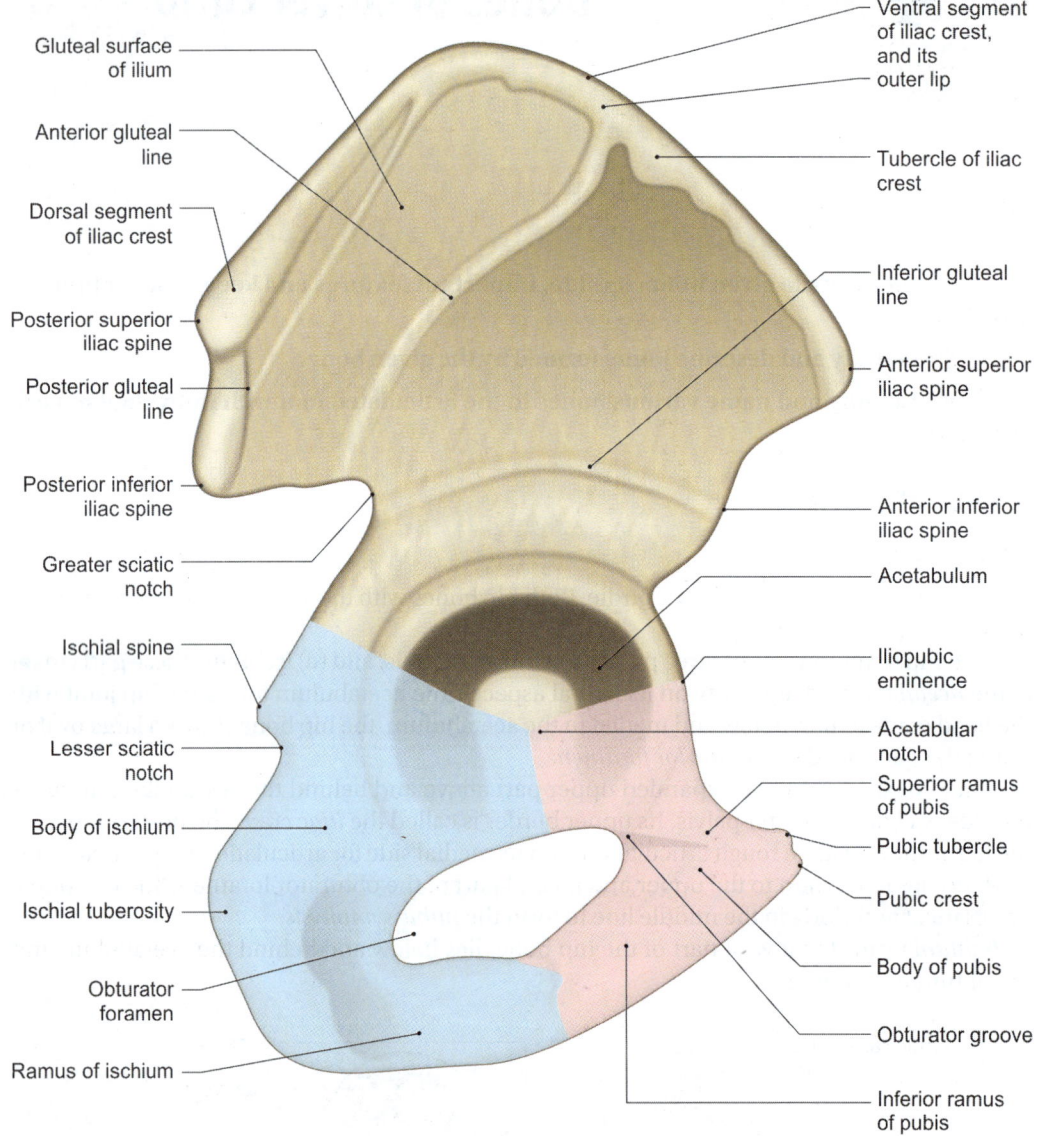

Fig. 4.2: Right hip bone: External aspect.

Anatomical Position

- *Coronal plane*: Anterior superior iliac spine (ASIS) and pubic tubercle
- *Sagittal plane*: Symphyseal surface of the body of the pubis
- *Horizontal plane*: Ischial spine and upper border of the superior ramus of the pubis.

Ilium

The anterior end of the iliac crest projects as the "ASIS". The posterior end of the crest also forms a projection called the *posterior superior iliac spine* (PSIS). The iliac crest is subdivided into a

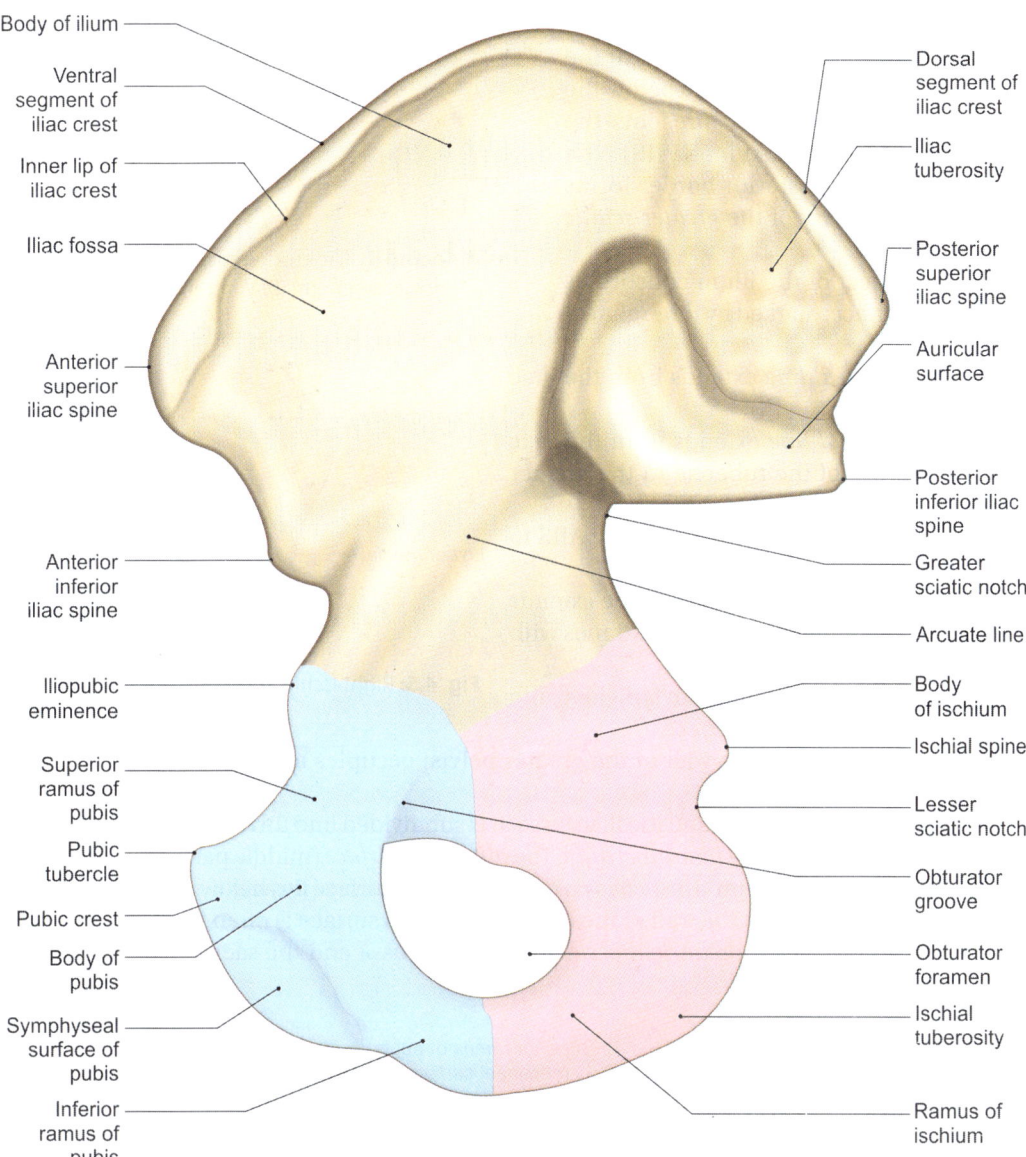

Fig. 4.3: Right hip bone: Internal aspect.

ventral segment (anterior two-thirds) and a *dorsal segment* (posterior one-third). The ventral segment shows a broad intermediate area; bounded by inner and outer lips. About 5 cm behind the ASIS the outer lip shows the *tubercle of the iliac crest*. The dorsal segment of the iliac crest has medial and lateral surfaces separated by a ridge **(Figs. 4.4 and 4.5)**.

The anterior border of the ilium extends from the ASIS to the acetabulum. Its lowest part presents the *anterior inferior iliac spine* (AIIS).

The posterior border of the ilium extends from the PSIS to the back of the acetabulum. A few centimeters below the PSIS the posterior border presents the *posterior inferior iliac spine* (PIIS). The lower part of the posterior border forms the upper boundary of the *greater sciatic notch*.

Lateral aspect of the ilium constitutes the gluteal surface; marked by three gluteal lines:
a. *Posterior gluteal line* extends from the iliac crest to the PIIS.
b. *Anterior gluteal line* extends from the iliac crest in front of the tubercle to the greater sciatic notch.
c. *Inferior gluteal line* extends from the AIIS to the greater sciatic notch.

The lower part of the gluteal surface extends behind the acetabulum where it continues with the ischium.

The medial surface of the ilium is divided into *iliac fossa* and *sacropelvic surface*.

The *iliac fossa* forms the wall of the greater pelvis; occupies anterior part of the medial surface.

Sacropelvic surface lies behind the iliac fossa. It is subdivided into three parts. The upper part is rough that constitutes the *iliac tuberosity*. The *auricular surface* (middle part) articulates with the lateral side of the sacrum. The *pelvic part* of the medial surface lies below and in front of the auricular surface. It forms the wall of the lesser pelvis. This surface is often marked in females by a rough groove called *preauricular sulcus*. The iliac fossa and the sacropelvic surface are

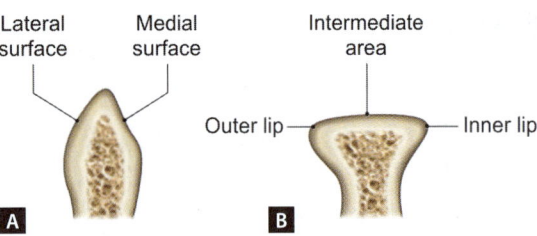

Figs. 4.4A and B: Iliac crest vertical section: (A) Across dorsal segment; (B) Ventral segment.

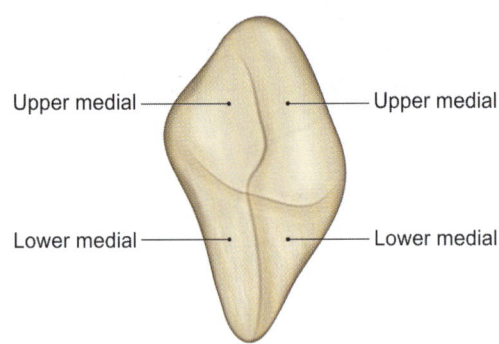

Fig. 4.5: Right ischial tuberosity from behind and below.

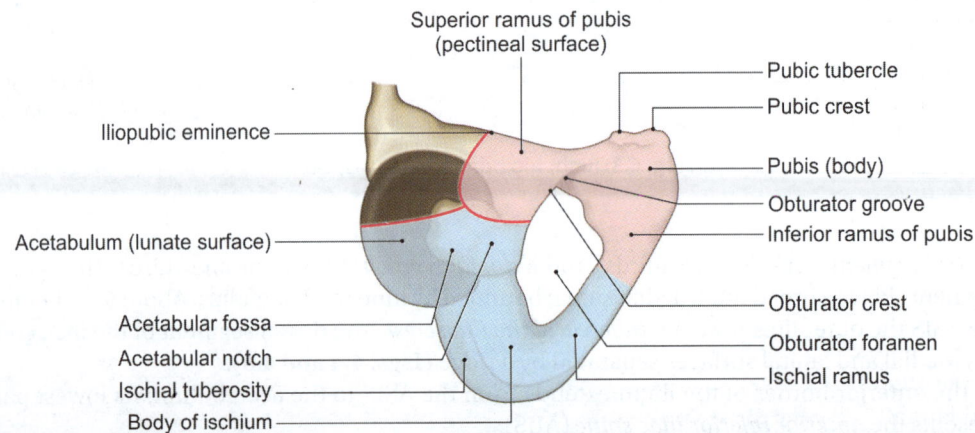

Fig. 4.6: Medial part of right hip bone: Anterosuperior aspect.

separated by the medial border of the ilium. This border is sharp in its upper part; separates the iliac fossa from the auricular surface. Its lower part is rounded and forms the *arcuate line*. The lower end of the arcuate line reaches the junction of the ilium and pubis; junction shows the *iliopubic eminence* **(Fig. 4.6)**.

Ischium

The ischium consists of the *body*, and a projection called the *ramus*. The lower part of the body has three surfaces: (a) dorsal, (b) femoral, and (c) pelvic. The lower part of the dorsal surface presents the *ischial tuberosity*; divided into upper and lower parts by a transverse ridge. Each part is further divided into medial and lateral parts. Superiorly, the dorsal surface of the ischium continues with the gluteal surface of the ilium. The posterior border of the dorsal surface of the ischium forms part of the lower margin of the *greater sciatic notch*. Just below this notch the border projects backward and medially as the *ischial spine*. Between the ischial spine and the upper border of the ischial tuberosity there is a shallow *lesser sciatic notch*.

The femoral surface of the ischium continues with the external surface of the *ramus of the ischium*. The ramus has anterior (external) and posterior (internal) surfaces.

Pubis

The pubis consists of a *body* and *superior* and *inferior rami*. The body forms the anterior and most medial part of the hip bone. It presents anterior and posterior surfaces. The upper border of the body forms a prominent ridge called the *pubic crest*. The crest ends laterally in the *pubic tubercle*.

Superior ramus runs upward, backward and laterally; meets the ilium at the iliopubic eminence. Superior ramus presents **(Figs. 4.7 and 4.8)**:

Three borders:
a. Anterior border is the *obturator crest*.
b. Sharp posterior border forms *pecten pubis* (pectineal line).
c. Sharp inferior border forms upper margin of the obturator foramen.

Three surfaces:
a. *Pectineal surface*: Between obturator crest and pecten pubis.
b. *Pelvic surface*: Between pecten pubis and inferior border.
c. *Obturator surface*: Between obturator crest and inferior border.

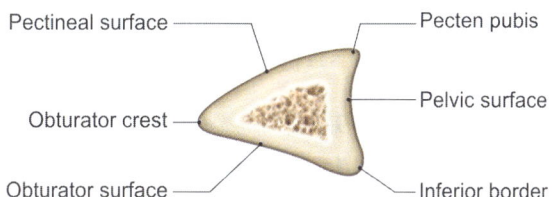

Fig. 4.7: Section at right angles to the long axis of the superior ramus of pubis.

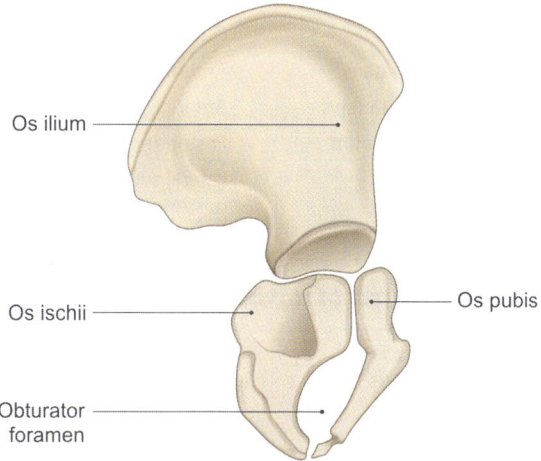

Fig. 4.8: Hip bone: Constituting parts.

The *obturator groove* runs forward and downward across it. *Inferior ramus* passes downward and laterally and joins the ischial ramus. This *conjoint ischiopubic ramus* forms the medial boundary of the obturator foramen.

In intact pelvis, the conjoined ischiopubic rami of both sides form the boundaries of the *pubic arch*. The inferior pubic ramus has anterior (outer) and posterior (inner) surfaces. These surfaces continue with corresponding surfaces of the ischial ramus.

Acetabulum

The acetabulum is directed laterally, downward and forward. The acetabular margin is deficient in the anteroinferior part; the gap in the margin is the *acetabular notch*. The floor of the acetabulum is partly articular and partly nonarticular. The articular area for the head of the femur is horseshoe shaped—the *lunate surface*. The inner border of the lunate surface forms the margin of the nonarticular part of the floor; the *acetabular fossa*. The contribution to the acetabulum is by:

- *Ilium*: Two-fifths superiorly
- *Ischium*: Two-fifths posteroinferiorly
- *Pubis*: One-fifth anteroinferiorly.

Obturator foramen is bounded by:
- *Above*: Superior ramus of pubis
- *Medially*: Body of pubis and conjoint ischiopubic rami
- *Laterally*: Body of ischium.

In the intact body, the foramen is covered by the *obturator membrane*. However, the membrane is deficient in the uppermost part of the foramen. Here the membrane has a free upper edge which is separated from the superior ramus of the pubis by a gap.

Attachments (Fig. 4.9)

Muscles Attached to Iliac Crest

Muscle	Attachment
Internal oblique abdominis	Intermediate area of the ventral segment (*origin*)
External oblique abdominis	Anterior two-thirds of the outer lip of ventral segment (*insertion*)
Latissimus dorsi	Outer lip of the iliac crest just behind its highest point (*origin*)
Tensor fasciae latae	Anterior part of the outer lip (*origin*)
Transversus abdominis	Anterior two-thirds of the inner lip of ventral segment (*origin*)
Quadratus lumborum	Posterior one-third of the inner lip of ventral segment (*origin*)
Gluteus maximus	Lateral surface of the dorsal segment and gluteal surface of ilium behind posterior gluteal line (*origin*)
Erector spinae	Medial surface of the dorsal segment

External Aspect of Hip Bone (Excluding Iliac Crest): Muscles Attachments

Muscle	Attachment
Gluteus maximus	See above
Gluteus medius	Gluteal surface of ilium between anterior and posterior gluteal lines (*origin*)
Gluteus minimus	Gluteal surface of ilium between anterior and inferior gluteal lines (*origin*)
Sartorius	Anterior superior iliac spine and small area below spine (*origin*)
Rectus femoris (*straight head*)	Anterior inferior iliac spine (*origin*)
Rectus femoris (*reflected head*)	Groove above acetabulum (*origin*)

(Contd...)

CHAPTER 4 ✦ Bones of Lower Limb

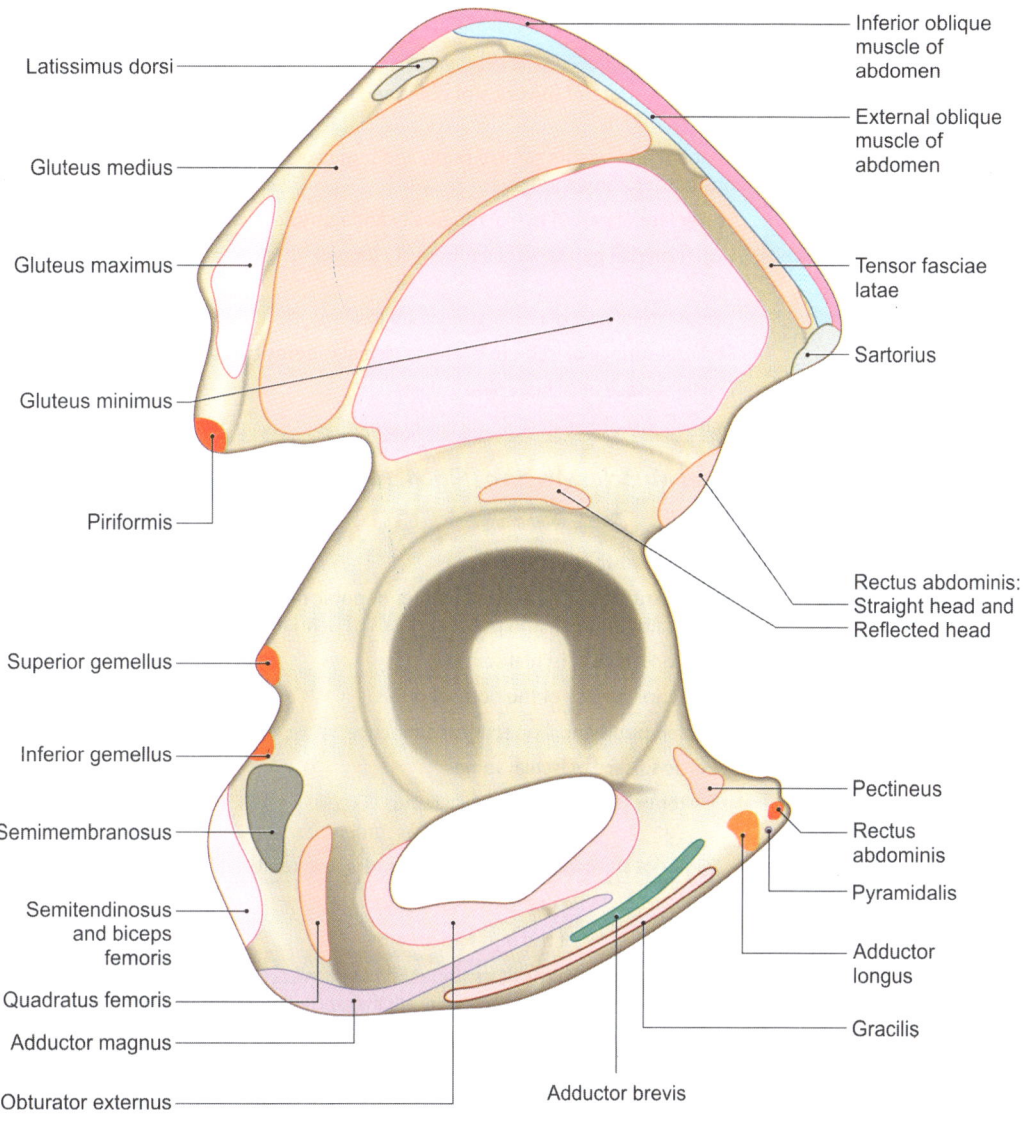

Fig. 4.9: Right hip bone attachments: External aspect.

(Contd...)

Muscle	Attachment
Piriformis	Upper border of greater sciatic notch near posterior inferior iliac spine (*insertion*)
Pectineus	Upper part of pectineal surface of superior ramus of pubis (*insertion*)
Rectus abdominis (*lateral head*)	Pubic crest (*origin*)
Pyramidalis and adductor longus	Anterior surface of the body of pubis (*origin*)
Gracilis	Anterior surface of the body of pubis and ischiopubic ramus (*origin*)

(Contd...)

(Contd...)

Muscle	Attachment
Adductor brevis	Anterior surface of the body of pubis and inferior ramus lateral to origin of gracilis (*origin*)
Obturator externus	Superior and inferior rami of pubis and ramus of ischium immediately around obturator foramen (*origin*)
Adductor magnus	Lower lateral part of ischial tuberosity and ramus of ischium (*origin*)
Semitendinosus and biceps femoris (LH)	Upper medial part of ischial tuberosity (*origin*)
Semimembranosus	Upper lateral part of ischial tuberosity (*origin*)
Quadratus femoris	Femoral surface of ischium lateral to ischial tuberosity (*origin*)
Superior gemellus	Dorsal surface of ischial spine (*origin*)
Inferior gemellus	Ischium just above ischial tuberosity (*origin*)

Internal Aspect of Hip Bone: Muscles Arising (Fig. 4.10)

Muscle	Attachments
Iliacus	Upper two-thirds of iliac fossa
Obturator internus	Pelvic surfaces of superior and inferior pubic rami, ramus of ischium, adjoining obturator foramen and pelvic surfaces of ischium and ilium
Levator ani (posterior fibers)	Pelvic surface of ischial spine
Levator ani (anterior fibers)	Posterior surface of the body of pubis
Psoas minor	Pecten pubis and iliopectineal eminence
Coccygeus	Pelvic surface of ischial spine
Superficial transversus perinei and ischiocavernosus	Posterior surface of the ischial ramus
Sphincter urethrae	Posterior surfaces of inferior pubic and ischial rami

Other Attachments

Structure	Attachment
Inguinal ligament	Pubic tubercle (medially) and anterior superior iliac spine (ASIS) (laterally)
Lacunar ligament (apex)	Pubic tubercle; posterior edge to medial part of pecten pubis
Conjoint tendon	Pubic crest and medial part of pecten pubis
Capsule of hip joint	Margin of acetabulum and acetabular labrum
Capsule of sacroiliac joint	Margin of the auricular surface
Deep fascia of thigh (fascia lata)	Outer lip of iliac crest; also attached to lower border of ischiopubic rami
Superior and inferior fasciae of urogenital diaphragm	Conjoined ischiopubic rami
Dorsal and interosseous sacroiliac ligaments	Iliac tuberosity
Sacrotuberous ligament (upper end)	Posterior superior and posterior inferior iliac spines and intervening part of posterior border of ilium
Sacrotuberous ligament (lower end)	Medial margin of ischial tuberosity; extends on ischial ramus—*falciform process*
Sacrospinous ligament	Apex of ischial spine

CHAPTER 4 ✦ Bones of Lower Limb

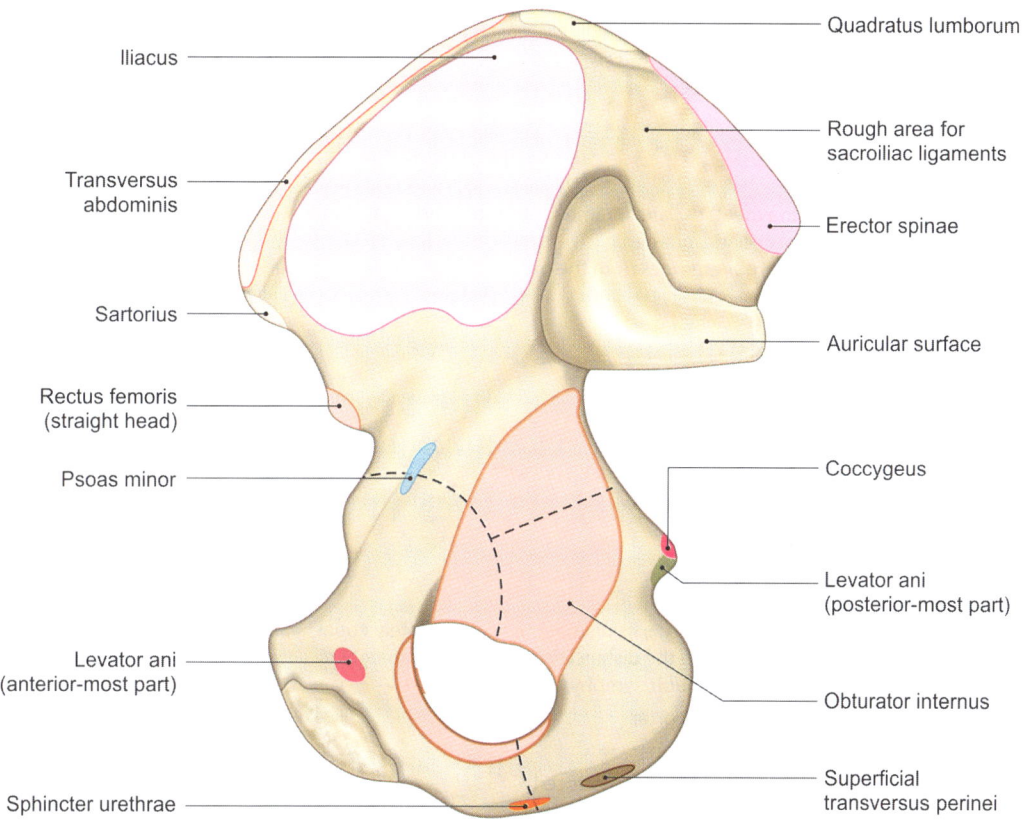

Fig. 4.10: Right hip bone attachments: Internal aspect.

Hip Bone: Relations

Part	Structure related
Posterior surface of the pubis	Urinary bladder
Right iliac fossa	Cecum and terminal ileum
Left iliac fossa	Terminal part of the descending colon

Greater and lesser sciatic notches are converted into respective foramina by the sacrotuberous and sacrospinous ligaments.

Foramen	Structure passing
Greater sciatic foramen	• Piriformis • Superior and inferior gluteal nerves and vessels • Internal pudendal vessels • Pudendal nerve • Sciatic nerve • Posterior cutaneous nerve of thigh • Nerves to obturator internus and quadratus femoris

(Contd...)

(Contd...)

Foramen	Structure passing
Lesser sciatic foramen	• Pudendal nerve • Nerve to obturator internus • Internal pudendal vessels • Tendon of obturator internus

- After emerging from the greater sciatic foramen these structures pass behind the ischial spine to enter the pelvis through the lesser sciatic foramen.
- Tendon of obturator internus emerges from the pelvis through the lesser sciatic foramen.

Sexual Differences

Feature	Male	Female
Subpubic angle	Acute 55°–60°	Obtuse 80–85°
Ischial spine	Inturned	
Preauricular sulcus		Marked
Ischiopubic rami (lower margin)	More everted	
Chilotic line		Pelvic part of chilotic line is longer than sacral part
Greater sciatic notch	About 50°	Wider: About 75°
Acetabulum	Large; its diameter is approximately equal to the distance from its anterior margin to pubic symphysis	Smaller
Pubic crest	Shorter	
Iliac fossa	Deeper	Shallow
Curvatures of the iliac crest	More pronounced	Less pronounced
Obturator foramen	Large and oval	Small and triangular

Development and Ossification (Fig. 4.11)

Hip bone ossifies from three primary centers: One each for ilium, ischium, and pubis. These centers appear in intrauterine life as follows:

❖ *For the ilium*: 8th week
❖ *For the ischium*: 3-4 months
❖ *For the pubis*: 4–5 months.

At birth the ilium, ischium and pubis are separated by a *Y-shaped cartilage* at the acetabulum. The three parts fuse completely after 18 years of age.

The conjoint ischiopubic ramus is separated by cartilage; both rami fuse with each other about the seventh year.

Secondary centers in the hip bone: Two in iliac crest, two in acetabular cartilage.

Occasional centers appear in: AIIS, lower part of acetabulum, pubic tubercle and pubic crest. These centers appear at puberty and fuse with the rest of the bone between 20 years and 25 years of age.

Clinical Anatomy

Pubic tubercle *as a landmark for*:

❖ *Saphenous opening*: Center of saphenous opening is situated about 1.5 inch below and lateral to the pubic tubercle.

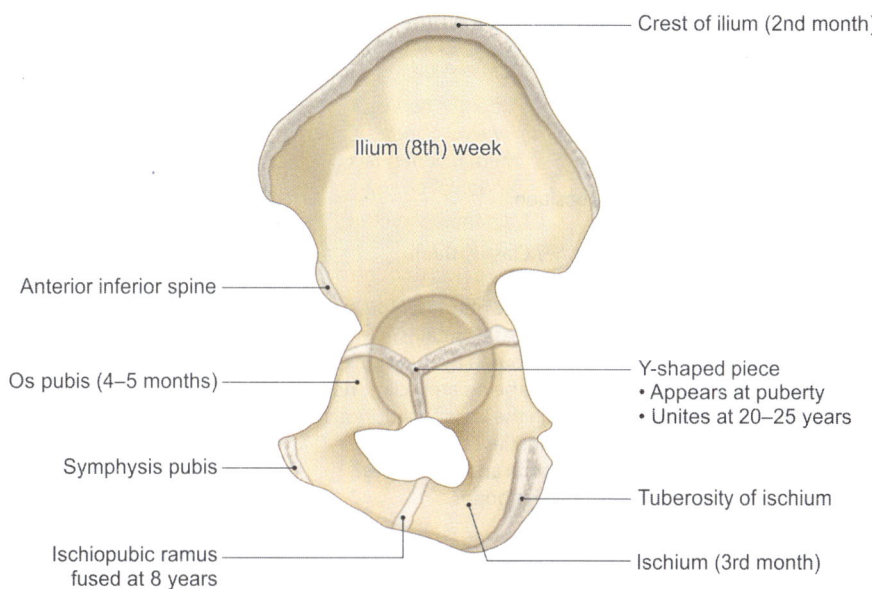

Fig. 4.11: Hip bone: Ossification.

- *Superficial inguinal ring*: It lies above and lateral to the pubic tubercle.
- *Spermatic cord*: It can be rolled medial to pubic tubercle as it crosses pubic crest.

Highest point on the iliac crest: A horizontal line drawn at the highest point of the iliac crest passes through the disc between L3 and L4 vertebrae. This is taken as a guideline for the lumbar puncture.

Bone marrow aspiration: Posterior superior iliac spine corresponds to the dimples in the skin. The bone marrow from the ilium is aspirated 1 cm below and lateral to the dimple.

Bone graft: These are required to treat some fractures. Iliac crest is one of the preferred sites to obtain pieces of the bone.

Fracture of the hip bone: Road traffic accidents (RTAs) may cause fractures of the hip bone. The pubic rami are commonly fractured due to anteroposterior compression **(Fig. 4.12)**. The acetabulum may be involved when the impact is from the lateral side.

Rider's bone: Rounded tendon of the adductor longus arises from the outer surface of the pubis in the angle area between the superior ramus and the body. At times tendon ossifies and appears as a thick bony spicule. This

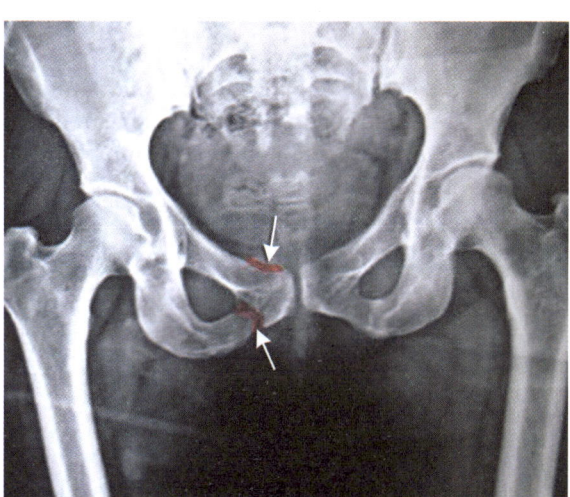

Fig. 4.12: Fracture of the hip bone.

may be commonly observed in horse riders where the adductor longus is active for keeping the thigh adducted against the saddle.

QUESTIONNAIRE

- Classify the bone.
- Side determination and anatomical position.
- Identify the parts of the hip bone.
- What are the joints associated with bone? Classify them.
- Identify the groove for the Iliopsoas.
- Enumerate the structures passing through the obturator foramen.
- What does nonarticular part of acetabular fossa contains?
- How much part of the acetabulum is contributed by the ilium, pubis, and ischium?
- Enumerate the structures passing through the greater sciatic notch.
- Enumerate the structures passing through the lesser sciatic notch.
- What are the features of the hamstring muscles?
- What are the joints associated with this bone and their types?
- Where sciatic nerve is directly related to this bone?
- Mark the attachments of:

Ligaments	Muscles
Sacrotuberous	On the iliac crest
Sacrospinous	On the ischial tuberosity
Inguinal	On the ischiopubic ramus
Sacroiliac	In relation to the gluteal lines
Ligaments of hip joint	

- What is falciform margin?
- Where is pudendal canal related? What are its contents?
- Why the hip dislocations occur posteriorly?
- Name the structures that pass through the obturator foramen.
- Comment on its ossification and development.

THE FEMUR

The femur (*longest bone*) presents a shaft and two ends (upper and lower). The upper end presents a rounded head that joins the shaft by an elongated neck. The head is directed medially; articulates with the acetabulum of the hip bone. The shaft is convex forward and its posterior aspect is marked by a prominent vertical ridge called the *linea aspera*.

Side Determination

- *Superiorly*: Head of femur.
- *Medially*: Head of femur.
- *Anteriorly*: Forward convexity of the shaft.

Anatomical Position (Figs. 4.13 to 4.16)

- Shaft is vertically placed.
- Femoral head faces upward, medially and forward.
- Femoral condyles touch horizontal plane.

Upper end: It presents the head, the neck, and two projections (*greater and lesser trochanters*).

Head (slightly more than half a sphere) is directed medially, upwards and somewhat forwards. Near the center of the head there is a pit (*fovea*).

Neck connects the head to the shaft. It joins the shaft at an angle of about 125°. The greater and lesser trochanters are situated near the junction of the neck with the shaft.

Greater trochanter is seen on the lateral aspect of the upper end of the femur. Its upper and posterior part projects upward beyond the level of the neck and presents a medial surface. On this surface a depressed area called *trochanteric fossa* is noted. The anterior aspect of the trochanter shows a large rough area for muscle attachments. The lateral surface is also marked by an area for muscle attachments.

Lesser trochanter (conical projection) is attached to the shaft where the lower border of the neck meets the shaft. It points medially and backward. The posterior parts of the greater and lesser trochanters are joined together by a prominent ridge called *intertrochanteric crest*. A little above its middle, the crest presents a rounded elevation —the *quadrate tubercle*. Anteriorly, the junction of the neck and the shaft is marked by the *intertrochanteric line*. The upper end of this line reaches the anterior and upper part of the greater trochanter; its lower end lies a little in front of the lesser trochanter. Here it continues with the *spiral line* which runs downward and backward across the medial aspect of the shaft to reach its posterior aspect.

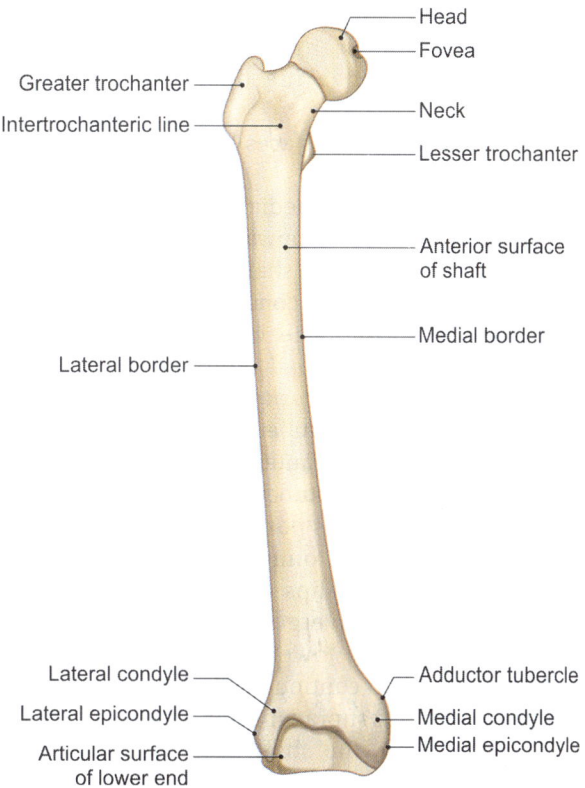

Fig. 4.13: Right femur: Anterior aspect.

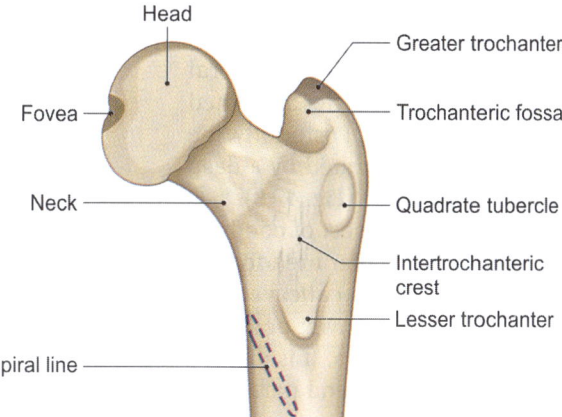

Fig. 4.14: Right femur: Posteromedial view of upper end.

Shaft: The shaft is smooth anteriorly; shows forward convexity. Its posterior aspect presents the *linea aspera*. The triangular shaft shows three borders (lateral, medial, and posterior) and three surfaces (anterior, lateral, and medial) **(Fig. 4.17)**.

- Lateral and medial borders are rounded.
- Posterior border is the linea aspera.
- Medial and lateral surfaces face backward.

The linea aspera has medial and lateral lips. When traced upward to the upper one-third of the shaft, the lips diverge. The medial lip continues with the spiral line. The lateral lip continues with a broad rough area— the *gluteal tuberosity*. The upper end of the gluteal tuberosity reaches the greater trochanter. The area between the gluteal tuberosity and the spiral line forms posterior surface at the upper one-third of the shaft. The two lips of the linea aspera also diverge from each other over the lower one-third of the shaft to continue with medial and lateral supracondylar lines. Here again, the shaft has an additional triangular surface directed posteriorly called the *popliteal surface*.

Lower end: The lower end consists of two large medial and lateral condyles. Both condyles are joined together anteriorly. Posteriorly, the condyles are separated by a deep *intercondylar notch* **(Fig. 4.18)**.

The anterior aspect of condyles presents an articular area for the patella. The area is concave from side to side for convex posterior surface of the patella. It is divided into medial and lateral parts. The lateral part is much larger.

Inferiorly, the condyles articulate with the tibia to form the knee joint. Each condyle bears a large convex articular surface which continues anteriorly with

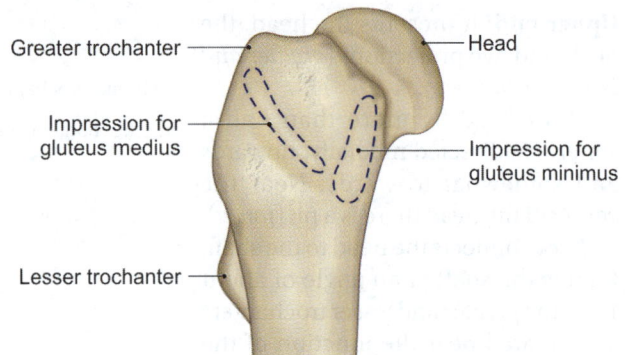

Fig. 4.15: Right femur: Lateral aspect of upper end.

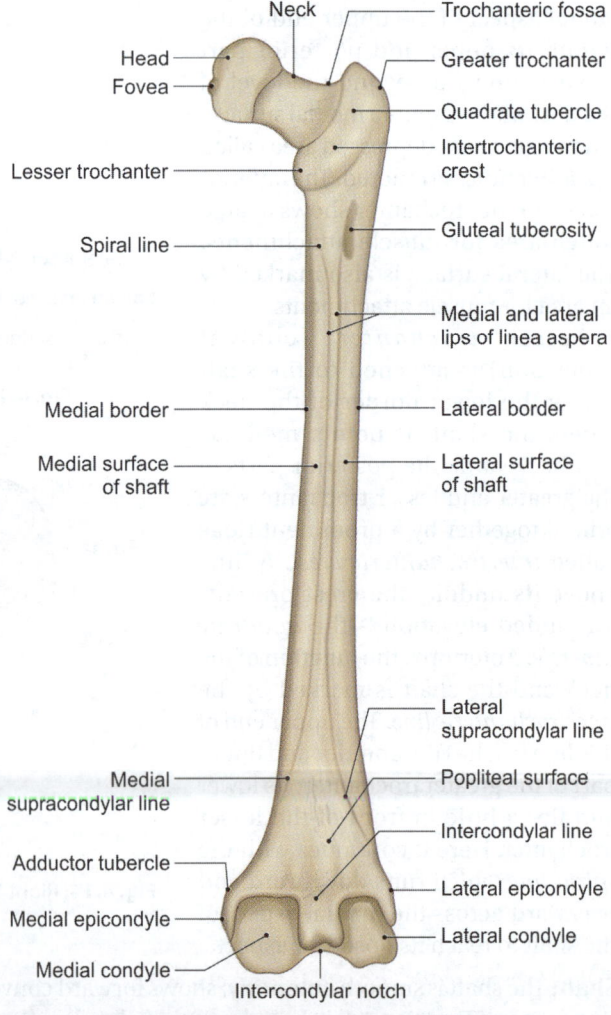

Fig. 4.16: Right femur: Posterior aspect.

the patellar surface. The articular surface covers the inferior and posterior aspects of each condyle **(Fig. 4.19)**.

When seen from the lateral aspect, the lateral femoral condyle is flat. A little behind the middle it is marked by a prominence called the *lateral epicondyle*. Behind and below the epicondyle there is a prominent groove for the tendon of popliteus.

When seen from the medial aspect, the medial condyle shows the *medial epicondyle*. The uppermost part of the medial condyle is marked by a prominence called the *adductor tubercle*. It lies above and behind the medial epicondyle; continues with the lower end of the medial supracondylar line.

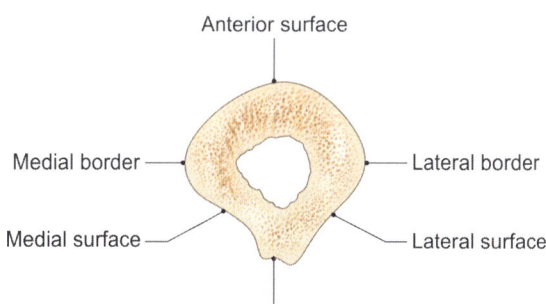

Fig. 4.17: Transverse section (TS) across the shaft of femur near its middle.

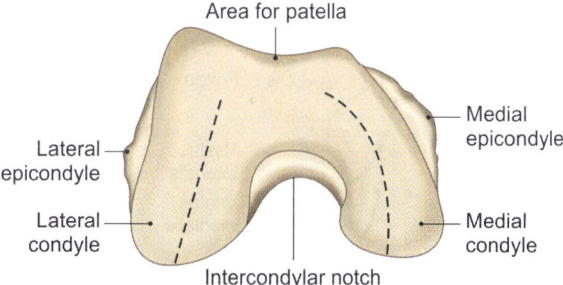

Fig. 4.18: Right femur, lower end: Viewed from below.

Attachments (Figs. 4.20 and 4.21)
Muscles Inserted

Muscle	Insertion
Gluteus minimus	Anterior aspect of the greater trochanter
Gluteus medius	Oblique strip downward and forward across the lateral surface of greater trochanter
Piriformis	Upper border of greater trochanter
Obturator internus and gemelli	Anterior part of the medial surface of greater trochanter
Obturator externus	Trochanteric fossa on the medial surface of greater trochanter
Psoas major	Medial part of the anterior surface of lesser trochanter
Iliacus	Medial side of the base of lesser trochanter and small area below it
Pectineus	Along a line from the root of lesser trochanter to upper end of linea aspera (between gluteal tuberosity and spiral line)
Quadratus femoris	Quadrate tubercle and a small area below it
Gluteus maximus (*deep fibers*)	Gluteal tuberosity
Adductor brevis (*upper part*)	Between insertions of pectineus (medially) and adductor magnus (laterally); lower part of the muscle is inserted into linea aspera
Adductor longus	Middle one-third of linea aspera
Adductor magnus	Medial margin of gluteal tuberosity, linea aspera and medial supracondylar line Hamstring part ends in a tendon attached to adductor tubercle

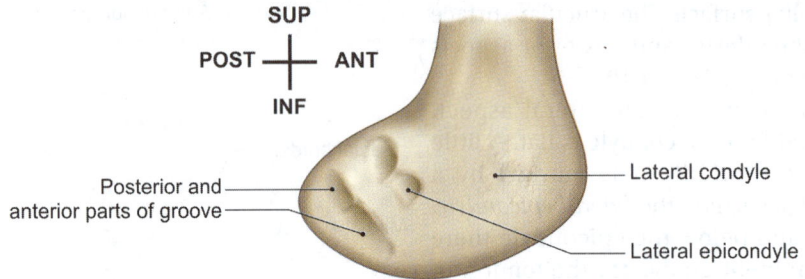

Fig. 4.19: Right femur, lower end: Seen from lateral side.

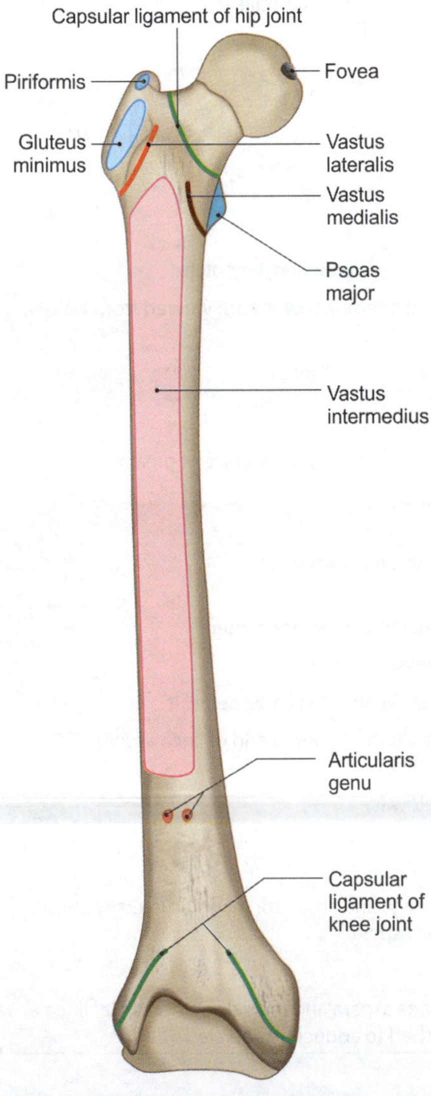

Fig. 4.20: Right femur attachments: From the front.

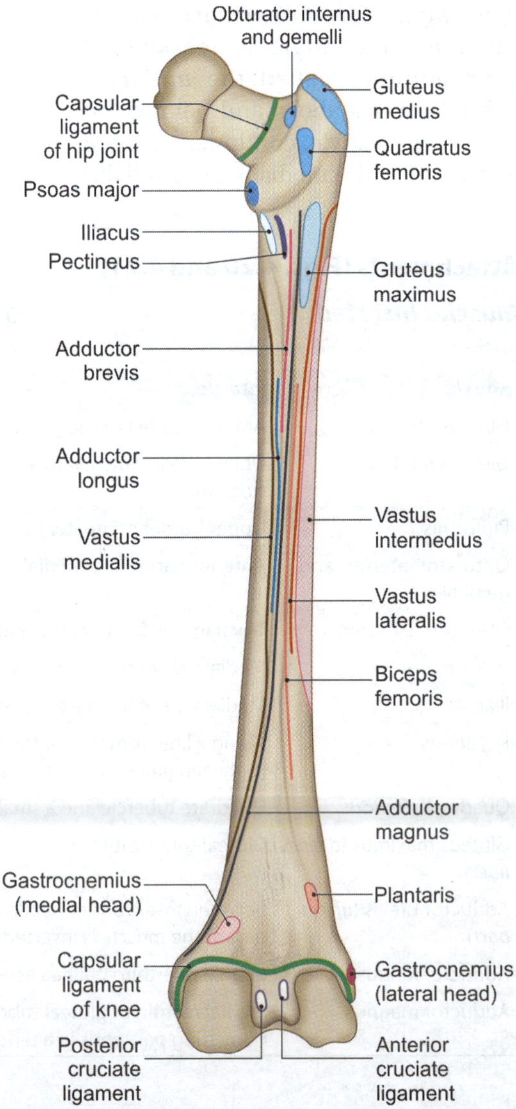

Fig. 4.21: Right femur attachments: From behind.

Muscles Arising

Muscle	Origin
Vastus lateralis	*Linear origin*: Upper end of intertrochanteric line, along anterior and lower borders of greater trochanter, lateral margin of gluteal tuberosity, and lateral lip of linea aspera
Vastus medialis	*Linear origin*: Lower part of intertrochanteric line, spiral line, medial lip of linea aspera, and medial supracondylar line up to adductor tubercle
Vastus intermedius	Upper three-fourths of anterior and lateral surfaces of the shaft
Articularis genu	Anterior surface of the shaft below origin of vastus intermedius
Biceps femoris (*short head*)	Linea aspera and upper part of lateral supracondylar line
Gastrocnemius (*medial head*)	Popliteal surface; above medial condyle
Gastrocnemius (*lateral head*)	Lateral surface of lateral condyle
Plantaris	Lower part of lateral supracondylar line
Popliteus	Anterior part of the groove on the lateral aspect of lateral condyle

Other Attachments

Structure	Attachment
Capsule of hip joint	Femoral neck (anteriorly) Intertrochanteric line (posteriorly): 1 cm medial to intertrochanteric crest
Ligament of the femoral head	Fovea on the femoral head
Capsule of knee joint	Femoral condyles and posterior margin of intercondylar fossa; on lateral condyle: above origin of popliteus, capsule is deficient anteriorly
Anterior cruciate ligament	Medial surface of lateral condyle
Posterior cruciate ligament	Lateral surface of medial condyle

Ossification (Fig. 4.22)

Femur is the second long bone in the body to start ossifying (*first being clavicle*). The primary center appears in the shaft during 7th week of intrauterine life; (femoral neck ossifies from the primary center).

Three secondary centers appear at the upper end of the bone, one each for:
1. Head (first year)
2. Greater trochanter (4th year)
3. Lesser trochanter (around 12th year).

Each center fuses independently with the shaft in the reverse order of appearance:
- Lesser trochanter at about 13 years
- Greater trochanter at about 14 years
- Head around 16 years.

One secondary center for the distal end appears before birth in the ninth month of fetal life. It fuses with the shaft between the 16th and 18th years.

AN 14.3 Describe the importance of ossification of lower end of femur and upper end of tibia.

The secondary centers of ossification for the lower end of femur and upper end at the tibia (*both growing* ends) appear at the ninth month of intrauterine life or at birth. The appearances of these centers signify that the fetus is viable. Hence, in the case of newborn found dead, X-ray of the knee region is carried out. Presence of ossification centers indicates that the fetus was viable and capable of survival. Thus the *medicolegal investigation* is conducted to rule out foul play (homicide).

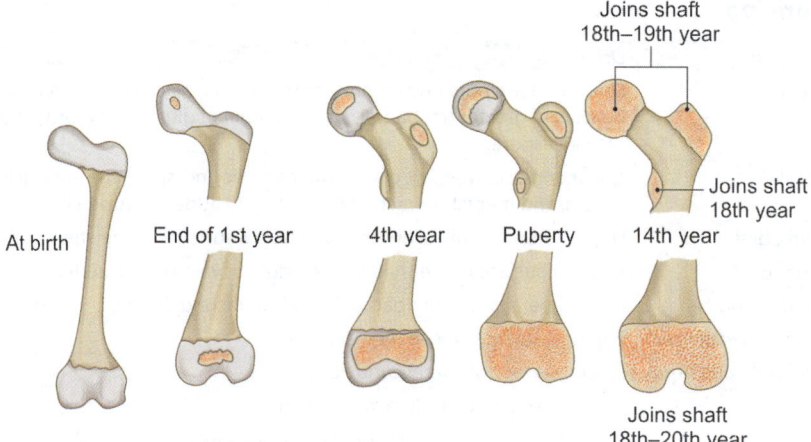

Fig. 4.22: Femur: Ossification.

Clinical Anatomy

❖ *Fracture of femoral head (Fig. 4.23):* It is caused by posterior hip dislocation in advanced age due to osteoporosis. It presents as shortened lower limb with medial rotation. It may require hip replacement.
❖ *Fracture of femoral neck:* It results in ischemic necrosis of the femoral head. The blood supply to the femoral head (by medial femoral circumflex artery) is affected. The distal fragment is pulled upward by the quadriceps femoris, adductors, and hamstrings. The affected lower limb is shortened and laterally rotated.
❖ *Pertrochanteric fracture:* It passes through the trochanters (extracapsular fracture). The pull of the quadriceps femoris, adductors, and hamstrings results in shortening and lateral rotation of the leg.
❖ *Fracture middle third of femoral shaft:* The proximal fragment is pulled by the quadriceps and the hamstrings, and the distal fragment is rotated backward by the gastrocnemius.
❖ *Coxa valga:* The neck-shaft angle of the femur exceeds 127° **(Fig. 4.24)**. The femoral neck becomes straighter.

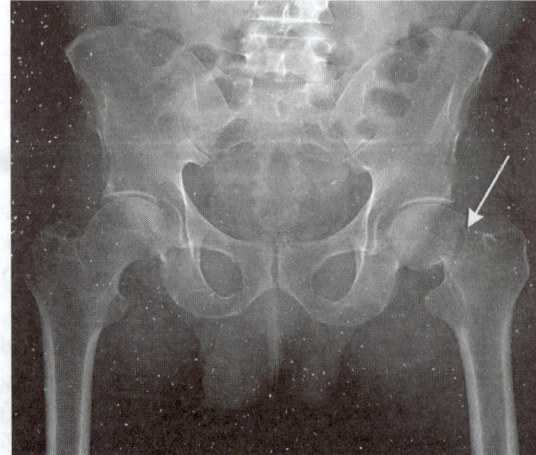

Fig. 4.23: Fracture femoral neck.

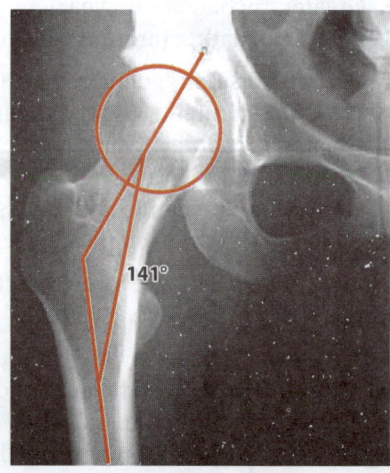

Fig. 4.24: Coxa valga.

❖ **Coxa vara:** The neck-shaft angle of the femur is less than 127° **(Fig. 4.25)**. The femoral neck becomes more horizontal.

QUESTIONNAIRE

- Classify the bone.
- Side determination and anatomical position.
- Enumerate the structures attached to the intertrochanteric line.
- Enumerate the structures attached to the linea aspera.
- Mark the attachments of:

Ligaments	Muscles
Capsule of hip joint	On the greater trochanter
Capsule of knee joint	On the lesser trochanter
Cruciate ligaments	On the gluteal tuberosity
Ligament of femoral head	Articularis genu
Tibial and fibular collateral ligaments	Gastrocnemius

- Identify the adductor tubercle. What is attached to it? What is its medicolegal significance?
- Identify the trochanters. What types of epiphyses they are?
- Identify the quadrate tubercle. What is attached to it?
- Where is the nutrient foramen directed? Which is the growing end of the bone?
- Mark the epiphyseal line at the lower end.
- Which structure is called the third trochanter?
- What is the blood supply to the head of the femur?
- Why avascular necrosis is common in intracapsular fracture of femoral neck?
- Where is femoral artery related to this bone? What is its applied importance?
- What is neck-shaft angle and its sexual variation?
- What is the position of the limb in the intracapsular and extracapsular fractures of femoral neck? Why?

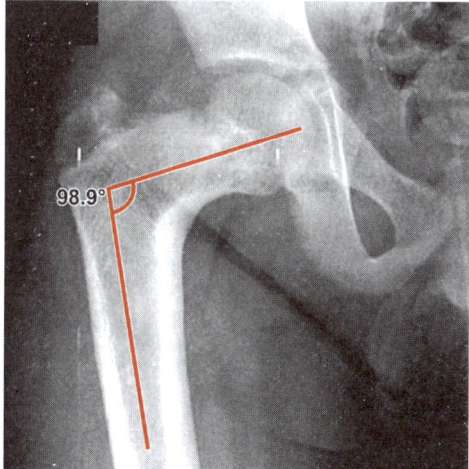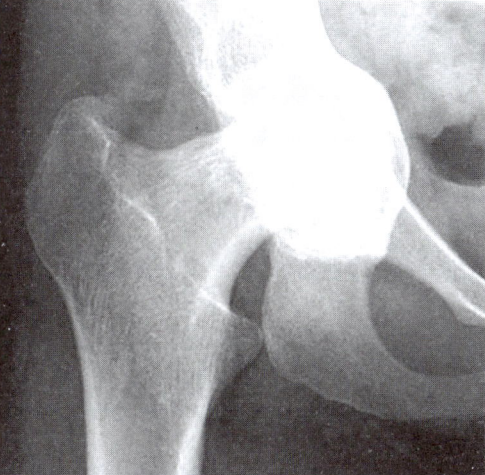

Fig. 4.25: Coxa vara.

THE PATELLA (KNEE CAP)

Sesamoid bones develop in certain tendons. The patella (*largest sesamoid bone*) develops in the tendon of the quadriceps femoris.

Side Determination

- Patella is triangular shaped; apex directed downward (apex is nonarticular posteriorly).
- Anterior surface is rough and nonarticular; upper three-fourths of posterior surface is smooth and articular.
- Posterior articular surface is divided into lateral (larger) and medial (small) areas by a vertical ridge.

Please note when the bone is laid on a table it rests on the broad lateral area.

The patella presents anterior and posterior surfaces separated by three (superior, medial, and lateral) borders. The superior border is the *base*. The inferior part of the bone shows the *apex*.

The *anterior surface* is rough. The upper part of the *posterior surface* is articular; it articulates with the patellar surface on the anterior aspect of the femoral condyles. It consists of a larger lateral part and a smaller medial part and these two parts are separated by a ridge. The most medial part articulates with the medial condyle of the femur only in extreme flexion of the knee joint. The lower part of the posterior surface is nonarticular. It is rough for attachment of the ligamentum patellae **(Figs. 4.26 and 4.27)**.

Attachments

Part	Structure
Superior border	Rectus femoris and vastus intermedius
Medial margin	Medial patellar retinaculum (expansion from vastus medialis tendon)
Lateral margin	Lateral patellar retinaculum (expansion from vastus lateralis tendon)
Apex	Ligamentum patellae

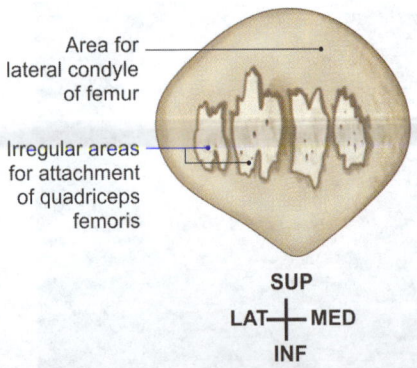

Fig. 4.26: Right patella: Anterior aspect.

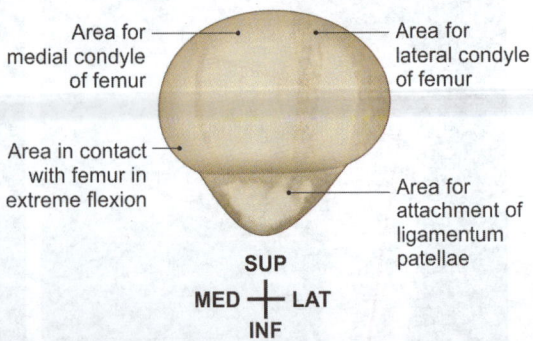

Fig. 4.27: Right patella: Posterior aspect.

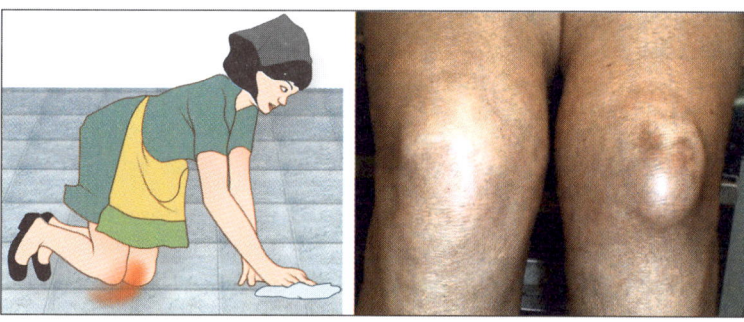

Fig. 4.28: Housemaid's knee.

Ossification

The patella ossifies from several centers that appear between the third and sixth years of life. The centers soon fuse with one another.

Clinical Anatomy

- ❖ *Transverse patellar fracture:* This results from a blow to the knee or from sudden contraction of the quadriceps femoris. The proximal fragment of the patella is pulled upward by the quadriceps tendon; distal fragment remains with the patellar ligament.
- ❖ *Housemaid's knee (prepatellar bursitis):* It is the chronic inflammation and swelling of the superficial prepatellar bursa **(Fig. 4.28)**. This bursa lies in front of the lower part of patella and upper part of ligamentum patellae. Chronic enlargement of this bursa is called *Housemaid's knee* because it commonly occurs in housemaids who have to kneel regularly for sweeping the floors.
- ❖ *Clergyman's knee (subcutaneous infrapatellar bursitis):* It is the chronic inflammation of the subcutaneous infrapatellar bursa **(Fig. 4.29)**. Its enlargement is called *clergyman's knee; often seen in persons who kneel* during prayers.

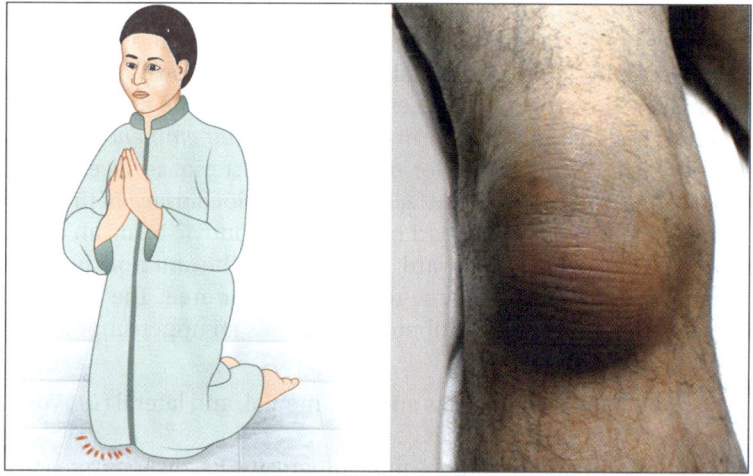

Fig. 4.29: Clergyman's knee.

> **QUESTIONNAIRE**
>
> - Classify the bone.
> - Side determination and anatomical position.
> - Enumerate the peculiarities of this bone.
> - Name the joint associated with this bone and its type.
> - Mark the attachments of:
>
> | Ligaments | Muscles |
> |---|---|
> | Ligamentum patellae | Quadriceps femoris components |
> | Medial and lateral patellar retinacula | |
>
> - Comment on its ossification.
> - What are the functions of patella?

▌THE TIBIA

The tibia (*long bone*) is the medial bone of the leg (*homologous with radius*). It has a shaft, and upper and lower ends. The upper end is much larger and expanded. The medial end has a prominent downward projection called *medial malleolus* on its medial side. The shaft is triangular in section and has a sharp anterior border.

Side Determination

- *Superior*: Upper expanded end.
- *Medial*: Medial malleolus.
- *Anterior*: Tibial tuberosity.

Anatomical Position (Figs. 4.30 to 4.32)

Vertically Placed

Upper end: The upper expanded end consists of medial and lateral condyles and separated by intercondylar area. The anterior aspect of the upper end presents the tibial tuberosity.

The upper surfaces of the medial and lateral condyles present large articular surfaces that take part in forming the knee joint. The medial articular surface is oval and larger; lateral surface is rounded and smaller. The articular surfaces are separated by the nonarticular *intercondylar area*. The intercondylar area is raised to form the *intercondylar eminence*.

The medial condyle shows rough anterior, medial, and posterior surfaces. The lateral condyle also has anterior, lateral, and posterior surfaces. The posterior surface of the medial condyle is marked by a groove. The posterolateral part of the lateral condyle bears an oval articular facet for the fibula; directed backward, downward, and laterally. The anterior surfaces of the medial and lateral condyles merge to form a large rough triangular area. The apex of the triangle is raised to form the *tibial tuberosity*. The tuberosity presents an upper smooth and lower rough parts.

Shaft: The shaft (triangular in section) has anterior, medial, and lateral (*interosseous*) borders; and medial, lateral, and posterior surfaces.

Anterior border runs downward from the tibial tuberosity. Its lower part reaches the anterior margin of the medial malleolus.

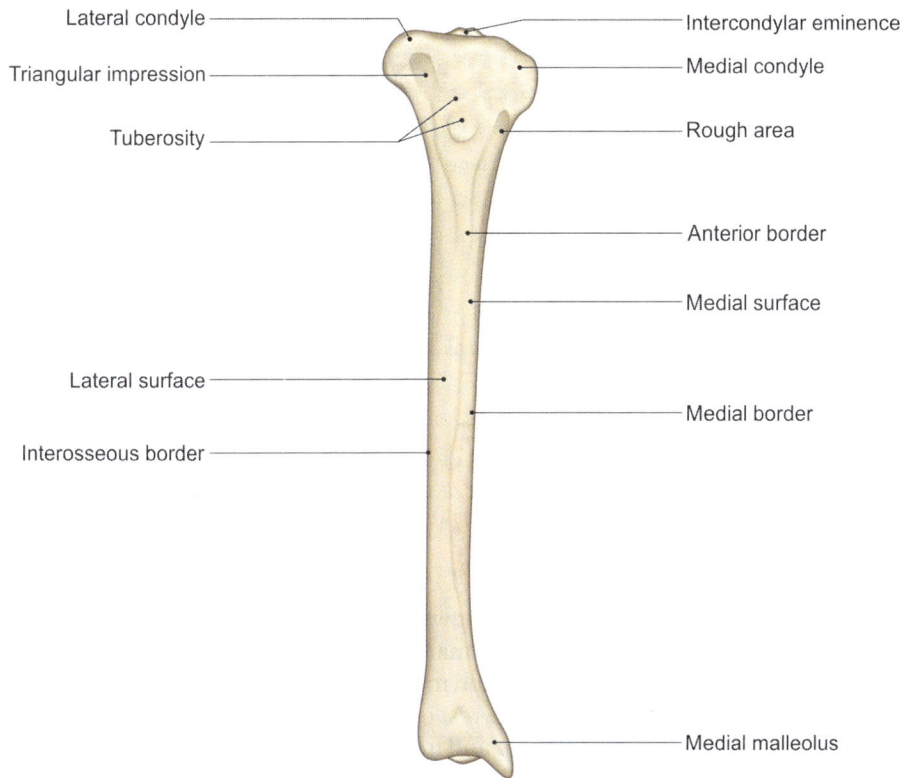

Fig. 4.30: Right tibia: Anterior aspect.

Interosseous (lateral) border begins below and in front of the articular facet for the fibula. It descends along the lateral aspect of the shaft. Its lower end forms the anterior margin of a rough triangular area on the lateral aspect of the lower end **(Fig. 4.33)**.

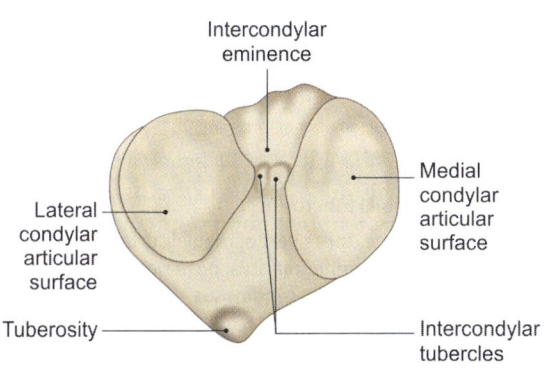

Fig. 4.31: Right tibia: From above.

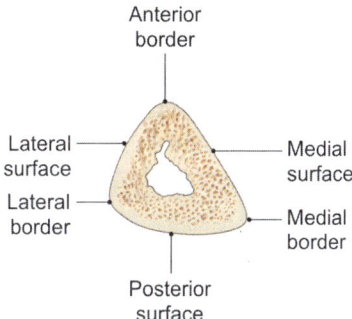

Fig. 4.32: Right tibia: Transverse section (TS) through the shaft viewed from below.

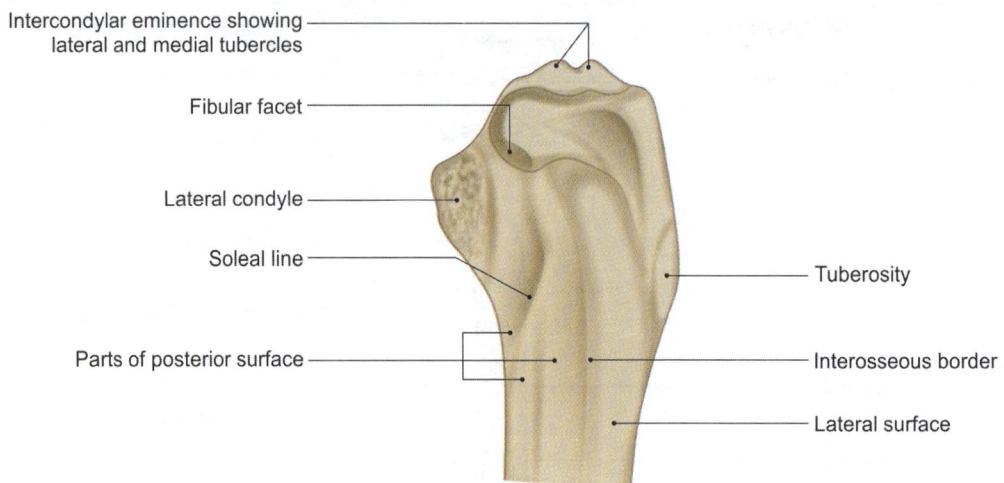

Fig. 4.33: Upper end of right tibia: Lateral aspect.

The upper end of the medial border lies below the most medial part of the medial condyle. Its lower end continues with the posterior margin of the medial malleolus.

Medial surface lies between the anterior and medial borders. The upper part of the surface is rough just in front of the medial border. The rest of the surface is smooth; can be felt.

Lateral surface lies between the anterior and interosseous borders.

Posterior surface is between the medial and interosseous borders. Over the upper one-third of the shaft it is marked by a ridge that runs downward and medially across it. This ridge is the *soleal line*. The part of the posterior surface above the soleal line is triangular. The part below the line is subdivided into medial and lateral parts by a faint vertical ridge **(Figs. 4.34 to 4.36)**.

Lower end: It is less expanded. Its medial part presents the *medial malleolus*. The posterior aspect of the malleolus shows a prominent groove. The lateral aspect of the lower end shows fibular notch for articulation with the fibula. The inferior surface of the lower end presents an articular area that articulates with the upper surface of the talus to form the ankle joint. The area continues with another articular area on the lateral aspect of the medial malleolus that articulates with the medial side of the talus.

Attachments (Figs. 4.37 and 4.38)
Muscles Inserted

Muscle	Insertion
Quadriceps femoris	Smooth upper part of tibial tuberosity
Sartorius, gracilis and semitendinosus	Linear vertical areas on the upper part of medial surface For sartorius: anterior; for semitendinosus: posterior; line for gracilis is higher than that for semitendinosus
Semimembranosus	Posterior and medial aspects of the medial condyle
Popliteus	Posterior surface of shaft on the triangular area above soleal line

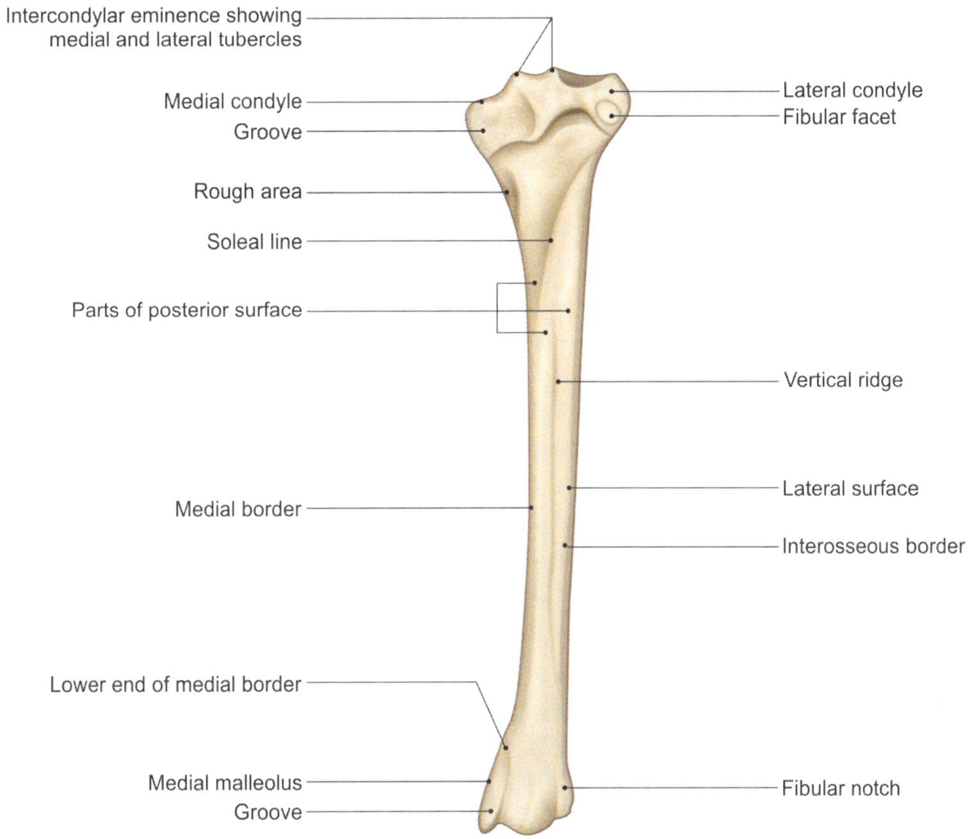

CHAPTER 4 ✦ Bones of Lower Limb

Fig. 4.34: Right tibia: Posterior aspect.

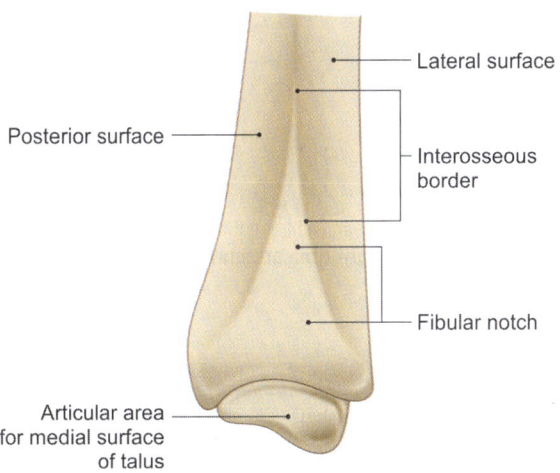

Fig. 4.35: Right tibia (lower end): From the lateral side.

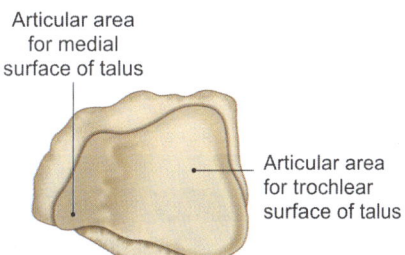

Fig. 4.36: Right tibia (lower end): From below.

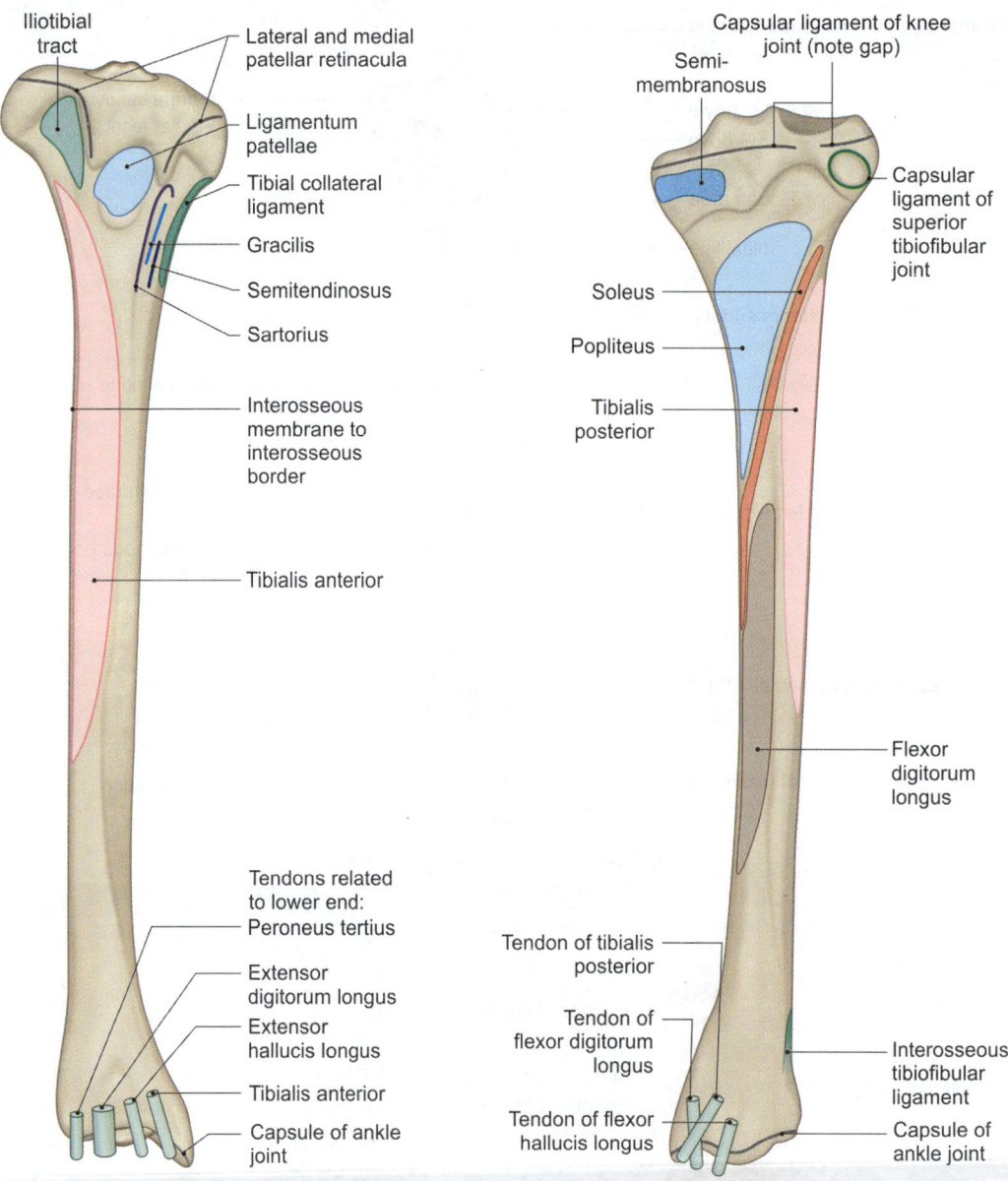

Fig. 4.37: Right tibia attachments from front.

Fig. 4.38: Right tibia attachments from behind.

Muscles Arising

Muscle	Origin
Tibialis anterior	Upper two-thirds of the lateral surface of the shaft
Soleus	Soleal line, and middle one-third of medial border of the shaft
Tibialis posterior	Upper two-thirds of lateral part of posterior surface of shaft, below soleal line
Flexor digitorum longus	Medial part of posterior surface of the shaft below soleal line

Other Attachments (Figs. 4.39 and 4.40)

Structure	Attachment
Capsule of knee joint	Condyles of tibia a little below the margins of the articular surfaces; posterolaterally, gap for passage of popliteus tendon
• Anteriorly and laterally, capsule of knee joint is represented by lateral patellar retinaculum • Anteriorly and medially, capsule is represented by medial patellar retinaculum • In the region of tuberosity, capsular attachment is replaced by ligamentum patellae	
• Anterior horn of medial meniscus • Anterior cruciate ligament • Anterior horn of lateral meniscus • Posterior horn of lateral meniscus • Posterior horn of medial meniscus • Posterior cruciate ligament	Intercondylar area: (before backward)
Capsule of superior tibiofibular joint	Margins of fibular facet
Iliotibial tract	Triangular impression on anterolateral part of lateral condyle
Tibial collateral ligament	Rough area on the medial surface adjoining the upper part of medial border
Interosseous membrane	Interosseous border
Interosseous tibiofibular ligament	Rough upper part of fibular notch
Articular capsule of ankle joint	Margins of the articular surface on the lower end
Medial end of superior extensor retinaculum of ankle	Anterior border of the shaft (near its lower end)
Upper "limb" of inferior extensor retinaculum	Anterior surface of medial malleolus
Flexor retinaculum	Posterior surface of medial malleolus

Tibia: Relations

❖ Anterior aspect of the lower end is crossed by tendons (from medial to lateral side):
  a. Tibialis anterior
  b. Extensor hallucis longus
  c. Extensor digitorum longus
  d. Peroneus tertius
❖ Anterior tibial vessels and deep peroneal nerve cross anterior aspect of the lower end between the tendons of extensor hallucis longus and extensor digitorum longus.
❖ Posterior aspect of the lower end of tibia is crossed by the tendons (*from medial to lateral side*):

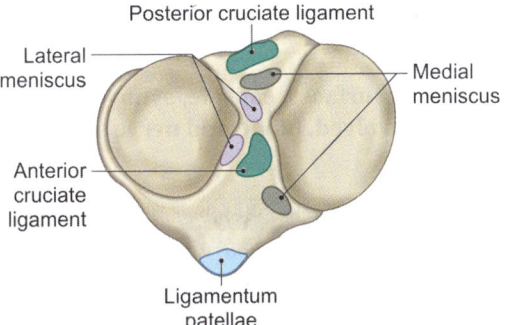

Fig. 4.39: Right tibia attachments from above.

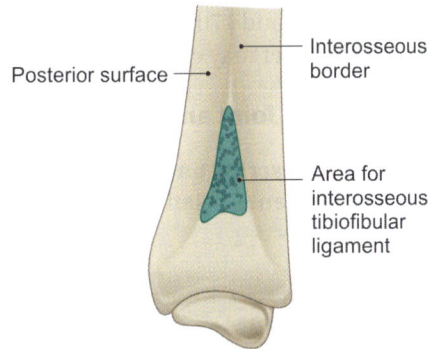

Fig. 4.40: Right tibia (lower end, lateral aspect): Area for interosseous tibiofibular ligament.

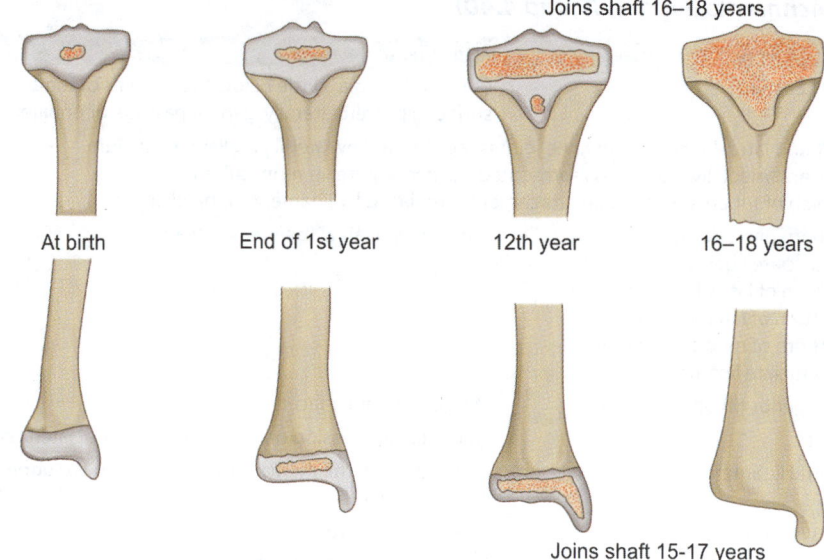

Fig. 4.41: Tibia: Ossification.

a. Tibialis posterior
b. Flexor digitorum longus
c. Flexor hallucis longus.
❖ Tendon of flexor digitorum longus crosses tibialis posterior tendon near the lower end.
❖ Posterior tibial vessels and nerve cross posterior aspect of the lower end; lying between the tendons of flexor digitorum longus and flexor hallucis longus.

Ossification (Fig. 4.41)

Tibia has three centers of ossification:
1. Primary center (for shaft): Appears in 7th week of fetal life.
2. Secondary center for upper end: Appears towards the end of fetal life; fuses with the shaft between 16th years and 18th years.
3. Secondary center for lower end: It appears during the first year; fuses with the shaft between 15th years and 17th years.

Separate center may exist for the tibial tuberosity.

Tibiofibular Joint and Ankle Joint

AN 20.1 Describe and demonstrate the type, articular surfaces, capsule, synovial membrane, ligaments, relations, movements and muscles involved, blood and nerve supply of ankle joint.

Superior tibiofibular joint	Middle tibiofibular joint	Inferior tibiofibular joint
Type: Synovial (plane)	Type: Fibrous (joined by interosseous membrane- syndesmosis)	Type: Fibrous (syndesmosis)
Between head of fibula and tibia	Between shafts of fibula and tibia	Between lower ends of fibula and tibia

(Contd...)

(Contd...)

Superior tibiofibular joint	Middle tibiofibular joint	Inferior tibiofibular joint
Little gliding movement	No movement	No movement
Blood supply: Anterior and posterior tibial recurrent tibial arteries	Blood supply: Branches from the adjoining arteries	Blood supply: Fibular artery, lateral malleolar branches from anterior and posterior tibial arteries
Nerve supply: Common fibular nerve, nerve to popliteus	Nerve supply: Nerve to popliteus	Nerve supply: Deep fibular nerve, sural nerve

Ankle (*Talocrural*) joint is a synovial joint (*hinge variety*) between tibia and fibula from above and the trochlear surface of the talus below. It is uniaxial (*transverse axis*) where dorsiflexion and plantar flexion takes place. It forms *tibiofibular mortise* from above by lower end of tibia and medial malleolus, lateral malleolus of fibula and inferior tibiofibular ligament which articulates with superior, medial and lateral surfaces of talus.

The articular capsule is thin anteriorly and posteriorly to allow movements. It is reinforced by strong collateral ligaments which prevents anterior and posterior slipping of the tibia and fibula on the talus.

Medial (Deltoid) ligament extends from the medial malleolus to the navicular bone, calcaneus, and talus. It has superficial (*tibionavicular, tibiocalcaneal and posterior tibiotalar ligaments*) and deep (*anterior tibiotalar ligament*) parts. It prevents over eversion and helps to maintain medial longitudinal arch.

Lateral ligament consists of anterior talofibular, posterior talofibular and calcaneofibular ligaments. It resists inversion of the foot.

Relations

Movement

Dorsiflexion	Plantar flexion
Tibialis anterior	Tendocalcaneus (*gastrocnemius initiates & soleus maintains*)
Extensor hallucis longus	Tibialis posterior
Extensor digitorum longus	Flexor hallucis longus
Peroneus tertius	Flexor digitorum longus
	Peroneus longus
	Peroneus brevis
	Plantaris

Clinical Anatomy

- Upper end of the tibia is one of the most common sites for **acute osteomyelitis**.
- **Fracture**: Tibia is commonly fractured at the junction of the upper two-thirds and lower one-third of the shaft (shaft is most slender) **(Fig. 4.42)**. These fractures unite slowly, or may not unite (non-union) as the blood supply to this part is poor.

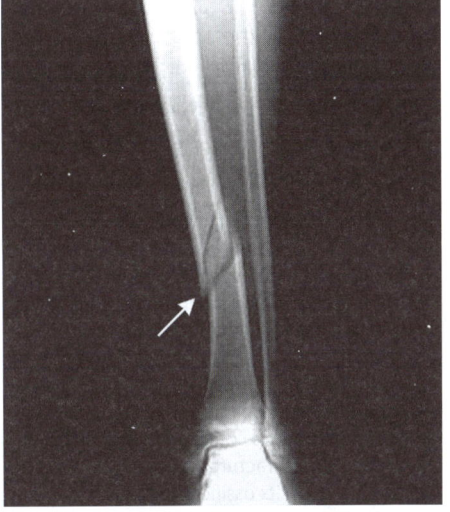

Fig. 4.42: Tibial fracture.

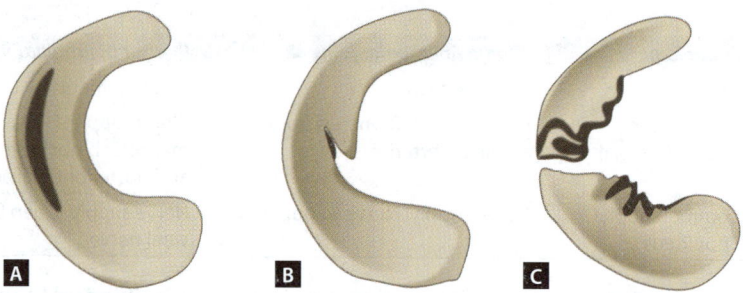

Figs. 4.43A to C: Meniscal tears: (A) Bucket handle tear; (B) Incomplete tear; (C) Complete tear.

- ***Tibia for bone graft:*** Bone pieces are obtained from the subcutaneous medial aspect of the tibia.
- ***Meniscal tears:*** A tear is caused by a twisting force with flexed knee. If meniscus does not move with femoral condyles it may be torn by the condyles. Most common injury is a longitudinal split of cartilage (*bucket-handle tear*) **(Figs. 4.43A to C)**. The central fragment is displaced in the middle of the joint where it limits full extension (locking); joint can still be flexed. Medial meniscus is torn more frequently because it is attached by tibial collateral ligament making it less mobile.

QUESTIONNAIRE

- Classify the bone.
- Side determination and anatomical position.
- Enumerate the structures attached to the soleal line.
- What are the joints associated with this bone and their types?
- What is attached to the subcutaneous anterior border of tibia?
- Mark the attachments of:

Ligaments	Muscles
Capsule of the knee joint	On medial side of shaft close to upper end
Medial and lateral menisci	On the lateral surface of the shaft
Anterior and posterior cruciate ligaments	On the posterior surface of the shaft
Tibial and fibular collateral ligaments of knee joint	Popliteus
Deltoid ligament of ankle joint	Semimembranosus and its expansions

- What is the mechanism of locking and unlocking at the knee joint?
- Mark the tendons related to the anterior aspects of the lower end of tibia.
- Which is the most vulnerable part of this bone? Why?
- What are the functions of cruciate ligaments?
- Enumerate the functions of menisci.
- What are the functions of iliotibial tract?
- Why nonunion is common in fracture of the lower end of tibia?
- What is Pott's fracture?
- Comment on its ossification. Which is the growing end?

THE FIBULA

The fibula (*long bone*) is the lateral bone of the leg; homologous with the ulna. It presents a shaft and two (upper and lower) ends. The upper end is expanded. The lower end is flattened from side to side and presents the *lateral malleolus*. The medial side of the malleolus shows a triangular articular surface (for talus). Just behind this articular surface the malleolus has a deep *malleolar fossa* (**Figs. 4.44 and 4.45**).

Side Determination

- *Superior*: Head with styloid process.
- *Lateral*: Lateral malleolus.
- *Anterior*: Triangular articular facet on the lateral malleolus.

Anatomical Position

Bone is vertically placed.

Upper end: The upper end of the fibula is the head. Its posterior and lateral part shows a projection called the *styloid process*. In front and medial to the styloid process, the head shows a circular facet for articulation for the tibia (*superior tibiofibular joint*). Immediately below the head is the neck of fibula.

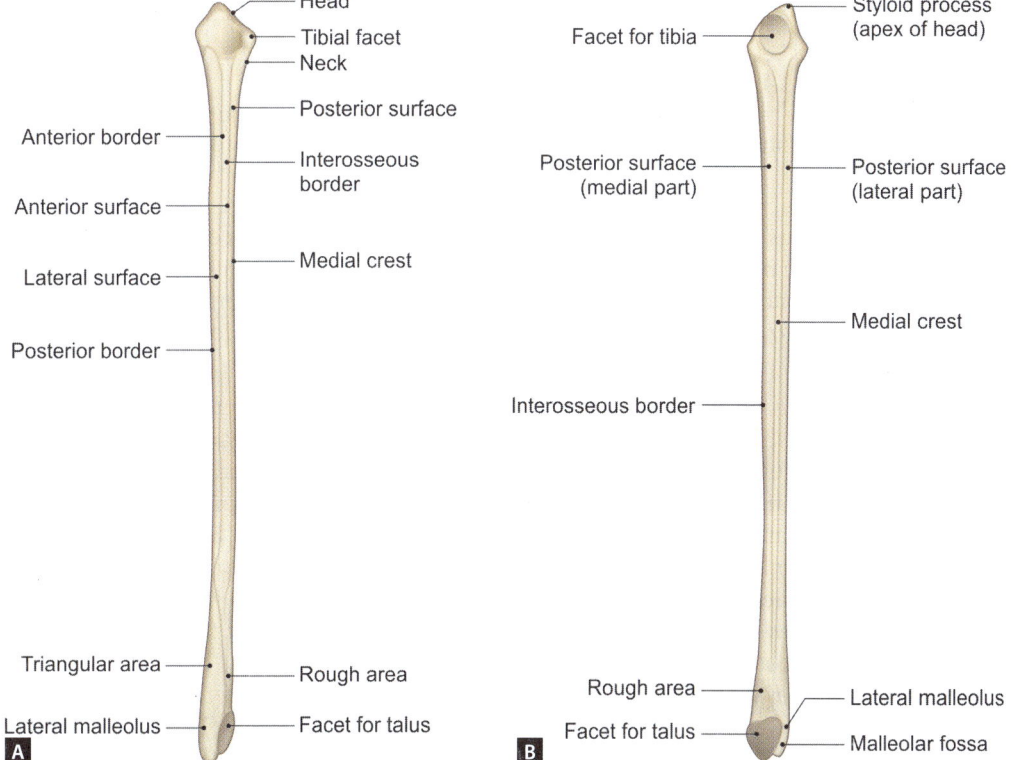

Figs. 4.44A and B: (A) Right fibula from the front; (B) Right fibula: Medial aspect.

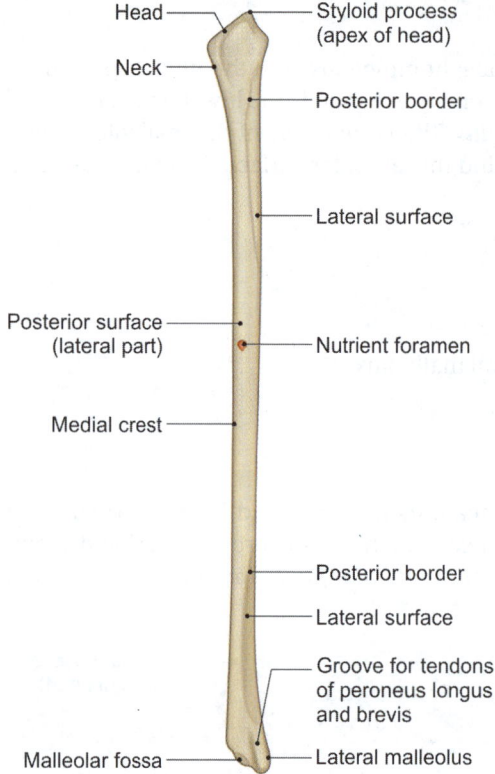

Fig. 4.45: Right fibula from behind.

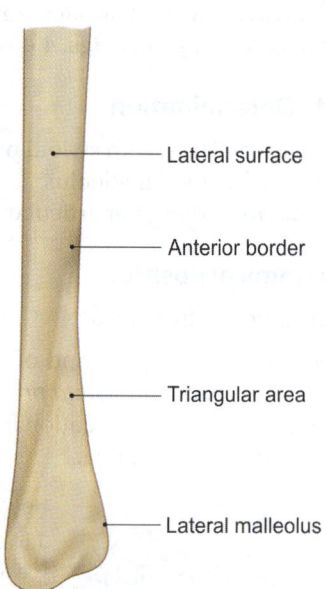

Fig. 4.46: Right fibula, lower part: Lateral aspect.

Lower end: It presents the lateral malleolus. It has a convex lateral surface that can be felt. The medial surface of the malleolus bears a triangular facet; articulates with the lateral surface of the talus and forms part of the ankle joint. Behind the facet the medial surface of the malleolus shows deep *malleolar fossa*. The lateral malleolus projects to a lower level than the medial malleolus.

Shaft: The shaft has three borders: (a) anterior, (b) posterior, and (c) interosseous (medial).

Anterior border is sharp. It begins below the anterior aspect of the head. Near its lower end it turns laterally and joins the apex of the triangular area above the lateral malleolus.

The upper end of the posterior border lies in line with the styloid process. Its lower end reaches the medial part of the posterior surface of the lateral malleolus **(Fig. 4.46)**.

Interosseous border lies near the anterior border. It merges with the upper part of the rough area above the talar facet of the lateral malleolus.

Lateral surface lies between the anterior and posterior borders. It faces backward and continues with the posterior aspect of the lateral malleolus.

Medial surface is between the anterior and interosseous borders. It is very narrow in the upper half of the shaft. Its lower broader part faces as much forward as medially **(Figs. 4.47A to B)**.

CHAPTER 4 ✦ Bones of Lower Limb

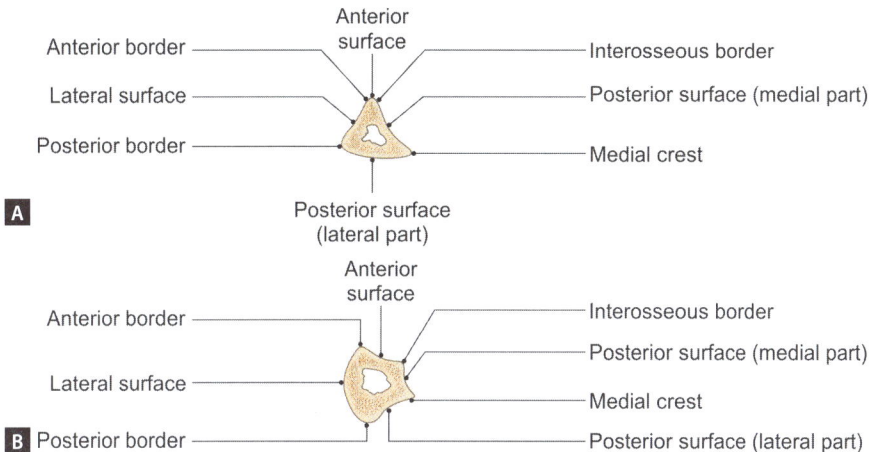

Figs. 4.47A and B: Transverse section (TS) shaft of right fibula: Borders and surfaces: (A) Through upper part; (B) Through lower part.

Posterior surface lies between the interosseous and posterior borders; occupying large area of the shaft. Over its upper three-fourths it is divided into medial and lateral parts by a vertical ridge called the *medial crest*. The medial part of the posterior surface is concave and faces forward and medially. The lateral part of the posterior surface faces posteriorly in its upper part and medially in its lower part. The lowest part of the posterior surface lies just above the talar facet of the lateral malleolus.

Attachments (Figs. 4.48 and 4.49)
Muscles

Muscle	Attachment
Biceps femoris	Head of fibula; through two separate slips separated by fibular collateral ligament of knee joint (*insertion*)
Extensor digitorum longus	Upper three-fourths of medial surface (*origin*)
Peroneus tertius	Medial surface below for extensor digitorum longus (*origin*)
Extensor hallucis longus	Middle two-fourths of medial surface, medial to origin of extensor digitorum longus (*origin*)
Peroneus longus	Upper two-thirds of lateral surface and lateral aspect of fibula head—common peroneal nerve is between two origins
Peroneus brevis	Lower two-thirds of lateral surface (*origin*)
Tibialis posterior	Upper two-thirds of medial part of posterior surface (*origin*)
Soleus	Posterior aspect of the head and upper one-fourth of lateral part of posterior surface (*origin*)
Flexor hallucis longus	Lower two-thirds of lateral part of posterior surface (*origin*)

Other Attachments

Structure	Area
Capsule of superior tibiofibular joint	Margins of tibial facet
Fibular collateral ligament of knee joint	Lateral aspect of the head (in between two slips of biceps femoris)
Interosseous membrane	Interosseous border
Interosseous ligament of inferior tibiofibular joint	Triangular area above malleolar articular surface
Posterior tibiofibular and posterior talofibular ligaments	Malleolar fossa
Superior extensor retinaculum of ankle	Anterior border of triangular area above lateral malleolus
Superior peroneal retinaculum	Posterior margin of lateral malleolus

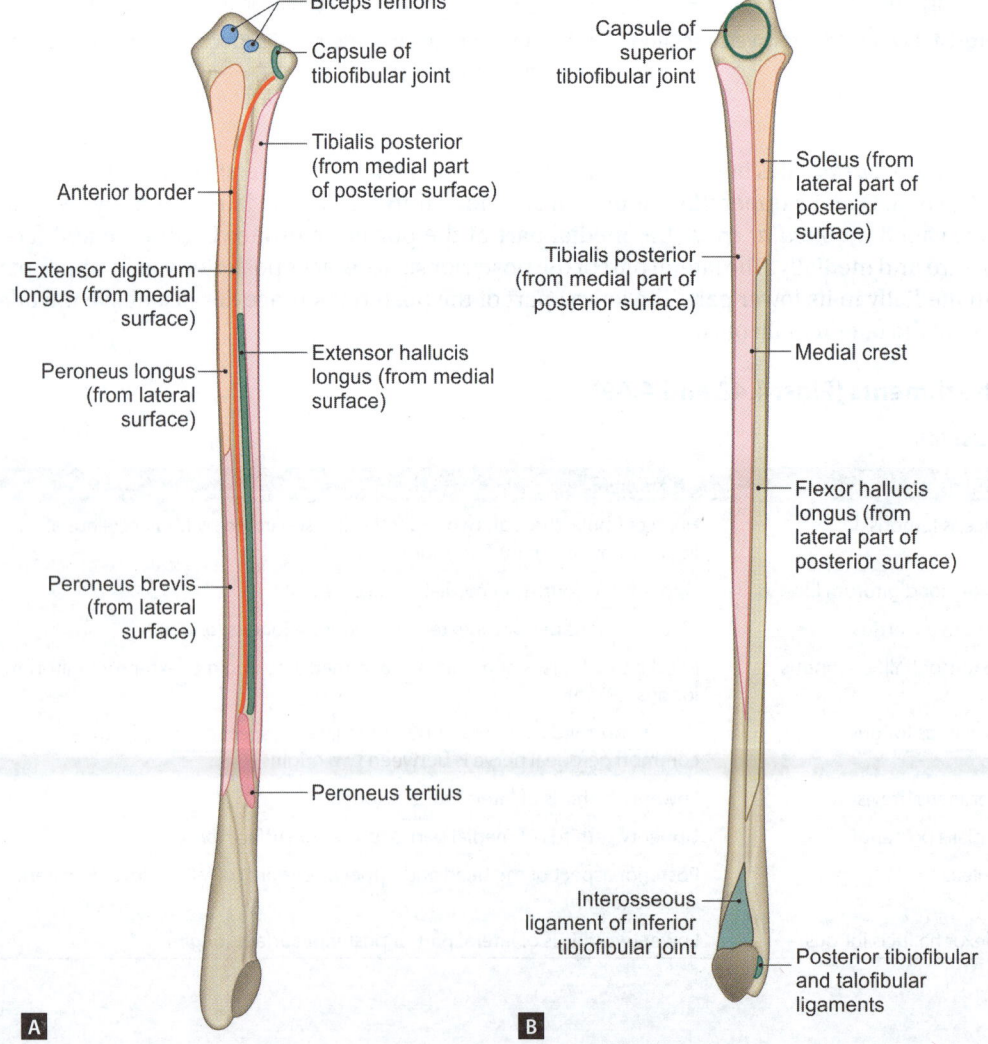

Figs. 4.48A and B: Right fibula attachments: (A) From front; (B) From medial side.

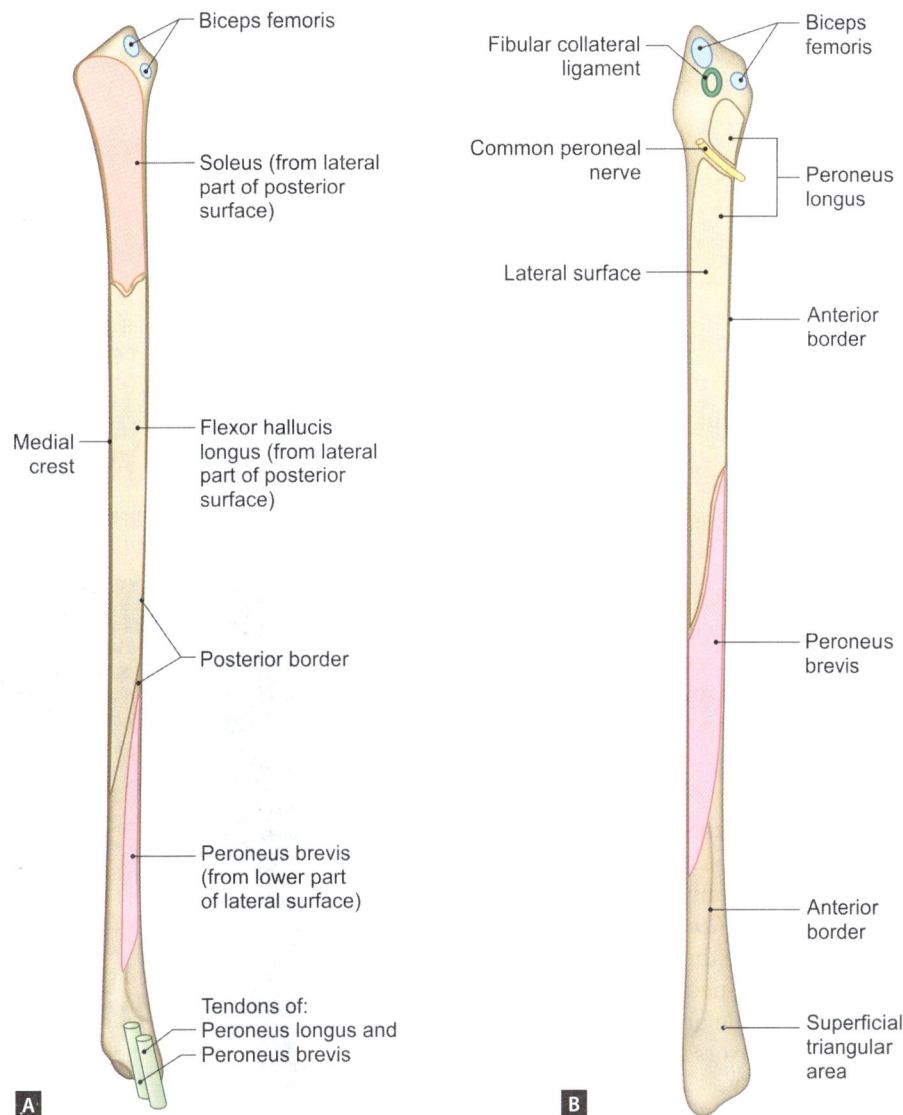

Figs. 4.49A and B: Right fibula attachments: (A) From behind; (B) From lateral side.

Fibula: Relations

❖ Common peroneal nerve winds round the lateral aspect of the neck of the fibula.
❖ Tendons of peroneus longus and brevis pass just behind lateral malleolus.

Ossification (Fig. 4.50)

Fibula has three centers of ossification:
1. Primary center (for shaft) appears in the 8th week of intrauterine life.
2. Secondary center for upper end appears in third or fourth year; fuses with the shaft between 17th and 19th years.

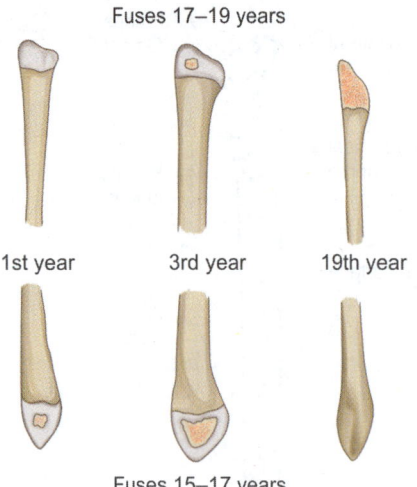

Fig. 4.50: Fibula: Ossification.

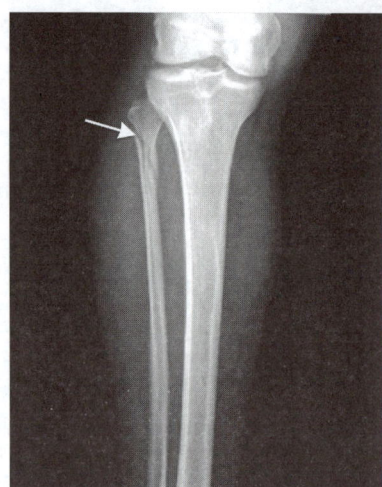

Fig. 4.51: Fracture neck of fibula.

3. Secondary center for lower end appears in first year; fuses with shaft between 15th and 17th years.
   Note: In long bones, secondary center appears first is last to fuse. Fibula is an *exception*—center appears first (*for lower end*) is also first to fuse.

Clinical Anatomy

- ❖ *Palpation of common peroneal nerve*: Common peroneal nerve can be rolled against the neck of the fibula; this nerve is commonly injured here.
- ❖ *Fractures neck of fibula and foot drop (Fig. 4.51)*: It may cause injury to the common peroneal nerve (winds laterally around the neck of fibula). This results in paralysis of all muscles in the anterior and lateral compartments of the leg (dorsiflexors and evertors of foot), causing foot drop.
  - Damage to superficial peroneal nerve causes loss of eversion of the foot.
  - Damage to deep peroneal nerve results in *foot drop* (loss of dorsiflexion).
- ❖ *Bone grafts*: Fibula is an ideal bone for a bone graft.
- ❖ *Pott's fracture*: It consists of the fracture of the lower end of fibula, fracture of medial malleolus, and rupture of deltoid ligament (**Fig. 4.52**). It is caused by forced eversion of the foot.

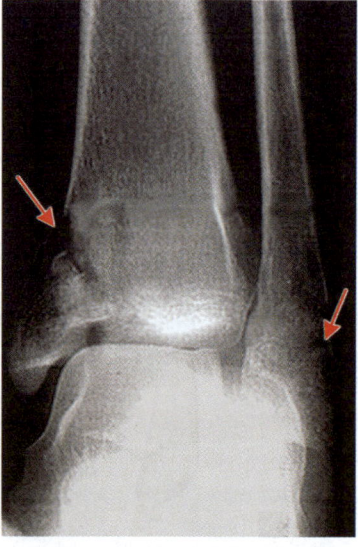

Fig. 4.52: Pott's fracture.

QUESTIONNAIRE

- Classify the bone. How does it differ from other long bones?
- Side determination and anatomical position.

- Enumerate the peculiarities of this bone.
- What are the joints associated with this bone and their types?
- Mark the attachments of:

Ligaments	Muscles
Fibular collateral ligament of knee joint	On the head
Lateral ligament of ankle joint	Peronei muscles
Interosseous membrane	On the posterior surface
Interosseous tibiofibular ligament	

- Which tendon is related to the lower end of fibula posteriorly?
- Mark the nerve palpable and related to this bone? Mention its clinical aspects.
- Explain the anatomical basis of foot drop.
- Comment on its ossification. Which is the growing end?

AN 14.4 Identify and name various bones in the articulated foot with individual muscle attachment

THE SKELETON OF THE FOOT

The posterior half of the foot is made up of seven *tarsal bones.* The largest tarsal bone is the *calcaneus;* forms the heel. Placed above the calcaneus is the *talus.* The talus articulates with the lower ends of the tibia and fibula to form the *ankle joint.* Anterior (distal) to the calcaneus and the talus there are the *navicular* (medially) and the *cuboid* (laterally). Distal to the navicular bone there are *medial cuneiform,* the *intermediate cuneiform,* and the *lateral cuneiform* bones **(Figs. 4.53 and 4.54)**.

Anterior to the tarsal bones are five *metatarsal bones.* Distal to the metatarsals there are *phalanges:* three (proximal, middle, and distal) for each digit except the great toe which has two phalanges—(a) proximal and (b) distal.

Calcaneus

Orientation and Side Determination

- Elongated anteroposteriorly—anterior aspect shows large articular facet; posterior aspect is nonarticular.
- Superior aspect presents three facets; inferior aspect is nonarticular.
- Medial aspect presents a prominent projection.

The calcaneus has anterior, posterior, superior, inferior, medial, and lateral surfaces.
- *Anterior surface* is covered by a large articular facet for the cuboid bone **(Figs. 4.55 and 4.56)**.
- *Posterior surface* is nonarticular; divided into upper, middle, and inferior parts.
- *Lateral surface* is flat. Its anterior part shows a small elevation called the *peroneal trochlea (tubercle).* The anterosuperior and the posteroinferior aspects of the tubercle are grooved.
- *Medial surface* presents the *sustentaculum tali*—projects medially from its anterior and upper part. The inferior aspect of the sustentaculum tali is marked by a groove.
- *Superior (dorsal) surface* bears anterior, middle, and posterior facets that articulate with corresponding facets on the talus. The middle facet lies on the upper surface of the

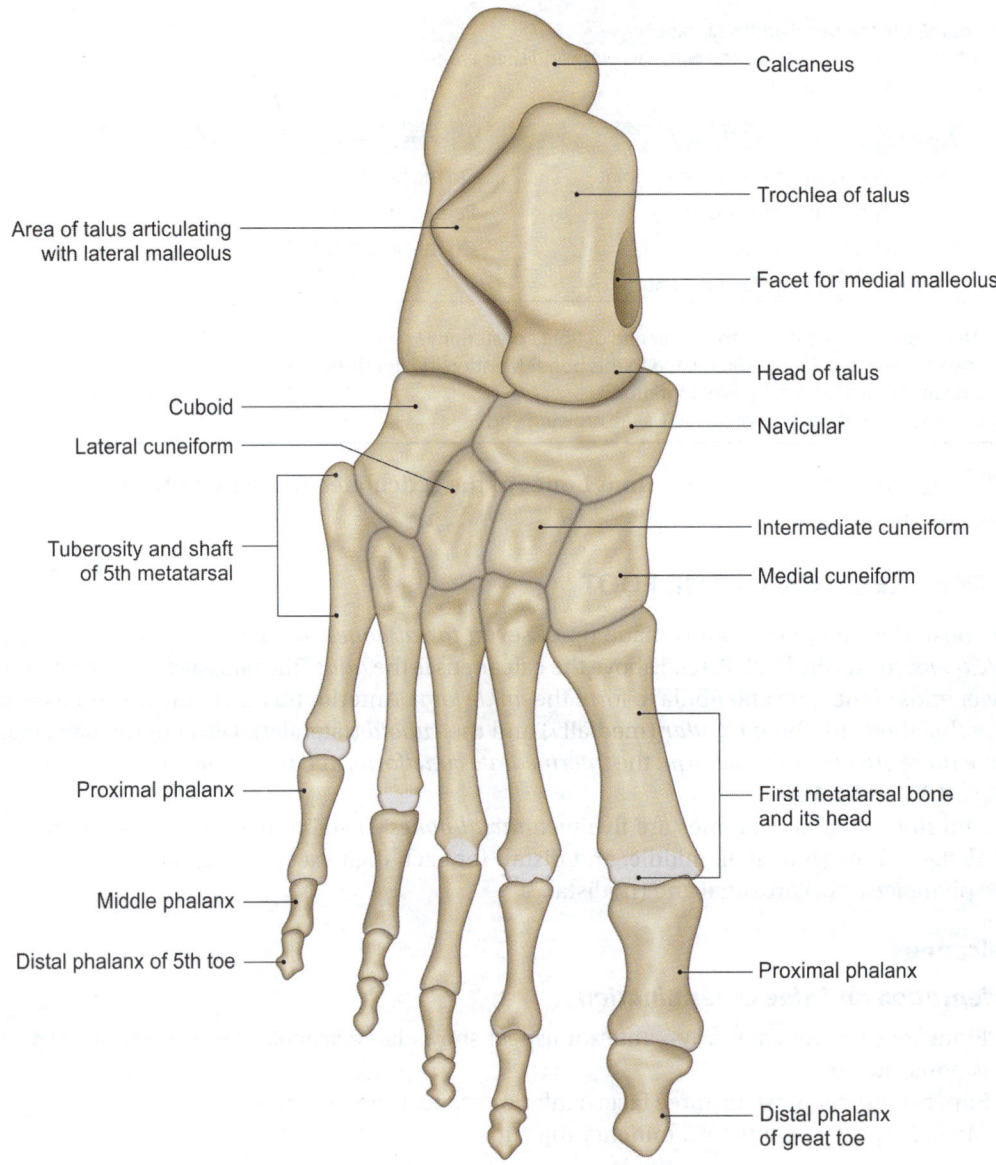

Fig. 4.53: Skeleton of the foot from above (dorsal aspect).

sustentaculum tali. It is separated from the posterior facet by a deep groove called the *sulcus calcanei*. In the articulated foot the sulcus calcanei comes into apposition with a similar groove on the talus (*sulcus tali*), to form the *sinus tarsi*.

Plantar (inferior) surface shows a prominence in its posterior part called the calcaneal tuberosity. The lateral and medial parts of it extend further forward called the *lateral and medial processes* of the tuberosity. The anterior part of the plantar surface shows another elevation called the *anterior tubercle*.

CHAPTER 4 ✦ Bones of Lower Limb

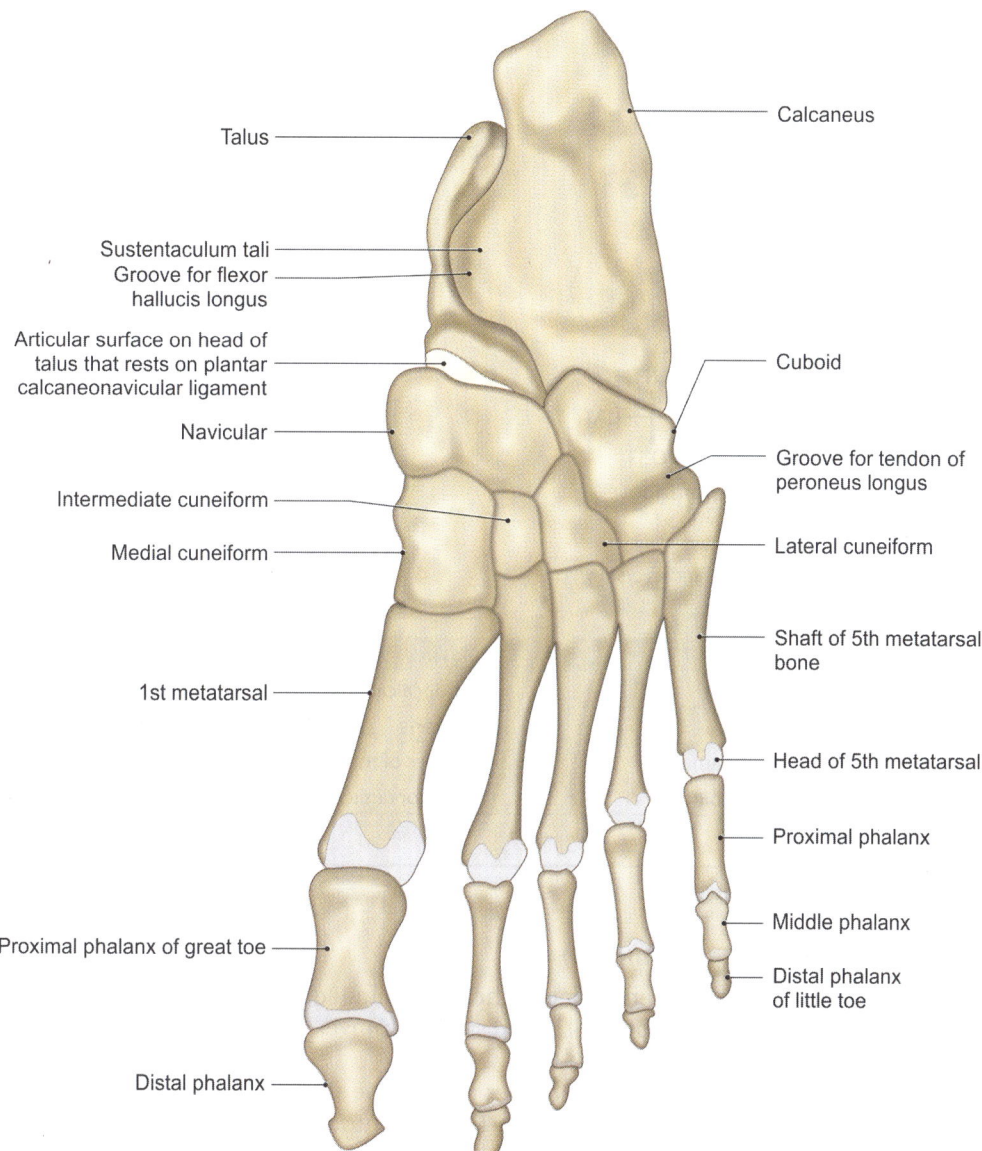

Fig. 4.54: Skeleton of the foot from below (plantar aspect).

QUESTIONNAIRE

- Side determination and anatomical position of the bone.
- What are the articulations of the calcaneus?
- Which tendon is directly related to this bone?
- Where does inversion begins and end?
- What is the sequence of movements bringing about inversion?
- How does the calcaneus moves under talus when none of the invertors or evertors are attached to it?

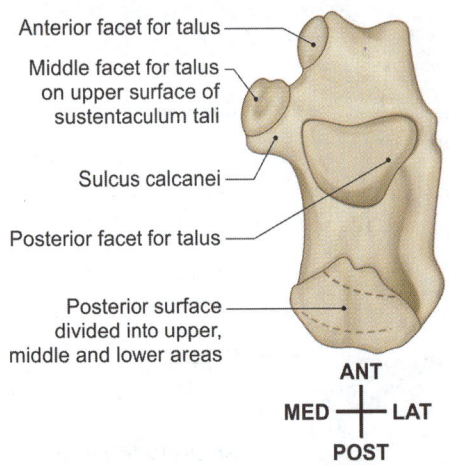

Fig. 4.55: Right calcaneus from above.

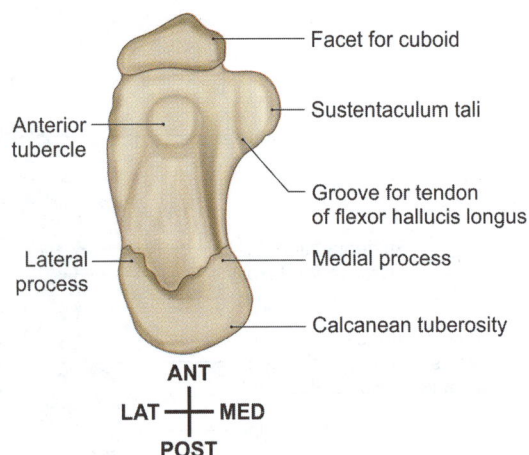

Fig. 4.56: Right calcaneus from below.

- What is the axis for inversion and eversion?
- Mark the attachments of:

Ligaments	Muscles
Spring ligament	Tendocalcaneus
Deltoid ligament	Plantaris
Long and short plantar ligaments	Muscles of the first layer of sole
Lateral ligament of ankle joint	Extensor digitorum brevis

- Comment on its ossification.

Talus

Orientation and Side Determination

❖ Elongated anteroposteriorly; anterior end (head) is rounded.
❖ Superior aspect bears a large pulley-shaped surface (convex upward); inferior aspect bears three facets.
❖ Lateral surface bears a large triangular facet; medial side shows a "comma-shaped" facet.

The talus presents a *head*, a *neck* and a *body*. The distal surface of the head has a large convex surface that articulates with the navicular bone. The upper surface of the body presents large *trochlear articular surface* which articulates with the lower end of the tibia **(Figs. 4.57 and 4.58)**.

Lateral surface bears a large triangular facet for articulation with the lateral malleolus of the fibula; while the *medial surface* bears a "comma-shaped" facet. This facet articulates with the medial malleolus of the tibia.

The lower and posterior part of the body projects backward. This projection is the *posterior process*. A groove divides this process into *medial* and *lateral tubercles*.

When the talus is viewed from below, the articular area on the head, for the navicular bone, extends on to the inferior aspect of the head. Behind this there are three facets (anterior, middle, and posterior) that articulate with corresponding facets on the upper surface of the calcaneus. The middle and posterior facets are separated by a deep groove called the sulcus tali. With sulcus

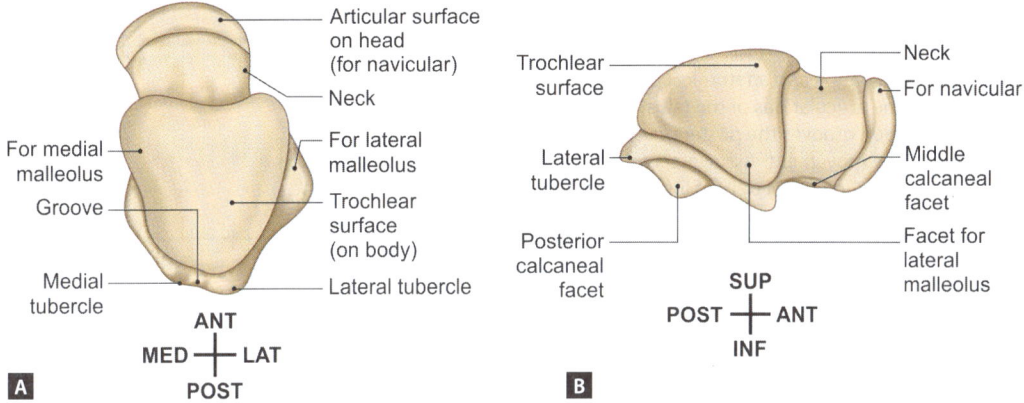

Figs. 4.57A and B: Right talus: (A) From above; (B) From the lateral side.

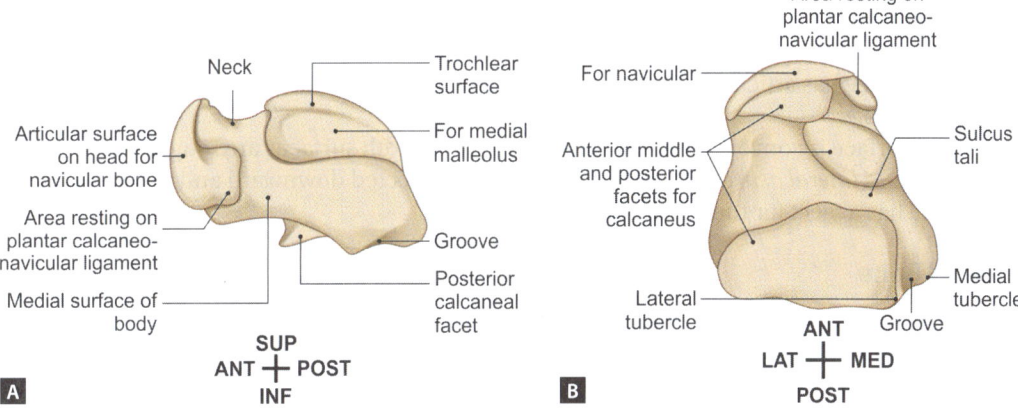

Figs. 4.58A and B: Right talus: (A) From the medial side; (B) From below.

calcanei, the sulcus tali form the *sinus tarsi*. Medial to the anterior calcaneal facet the lower aspect of the head of the talus has an area that rests on the plantar calcaneonavicular ligament.

Subtalar Joints

AN 20.2 **Describe the subtalar joints.**

Subtalar joints are anterior and posterior talocalcaneal joints. The movements of *inversion and eversion* occur at subtalar joints. These movements are essential for walking on slippery and uneven ground.

The axis is oblique that runs from back of calcaneus; passes through sinus tarsi to emerge at superomedial aspect of the neck of talus. This obliquity is responsible for adduction and plantar flexion with inversion and abduction and dorsiflexion associate with eversion.

Inversion is the movements of foot where medial border of sole is raised and sole faces inwards caused by tibialis anterior and posterior assisted by long extensor and flexor tendons of big toe.

Eversion is the movement where lateral border of sole is raised and sole faces outwards; caused by peroneus longus and brevis assisted by peroneus tertius.

> **QUESTIONNAIRE**
> - Side determination and anatomical position of talus.
> - What are the articulations of the talus? Classify them.
> - Which tendon grooves the posterior aspect of the talus?
> - What are the movements associated with talus?
> - Mark the attachments of deltoid ligament and lateral ligament of ankle joint.
> - What is the sequence of movements bringing about inversion?

Navicular Bone

Navicular bone articulates:
- Proximally with the head of talus
- Distally with three cuneiforms
- Laterally with cuboid.

The medial part of the bone presents *navicular tuberosity* **(Figs. 4.59A and B)**.

Side Determination

- Proximal surface presents single large concave articular facet for the head of the talus; distal surface has articular surface subdivided by ridges into three triangular areas for three cuneiforms.
- Dorsal surface is convex; plantar surface is concave (both surfaces are rough).
- *Medial and lateral aspects*: Navicular tuberosity is directed downward and medially; lateral surface has a facet for the cuboid bone.

Cuboid Bone

Cuboid articulates:
- Proximally with calcaneus.
- Distally with fourth and fifth metatarsals.
- Medially with navicular and lateral cuneiform.

The lateral and plantar aspects show a groove; limited posteriorly by a ridge. The lateral end of this ridge forms a projection called the *tuberosity*.

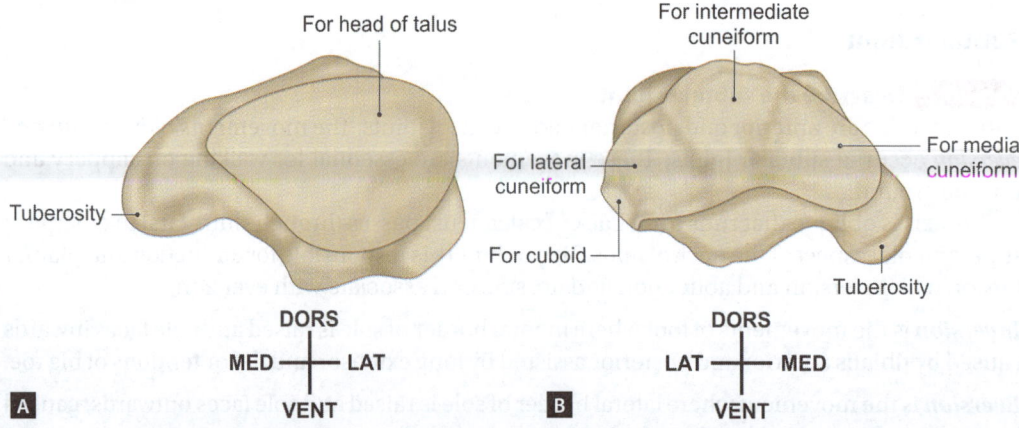

Figs. 4.59A and B: Right navicular bone: (A) Proximal aspect; (B) Distal aspect.

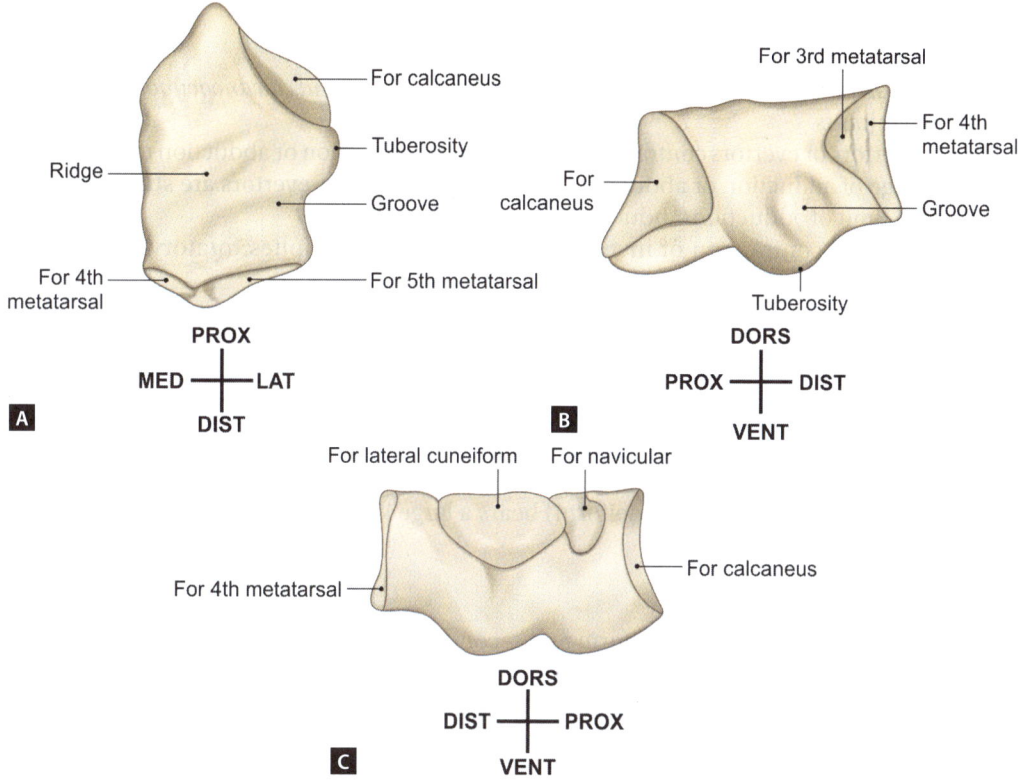

Figs. 4.60A to C: Right cuboid bone: (A) Plantar aspect; (B) Lateral aspect; (C) Medial aspect.

Side Determination (Figs. 4.60A to C)
- Proximal end presents large concavo-convex facet for calcaneus; distal end bears articular surface that is divided into two parts for fourth and fifth metatarsals.
- Plantar (inferior) surface shows a deep groove; limited posteriorly by a ridge.
- *Lateral aspect*: Groove on the plantar surface extends onto the lateral surface also; lateral end of the ridge is enlarged to form the tuberosity, medial surface bears a facet for the lateral cuneiform bone.

Transverse Tarsal Joints

AN 20.2 Describe the transverse tarsal joints.

Transverse tarsal (midtarsal) joints consist of *talonavicular and calcaneocuboid joints* that act together functionally.

All muscles causing inversion and eversion are attached to forefoot anterior to midtarsal joints. Inversion and eversion initiates at midtarsal joints. Once ligaments of midtarsal joints become tense, rotatory force is transmitted passively to subtalar joints where these movements are completed.

Sequence of Movements

- Invertors and evertors are attached to forefoot bones
- Inversion or eversion starts at midtarsal joints (*talonavicular and calcaneocuboid*); complete at subtalar joints
- When invertors or evertors contract, first movement is adduction or abduction of the forefoot
- Since range of adduction or abduction is limited, invertors or evertors are still contracting when full limit of adduction/abduction has been reached
- The continued contraction of invertors and evertors now applies rotatory force on the ligaments
- This rotatory force is transmitted back to calcaneus via spring ligament, long and short plantar ligaments
- Since talus is firmly wedged in tibiofibular mortise, calcaneus rotates under talus; rotates laterally during inversion and medially during eversion.

Medial Cuneiform

Medial cuneiform bone (largest cuneiform) bears a large kidney-shaped facet on one side. It articulates:
- Proximally with navicular bone.
- Distally with first metatarsal.
- Laterally with intermediate cuneiform and second metatarsal.

Side Determination (Figs. 4.61A and B)

- Dorsal surface is narrower than the plantar surface (both are nonarticular).
- Proximal end bears piriform facet (for navicular); distal surface presents a kidney-shaped facet (for first metatarsal).
- Medial surface is nonarticular; lateral surface bears articular areas for intermediate cuneiform and second metatarsal.

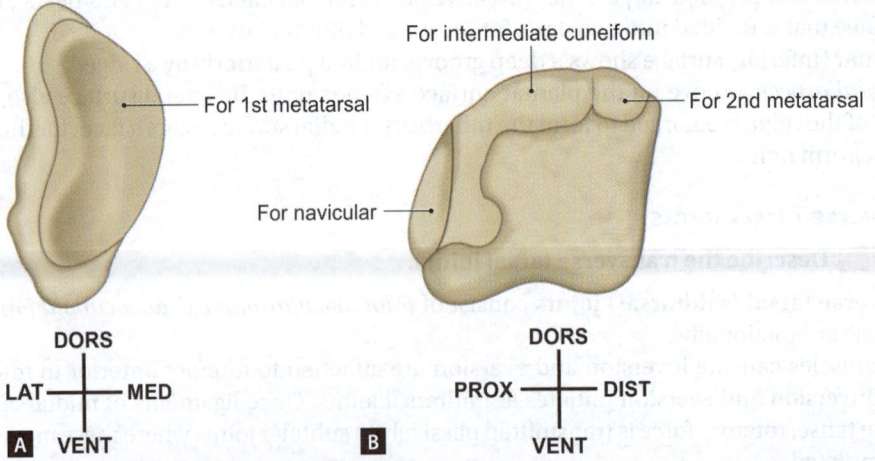

Figs. 4.61A and B: Right medial cuneiform bone: (A) Distal aspect; (B) Lateral aspect.

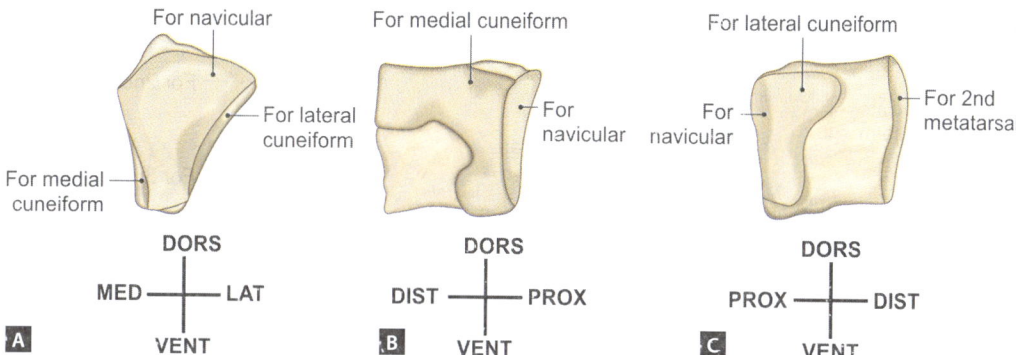

Figs. 4.62A to C: Right intermediate cuneiform bone: (A) Proximal aspect; (B) Medial aspect; (C) Lateral aspect.

Intermediate Cuneiform

The intermediate cuneiform (*smallest cuneiform*) is typical wedge shaped. It articulates:
* Proximally with navicular bone
* Distally with second metatarsal
* Medially with medial cuneiform
* Laterally with lateral cuneiform.

Side Determination (Figs. 4.62A to C)
* Dorsal surface is wide; plantar surface is narrow.
* Medial surface bears L-shaped facet (for medial cuneiform); lateral side bears vertical facet (for lateral cuneiform).
* *Proximal and distal aspects (both present triangular facets)*: Proximal aspect can be distinguished by looking at the lateral surface; vertical facet for the lateral cuneiform is placed along the proximal margin of this surface. Distal part of the lateral surface is nonarticular.

Lateral Cuneiform

Lateral cuneiform articulates:
* Proximally with navicular bone
* Distally with third metatarsal
* Medially with intermediate cuneiform and second metatarsal
* Laterally with cuboid and fourth metatarsal.

Side Determination
* Dorsal surface is wider than the plantar surface.
* *Proximal and distal surfaces*: Entire distal surface is covered by a triangular facet (for third metatarsal); proximal surface is covered by a smaller facet (for navicular) on the dorsal two-third of the surface.
* Both medial and lateral surfaces bear facets; larger and more prominent on the medial aspect **(Figs. 4.63A to D)**.

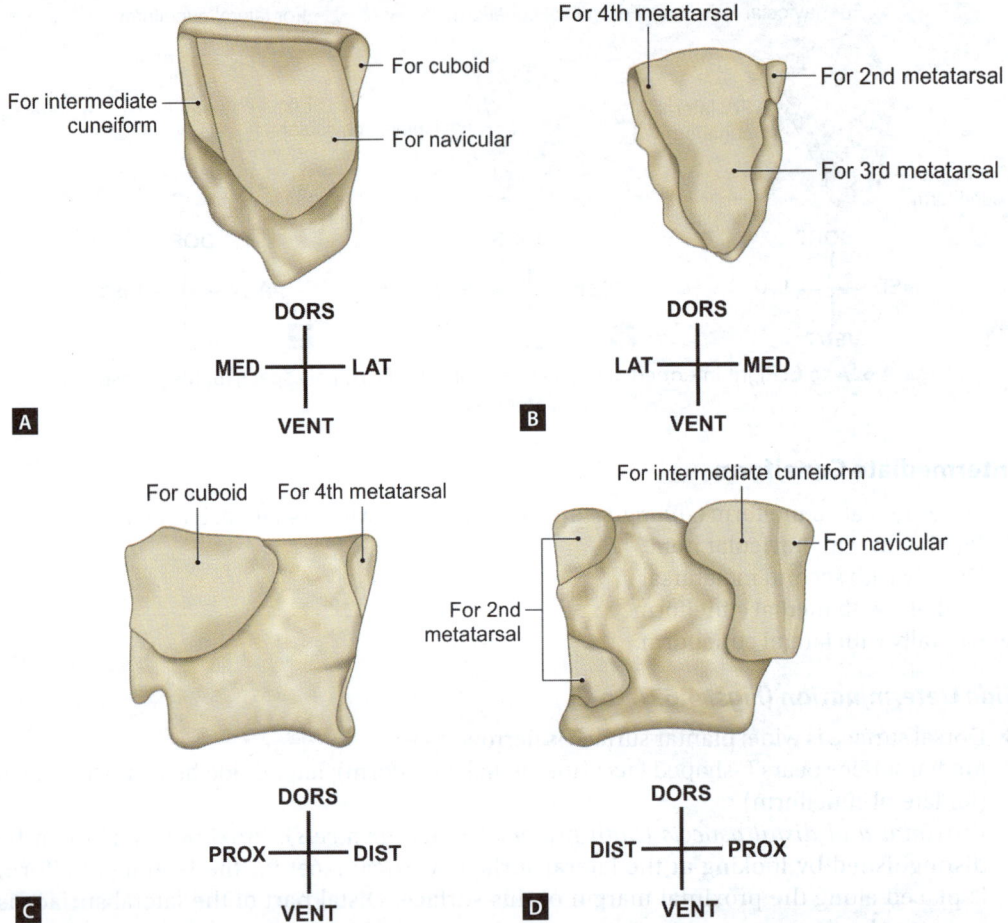

Figs. 4.63A to D: Right lateral cuneiform bone: (A) Proximal aspect; (B) Distal aspect; (C) Lateral aspect; (D) Medial aspect.

Metatarsals

The metatarsal bones (five in number) are numbered from medial to lateral side (metacarpals: numbered from lateral to medial side). Structurally both metatarsals and metacarpals are similar. Each metatarsal has a distal end (head); a proximal end (base), and an intervening shaft. The head is rounded. The base is enlarged with proximal, dorsal, plantar, medial, and lateral surfaces. The shaft is slightly convex on its dorsal side and concave on the plantar side **(Fig. 4.64)**.

Metatarsals: Articulations (Figs. 4.65 to 4.69)

Head of each metatarsal articulates with the proximal phalanx of the corresponding digit. The articulations of the bases of the metatarsals are as follows:

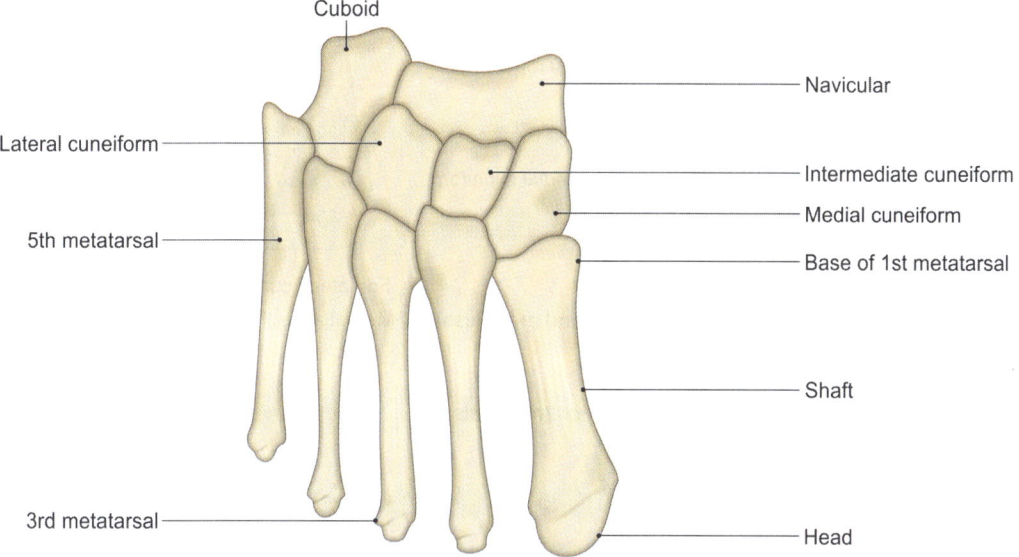

Fig. 4.64: Articulations of the metatarsal bones.

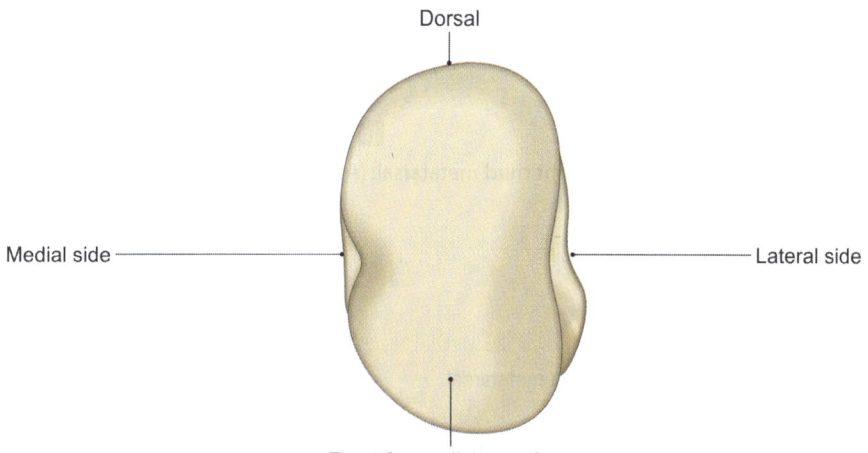

Fig. 4.65: Right first metatarsal: Proximal end.

Base of 1st metatarsal	Base of 2nd metatarsal	Base of 3rd metatarsal	Base of 4th metatarsal	Base of 5th metatarsal
• Medial cuneiform • Base of second metacarpal	• Intermediate cuneiform • Medial cuneiform • Lateral cuneiform	• Lateral cuneiform • Second metatarsal • Fourth metatarsal	• Cuboid • Lateral cuneiform • Base of third metatarsal • Laterally with base of fifth metatarsal	• Cuboid • Fourth metatarsal

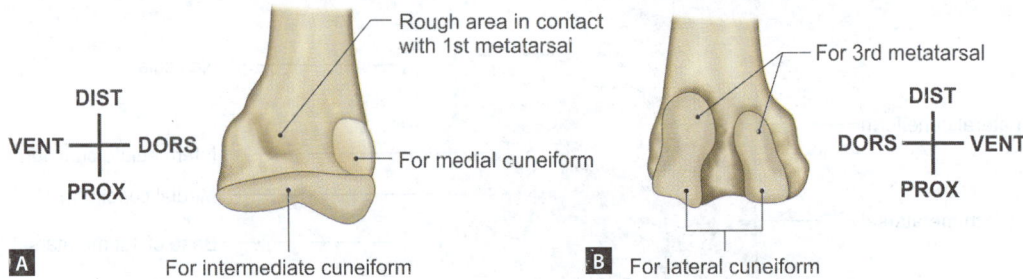

Figs. 4.66A and B: Base of right second metatarsal: (A) Medial aspect; (B) Lateral aspect.

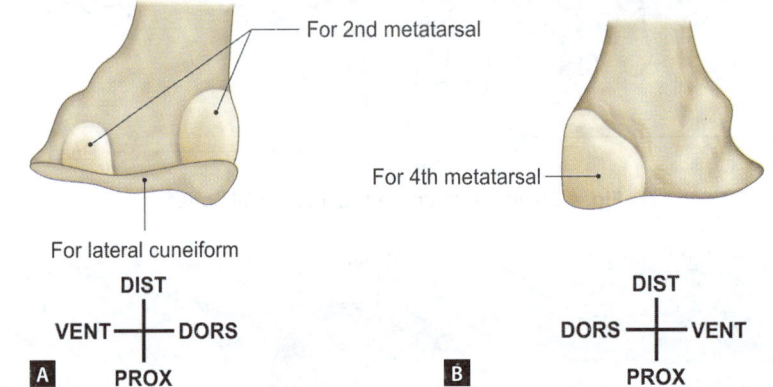

Figs. 4.67A and B: Base of right third metatarsal: (A) Medial aspect; (B) Lateral aspect.

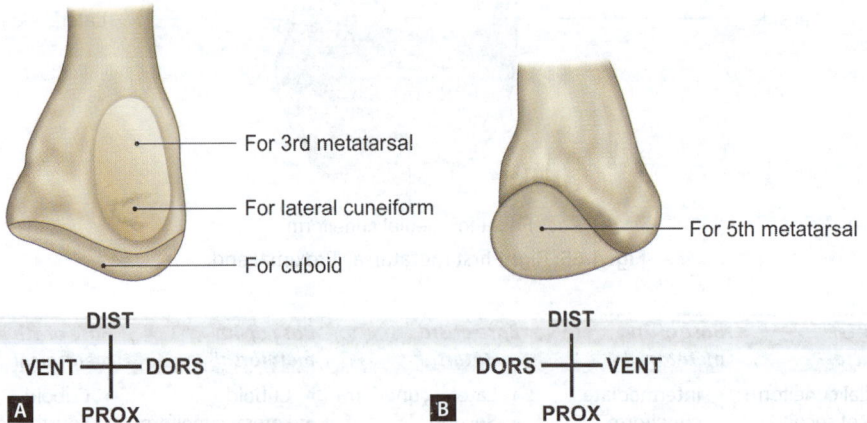

Figs. 4.68A and B: Base of right fourth metatarsal: (A) Medial aspect; (B) Lateral aspect.

Identification of Metatarsals

First metatarsal:
- Short and thick
- Large kidney-shaped facet on the proximal surface of the base.

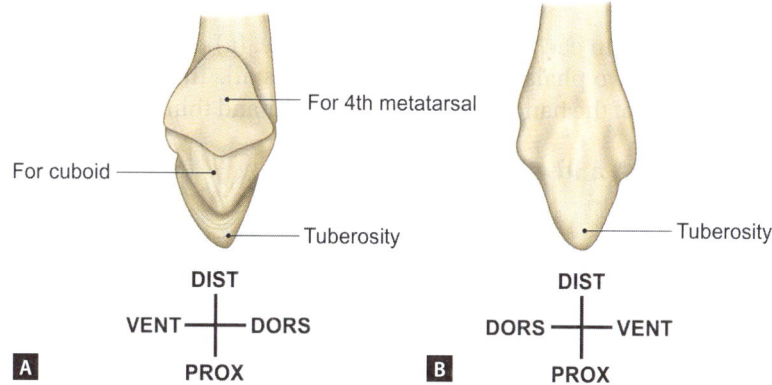

Figs. 4.69A and B: Base of right fifth metatarsal: (A) Medial aspect; (B) Lateral aspect.

Fifth metatarsal: Only metatarsal having a tuberosity (on lateral side of its base).
Second, third and fourth metatarsals distinguished from their bases:
- Facet on the proximal surface of the base of fourth metatarsal is quadrangular; facets on the second and third metatarsals are triangular.
- Triangular facet on the proximal surface of the base of third metatarsal is flat; on the second metatarsal is concave.

Additional confirmation about the medial and lateral sides of the metatarsals can be obtained by examining facets present on the medial and lateral sides of their bases. It is noted that these facets are subject to variations.

Side Determination of Metatarsals

Proximal end of a metacarpal forms enlarged base; distal end bears a rounded head. Plantar aspect of the shaft is concave. Thus, side of the metatarsal can be determined by distinguishing between the medial and lateral aspects of the bone.

First metatarsal: Medial and lateral sides distinguished by examining the kidney-shaped facet on its base; is directed laterally.

Second metatarsal: Medial and lateral aspects distinguished by examining the dorsal side of the base; proximal end of the base is placed oblique to the long axis of the shaft, and the lateral side of the base extends proximally for a greater distance than the medial side.

Distinguishing Metacarpals and Metatarsals from Each Other (Fig. 4.70)

Distinguished by comparing the relative size of the head and the base:
- Approximately equal in metacarpals
- In metatarsals, base is much larger than the head.

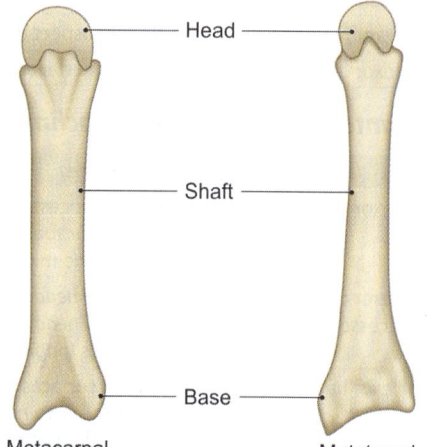

Fig. 4.70: Metacarpals and metatarsals: Comparison.

Phalanges of the Foot

There are three phalanges in each toe except the great toe: (a) proximal, (b) middle, and (c) distal. The great toe has two phalanges (proximal and distal). The phalanges of the foot are similar in shape to those of the hand, but are much shorter and thinner than the latter.

Attachments (Figs. 4.71 and 4.72)

On the Dorsal Aspect

Muscle	Attachment
Gastrocnemius, soleus and plantaris	By tendocalcaneus into middle of posterior surface of calcaneus (*insertion*)
Peroneus brevis	Lateral side of the base of fifth metatarsal (*insertion*)
Peroneus tertius	Dorsal surface of the base of fifth metatarsal (*insertion*)
Extensor digitorum longus	Tendon for each digit ends in three slips (one intermediate and two collateral); intermediate slip into base of middle phalanx; collateral slips into base of distal phalanx (*insertion*)
Extensor hallucis longus	Dorsal aspect of the base of distal phalanx of great toe (*insertion*)
Extensor digitorum brevis	Anterior part of superior and lateral aspects of calcaneus (*origin*)
Extensor hallucis brevis	(Part of extensor digitorum brevis) dorsal surface of the base of the proximal phalanx of great toe (*insertion*)

Plantar Aspect of Foot: Insertion of Leg Tendons

Tendon	Insertion
Tibialis posterior	Tuberosity of navicular and medial cuneiform; slips from tendon also reach sustentaculum tali, intermediate cuneiform, lateral cuneiform, cuboid and bases of second, third and fourth metatarsals
Tibialis anterior	Medial cuneiform (medial and plantar aspects) and medial side of the base of first metatarsal
Peroneus longus	Lateral side of medial cuneiform, and lateral side of base of 1st metatarsal
Peroneus brevis	See above
Flexor hallucis longus	Plantar aspect of the base of the distal phalanx of great toe
Flexor digitorum longus	Plantar surfaces of the bases of distal phalanges of all digits except great toe

Plantar Aspect of Foot: Attachments of Intrinsic Muscles (Excluding Interossei)

Muscle	Attachment
Flexor digitorum brevis	Medial process of calcaneal tuberosity (*origin*); muscle ends in four tendons (for lateral four toes); each tendon divides into two slips attached to medial and lateral sides of the middle phalanx of the concerned digit
Flexor digitorum accessorius	• *Lateral head*: Lateral process of calcaneal tuberosity • *Medial head*: Medial surface, inferior to groove for the tendon of flexor hallucis longus (*origin*)
Flexor hallucis brevis	Plantar surfaces of cuboid and lateral cuneiform (*origin*); at insertion muscle divides into two parts: *medial and lateral*—attached to corresponding sides of the base of proximal phalanx of great toe
Abductor hallucis	Medial process of calcaneal tuberosity; inserted into medial side of the base of proximal phalanx of great toe (with medial part of flexor hallucis brevis)

(Contd...)

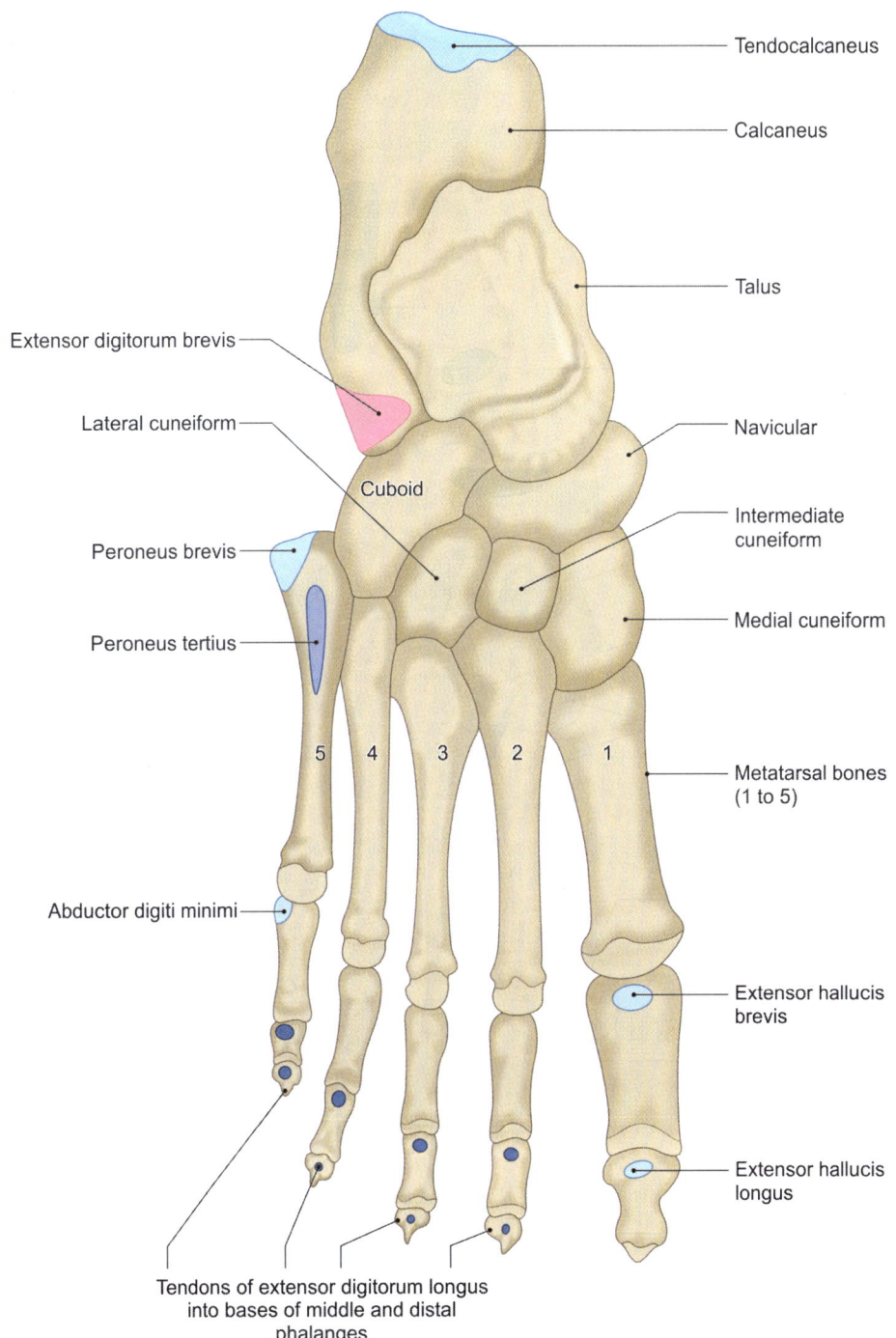

Fig. 4.71: Skeleton of the right foot: Attachments on the dorsal aspect.

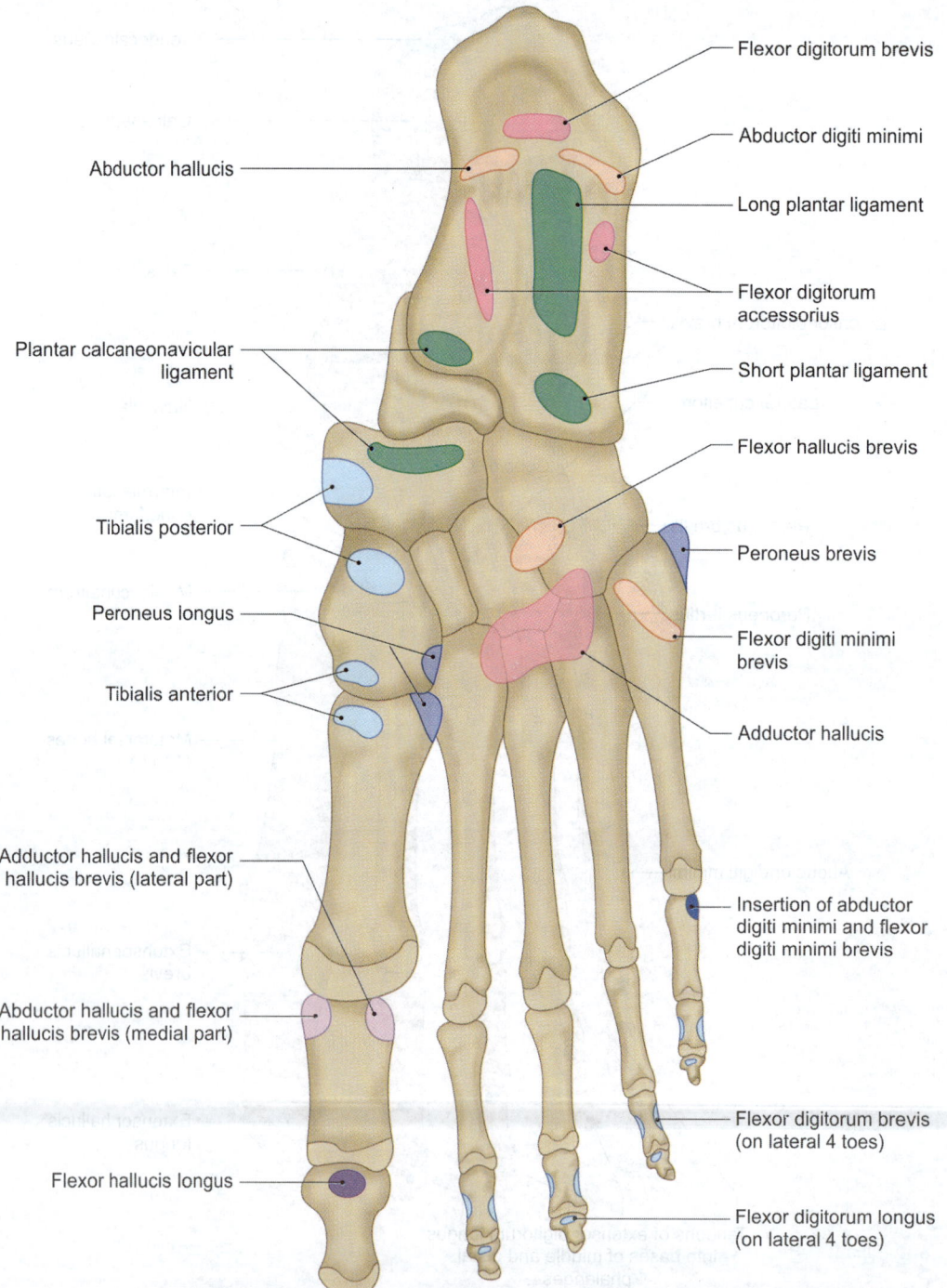

Fig. 4.72: Skeleton of the right foot: Attachments on the ventral aspect.

(Contd...)

Muscle	Attachment
Adductor hallucis (oblique head)	• Origin: Bases of second, third and fourth metatarsals (*transverse head*—no bony origin;. arises from ligaments on the plantar aspect of metatarsophalangeal joints of second, third and fourth toes) • Insertion: Lateral side of the base of proximal phalanx of great toe (with lateral part of flexor hallucis brevis)
Flexor digitorum longus	Plantar surfaces of the bases of the distal phalanges of all digits except great toe (insertion)
Abductor digiti minimi	• Origin: Lateral and medial processes of calcaneal tuberosity • Insertion: Lateral side of proximal phalanx of 5th toe (with flexor digiti minimi brevis)
Flexor digiti minimi brevis	• Origin: Plantar surface of the base of fifth metatarsal • Insertion—into lateral side of the proximal phalanx of fifth toe (with abductor digiti minimi)

Interossei: Attachments (Figs. 4.73 and 4.74)

Plantar interossei	
Origin	**Insertion**
• *First plantar interosseous*: Plantar aspect of the shaft of third metatarsal • *Second plantar*: Plantar aspect of the shaft of fourth metatarsal • *Third plantar*: Plantar aspect of the shaft of fifth metatarsal	Medial side of the base of the proximal phalanx of the corresponding digit (*also into dorsal digital expansion*)
Dorsal interossei	
Origin	**Insertion**
• Each dorsal interosseous arises from the adjacent sides of the shafts of two metatarsals • *First muscle*: First and second metatarsals • *Second muscle*: Second and third metatarsals • *Third muscle*: Third and fourth metatarsals • *Fourth muscle*: Fourth and fifth metatarsals	• *First muscle*: Medial side of the base of the proximal phalanx of 2nd digit • *Second muscle*: Lateral side of the base of the proximal phalanx of 2nd digit • *Third muscle*: Lateral side of the base of the proximal phalanx of 3rd digit • *Fourth muscle*: Lateral side of the base of the proximal phalanx of 4th digit

Other Attachments

Provide attachment to many ligaments connected with the ankle, intertarsal, and tarsometatarsal joints; and with interphalangeal joints. Important ligaments are:

Ligament	Attachment
Anterior and posterior talofibular ligaments	Lateral side of talus
Anterior and posterior tibiotalar ligaments	Medial side of talus
Calcaneofibular ligament	Lateral surface of calcaneus
Cervical ligament	Above to inferolateral aspect of neck of talus; below to superior surface of calcaneus

(Contd...)

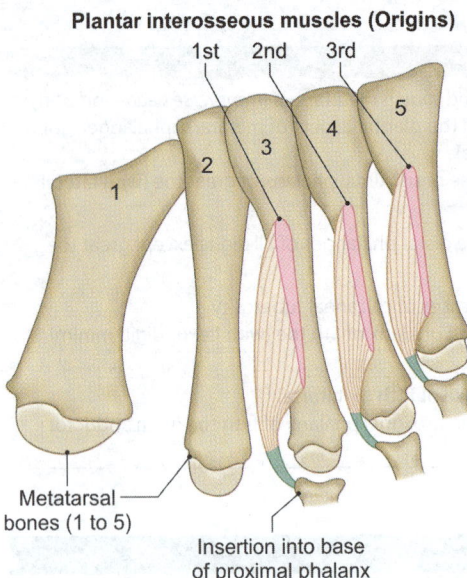

Fig. 4.73: Metatarsals: Attachments of plantar interossei.

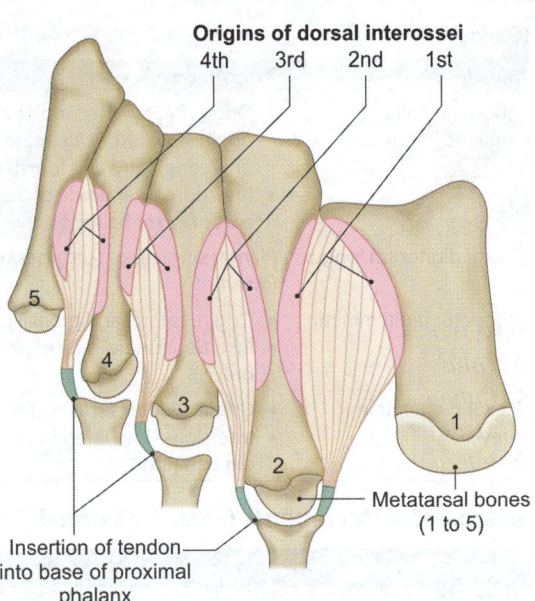

Fig. 4.74: Attachments of dorsal interossei on the metatarsals.

Ligament	Attachment
Long plantar ligament	Posteriorly to plantar surface (tuberosity) of calcaneus; anteriorly to plantar surface of cuboid distal to groove for peroneus longus; fibers reach bases of second, third and fourth metatarsals
Short plantar ligament	Anterior tubercle of calcaneus to cuboid (proximal to groove for peroneus longus)
Plantar calcaneonavicular ligament (*Spring ligament*)	Anterior margin of sustentaculum tali to plantar surface of navicular
bifurcate ligament (Y-shaped)	*Stem*: Upper surface of calcaneus *Limbs*: Dorsal aspect of cuboid and navicular
Interosseous talocalcaneal ligament	Passes from sulcus tali to sulcus calcanei

Structure	Attachment
Inferior extensor retinaculum (lateral end)	Upper surface of calcaneus
Flexor retinaculum (lower end)	Medial surface of calcaneus
Peroneal retinacula	Lateral surface of calcaneus
Fibrous flexor sheath of each digit	Sides of the phalanges on the plantar aspect

Ossification

Calcaneus has one primary center of ossification that appears in the third fetal month; and a secondary center (for scale-like epiphysis covering its posterior part) that appears in the sixth to eight years.

CHAPTER 4 ✦ Bones of Lower Limb

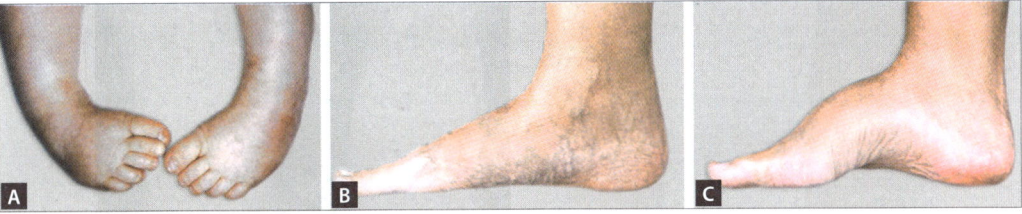

Figs. 4.75A to C: Deformities of foot: (A) Club foot; (B) Flat foot; (C) Claw foot.

Other tarsal bones normally have one center; appears as follows:
- *Talus*: 6th fetal month
- *Cuboid*: Just before or after birth
- *Medial cuneiform*: Third year
- *Intermediate cuneiform*: First year
- *Lateral cuneiform*: First year
- *Navicular*: Third year.

Each metatarsal has a primary center for the shaft that appears in the 9th or 10th fetal week. The first metatarsal has a secondary center for its base; appears in the third year. Other metatarsals have secondary centers for their heads (not bases) which appear in the third or fourth year. The secondary centers unite with the shafts between the 17th and 20th years.

Each phalanx has a primary center for the shaft (appears in 7th to 15th fetal weeks); and a secondary center for the base (appears between second to eight years) which unites with the shaft by the 18th year.

Clinical Anatomy

Deformities of the Foot (Figs. 4.75A to C)
- Talipes equinus—person walks on the toes.
- Talipes calcaneus—person walks on the heel.
- Talipes varus—person walks on the lateral border of the foot.
- Talipes valgus—person walks on the medial border of the foot.

Talipes equinovarus (club foot): In this congenital deformity of the foot the foot is plantarflexed, inverted, and adducted. It involves a deformity in which the foot is plantarflexed (equinus) and the heel is elevated and turned medially (equinovarus) **(Fig. 4.75A)**.

Flat foot (pes planus): Loss of arches of the foot **(Fig. 4.75B)**.

Claw foot (pes cavus): Exaggerated arched foot **(Fig. 4.75C)**.

March fracture (stress fracture) (Fig. 4.76): It is a fatigue fracture of one of the metatarsals, which may result from prolonged walking.

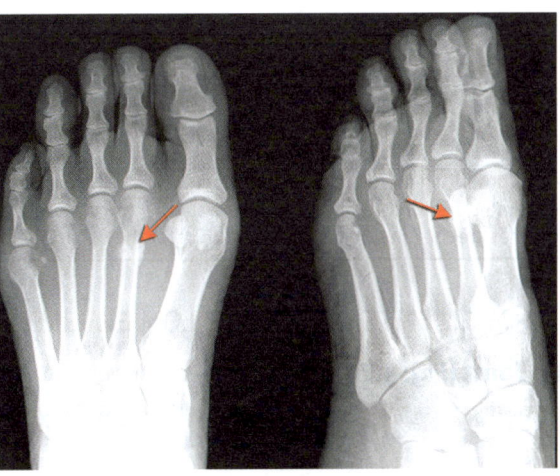

Fig. 4.76: March fracture.

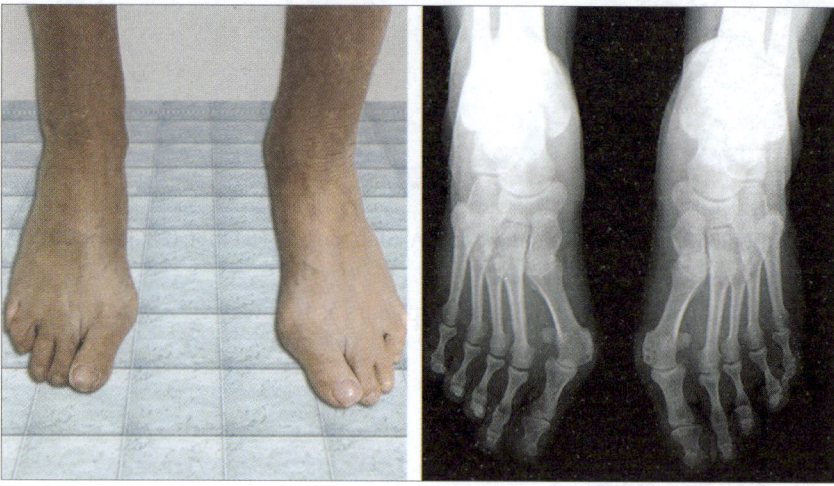

Fig. 4.77: Hallux valgus.

Hallux valgus (Fig. 4.77): It is the lateral deviation of the big toe; accompanied by swelling on the medial aspect of the first metatarsophalangeal joint.

Hallux varus: It is the medial deviation of the big toe.

Bunion: It is a localized swelling at the medial side of the first metatarsophalangeal joint; caused by an inflamed bursa. It is unusually associated with hallux valgus.

QUESTIONNAIRE

- Classify the metatarsals. How does it differ from other long bones?
- Side determination and anatomical position of calcaneus.
- What are the joints associated with inversion and eversion and their types?
- Mark the attachments of:

Ligaments	Muscles
Deltoid ligament	Plantar interossei
Slips of lateral ligament of ankle joint	Dorsal interossei
Long and short plantar ligaments	Peronei (longus, brevis, and tertius)
Spring ligament	Tibialis anterior and posterior

- Comment on metatarsals' ossification. Which is the growing end?
- Name the structures attached to the styloid process of the fifth metatarsal?
- What are the anatomical considerations for the collapse of the medial longitudinal arch?

MOVEMENTS AT MAJOR LOWER LIMB JOINTS

Hip Joint (Fig. 4.78)

Type	Axis	Movements
Ball and socket	Multiaxial	Flexion and extension, Abduction and adduction, Medial and lateral rotations and Circumduction

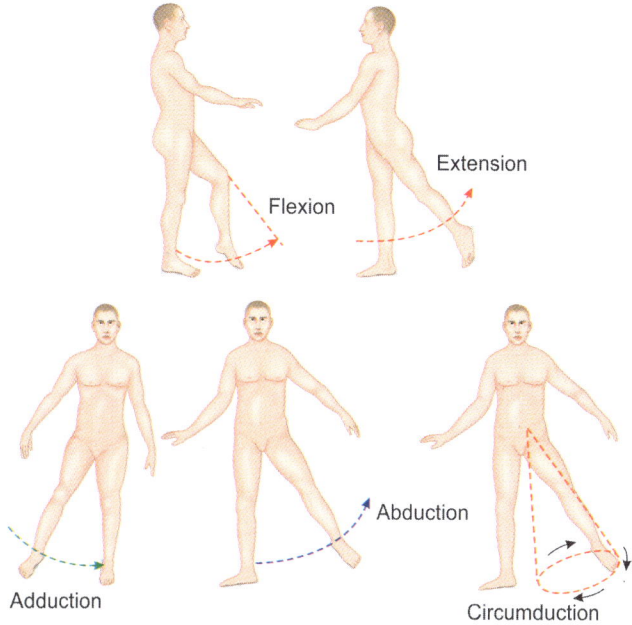

Fig. 4.78: Movements at hip joint.

Knee Joint (Fig. 4.79)

Type	Axis	Movements
Modified hinge	Biaxial	Flexion and extension, Medial and lateral rotations

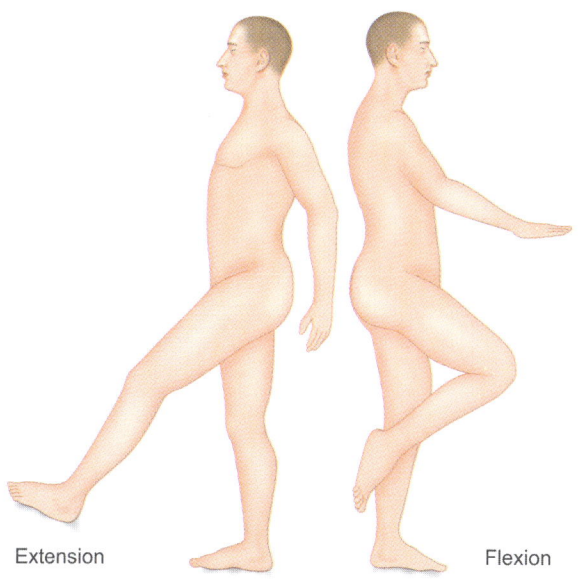

Fig. 4.79: Movements at knee joint.

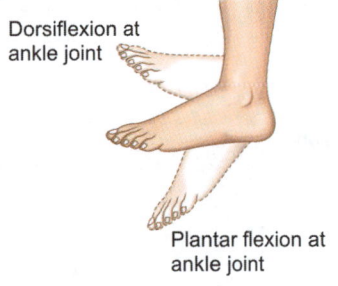

Fig. 4.80: Movements at ankle joint.

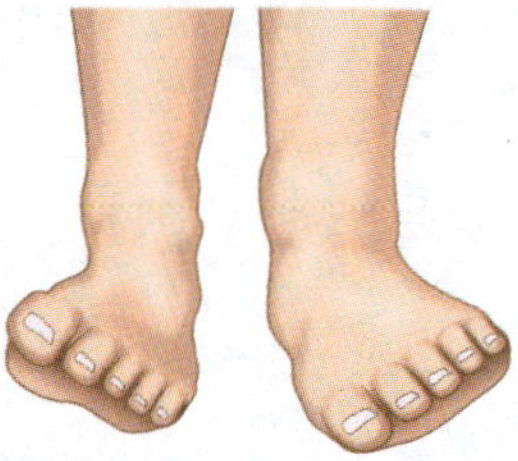

Fig. 4.81: Movements at subtalar joints.

Ankle Joint (Fig. 4.80)

Type	Axis	Movements
Hinge	Uniaxial	Flexion and extension

Subtalar Joints (Fig. 4.81)

Type	Axis	Movements
Plane	Modified multiaxial	Inversion and eversion

Metacarpophalangeal Joints

Type	Axis	Movements
Condylar	Biaxial	Flexion and extension, Abduction and adduction

Interphalangeal Joints

Type	Axis	Movements
Hinge	Uniaxial	Flexion and extension

ATLAS OF MUSCLE ATTACHMENTS: LOWER LIMB

Plate 1

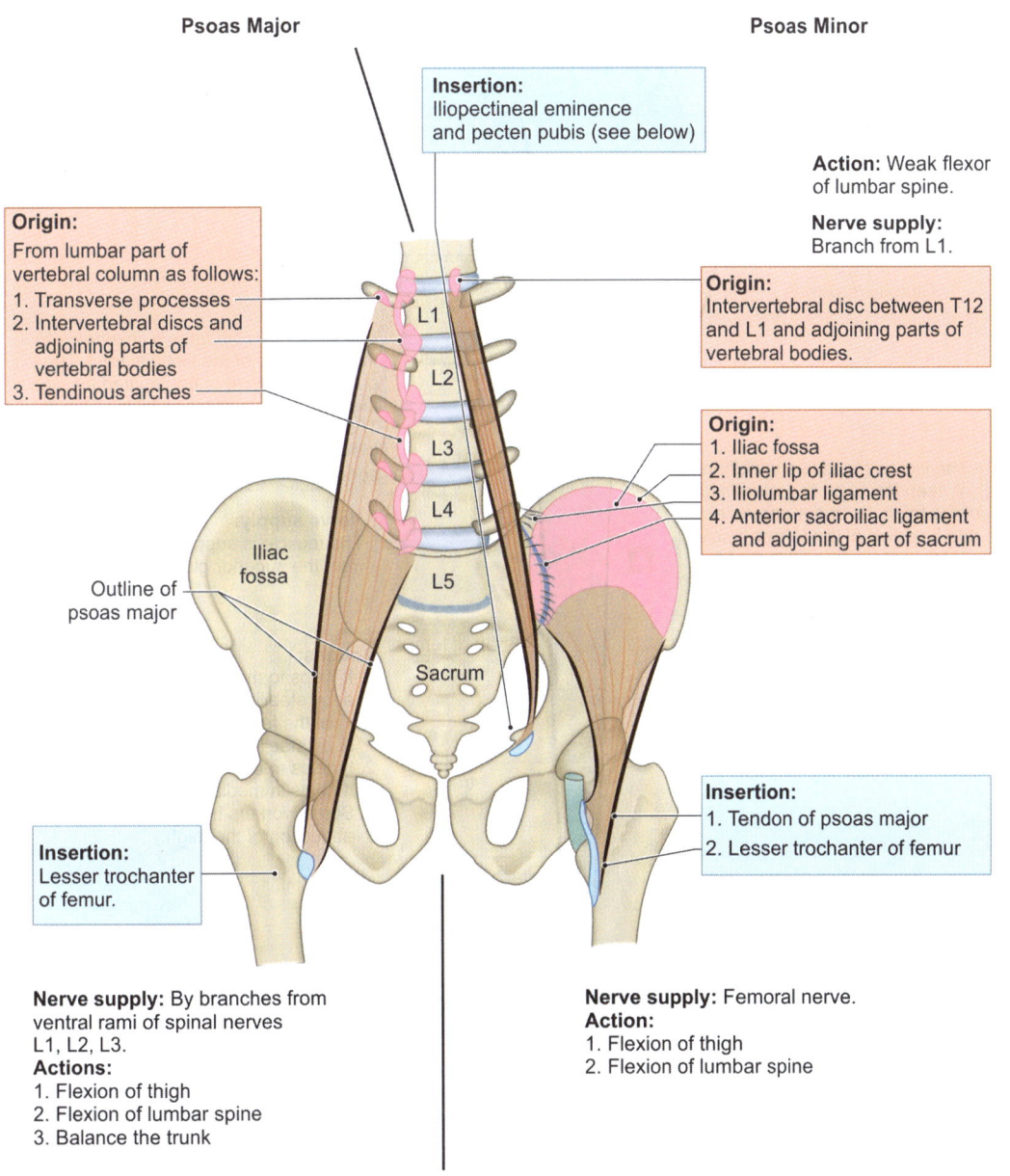

Psoas Major

Insertion: Iliopectineal eminence and pecten pubis (see below)

Origin: From lumbar part of vertebral column as follows:
1. Transverse processes
2. Intervertebral discs and adjoining parts of vertebral bodies
3. Tendinous arches

Outline of psoas major

Iliac fossa

Sacrum

Insertion: Lesser trochanter of femur.

Nerve supply: By branches from ventral rami of spinal nerves L1, L2, L3.
Actions:
1. Flexion of thigh
2. Flexion of lumbar spine
3. Balance the trunk

Psoas Minor

Action: Weak flexor of lumbar spine.

Nerve supply: Branch from L1.

Origin: Intervertebral disc between T12 and L1 and adjoining parts of vertebral bodies.

Origin:
1. Iliac fossa
2. Inner lip of iliac crest
3. Iliolumbar ligament
4. Anterior sacroiliac ligament and adjoining part of sacrum

Insertion:
1. Tendon of psoas major
2. Lesser trochanter of femur

Nerve supply: Femoral nerve.
Action:
1. Flexion of thigh
2. Flexion of lumbar spine

Atlas of Muscle Attachments: Lower Limb

Plate 2

Iliotibial Tract

Tensor Fasciae Latae

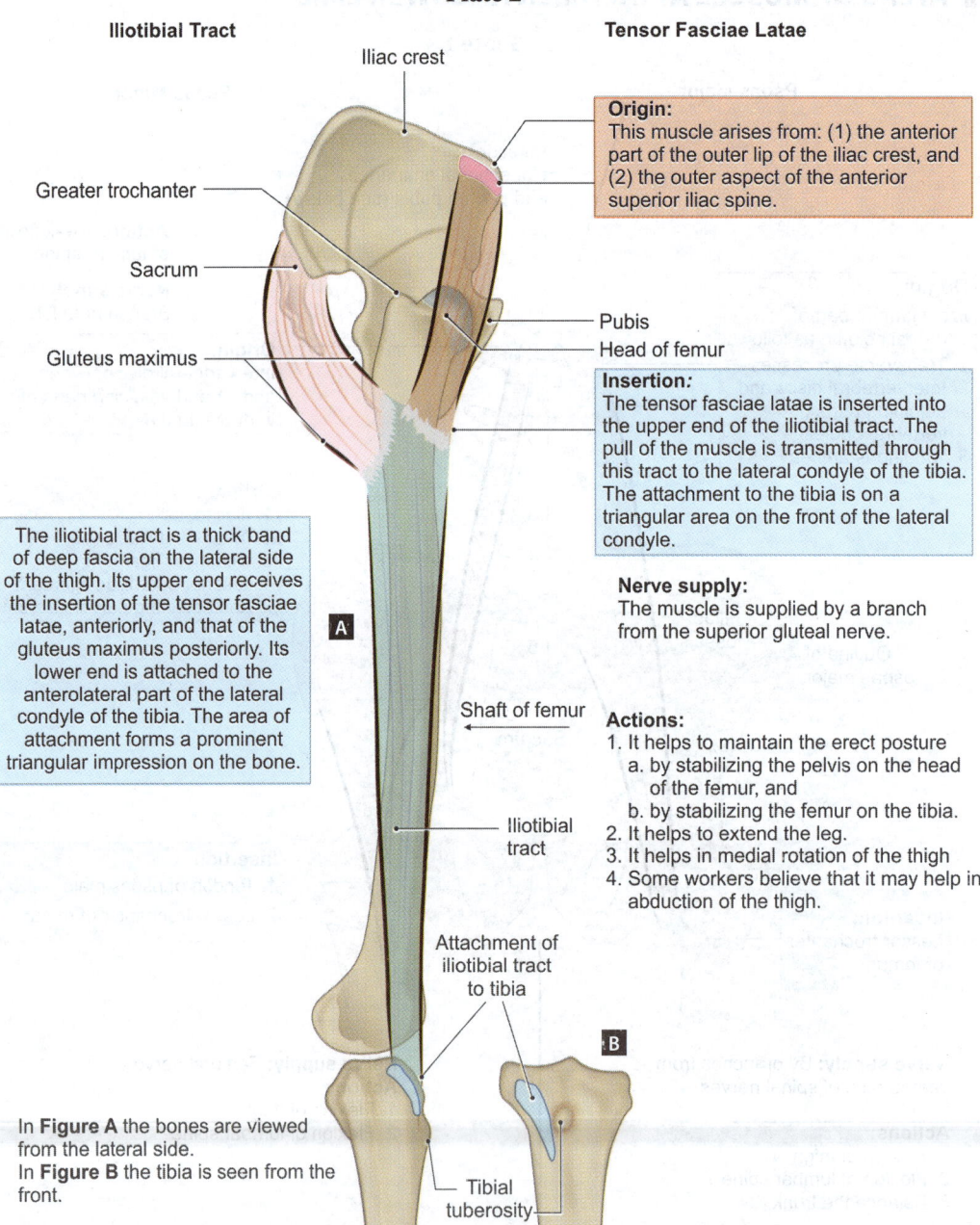

Origin:
This muscle arises from: (1) the anterior part of the outer lip of the iliac crest, and (2) the outer aspect of the anterior superior iliac spine.

Insertion:
The tensor fasciae latae is inserted into the upper end of the iliotibial tract. The pull of the muscle is transmitted through this tract to the lateral condyle of the tibia. The attachment to the tibia is on a triangular area on the front of the lateral condyle.

Nerve supply:
The muscle is supplied by a branch from the superior gluteal nerve.

Actions:
1. It helps to maintain the erect posture
   a. by stabilizing the pelvis on the head of the femur, and
   b. by stabilizing the femur on the tibia.
2. It helps to extend the leg.
3. It helps in medial rotation of the thigh.
4. Some workers believe that it may help in abduction of the thigh.

The iliotibial tract is a thick band of deep fascia on the lateral side of the thigh. Its upper end receives the insertion of the tensor fasciae latae, anteriorly, and that of the gluteus maximus posteriorly. Its lower end is attached to the anterolateral part of the lateral condyle of the tibia. The area of attachment forms a prominent triangular impression on the bone.

In **Figure A** the bones are viewed from the lateral side.
In **Figure B** the tibia is seen from the front.

Atlas of Muscle Attachments: Lower Limb

Plate 3
Sartorius

Inguinal ligament

Sacrum

Origin:
The sartorius arises from the anterior superior iliac spine (and a small area below it).

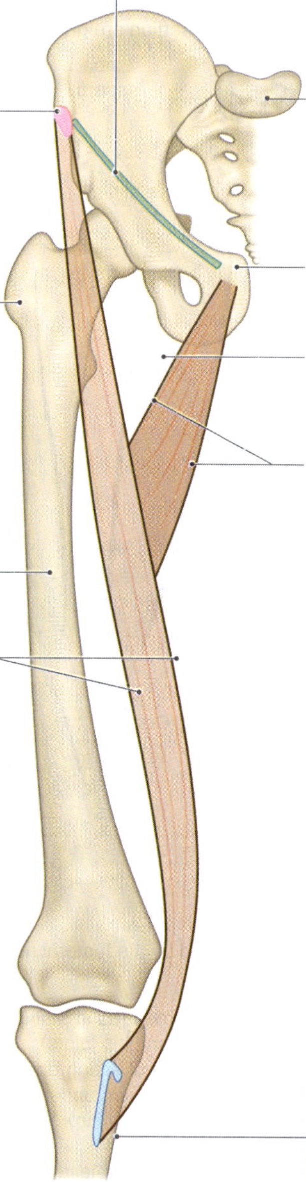

Pubis

Greater trochanter

Femoral triangle

Nerve supply:
Femoral nerve

Outline of adductor longus

Shaft of femur

Note:
1. The medial border of the upper part of the sartorius forms the lateral boundary of the femoral triangle.
2. In the middle one-third of the thigh the muscle forms the roof of the adductor canal.

Outline of sartorius

Actions:
The sartorius helps in:
1. Flexion of the leg (at knee joint)
2. Flexion of the thigh (at hip joint)
3. Abduction of thigh
4. Lateral rotation of thigh

Insertion:
The muscle runs downward and medially across the front of the thigh to reach the upper end of the tibia. It is inserted along a vertical line on the upper part of the medial surface of this bone. The insertion is anterior to that of the gracilis and of the semitendinosus.

Plate 4

Quadriceps Femoris

This muscle consists of four parts. These are the rectus femoris and three vasti (vastus lateralis, vastus medialis, and vastus intermedius). The relative positions of these can be understood from the figure below in which the upper parts of the rectus femoris, the vastus lateralis and the vastus medialis have been removed. For details of origin of each part see the next page. Details of insertion are given below.

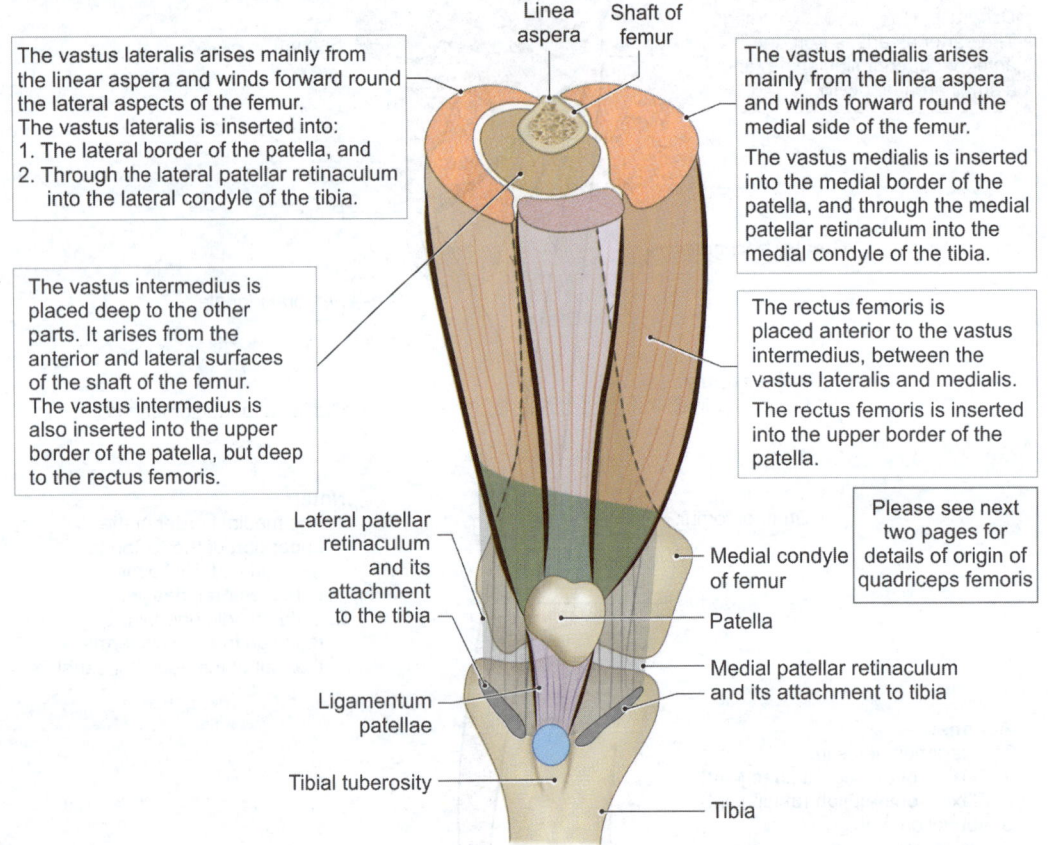

The vastus lateralis arises mainly from the linear aspera and winds forward round the lateral aspects of the femur.
The vastus lateralis is inserted into:
1. The lateral border of the patella, and
2. Through the lateral patellar retinaculum into the lateral condyle of the tibia.

The vastus intermedius is placed deep to the other parts. It arises from the anterior and lateral surfaces of the shaft of the femur.
The vastus intermedius is also inserted into the upper border of the patella, but deep to the rectus femoris.

The vastus medialis arises mainly from the linea aspera and winds forward round the medial side of the femur.
The vastus medialis is inserted into the medial border of the patella, and through the medial patellar retinaculum into the medial condyle of the tibia.

The rectus femoris is placed anterior to the vastus intermedius, between the vastus lateralis and medialis.
The rectus femoris is inserted into the upper border of the patella.

Please see next two pages for details of origin of quadriceps femoris

Nerve supply: The quadriceps femoris is supplied by the femoral nerve.

Actions:
The muscle straightens the lower extremity at the knee (as in standing up from a sitting position). This involves extension of both the leg and the thigh (at the knee and hip joints).
The muscle is also active in the opposite movement of sitting down. Here its gradual relaxation allows proper control of flexion of the knee (i.e. it prevents sudden flexion under the influence of gravity).
The rectus femoris can produce flexion of the thigh (at the hip). With the thigh fixed (as in standing) it can rotate the pelvis forward on the head of the femur.
The vastus medialis prevents lateral displacement of the patella during extension of the knee.

Note: The muscle is not active while standing upright because the knee is locked when the knee is fully extended.

Atlas of Muscle Attachments: Lower Limb

Plate 5
Quadriceps Femoris

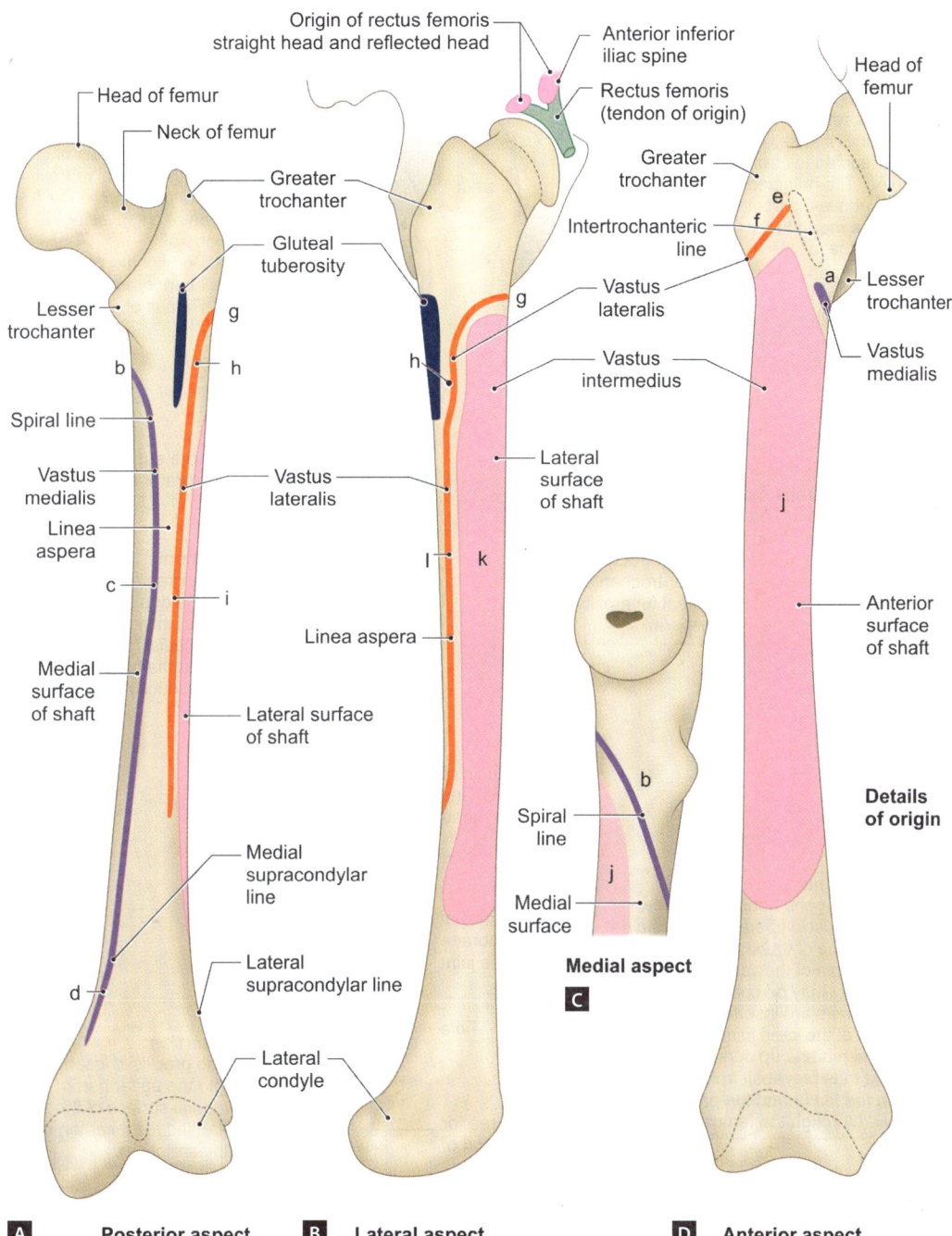

Atlas of Muscle Attachments: Lower Limb

Plate 6
Gracilis

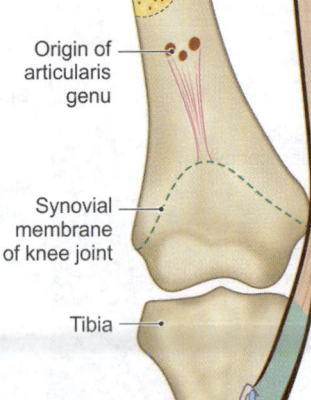

Quadriceps Femoris (Continued)

Details of origin are as follows:
The **rectus femoris** has a tendinous origin from the hip bone. It arises by two heads. The straight head arises from the anterior inferior iliac spine. The reflected heads arises from the ilium just above the acetabulum.
The **vastus medialis** has a long linear origin from the following:
1. The lower part of intertrochanteric line.
2. The spiral line
3. The medial lip of the linea aspera.
4. The medial supracondylar line.

The **vastus intermedius** arises from a large area extending onto the following:
1. Anterior surface of shaft
2. Lateral surface of shaft. The medial surface of the shaft does not give origin to the muscle but is covered by it.

The **vastus lateralis** has a long linear origin from the following:
1. The upper end of the intertrochanteric line.
2. The interior border of the greater trochanter.
3. The lower border of the greater trochanter.
4. The lateral margin of the gluteal tuberosity.
5. The lateral lip of the linea aspera.

Origin:
This muscle takes origin from the medial margin of the pubic arch. The area of origin includes parts of:
1. Body of the pubis.
2. Inferior ramus of pubis.
3. Ramus of ischium.

Nerve supply:
Obturator nerve.

Actions:
The gracilis helps in:
1. Flexion of the leg (at the knee joint).
2. Medial rotation of thigh (at the hip joint).
3. Adduction of the thigh.

Articularis Genu
The articularis genu consists of a few fascicles of muscle fibers arising from the anterior surface of the shaft of the femur, below the origin of the vastus intermedius (of which they may be considered a separated part). The fibers are inserted into the synovial membrane of the knee joint. The fibers pull the synovial membrane up during extension of the knee, and thus prevent it from being pinched between the femur and the patella. The muscle is supplied through the femoral nerve.

Insertion:
The gracilis is inserted into the upper part of the medial surface of the tibia (behind the insertion of the sartorius).

Atlas of Muscle Attachments: Lower Limb

Plate 7
Pectineus

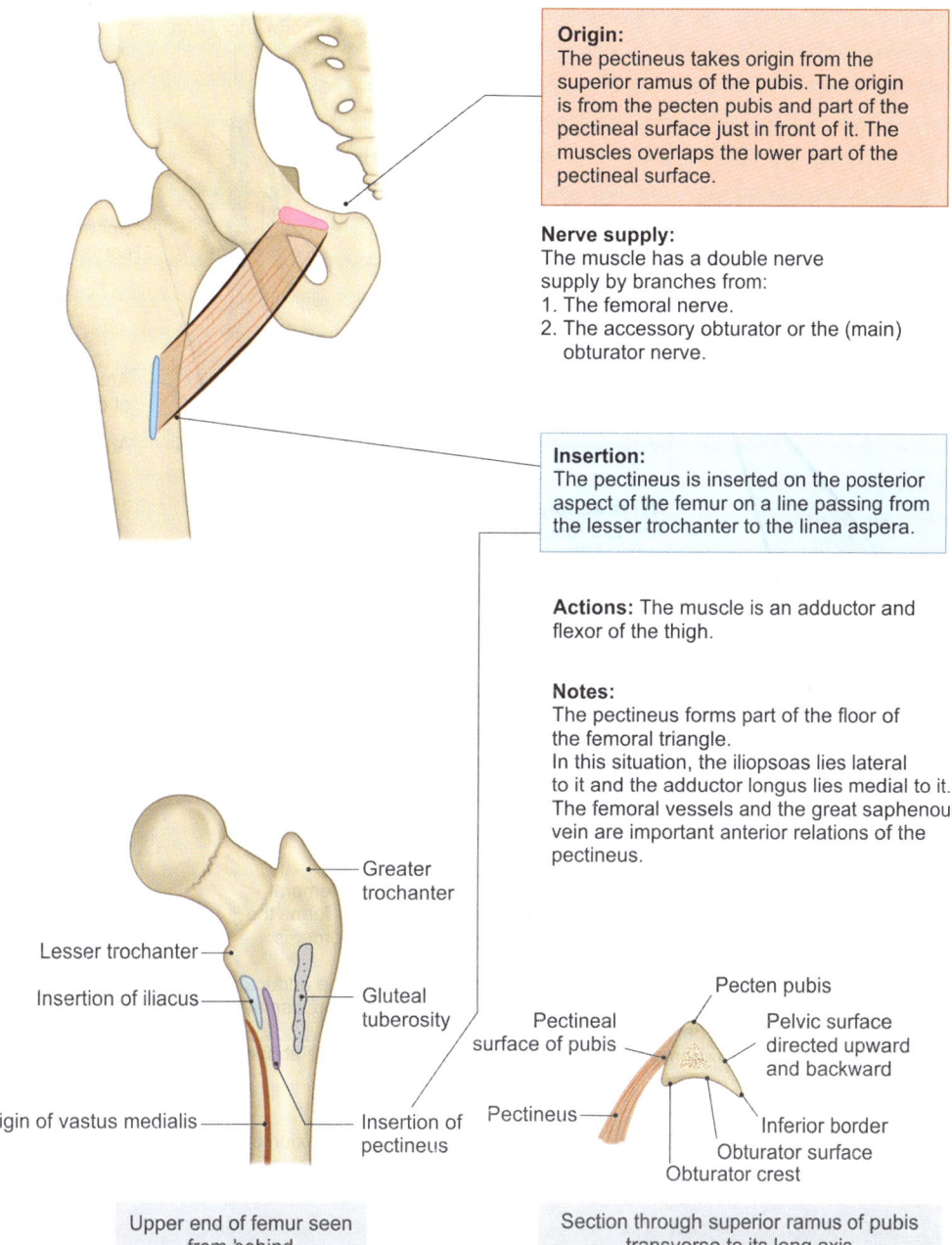

Origin:
The pectineus takes origin from the superior ramus of the pubis. The origin is from the pecten pubis and part of the pectineal surface just in front of it. The muscles overlaps the lower part of the pectineal surface.

Nerve supply:
The muscle has a double nerve supply by branches from:
1. The femoral nerve.
2. The accessory obturator or the (main) obturator nerve.

Insertion:
The pectineus is inserted on the posterior aspect of the femur on a line passing from the lesser trochanter to the linea aspera.

Actions: The muscle is an adductor and flexor of the thigh.

Notes:
The pectineus forms part of the floor of the femoral triangle.
In this situation, the iliopsoas lies lateral to it and the adductor longus lies medial to it. The femoral vessels and the great saphenous vein are important anterior relations of the pectineus.

Atlas of Muscle Attachments: Lower Limb

Plate 8
Adductor Longus

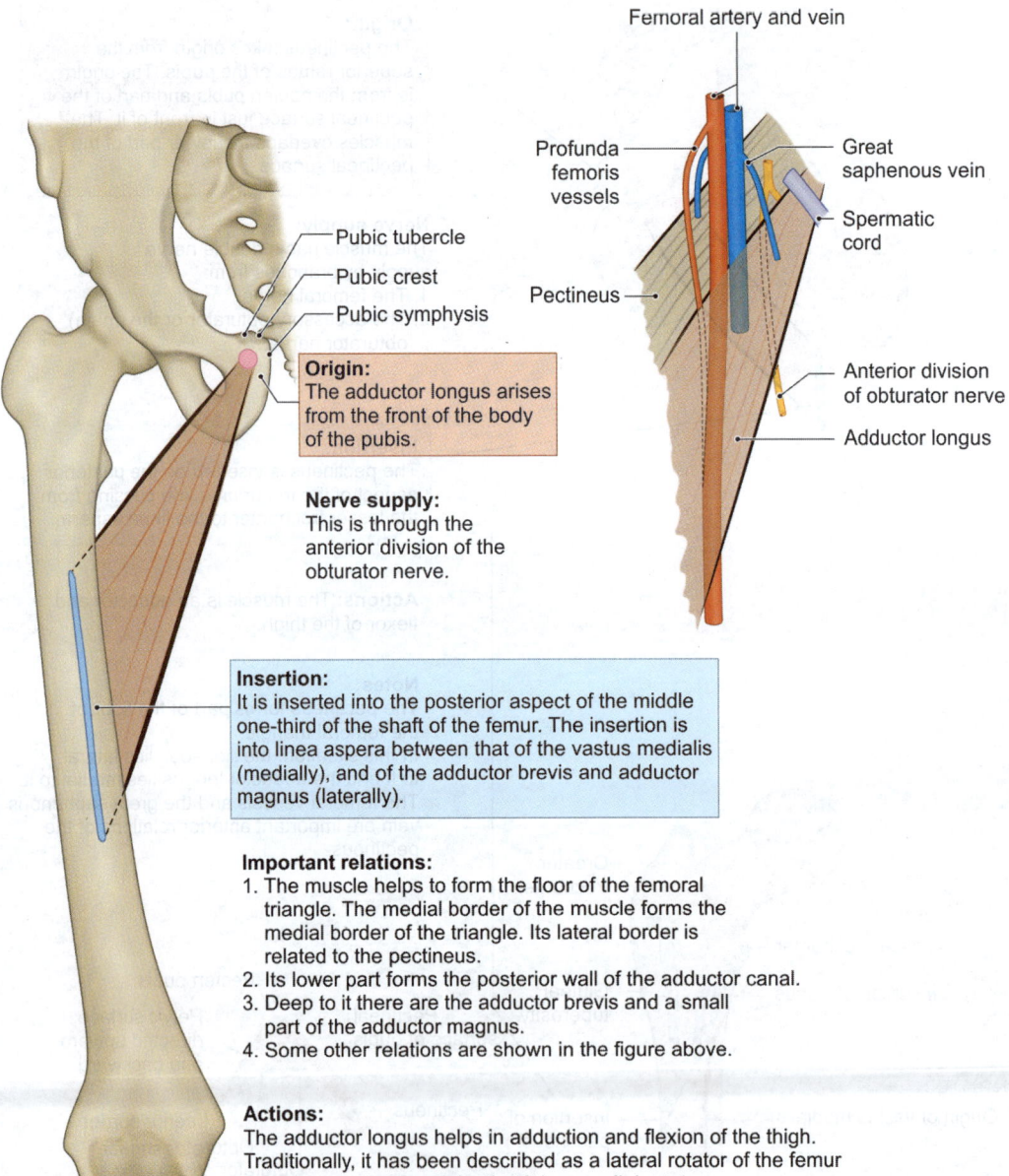

Origin:
The adductor longus arises from the front of the body of the pubis.

Nerve supply:
This is through the anterior division of the obturator nerve.

Insertion:
It is inserted into the posterior aspect of the middle one-third of the shaft of the femur. The insertion is into linea aspera between that of the vastus medialis (medially), and of the adductor brevis and adductor magnus (laterally).

Important relations:
1. The muscle helps to form the floor of the femoral triangle. The medial border of the muscle forms the medial border of the triangle. Its lateral border is related to the pectineus.
2. Its lower part forms the posterior wall of the adductor canal.
3. Deep to it there are the adductor brevis and a small part of the adductor magnus.
4. Some other relations are shown in the figure above.

Actions:
The adductor longus helps in adduction and flexion of the thigh. Traditionally, it has been described as a lateral rotator of the femur but some authorities claim that it is a medial rotator.

Atlas of Muscle Attachments: Lower Limb

Plate 9

Attachments to the Posterior Aspect of the Shaft of the Femur

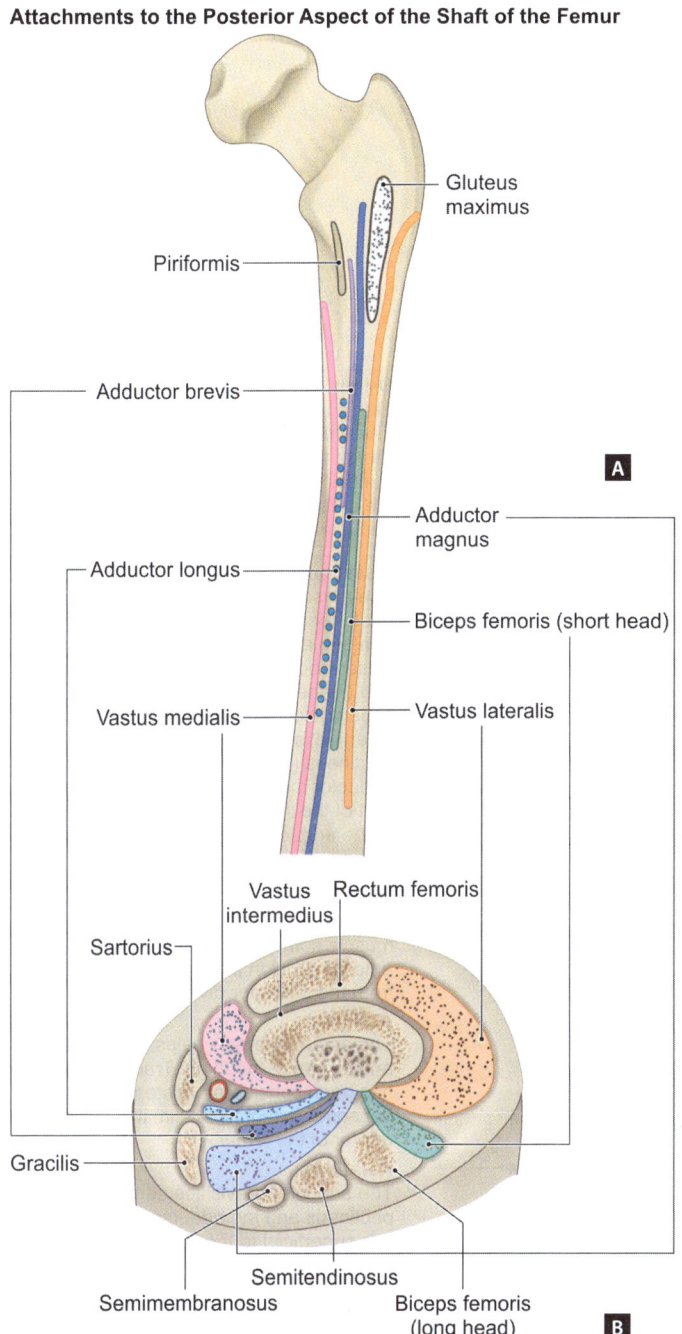

The posterior border of the shaft of the femur is in the form of a broad rough ridge called the **linea aspera**. Several muscles are attached to this ridge. From lateral to medial side these are:
1. Origin of vastus lateralis
2. Origin of short head of biceps femoris
3. Insertion of adductor magnus
4. Insertion of adductor brevis
5. Insertion of adductor longus
6. Origin of vastus medialis.

The logic for this sequence is easily understood when the relative position of the muscles as seen in a transverse section through the thigh is kept in mind.

In **Figure B** note the femoral vessels. The triangular space in which they lie is the **adductor canal**. The canal is bounded anteriorly and laterally by the vastus medialis, behind by the adductor longus (and at a lower level by the adductor magnus) and medially by the sartorius. (Note that the adductor brevis is shown schematically and would not be seen in a section at this level).

Plate 10

Adductor Brevis

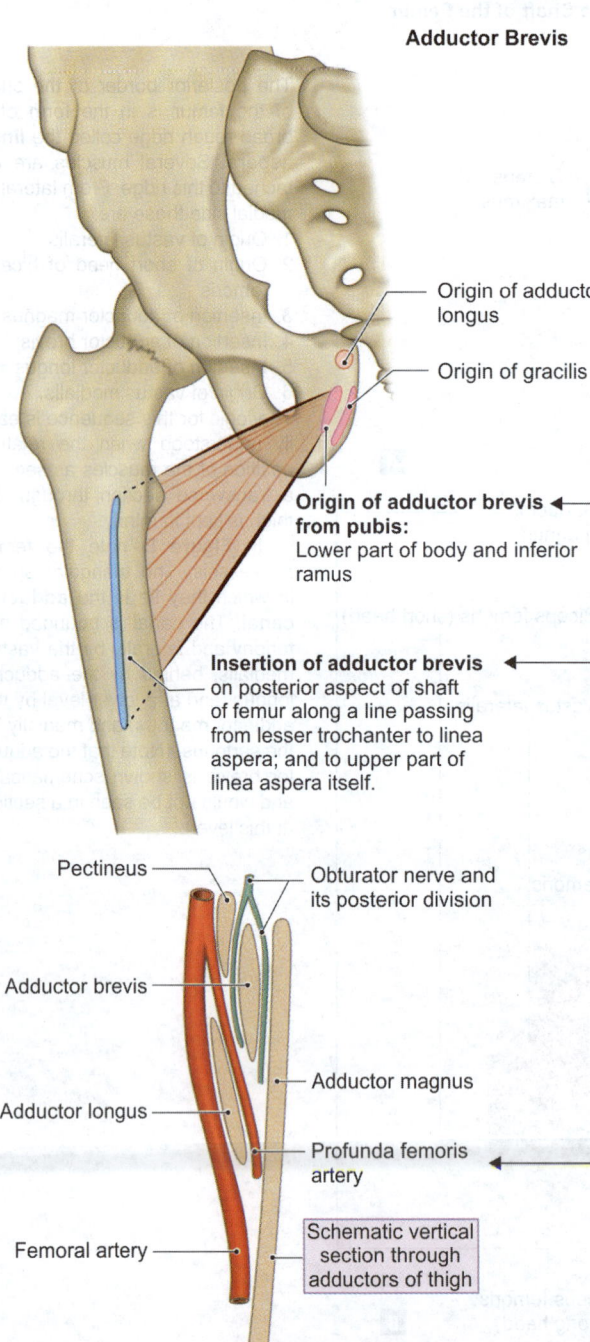

Origin of adductor longus

Origin of gracilis

Origin of adductor brevis from pubis: Lower part of body and inferior ramus

Insertion of adductor brevis on posterior aspect of shaft of femur along a line passing from lesser trochanter to linea aspera; and to upper part of linea aspera itself.

Pectineus

Obturator nerve and its posterior division

Adductor brevis

Adductor magnus

Adductor longus

Profunda femoris artery

Femoral artery

Schematic vertical section through adductors of thigh

Origin:
This muscle arises from the pubis: The area of origin includes the lower part of the body and the inferior ramus. The origin is lateral to that of the gracilis and below that of the adductor longus.

Insertion:
The muscle is inserted on the posterior aspect of the femur (i) along a line passing from the lesser trochanter to the linea aspera, and (ii) the upper part of the linea aspera itself. The upper end of the insertion is between those of the pectineus (medially), and of the adductor magnus (laterally). The lower part of the insertion is between those of the adductor longus (medially) and of the adductor magnus.

Nerve supply:
Obturator nerve. The branch to the muscle sometimes arises from the anterior division and sometimes from the posterior division.

Actions:
The adductor brevis helps in adduction and flexion of the thigh. Traditionally, it has been considered a lateral rotator but some authorities claim it is a medial rotator of the femur.

Relations:
The adductor brevis lies deep to the pectineus and the adductor longus. It is superficial to the adductor magnus. The profunda femoris vessels and the anterior division of the obturator nerve run downward anterior to it. The posterior division of the obturator nerve is deep (i.e. posterior) to it.

Atlas of Muscle Attachments: Lower Limb

Plate 11

Adductor Magnus

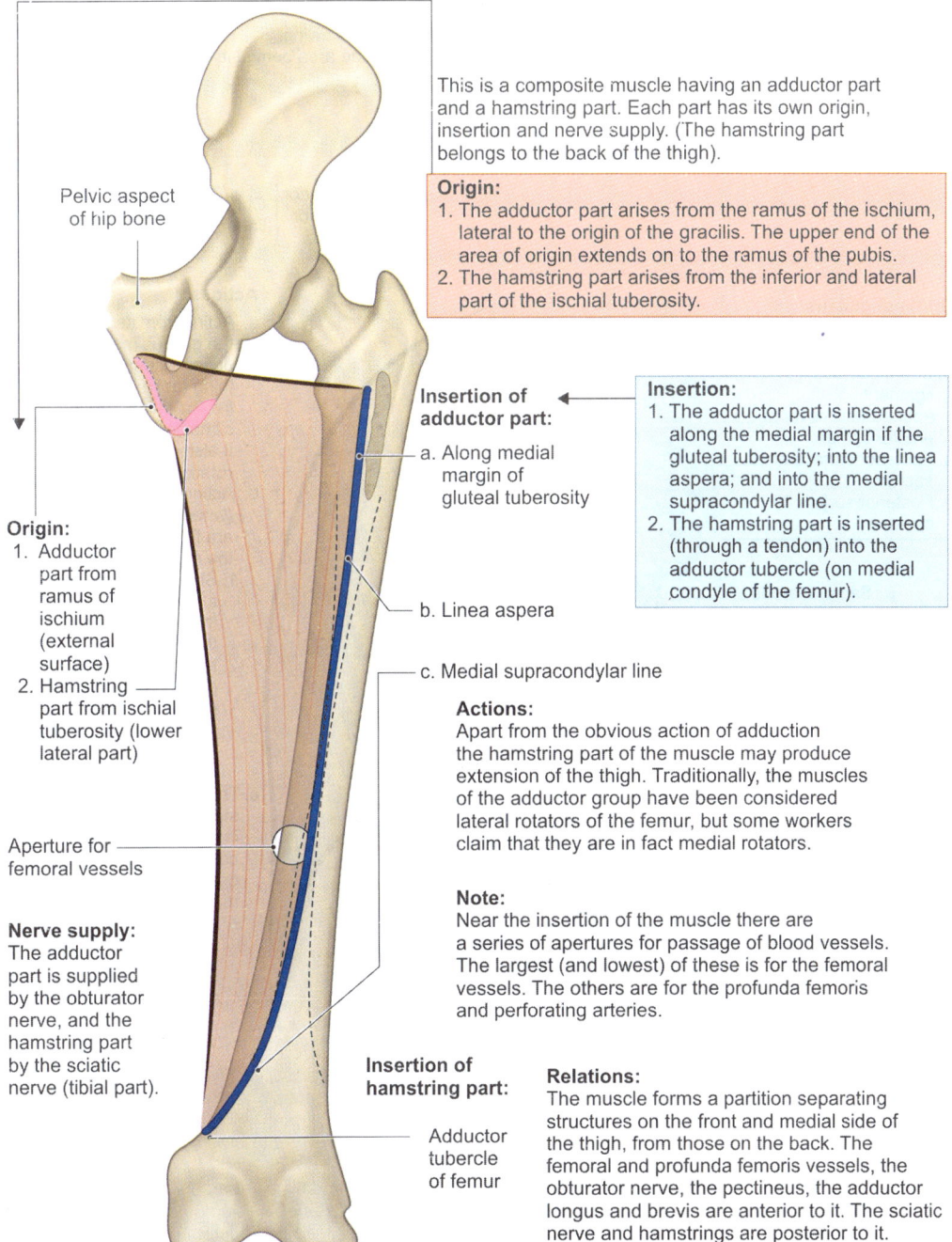

This is a composite muscle having an adductor part and a hamstring part. Each part has its own origin, insertion and nerve supply. (The hamstring part belongs to the back of the thigh).

Origin:
1. The adductor part arises from the ramus of the ischium, lateral to the origin of the gracilis. The upper end of the area of origin extends on to the ramus of the pubis.
2. The hamstring part arises from the inferior and lateral part of the ischial tuberosity.

Insertion:
1. The adductor part is inserted along the medial margin if the gluteal tuberosity; into the linea aspera; and into the medial supracondylar line.
2. The hamstring part is inserted (through a tendon) into the adductor tubercle (on medial condyle of the femur).

Actions:
Apart from the obvious action of adduction the hamstring part of the muscle may produce extension of the thigh. Traditionally, the muscles of the adductor group have been considered lateral rotators of the femur, but some workers claim that they are in fact medial rotators.

Note:
Near the insertion of the muscle there are a series of apertures for passage of blood vessels. The largest (and lowest) of these is for the femoral vessels. The others are for the profunda femoris and perforating arteries.

Relations:
The muscle forms a partition separating structures on the front and medial side of the thigh, from those on the back. The femoral and profunda femoris vessels, the obturator nerve, the pectineus, the adductor longus and brevis are anterior to it. The sciatic nerve and hamstrings are posterior to it.

Labels on figure:
- Pelvic aspect of hip bone
- Origin:
  1. Adductor part from ramus of ischium (external surface)
  2. Hamstring part from ischial tuberosity (lower lateral part)
- Aperture for femoral vessels
- Nerve supply: The adductor part is supplied by the obturator nerve, and the hamstring part by the sciatic nerve (tibial part).
- Insertion of adductor part:
  a. Along medial margin of gluteal tuberosity
  b. Linea aspera
  c. Medial supracondylar line
- Insertion of hamstring part: Adductor tubercle of femur

174 Atlas of Muscle Attachments: Lower Limb

Plate 12
Gluteus Maximus

Origin:
The gluteus maximus arises from one large area that extends onto the following:
1. External surface of the ilium including the posterior gluteal line and the area behind it.
2. The sacrotuberous ligament.
3. The aponeurosis covering the erector spinae.
4. The lower lateral part of the posterior surface of the sacrum.
5. The lateral part of the posterior surface of the coccyx.

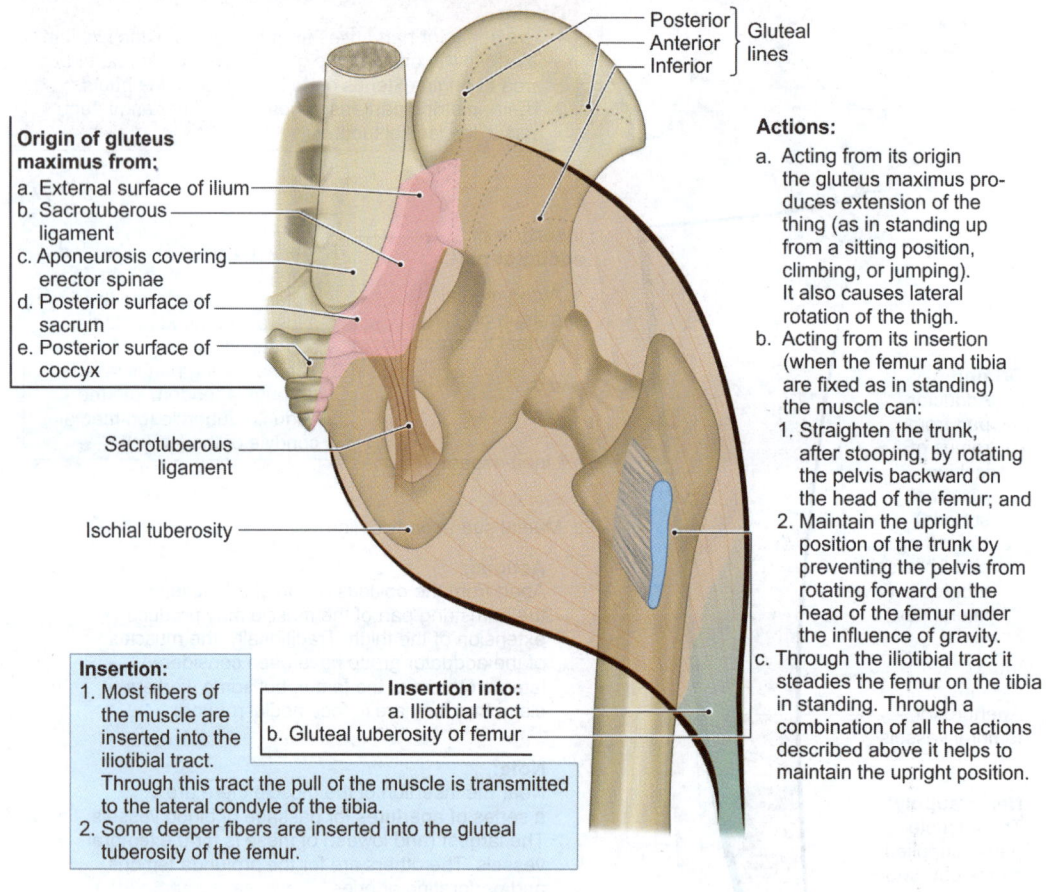

Origin of gluteus maximus from:
a. External surface of ilium
b. Sacrotuberous ligament
c. Aponeurosis covering erector spinae
d. Posterior surface of sacrum
e. Posterior surface of coccyx

Sacrotuberous ligament

Ischial tuberosity

Posterior / Anterior / Inferior — Gluteal lines

Insertion into:
a. Iliotibial tract
b. Gluteal tuberosity of femur

Actions:
a. Acting from its origin the gluteus maximus produces extension of the thing (as in standing up from a sitting position, climbing, or jumping). It also causes lateral rotation of the thigh.
b. Acting from its insertion (when the femur and tibia are fixed as in standing) the muscle can:
   1. Straighten the trunk, after stooping, by rotating the pelvis backward on the head of the femur; and
   2. Maintain the upright position of the trunk by preventing the pelvis from rotating forward on the head of the femur under the influence of gravity.
c. Through the iliotibial tract it steadies the femur on the tibia in standing. Through a combination of all the actions described above it helps to maintain the upright position.

Insertion:
1. Most fibers of the muscle are inserted into the iliotibial tract. Through this tract the pull of the muscle is transmitted to the lateral condyle of the tibia.
2. Some deeper fibers are inserted into the gluteal tuberosity of the femur.

Nerve supply:
This is through the inferior gluteal nerve (L5, S1, S2).

Atlas of Muscle Attachments: Lower Limb 175

Plate 13

Structures Deep to the Gluteus Maximus

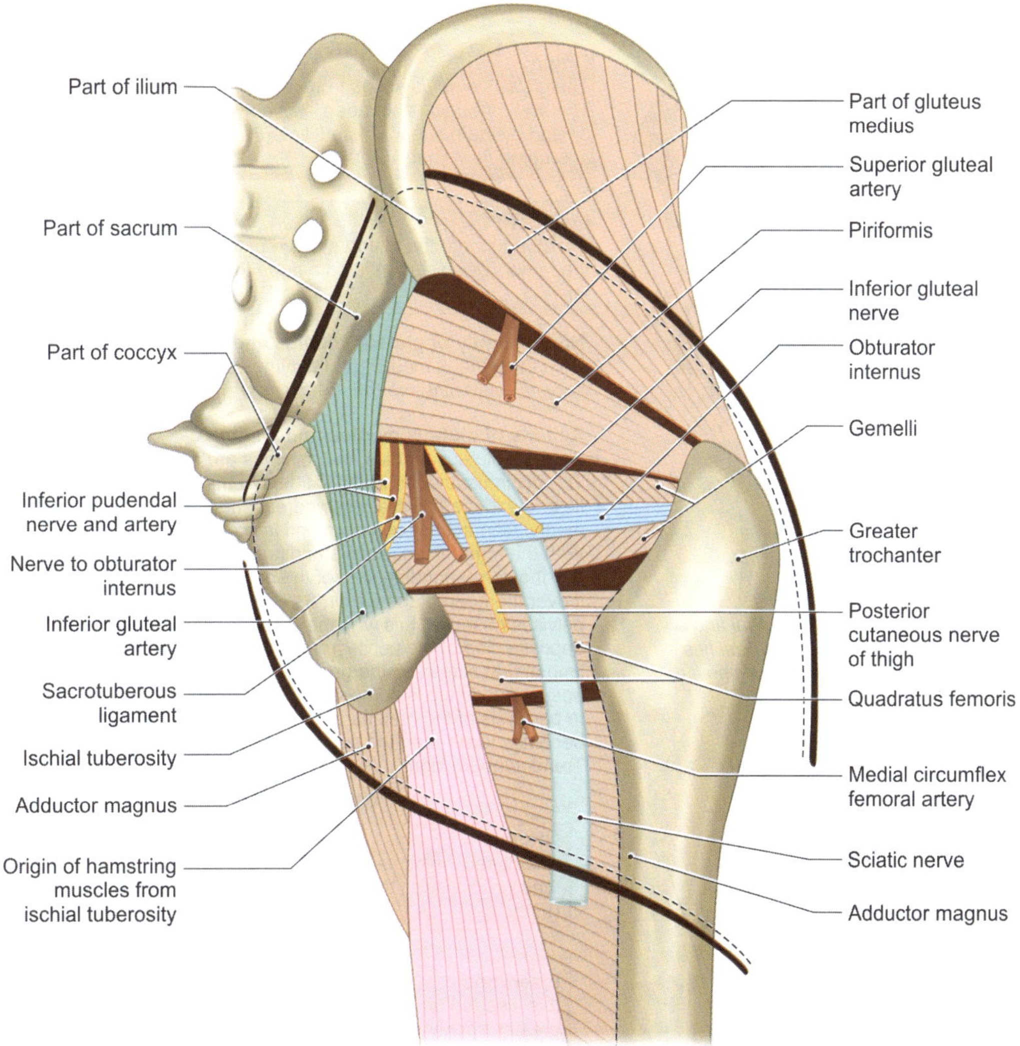

- Part of ilium
- Part of sacrum
- Part of coccyx
- Inferior pudendal nerve and artery
- Nerve to obturator internus
- Inferior gluteal artery
- Sacrotuberous ligament
- Ischial tuberosity
- Adductor magnus
- Origin of hamstring muscles from ischial tuberosity

- Part of gluteus medius
- Superior gluteal artery
- Piriformis
- Inferior gluteal nerve
- Obturator internus
- Gemelli
- Greater trochanter
- Posterior cutaneous nerve of thigh
- Quadratus femoris
- Medial circumflex femoral artery
- Sciatic nerve
- Adductor magnus

The outline of the gluteus maximus is shown in thick brown line.

Plate 14

Gluteus Medius

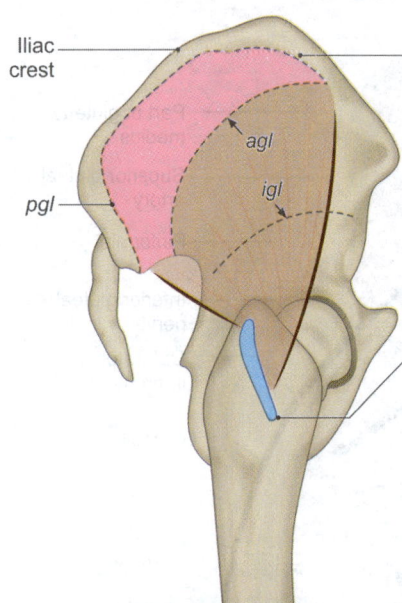

Origin:
The gluteus medius arises from the outer surface of the ilium. The area of origin is bounded above by the iliac crest, behind by the posterior gluteal line (PGL), and in front by the anterior gluteal line (AGL).

Insertion:
It is inserted into the lateral surface of the greater trochanter of the femur. The insertion is on a ridge that runs downward and forward.

Nerve supply of gluteus medius and minimus:
Both the gluteus medius and minimus are supplied by the superior gluteal nerve (L5, S1).

Actions of gluteus medius and minimus:
Both the gluteus medius and minimus are abductors of the thigh. The minimus and the anterior fibers of the medius can act as flexors and medial rotators, whereas the posterior fibers of the medius can act as extensors and lateral rotators of the thigh. With the femur fixed (as in standing) the medius and minimus pull the corresponding side of the pelvis downward by rotating it over the head of the femur. As a result the opposite side of the pelvis is raised. In this way the muscles of one side prevent the opposite side of the pelvis from sinking downward when the limb of that side is off the ground. In fact the pelvis on the unsupported side is somewhat higher than on the supported side. In paralysis of the medius and minimus the unsupported side becomes lower than the supported side. This is referred to as the Trendelenburg sign.

agl = Anterior gluteal line
pgl = Posterior gluteal line
igl = Inferior gluteal line

Gluteus Minimus

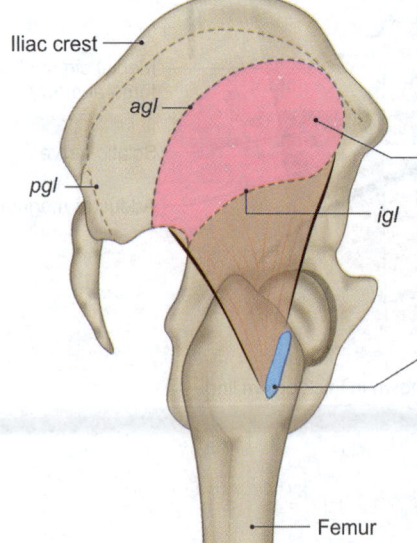

Origin:
The gluteus minimus arises from the outer surface of the ilium between the anterior and inferior gluteal lines (IGL).

Insertion:
It is inserted on the ridge on the anterior aspect of the greater trochanter of the femur.

Nerve supply and action: See under gluteus medius.

Atlas of Muscle Attachments: Lower Limb

Plate 15

Piriformis

Origin
From anterior surface of sacrum (lateral part)

The muscle arises within pelvis. It leaves the pelvis through the greater sciatic foramen to reach the gluteal region.

Origin:
The piriformis from the lateral part of the anterior (or pelvic) aspect of the sacrum. The origin is by three digitations each of which arises from the area between two sacral foramina. A few fibers arise from the ilium (outer surface) near the posterior inferior iliac spine.

Insertion:
The muscle is inserted into the upper border of the greater trochanter of the femur.

Nerve supply:
The muscle is innervated by direct branches from L5, S1, S2.

Action:
The piriformis is a lateral rotator of the femur.

A — Sacrum: Anterior aspects

Sacrum and hip: Posterior aspects

B — Insertion: Greater trochanter of femur, on its upper border

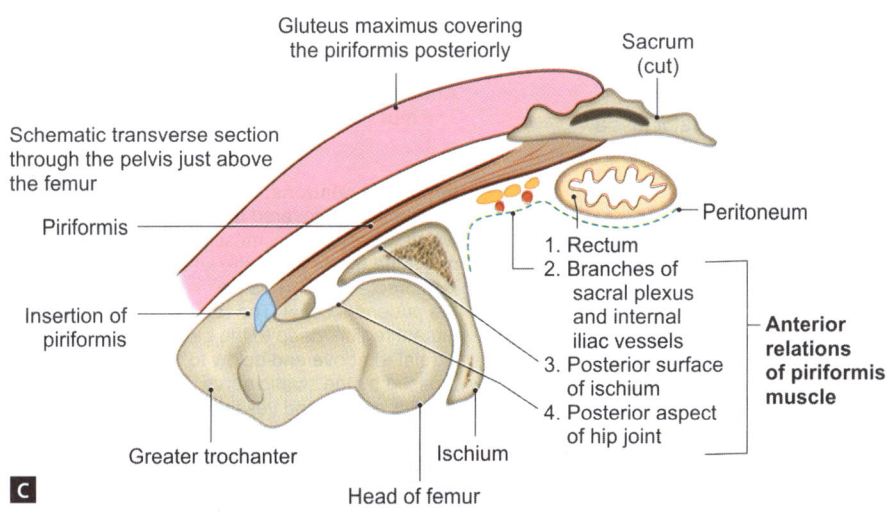

Schematic transverse section through the pelvis just above the femur

- Piriformis
- Insertion of piriformis
- Greater trochanter
- Ischium
- Head of femur
- Gluteus maximus covering the piriformis posteriorly
- Sacrum (cut)
- Peritoneum

Anterior relations of piriformis muscle:
1. Rectum
2. Branches of sacral plexus and internal iliac vessels
3. Posterior surface of ischium
4. Posterior aspect of hip joint

C

Plate 16
Obturator Internus

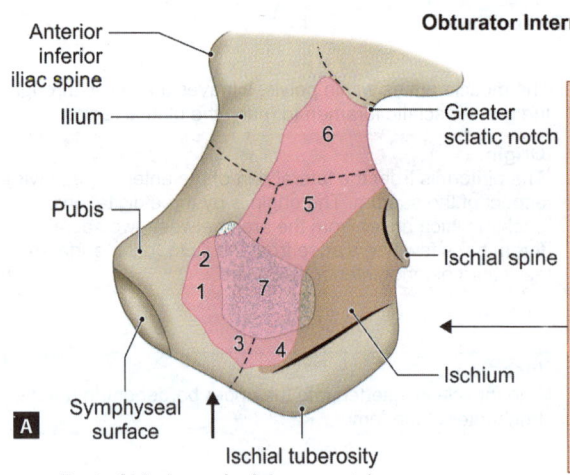

A. Part of hip bone (pelvic aspects)

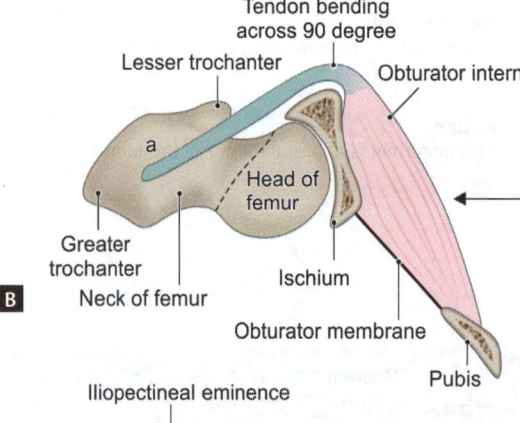

B.

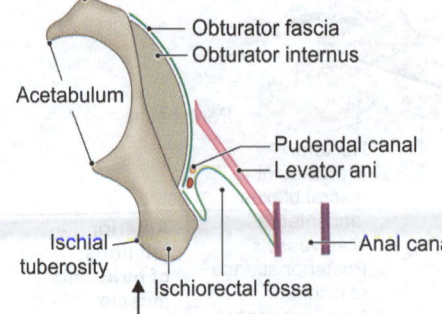

C. Vertical section through anterior and inferior part of hip bone

Origin:
This muscle arises from the inner (pelvic) surface of the hip bone and from the pelvic surface of the obturator membrane. The area of origin covers the following parts of the hip bone. Body (1), the superior ramus (2), and the inferior ramus (3) of the pubis; ramus (4) and body (5) of the ischium; and part of the pelvic surface of the ilium (6). The obturator membrane is shown at 7. The fibers of the muscle converge toward a tendon which leaves the pelvis through the lesser sciatic foramen to enter the gluteal region. The tendon turns through 90 degrees and runs laterally behind the hip joint to reach its insertion.

Nerve supply:
The muscle is supplied by the nerve to obturator internus (L5, S1).

Scheme to show arrangement of the obturator internus. The upper part of the pelvis has been removed by cutting transversely across the ischium and pubis, The femur is seen from above.

Insertion:
The tendon is inserted into anterior part of the medial surface of the greater trochanter of the femur. The insertion is above and in front of the trochanteric fossa ('a' in Fig. B) (into which the obturator externus is inserted).

Actions:
The muscle is a lateral rotator of the femur.

Important relations:
The muscle is covered by obturator fascia from which the levator ani muscle arises. Below this origin the fascia forms the lateral wall of the ischiorectal fossa. This wall is closely related to the pudendal canal. The tendon runs across the gluteal region, deep to the gluteus maximus. It is related above and below to the gemelli. It is crossed by the sciatic nerve, and by several smaller nerves and vessels.

Plate 17

Gemelli

These are two small muscles situated in the gluteal region, above and below the tendon of the obturator internus.

Origin:
The superior gemellus arises from the posterior aspect of the ischial spine. The inferior gemellus takes origin from the uppermost part of the ischial tuberosity.

Insertion:
The gemelli are inserted into the tendon of the obturator internus (and exert their pull through it on the greater trochanter of the femur).

Nerve supply:
The superior gemellus is supplied by the nerve to the obturator internus (L5, S1). The inferior gemellus is supplied by a branch from the nerve to the quadratus femoris (L5, S1).

Action:
The gemelli help in lateral rotation of the femur.

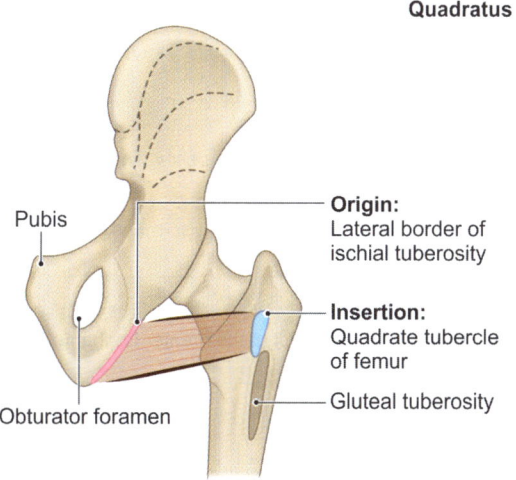

Quadratus Femoris

Origin:
The quadratus femoris takes origin from the lateral border of the ischial tuberosity.

Insertion:
It is inserted into the quadrate tubercle. This is a bony elevation present on the upper part of the trochanteric crest of the femur.

Nerve supply:
The nerve to the quadratus femoris is a branch from the sacral plexus (L4, L5, S1).

Action:
The quadratus femoris is a lateral rotator of the femur.

Atlas of Muscle Attachments: Lower Limb

Plate 18
Obturator Externus

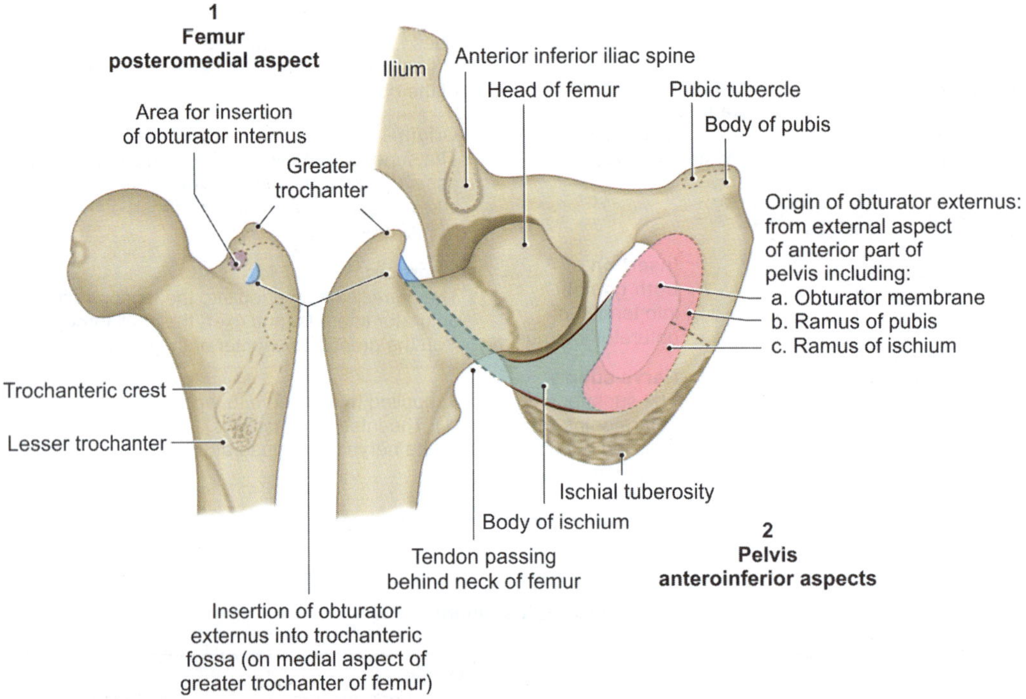

1 Femur posteromedial aspect

- Area for insertion of obturator internus
- Greater trochanter
- Ilium
- Anterior inferior iliac spine
- Head of femur
- Pubic tubercle
- Body of pubis
- Origin of obturator externus: from external aspect of anterior part of pelvis including:
  a. Obturator membrane
  b. Ramus of pubis
  c. Ramus of ischium
- Trochanteric crest
- Lesser trochanter
- Ischial tuberosity
- Body of ischium
- Tendon passing behind neck of femur
- Insertion of obturator externus into trochanteric fossa (on medial aspect of greater trochanter of femur)

2 Pelvis anteroinferior aspects

Origin:
The obturator externus takes origin from the external surface of the anterior part of the pelvis. The area of origin covers parts of the following:
1. Ramus of ischium, 2. Ramus of pubis, 3. Obturator membrane (medial two-thirds).
The muscle ends in a tendon that runs upward and laterally behind the neck of the femur to reach the gluteal region.

Insertion:
The tendon is inserted into the trochanteric fossa (situated on the medial aspect of the greater trochanter) of the femur.

Nerve supply:
The muscle is supplied by a branch from the obturator nerve (L3, L4).

Actions:
It is a lateral rotator of the femur.

Note on actions of small muscles around the hip joint.
Although the various small muscles related to the hip joint are described as medial or lateral rotators, their main action is to stabilize the joint. In performing this action they have an advantage over ligaments in that they can fix the joint in any position, whereas a ligament can do so only when fully stretched. Such muscles are, therefore, sometimes referred to as extensible or adjustable ligaments.

Atlas of Muscle Attachments: Lower Limb

Plate 19

Semitendinosus

The muscle is so called because its lower half is tendinous. It belongs to the hamstring group of muscles.

Origin:
The semitendinosus arises from the upper and medial part of the ischial tuberosity, in common with the biceps femoris.

Insertion:
On reaching the knee the tendon of the semitendinosus runs forward across the tibial collateral ligament to be inserted into the upper part of the medial surface of the shaft of the tibia. The area of insertion is behind that of the sartorius, and below and behind that for the gracilis.

Nerve supply:
Tibial part of sciatic nerve.

Actions:
(Common to all hamstring muscles)
1. Acting from their origin (i.e. when the pelvis is fixed) the hamstring muscles flex the leg at the knee joint.
2. Acting from their insertion (i.e. when the knee is fixed, as in standing upright) they exert a downward pull on the ischial tuberosity. This is useful:
   a. In preventing the pelvis from rolling forward on the head of the femur, and
   b. In straightening the trunk after bending forward.

Hamstrings
The long muscles of the back of the thigh that take origin from the ischial tuberosity (i.e. biceps femoris, semitendinosus, semimembranosus) are called the hamstring muscles. Their common actions have been given above.

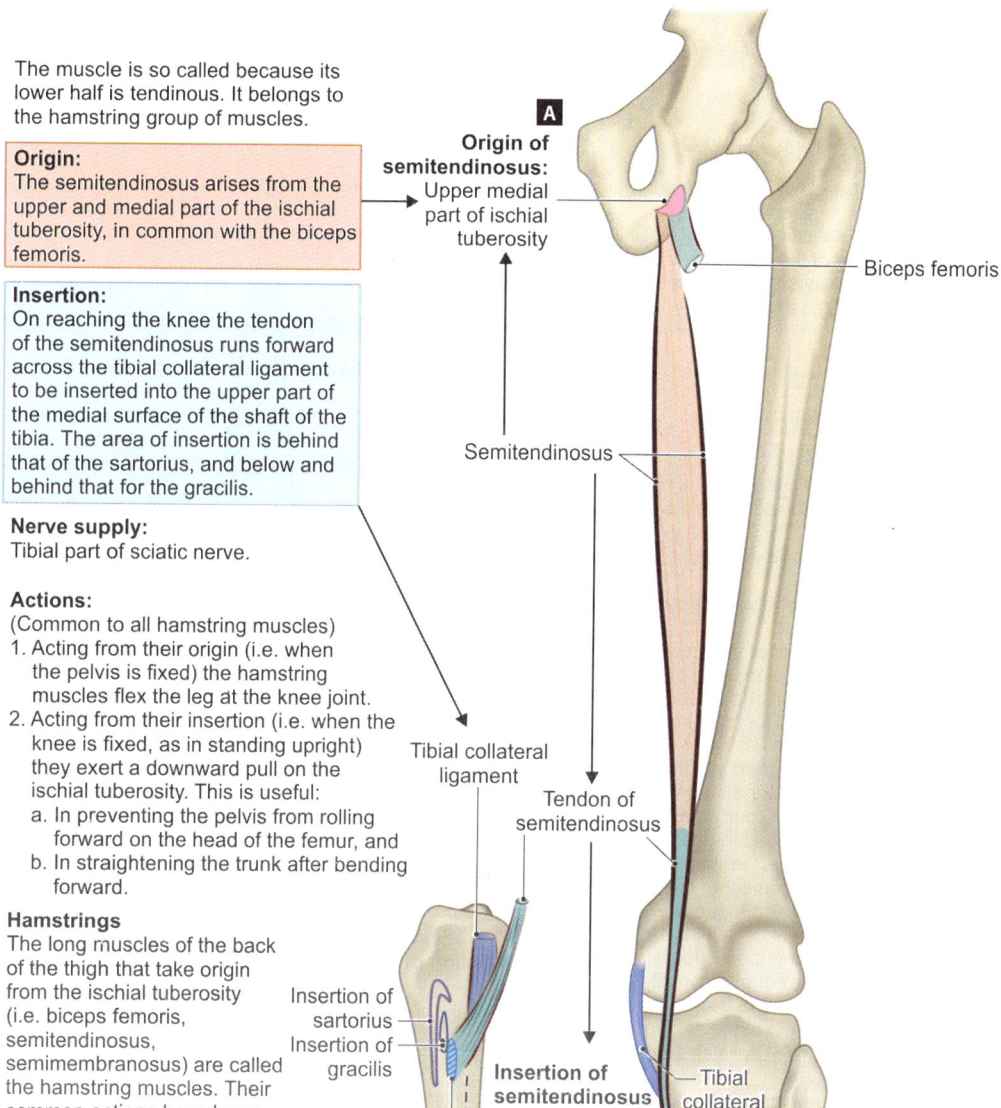

Atlas of Muscle Attachments: Lower Limb

Plate 20

Semimembranosus

This is a muscle of the hamstring group. The muscle is so called because its upper part is membranous. (Compare with semitendinosus). The membranous part of the muscle lies under cover of the biceps femoris. The origin of the muscle is tendinous. The lower part is fleshy.

Origin:
The muscle arises from the upper lateral part of the ischial tuberosity.

Insertion:
The fleshy fibers of the muscle end in a tendon which is placed along the medial edge of the muscle. This tendon is inserted into the medial condyle of the tibia.

The following points should be noted about the insertion.
1. The posterior aspect of the medial condyle of the tibia is marked by a groove, at the lateral end of which there is a tubercle. The main insertion is into this tubercle.
2. Some fibers are inserted into the groove itself, and extend onto the medial aspect of the condyle as well.
3. Some fibers of the tendon pass upward and laterally (forming the oblique popliteal ligament of the knee joint) and get attached to the lateral condyle of the femur.
4. Some fibers become continuous with the fascia covering the popliteus.
5. Some fibers descend to be attached to the medial margin of the shaft of the tibia behind the tibial collateral ligament.

Nerve supply:
The muscle is supplied by a branch from the tibial part of the sciatic nerve.

Actions:
See under semitendinosus.

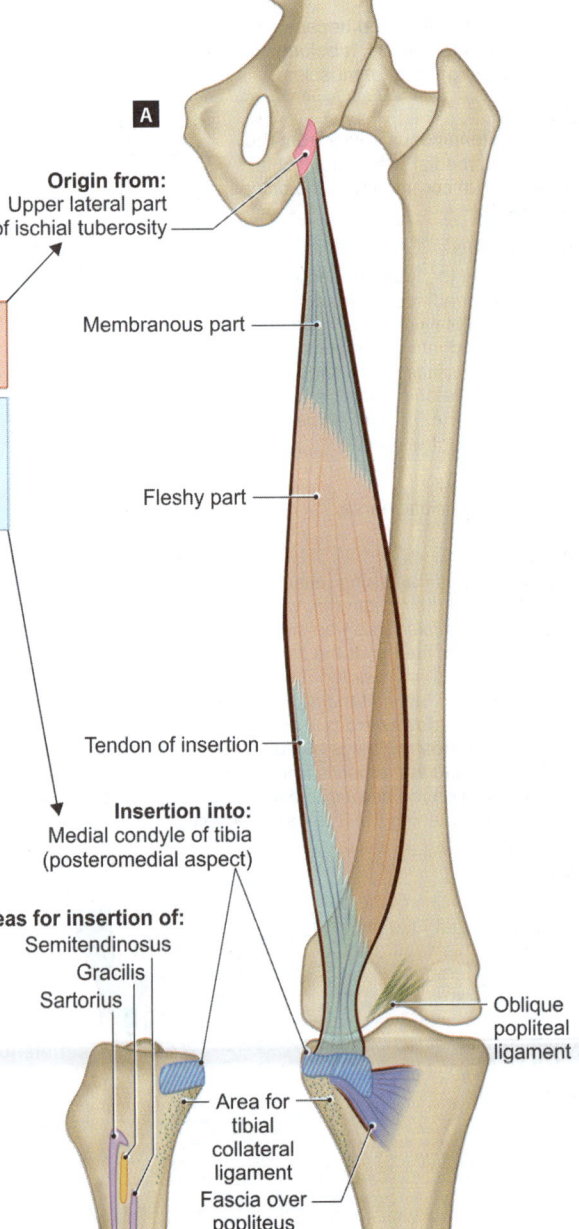

Atlas of Muscle Attachments: Lower Limb

Plate 21

Biceps Femoris

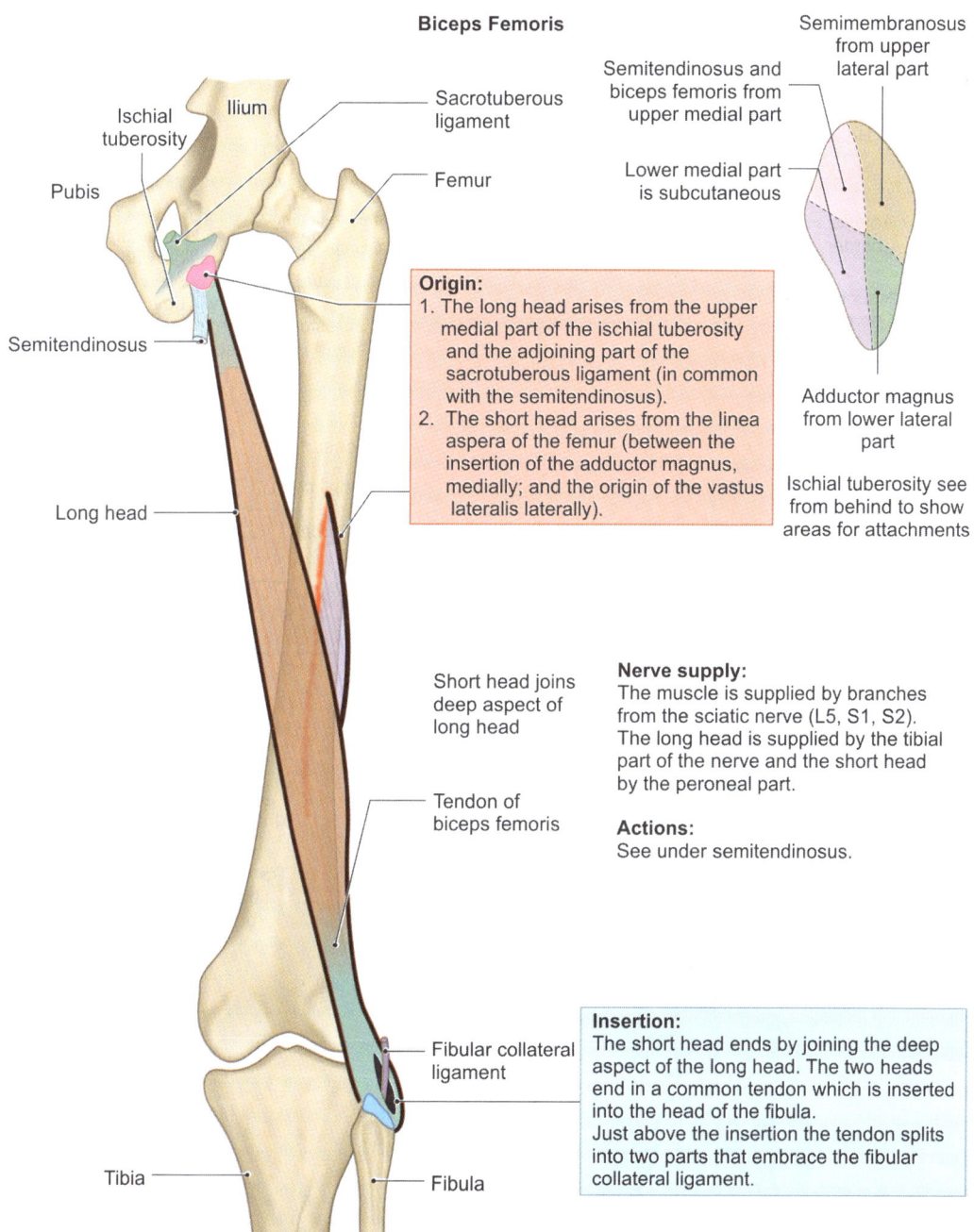

Origin:
1. The long head arises from the upper medial part of the ischial tuberosity and the adjoining part of the sacrotuberous ligament (in common with the semitendinosus).
2. The short head arises from the linea aspera of the femur (between the insertion of the adductor magnus, medially; and the origin of the vastus lateralis laterally).

Nerve supply:
The muscle is supplied by branches from the sciatic nerve (L5, S1, S2). The long head is supplied by the tibial part of the nerve and the short head by the peroneal part.

Actions:
See under semitendinosus.

Insertion:
The short head ends by joining the deep aspect of the long head. The two heads end in a common tendon which is inserted into the head of the fibula.
Just above the insertion the tendon splits into two parts that embrace the fibular collateral ligament.

Atlas of Muscle Attachments: Lower Limb

Plate 22

Bony Landmarks on Front of the Leg and Foot

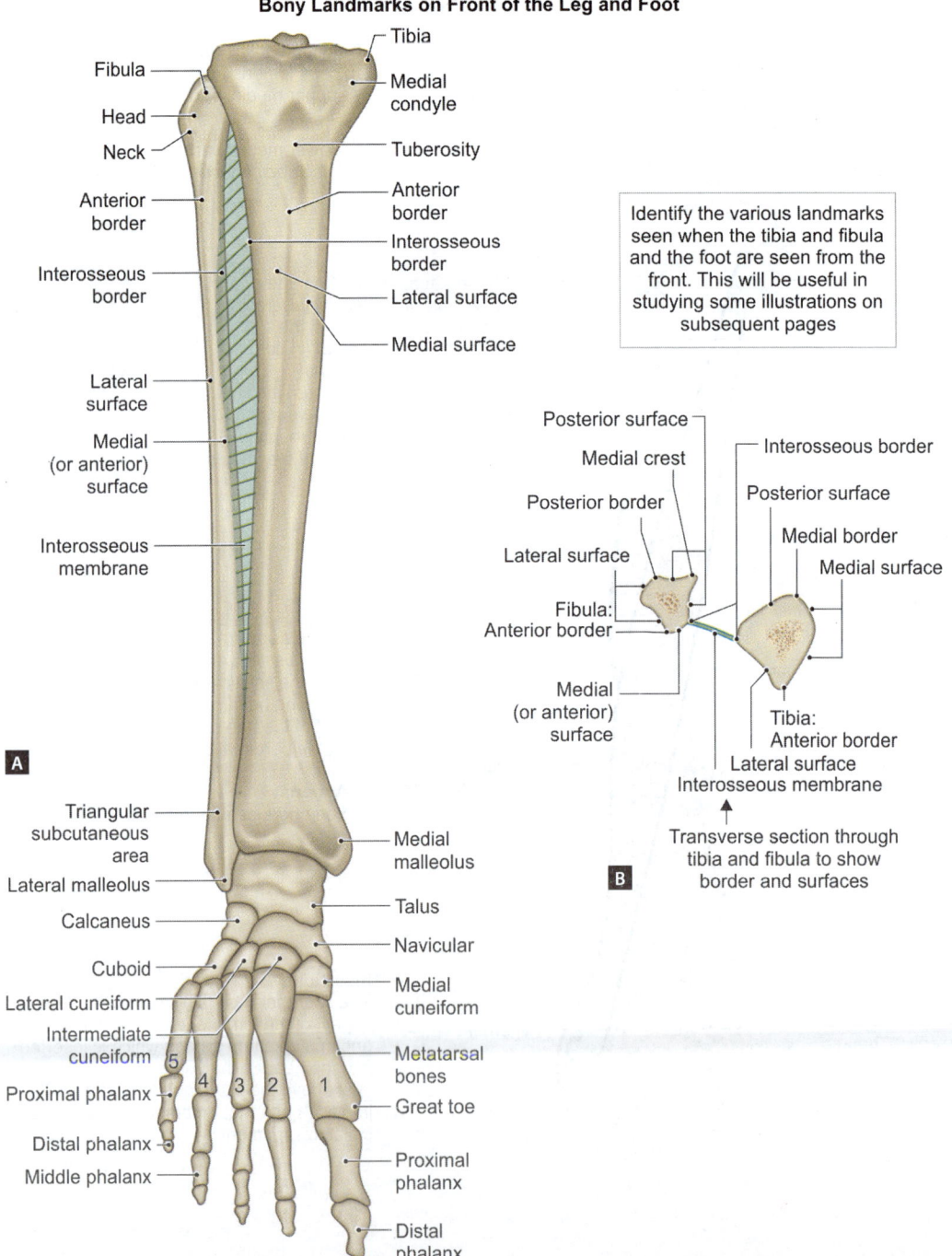

Plate 23

Tibialis Anterior

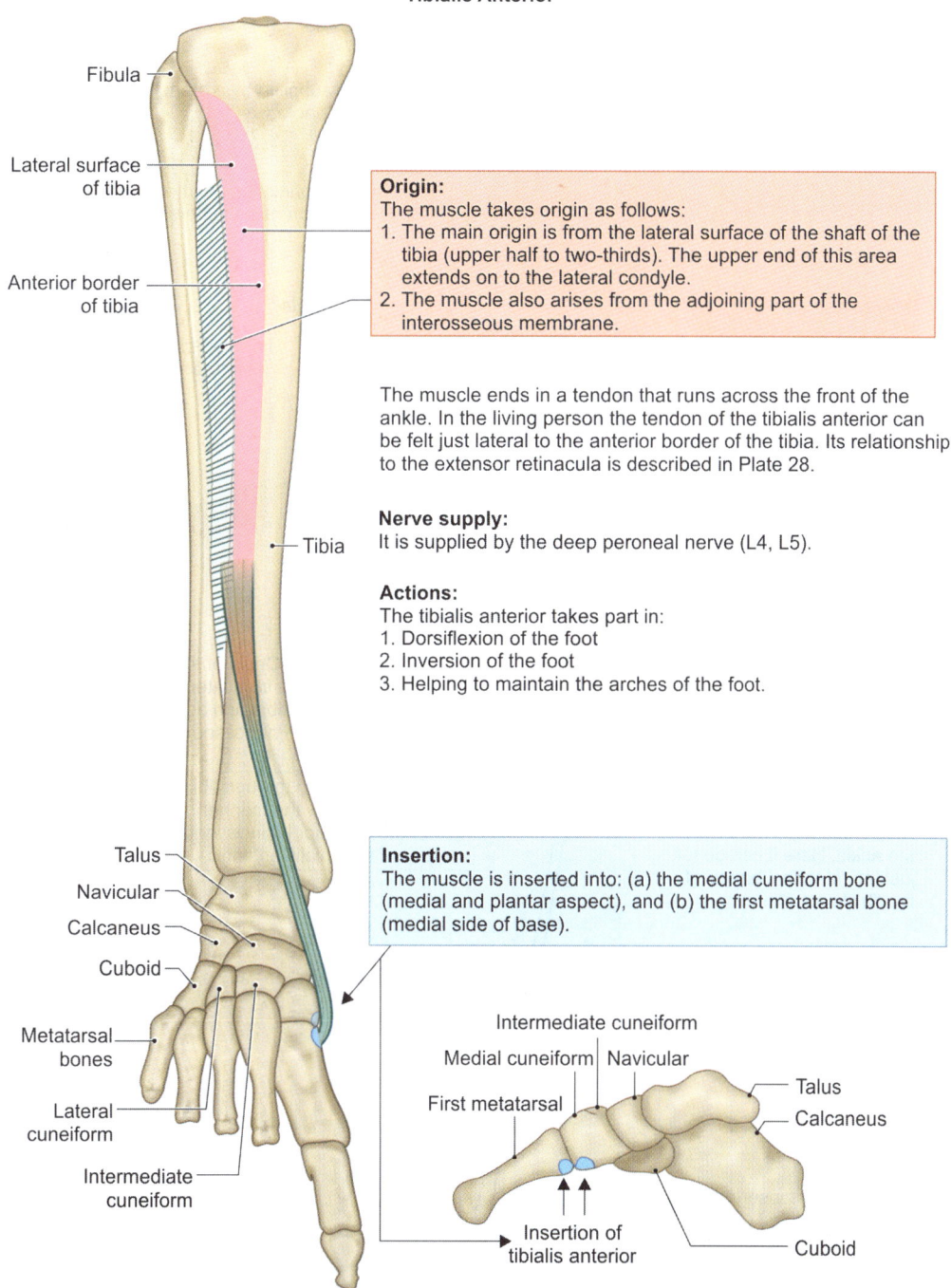

Origin:
The muscle takes origin as follows:
1. The main origin is from the lateral surface of the shaft of the tibia (upper half to two-thirds). The upper end of this area extends on to the lateral condyle.
2. The muscle also arises from the adjoining part of the interosseous membrane.

The muscle ends in a tendon that runs across the front of the ankle. In the living person the tendon of the tibialis anterior can be felt just lateral to the anterior border of the tibia. Its relationship to the extensor retinacula is described in Plate 28.

Nerve supply:
It is supplied by the deep peroneal nerve (L4, L5).

Actions:
The tibialis anterior takes part in:
1. Dorsiflexion of the foot
2. Inversion of the foot
3. Helping to maintain the arches of the foot.

Insertion:
The muscle is inserted into: (a) the medial cuneiform bone (medial and plantar aspect), and (b) the first metatarsal bone (medial side of base).

Atlas of Muscle Attachments: Lower Limb

Plate 24

Extensor Hallucis Longus

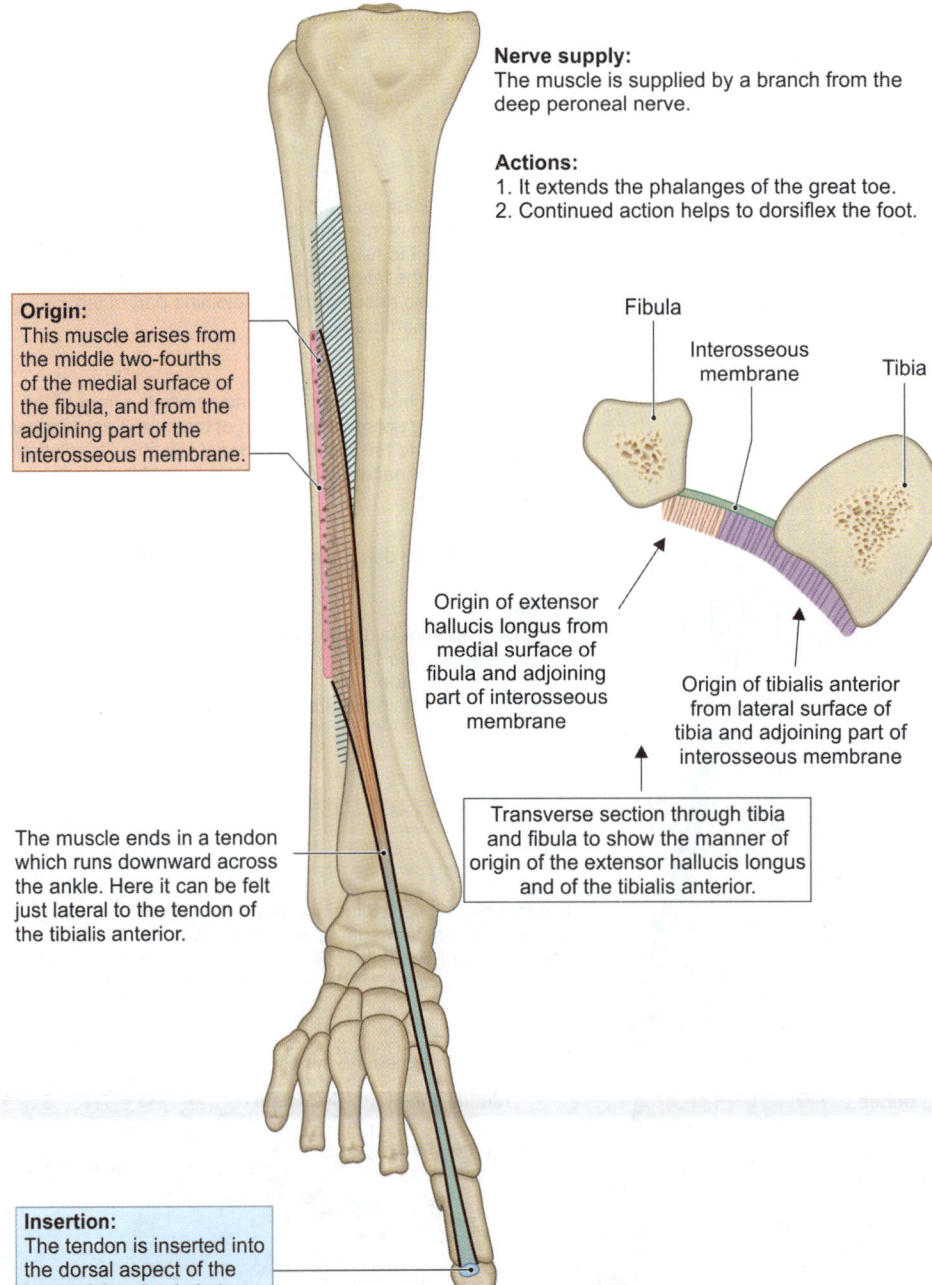

Nerve supply:
The muscle is supplied by a branch from the deep peroneal nerve.

Actions:
1. It extends the phalanges of the great toe.
2. Continued action helps to dorsiflex the foot.

Origin:
This muscle arises from the middle two-fourths of the medial surface of the fibula, and from the adjoining part of the interosseous membrane.

Origin of extensor hallucis longus from medial surface of fibula and adjoining part of interosseous membrane

Origin of tibialis anterior from lateral surface of tibia and adjoining part of interosseous membrane

Transverse section through tibia and fibula to show the manner of origin of the extensor hallucis longus and of the tibialis anterior.

The muscle ends in a tendon which runs downward across the ankle. Here it can be felt just lateral to the tendon of the tibialis anterior.

Insertion:
The tendon is inserted into the dorsal aspect of the base of the distal phalanx of the great toe.

Atlas of Muscle Attachments: Lower Limb

Plate 25
Extensor Digitorum Longus

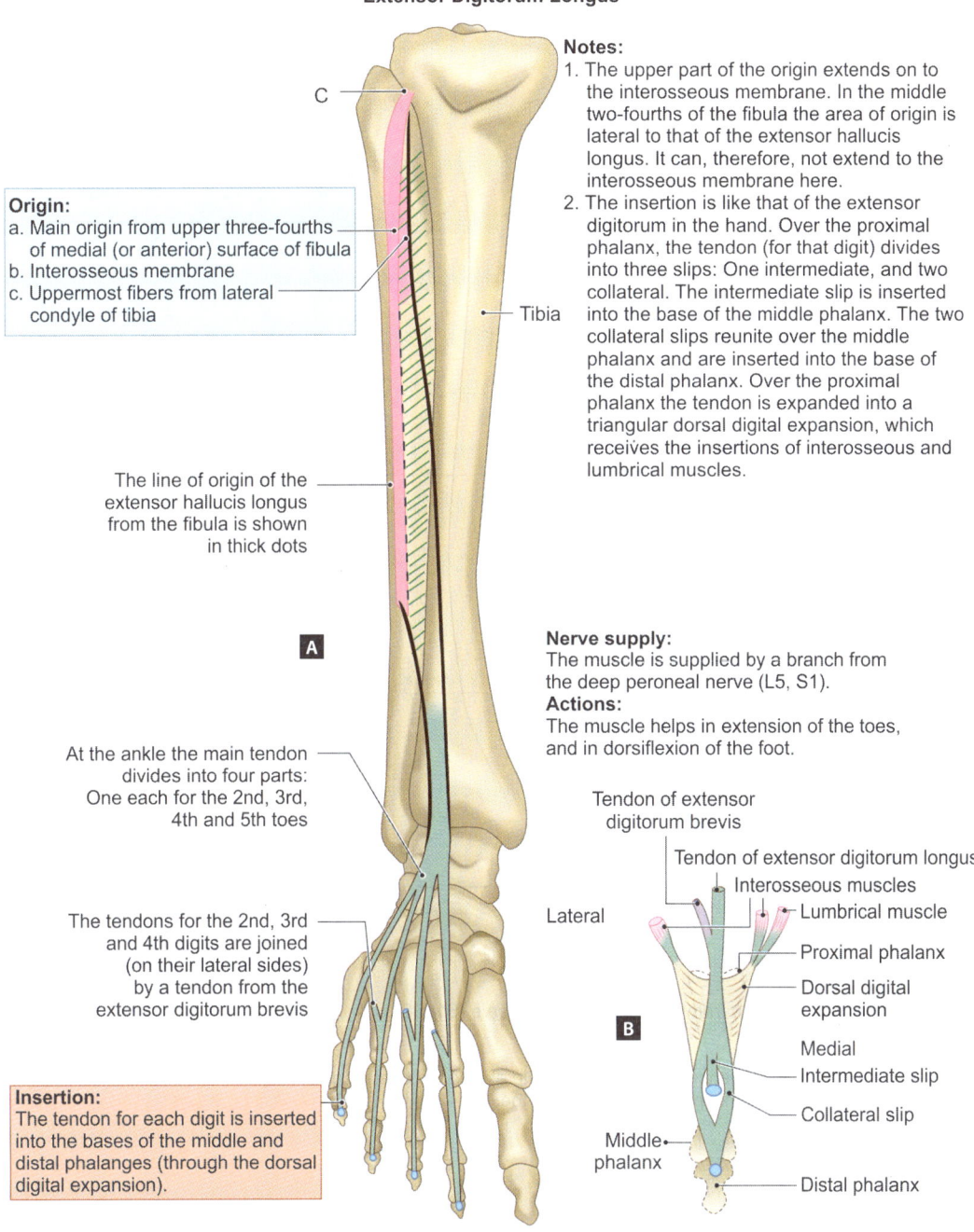

Origin:
a. Main origin from upper three-fourths of medial (or anterior) surface of fibula
b. Interosseous membrane
c. Uppermost fibers from lateral condyle of tibia

The line of origin of the extensor hallucis longus from the fibula is shown in thick dots

At the ankle the main tendon divides into four parts: One each for the 2nd, 3rd, 4th and 5th toes

The tendons for the 2nd, 3rd and 4th digits are joined (on their lateral sides) by a tendon from the extensor digitorum brevis

Insertion:
The tendon for each digit is inserted into the bases of the middle and distal phalanges (through the dorsal digital expansion).

Notes:
1. The upper part of the origin extends on to the interosseous membrane. In the middle two-fourths of the fibula the area of origin is lateral to that of the extensor hallucis longus. It can, therefore, not extend to the interosseous membrane here.
2. The insertion is like that of the extensor digitorum in the hand. Over the proximal phalanx, the tendon (for that digit) divides into three slips: One intermediate, and two collateral. The intermediate slip is inserted into the base of the middle phalanx. The two collateral slips reunite over the middle phalanx and are inserted into the base of the distal phalanx. Over the proximal phalanx the tendon is expanded into a triangular dorsal digital expansion, which receives the insertions of interosseous and lumbrical muscles.

Nerve supply:
The muscle is supplied by a branch from the deep peroneal nerve (L5, S1).
Actions:
The muscle helps in extension of the toes, and in dorsiflexion of the foot.

Atlas of Muscle Attachments: Lower Limb

Plate 26
Extensor Digitorum Brevis

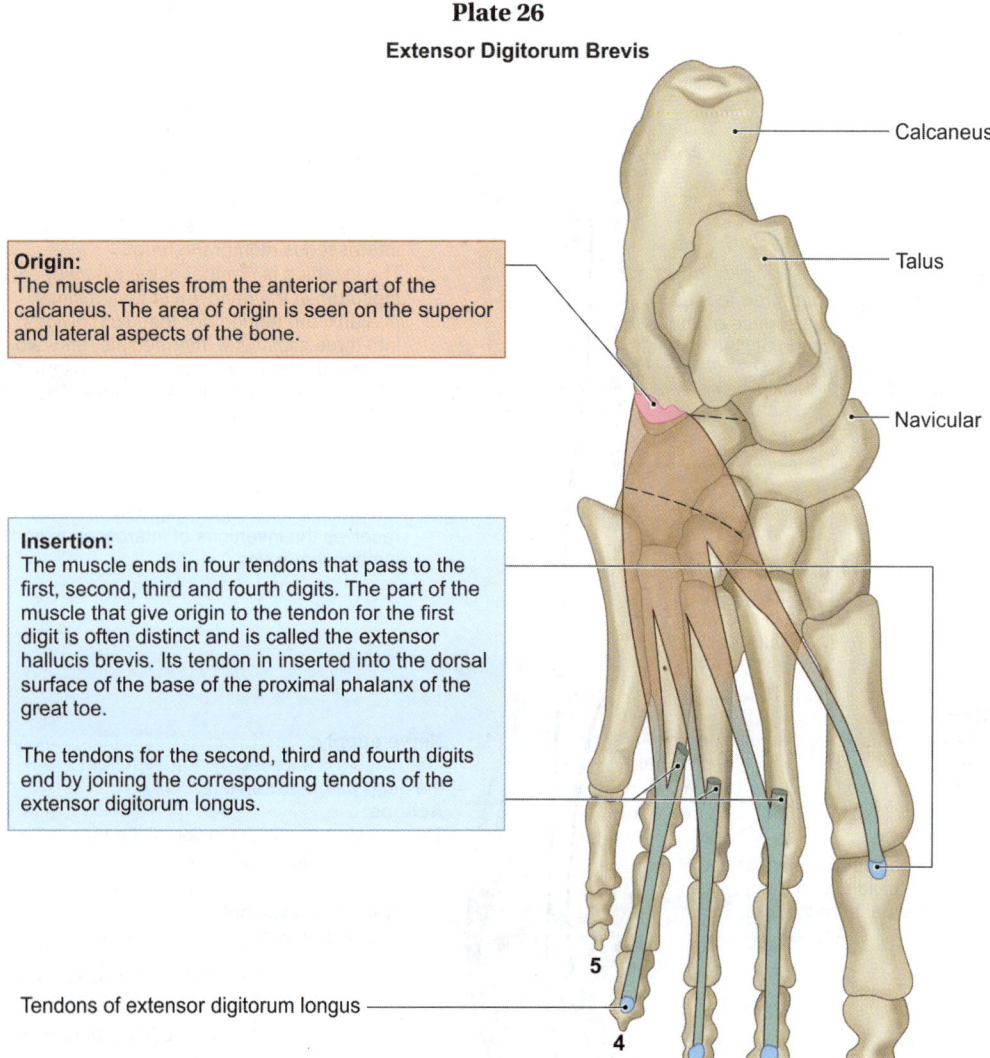

Origin:
The muscle arises from the anterior part of the calcaneus. The area of origin is seen on the superior and lateral aspects of the bone.

Insertion:
The muscle ends in four tendons that pass to the first, second, third and fourth digits. The part of the muscle that give origin to the tendon for the first digit is often distinct and is called the extensor hallucis brevis. Its tendon in inserted into the dorsal surface of the base of the proximal phalanx of the great toe.

The tendons for the second, third and fourth digits end by joining the corresponding tendons of the extensor digitorum longus.

Nerve supply:
It is supplied by a branch from the deep peroneal nerve (S1, S2).

Action:
The muscle helps the extensor digitorum longus to extend the phalanges of the foot. The extensor hallucis brevis extends the proximal phalanx of the great toe.

Atlas of Muscle Attachments: Lower Limb

Plate 27
Peroneus Tertius

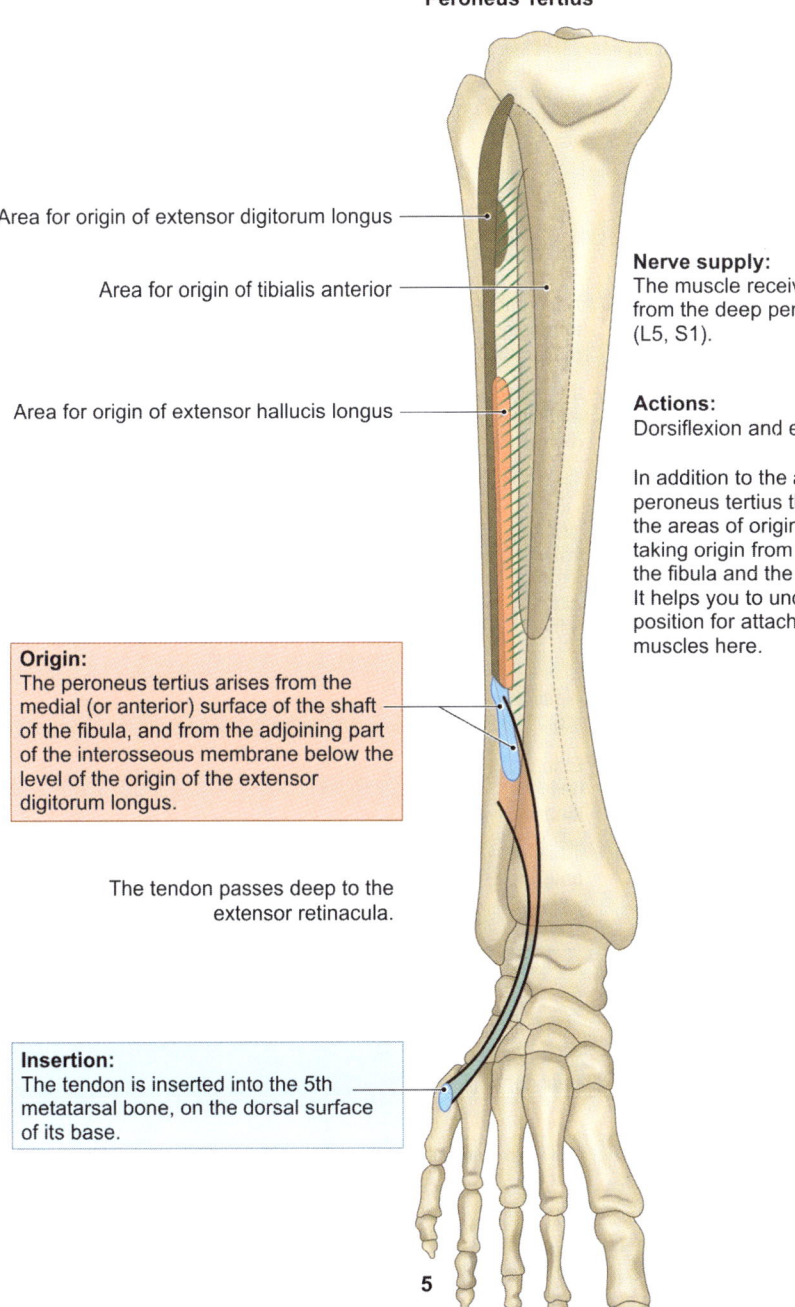

Area for origin of extensor digitorum longus

Area for origin of tibialis anterior

Area for origin of extensor hallucis longus

Nerve supply:
The muscle receives a branch from the deep peroneal nerve (L5, S1).

Actions:
Dorsiflexion and eversion of the foot.

In addition to the attachments of the peroneus tertius this figure also shows the areas of origin of other muscles taking origin from the front of the tibia, the fibula and the interosseous membrane. It helps you to understand the relative position for attachment of the various muscles here.

Origin:
The peroneus tertius arises from the medial (or anterior) surface of the shaft of the fibula, and from the adjoining part of the interosseous membrane below the level of the origin of the extensor digitorum longus.

The tendon passes deep to the extensor retinacula.

Insertion:
The tendon is inserted into the 5th metatarsal bone, on the dorsal surface of its base.

Plate 28
Extensor Retinacula

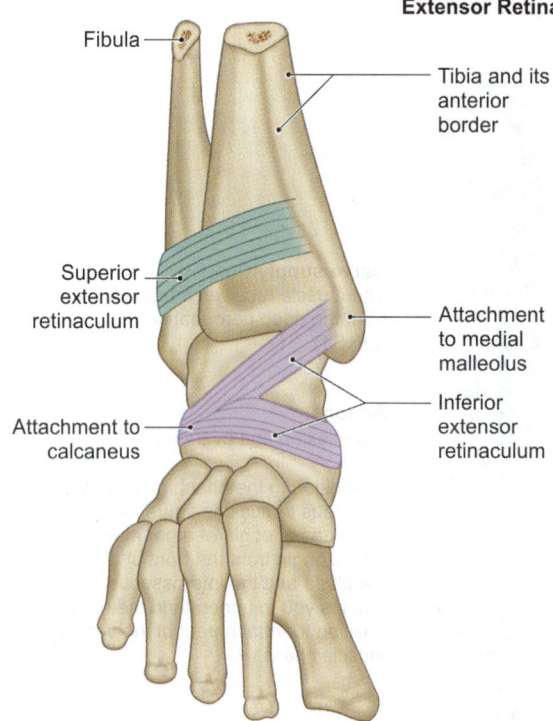

Superior Extensor Retinaculum
The superior extensor retinaculum is attached (a) medially to the anterior border of the tibia, and (b) laterally to the anterior aspect of the fibula.

Inferior Extensor Retinaculum
The inferior extensor retinaculum is shaped like the letter 'Y' placed on its side; the stem of the 'Y' is directed laterally and the two limbs pass medially. The stem of the 'Y' is attached to the upper surface of the calcaneus. The upper limb of the 'Y' is attached to the medial malleolus.
The lower limb of the 'Y' winds round the medial side of the foot to become continuous with the plantar aponeurosis.

Tendons Passing Under Cover of Extensor Retinacula
The tendons passing under cover of the extensor retinacula are from medial to lateral side those of the tibialis anterior, the extensor hallucis longus, the extensor digitorum longus, and the peroneus tertius.
The superior extensor retinaculum is superficial to all the tendons. The relationship of the inferior extensor retinaculum to the tendons is as follows, The stem is in the form of a loop through which the tendons of the extensor digitorum and peroneus tertius pass. The superior limb has two layers one passing superficial to the extensor hallucis and the tibialis anterior, and the other deep to them. The inferior limb is superficial to these tendons; it may sometimes have an additional layer deep to the tendons. As they pass under the retinacula the extensor tendons are surrounded by synovial sheaths. There is one sheath each for the tibialis anterior and for the extensor hallucis. The extensor digitorum and the peroneus tertius have a common sheath.

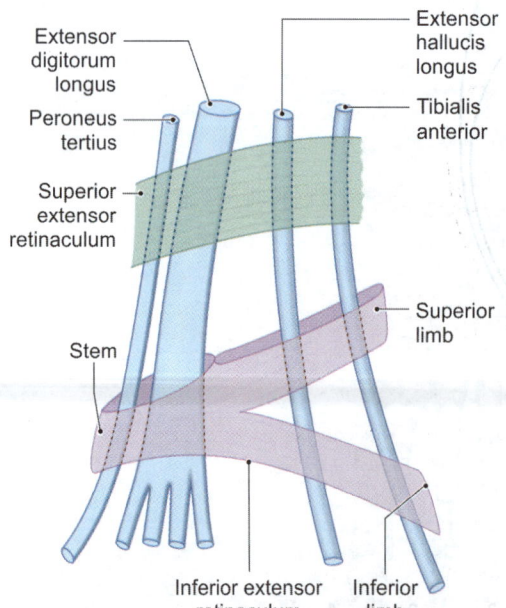

Atlas of Muscle Attachments: Lower Limb

Plate 29

Peroneus Longus

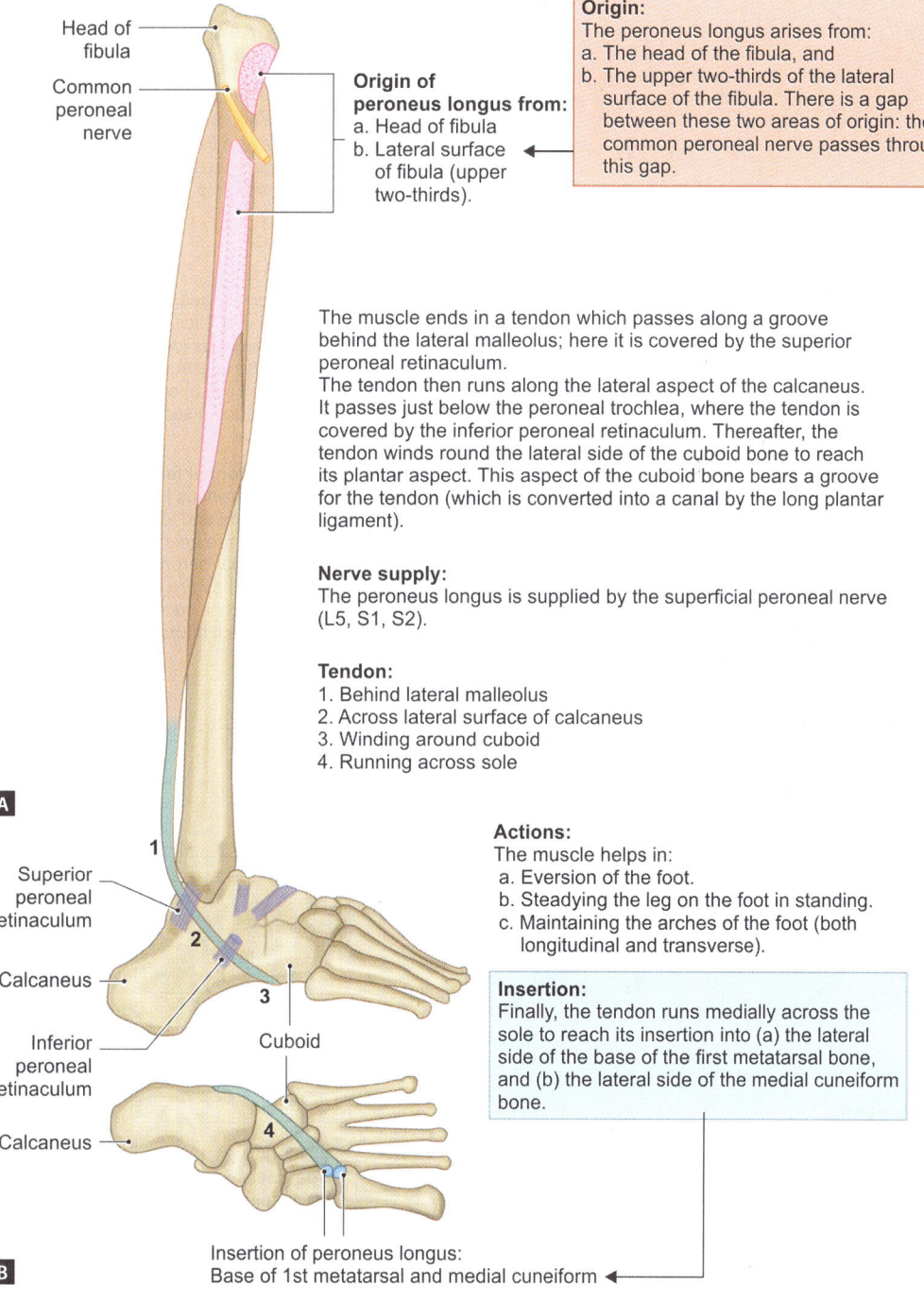

Origin:
The peroneus longus arises from:
a. The head of the fibula, and
b. The upper two-thirds of the lateral surface of the fibula. There is a gap between these two areas of origin: the common peroneal nerve passes through this gap.

The muscle ends in a tendon which passes along a groove behind the lateral malleolus; here it is covered by the superior peroneal retinaculum.
The tendon then runs along the lateral aspect of the calcaneus. It passes just below the peroneal trochlea, where the tendon is covered by the inferior peroneal retinaculum. Thereafter, the tendon winds round the lateral side of the cuboid bone to reach its plantar aspect. This aspect of the cuboid bone bears a groove for the tendon (which is converted into a canal by the long plantar ligament).

Nerve supply:
The peroneus longus is supplied by the superficial peroneal nerve (L5, S1, S2).

Tendon:
1. Behind lateral malleolus
2. Across lateral surface of calcaneus
3. Winding around cuboid
4. Running across sole

Actions:
The muscle helps in:
a. Eversion of the foot.
b. Steadying the leg on the foot in standing.
c. Maintaining the arches of the foot (both longitudinal and transverse).

Insertion:
Finally, the tendon runs medially across the sole to reach its insertion into (a) the lateral side of the base of the first metatarsal bone, and (b) the lateral side of the medial cuneiform bone.

Plate 30
Peroneus Brevis

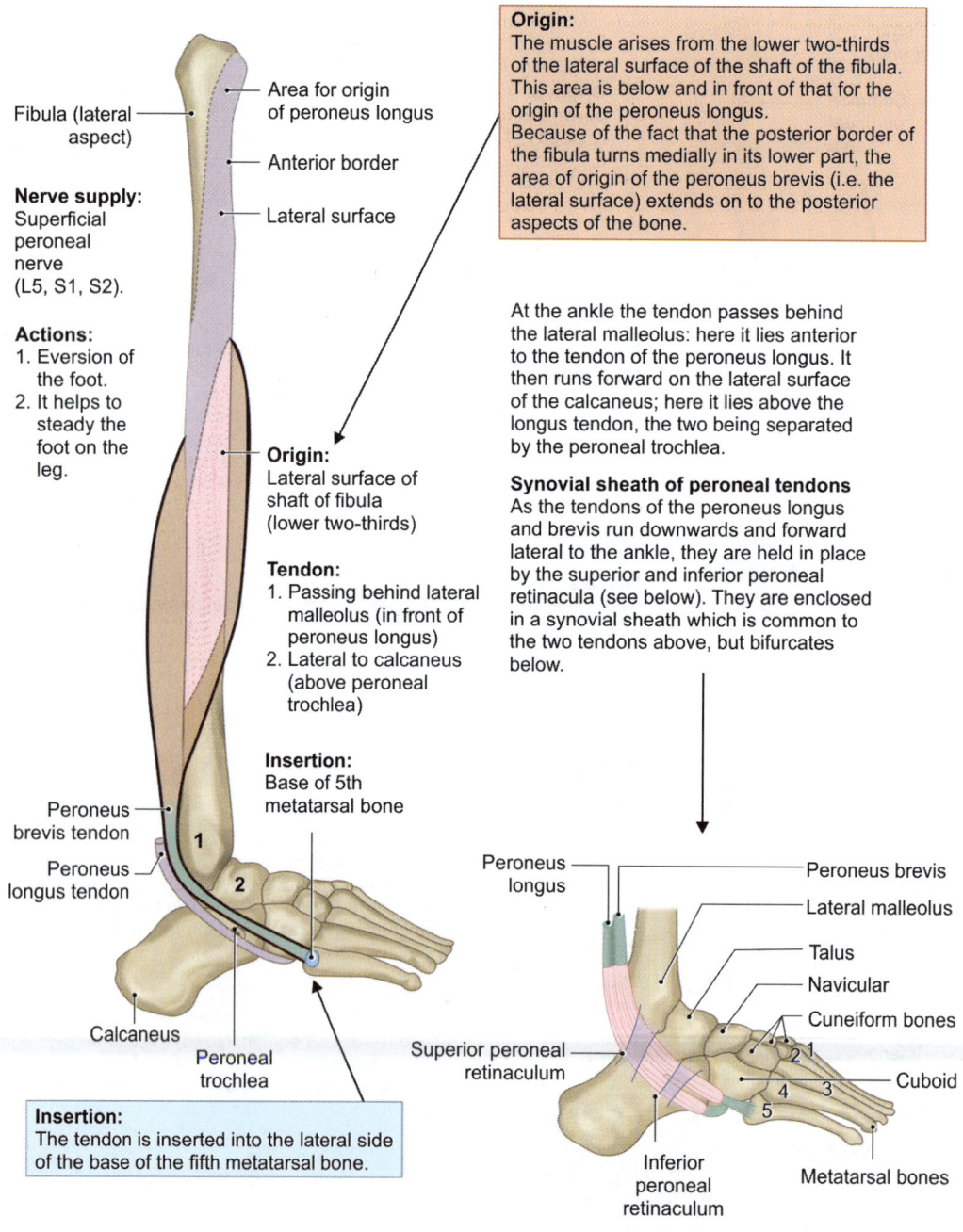

Fibula (lateral aspect)

Area for origin of peroneus longus
Anterior border
Lateral surface

Nerve supply: Superficial peroneal nerve (L5, S1, S2).

Actions:
1. Eversion of the foot.
2. It helps to steady the foot on the leg.

Origin:
The muscle arises from the lower two-thirds of the lateral surface of the shaft of the fibula. This area is below and in front of that for the origin of the peroneus longus.
Because of the fact that the posterior border of the fibula turns medially in its lower part, the area of origin of the peroneus brevis (i.e. the lateral surface) extends on to the posterior aspects of the bone.

Origin: Lateral surface of shaft of fibula (lower two-thirds)

Tendon:
1. Passing behind lateral malleolus (in front of peroneus longus)
2. Lateral to calcaneus (above peroneal trochlea)

Insertion: Base of 5th metatarsal bone

At the ankle the tendon passes behind the lateral malleolus: here it lies anterior to the tendon of the peroneus longus. It then runs forward on the lateral surface of the calcaneus; here it lies above the longus tendon, the two being separated by the peroneal trochlea.

Synovial sheath of peroneal tendons
As the tendons of the peroneus longus and brevis run downwards and forward lateral to the ankle, they are held in place by the superior and inferior peroneal retinacula (see below). They are enclosed in a synovial sheath which is common to the two tendons above, but bifurcates below.

Peroneus brevis tendon
Peroneus longus tendon
Calcaneus
Peroneal trochlea

Peroneus longus
Superior peroneal retinaculum
Inferior peroneal retinaculum

Peroneus brevis
Lateral malleolus
Talus
Navicular
Cuneiform bones
Cuboid
Metatarsal bones

Insertion:
The tendon is inserted into the lateral side of the base of the fifth metatarsal bone.

Plate 31
Gastrocnemius

Origin:
Medial head from medial condyle of femur; and adjoining part of posterior surface of shaft

Lateral head from lateral condyle of femur (lateral aspect)

Origin:
The gastrocnemius arises from the femur by two heads. The medial head arises from the posterior aspects of the medical condyle, and from the adjoining part of the posterior surface. The lateral head arises from the lateral surface of the lateral condyle.

Nerve supply:
The muscle is supplied by a branch from the tibial nerve (S1, S2).

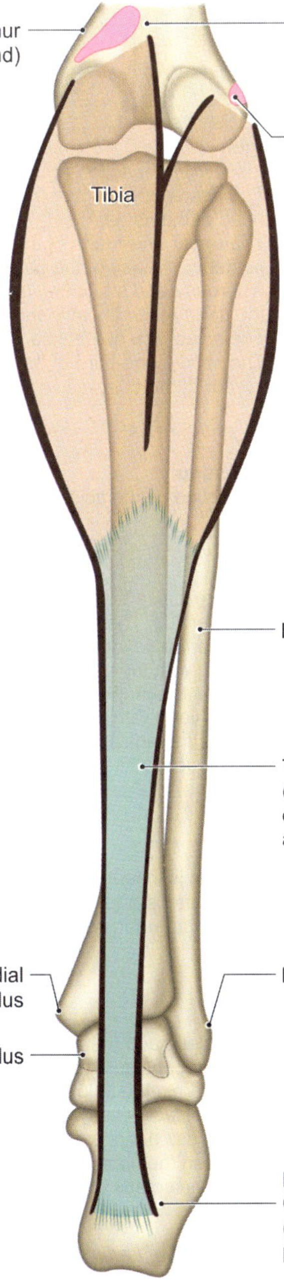

At about the middle of the leg the muscle fibers end in an aponeurosis. This aponeurosis receives the insertion of the soleus muscle on its deep surface. Lower down the aponeurosis becomes continuous with the tendocalcaneus.

Notes:
1. The gastrocnemius and the soleus are together called the triceps surae.
2. The uppermost parts of the medial and lateral heads form the boundaries of the lower part of the popliteal fossa.

Actions:
1. The muscle is a strong plantar flexor of the foot. This movement provides the propelling force in walking, running or jumping.
2. As the upper part of the muscle crosses the knee joint, it helps in flexion of that joint.
3. Along with other muscles that cross the ankle joint, it helps to steady the leg on the foot.

Insertion:
The tendocalcaneus is the common tendon of insertion of both the gastrocnemius and the soleus. It is the strongest tendon in the body. It is attached below to the middle of the posterior surface of the calcaneus.

Insertion:
Calcaneus (middle part of posterior surface)

Labels: Femur (lower end), Tibia, Fibula, Tendocalcaneus (common tendon of gastrocnemius and soleus), Medial malleolus, Talus, Lateral malleolus

Atlas of Muscle Attachments: Lower Limb

Plate 32

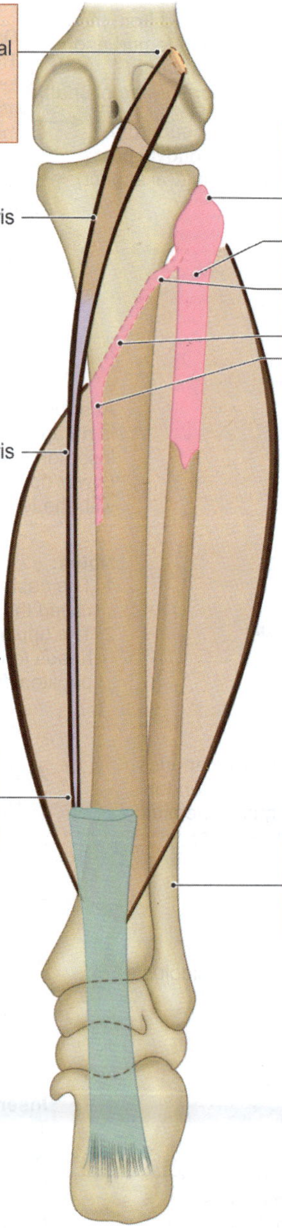

Plantaris

Origin:
It arises from the lower part of the lateral supracondylar line of the femur. (The origin is just above that of the lateral head of the gastrocnemius).

Muscle belly of plantaris

Tendon of plantaris

Nerve supply:
It is supplied by the tibial nerve (S1, S2).

Actions:
These are similar to those of the gastrocnemius and soleus. However, because of its small size it is of little functional importance.

Insertion:
The plantaris is inserted into the medial margin of the tendocalcaneus.

The muscle belly, which is only a few centimeters long, ends in a long thin tendon which runs downward between the gastrocnemius and the soleus. The plantar is a vestigeal remnant of a large muscle which was originally attached, below, to the plantar aponeurosis. (Compare with the palmaris longus).

Soleus

Origin:
It arises from the following:
1. The posterior aspect of the head of the fibula.
2. The upper one-fourth of the posterior surface of the fibula.
3. A fibrous band stretching from the head of the fibula to the tibia
4. The soleal line of the tibia.
5. The middle one-third of the medial border of the tibia.

Nerve supply:
It is supplied by the tibial nerve (S1, S2).

Actions:
These are similar to those of the gastrocnemius. The muscle is a strong plantar flexor of the foot, and along with the gastrocnemius it provides the propelling force in walking. Along with other muscles that cross the ankle it steadies the leg on the foot while standing.

Insertion:
The soleus is inserted into the tendocalcaneus and through it onto the posterior surface of the calcaneus.

Notes:
1. The soleus and the gastrocnemius together constitute the triceps surae, which forms the bulging of the calf.
2. The popliteal vessels and the tibial nerve pass deep to the fibrous band (between the fibula and the tibia) from which the soleus takes origin.

Atlas of Muscle Attachments: Lower Limb

Plate 33
Popliteus

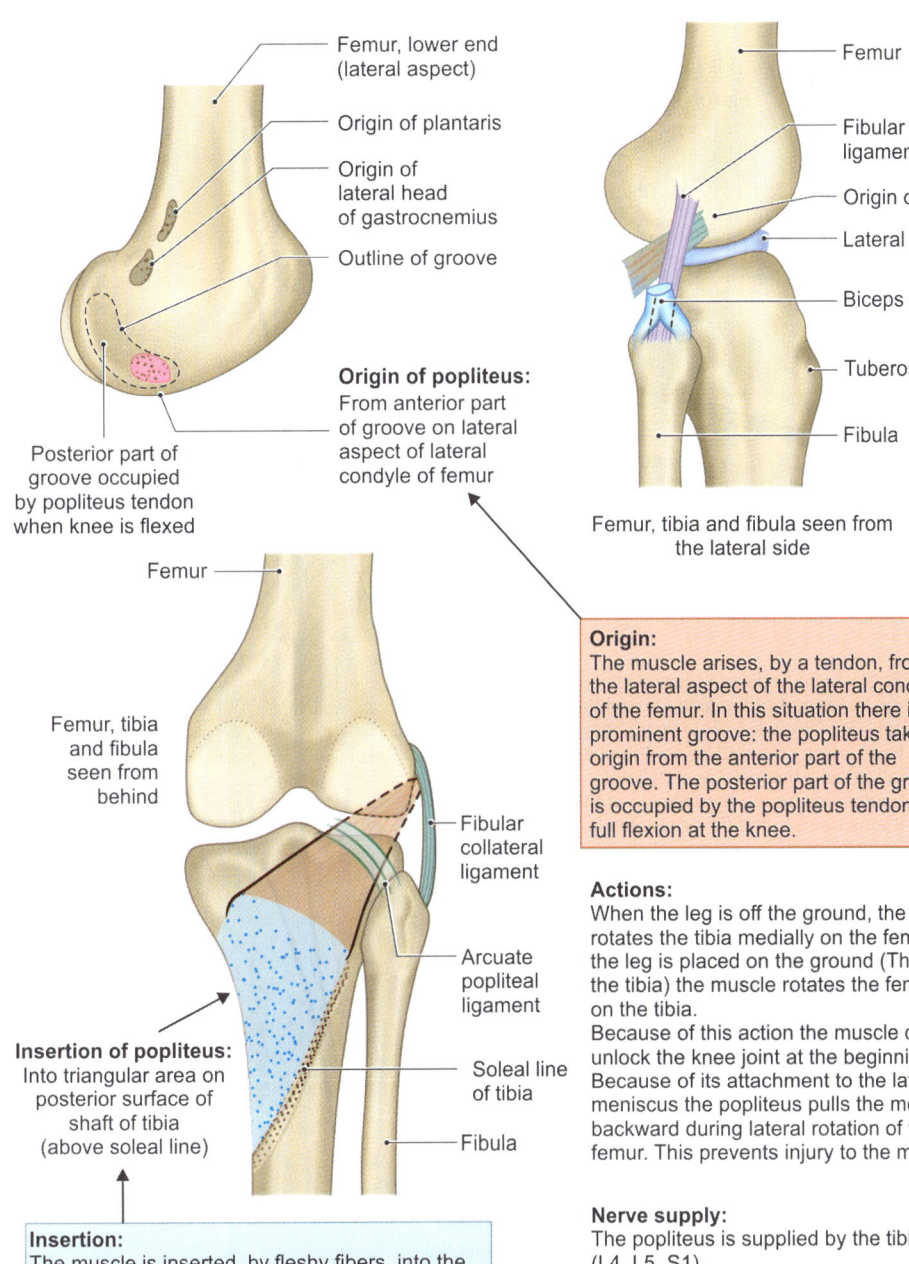

Origin of popliteus:
From anterior part of groove on lateral aspect of lateral condyle of femur

Femur, tibia and fibula seen from the lateral side

Insertion of popliteus:
Into triangular area on posterior surface of shaft of tibia (above soleal line)

Insertion:
The muscle is inserted, by fleshy fibers, into the posterior surface of the shaft of the tibia. The area of insertion is triangular.

Origin:
The muscle arises, by a tendon, from the lateral aspect of the lateral condyle of the femur. In this situation there is a prominent groove: the popliteus takes origin from the anterior part of the groove. The posterior part of the groove is occupied by the popliteus tendon in full flexion at the knee.

Actions:
When the leg is off the ground, the popliteus rotates the tibia medially on the femur. When the leg is placed on the ground (Thus fixing the tibia) the muscle rotates the femur laterally on the tibia.
Because of this action the muscle can unlock the knee joint at the beginning of flexion. Because of its attachment to the lateral meniscus the popliteus pulls the meniscus backward during lateral rotation of the femur. This prevents injury to the meniscus.

Nerve supply:
The popliteus is supplied by the tibial nerve (L4, L5, S1).

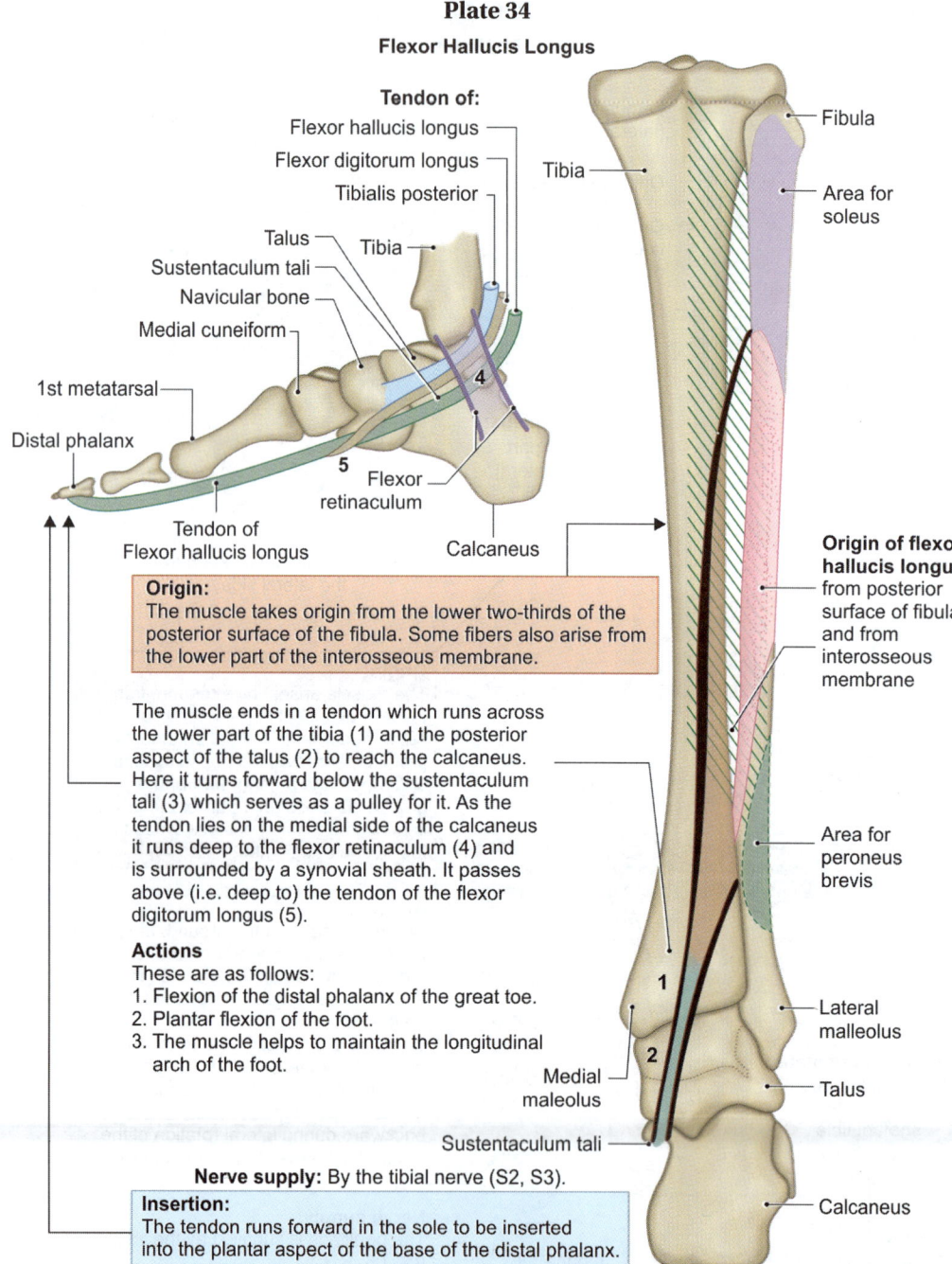

Plate 34
Flexor Hallucis Longus

Origin:
The muscle takes origin from the lower two-thirds of the posterior surface of the fibula. Some fibers also arise from the lower part of the interosseous membrane.

The muscle ends in a tendon which runs across the lower part of the tibia (1) and the posterior aspect of the talus (2) to reach the calcaneus. Here it turns forward below the sustentaculum tali (3) which serves as a pulley for it. As the tendon lies on the medial side of the calcaneus it runs deep to the flexor retinaculum (4) and is surrounded by a synovial sheath. It passes above (i.e. deep to) the tendon of the flexor digitorum longus (5).

Actions
These are as follows:
1. Flexion of the distal phalanx of the great toe.
2. Plantar flexion of the foot.
3. The muscle helps to maintain the longitudinal arch of the foot.

Nerve supply: By the tibial nerve (S2, S3).

Insertion:
The tendon runs forward in the sole to be inserted into the plantar aspect of the base of the distal phalanx.

Plate 35

Flexor Digitorum Longus

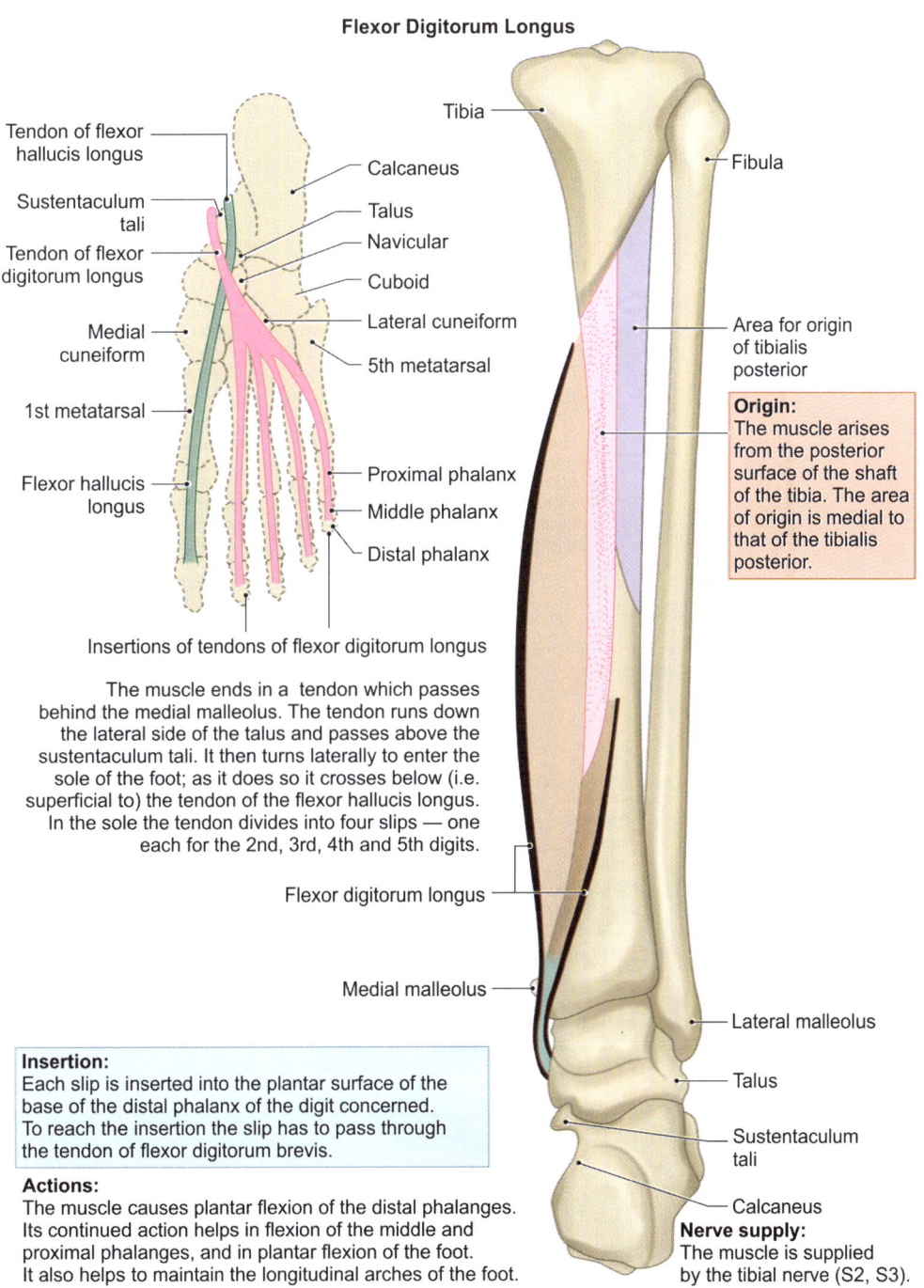

Origin:
The muscle arises from the posterior surface of the shaft of the tibia. The area of origin is medial to that of the tibialis posterior.

The muscle ends in a tendon which passes behind the medial malleolus. The tendon runs down the lateral side of the talus and passes above the sustentaculum tali. It then turns laterally to enter the sole of the foot; as it does so it crosses below (i.e. superficial to) the tendon of the flexor hallucis longus. In the sole the tendon divides into four slips — one each for the 2nd, 3rd, 4th and 5th digits.

Insertion:
Each slip is inserted into the plantar surface of the base of the distal phalanx of the digit concerned. To reach the insertion the slip has to pass through the tendon of flexor digitorum brevis.

Actions:
The muscle causes plantar flexion of the distal phalanges. Its continued action helps in flexion of the middle and proximal phalanges, and in plantar flexion of the foot. It also helps to maintain the longitudinal arches of the foot.

Nerve supply:
The muscle is supplied by the tibial nerve (S2, S3).

Atlas of Muscle Attachments: Lower Limb

Plate 36
Tibialis Posterior

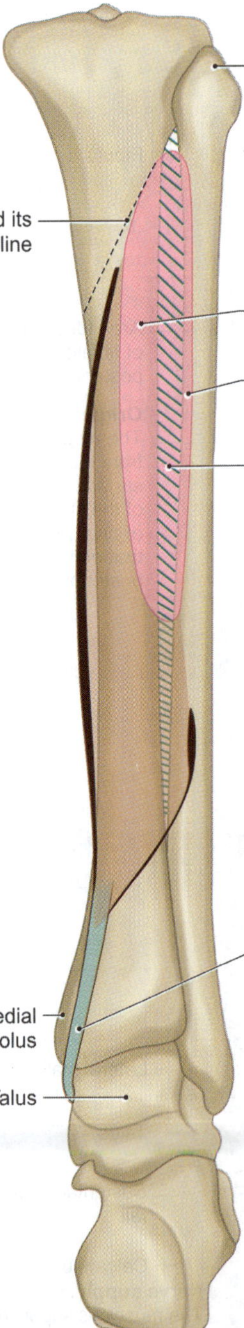

Origin:
This muscle arises from:
1. The upper two-thirds of the lateral part of the posterior surface of the shaft of the tibia: the upper part of the area of origin lies below the soleal line.
2. The upper two-thirds of the medial part of the posterior surface of the fibula. (This surface cannot be seen from the posterior aspect. The bone has to be viewed from the medial aspect to see it).
3. Between the tibia and the fibula the muscle arises from the interosseous membrane.

The muscle ends in a tendon which passes behind the medial malleolus; and then deep to the flexor retinaculum to reach the sole of the foot.

Insertion:
The tendon divides into a number of slips. The main slip is inserted into the tuberosity of the navicular bone (1). and the medial cuneiform bone (2). Other slips are inserted into the sustentaculum tali of the calcaneus (3); the intermediate cuneiform (4); and the bases of the 2nd, 3rd and 4th metatarsals (5). Occasionally some slips may reach the lateral cuneiform (6). and cuboid (7) bones.

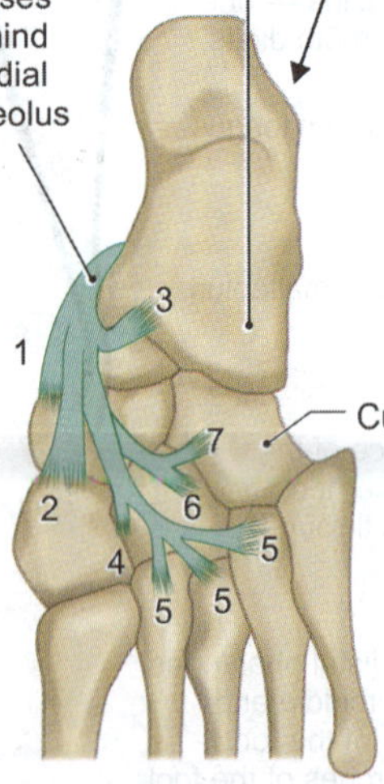

Nerve supply:
The tibialis posterior is supplied by the tibial nerve (L4, L5).

Actions:
The muscle causes inversion of the foot. It also helps to maintain the longitudinal arches of the foot.

Plate 37
Flexor Retinaculum

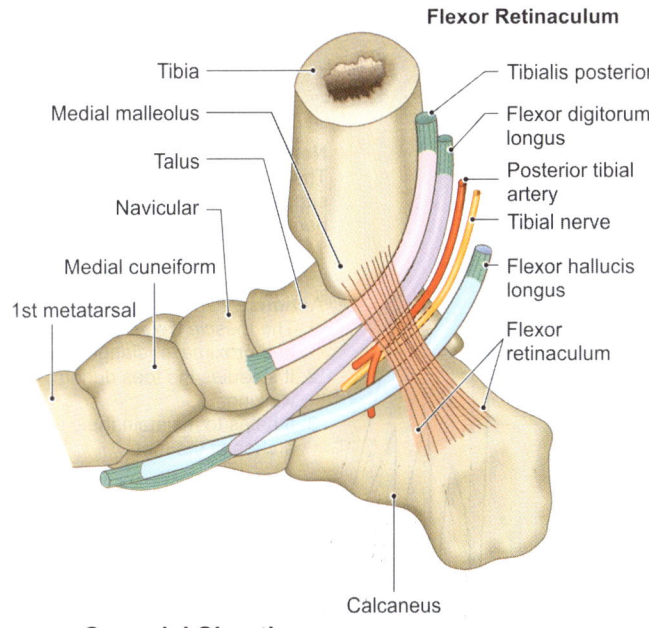

The flexor retinaculum is a thickened band of deep fascia present on the medial side of the ankle. It is attached above to the medial malleolus and below to the medial surface of the calcaneus. It is directed downward, backward and laterally. The structures passing under cover of it are as follows (from above downward, and also from medial to lateral side):
1. Tendon of the tibialis posterior
2. Tendon of the flexor digitorum longus
3. The posterior tibial vessels
4. The tibial nerve, and
5. The tendon of the flexor hallucis longus.

Synovial Sheaths

The three tendons passing deep to the flexor retinaculum are surrounded by synovial sheaths which extend for some distance proximal to the retinaculum. Their distal extent is variable. The sheath for the tibialis posterior extends almost to the insertion of the muscle. The sheath for the flexor hallucis longus may end near the base of the 1st metatarsal, or may extend right up to the insertion into the terminal phalanx.
The sheath for the flexor digitorum longus may end near the navicular bone; or may expand to enclose the proximal parts of the tendons for the digits.
The distal parts of the tendons for the 2nd, 3rd and 4th digits have independent synovial sheaths, which facilitate their movement through osseoaponeurotic canals. The 5th digit has a similar sheath which is continuous proximally with the sheath for the tendon of the flexor digitorum longus.

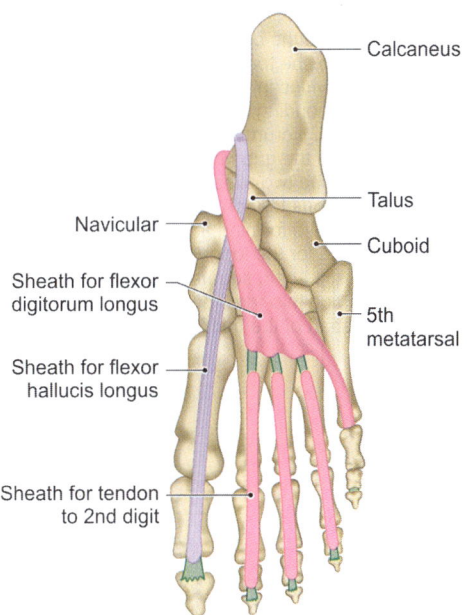

Plate 38

Flexor Digitorum Brevis

Origin:
The muscle arises (by a tendon) from the medial process of the tuberosity of the calcaneus.

Nerve supply:
The flexor digitorum brevis is supplied by the medial plantar nerve (S2, S3).

Actions:
1. The muscle flexes the middle and proximal phalanges.
2. It steadies the toes during walking.
3. It helps to maintain the arches of the foot.

The muscle ends in four tendons; one each for the 2nd, 3rd, 4th and 5th digits

Insertion:
Opposite the base of the proximal phalanx the tendon for each digit divides into two slip: the corresponding tendon of the flexor digitorum longus passes through the gap between the two slips. The two slips reunite deep to the longus tendon, and partially decussate forming a grooved surface for the longus tendon. The slip again separate to gain insertion into the sides of the shaft of the middle phalanx.

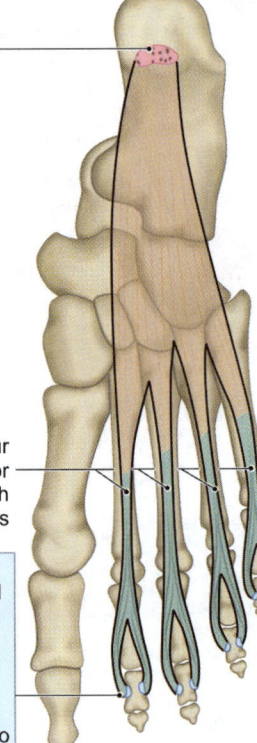

Note that the mode of insertion of the flexor digitorum brevis corresponds to that of the flexor digitorum superficialis in the hand.

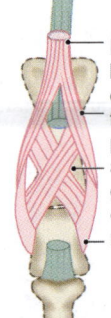

Flexor digitorum longus tendon

Insertion of flexor digitorum longus terminal phalanx

Flexor digitorum brevis tendon dividing into two slips that partly decussate and then gain insertion on sides of middle phalanx

Atlas of Muscle Attachments: Lower Limb

Plate 39

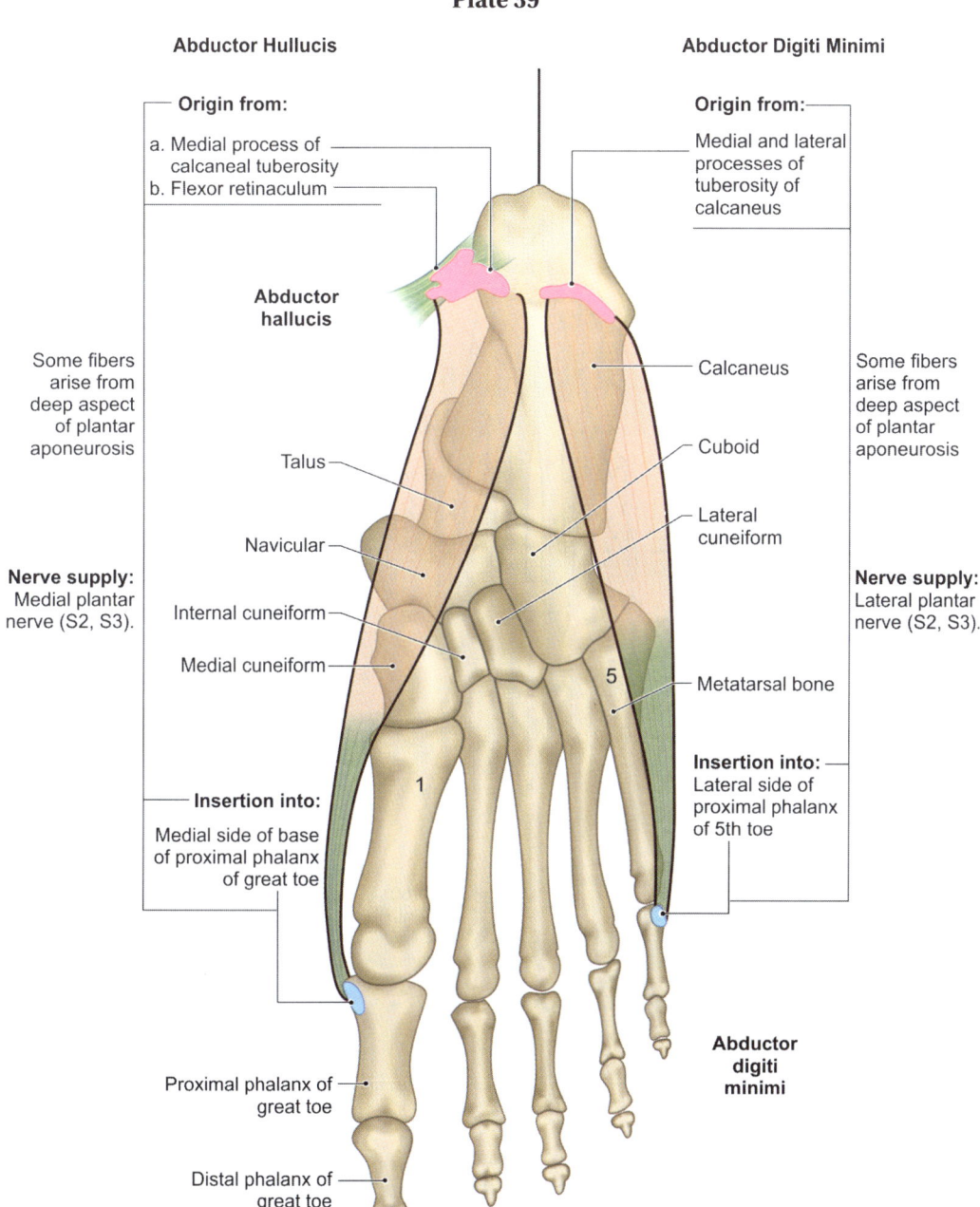

Abductor Hullucis

Origin from:
a. Medial process of calcaneal tuberosity
b. Flexor retinaculum

Some fibers arise from deep aspect of plantar aponeurosis

Nerve supply: Medial plantar nerve (S2, S3).

Insertion into:
Medial side of base of proximal phalanx of great toe

Abductor Digiti Minimi

Origin from:
Medial and lateral processes of tuberosity of calcaneus

Some fibers arise from deep aspect of plantar aponeurosis

Nerve supply: Lateral plantar nerve (S2, S3).

Insertion into:
Lateral side of proximal phalanx of 5th toe

Actions:
The abductor hallucis abducts the great toe, and helps to flex it. The abductor digiti minimi abducts the 5th toe. However, the main function of these muscles (and of other short muscles of the foot) is to stabilize the toes while walking. This is necessary as the propulsive force is transmitted to the ground through the toes. These muscles also play an important part in maintaining the arches of the foot.

Plate 40

Plantar Aponeurosis

Underlying the skin of the sole there is a thick layer of deep fascia which is given the name plantar aponeurosis. It consists of central, medial and lateral parts.

The medial and lateral parts of the aponeurosis are relatively thin. They cover the abductor hallucis and the abductor digiti minimi respectively.

The central part is the thickest and strongest. It overlies the flexor digitorum brevis. (Some authors describe this part alone as the plantar aponeurosis). It consists of longitudinal fibers that are attached posteriorly to the medial process of the calcaneal tuberosity. Traced distally the aponeurosis broadens and divides into five processes, one for each digit.

Near the head of the corresponding metatarsal bone, each process divides into two slips which pass round the sides of the flexor tendons of the digit and get attached to the deep transverse metatarsal ligaments (which stretch between the heads of the metatarsals). Distally, the two slips of each process become continuous with the proximal end of the fibrous flexor sheath of the digit.

Fibrous Flexor Sheaths

Over each toe the deep fascia (which is thick) winds round the sides of the flexor tendons of the digit to get attached to the lateral margins of the phalanges. The fascia constitutes the fibrous flexor sheath. The tendons are thus enclosed in an osseoaponeurotic canal. This canal is lined by a synovial sheath to permit smooth movement of the tendons. The fibrous sheath is closed distally by attachment to the base of the terminal phalanx. Proximally the fibrous sheath is continuous with the distal margins of the slips of the plantar aponeurosis.

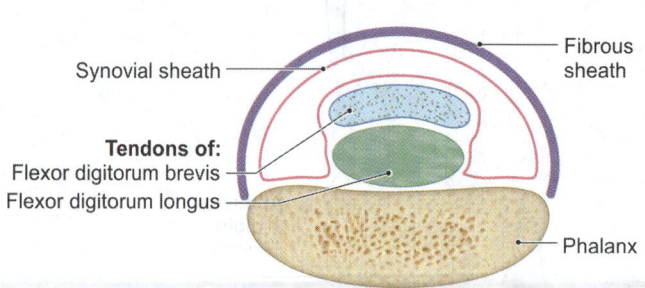

Transverse section across a digit to show the placing of tendons and of sheaths.

Plate 41

Flexor Digitorum Accessorius

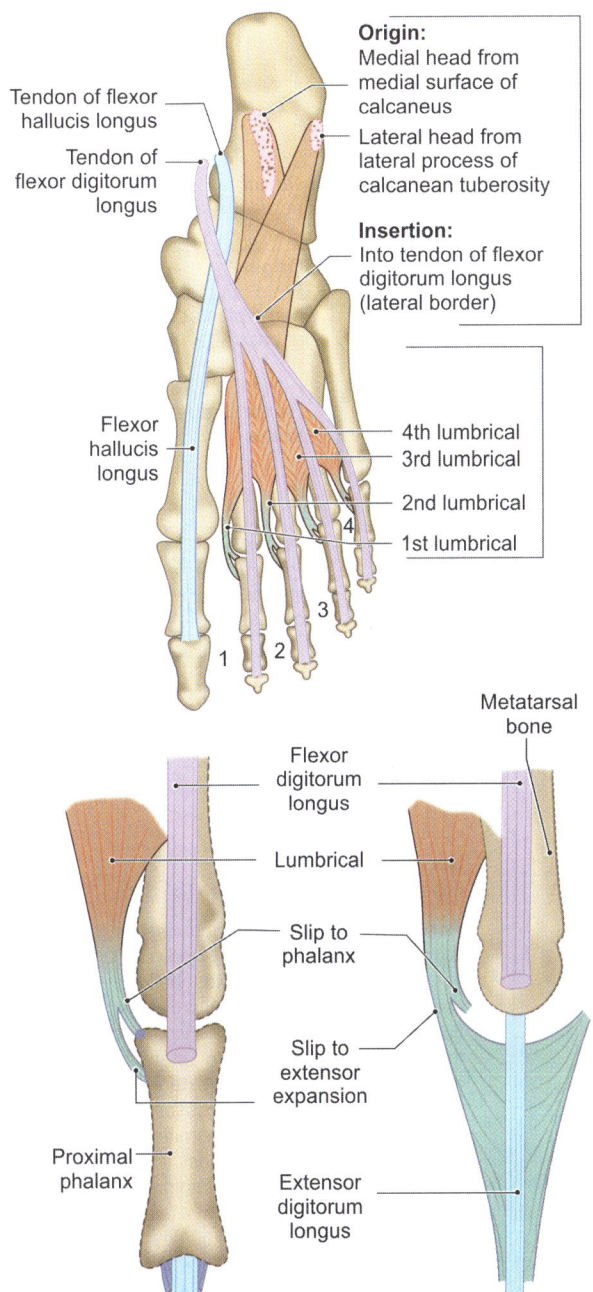

Origin:
Medial head from medial surface of calcaneus
Lateral head from lateral process of calcanean tuberosity

Insertion:
Into tendon of flexor digitorum longus (lateral border)

Nerve supply:
Lateral plantar nerve (S2, S3).

Actions:
This muscle straightens the oblique pull of the flexor digitorum longus. Acting through the tendons of the flexor digitorum longus it can flex the toes.

Lumbrical Muscles of the Foot

These are four slender muscles numbered from the medial to the lateral side.

Origin:
The lumbrical muscles take origin from the digital tendons of the flexor digitorum longus. The first lumbrical arises from the medial side of the tendon to the 2nd toe. The 2nd, 3rd and 4th muscles arise from the contiguous sides of the four tendons.

Insertion:
Each muscle ends in a tendon which curves round the medial side of the corresponding metatarsophalangeal joint. It is inserted partly into the base of the proximal phalanx, and partly into the extensor expansion. The insertion is similar to that of the lumbricals of the hand.

Nerve supply: The first lumbrical by the medial plantar nerve, all others by the lateral plantar nerve (S2, S3).

Action: These muscles maintain extension of interphalangeal joints of toes.

Atlas of Muscle Attachments: Lower Limb

Plate 42

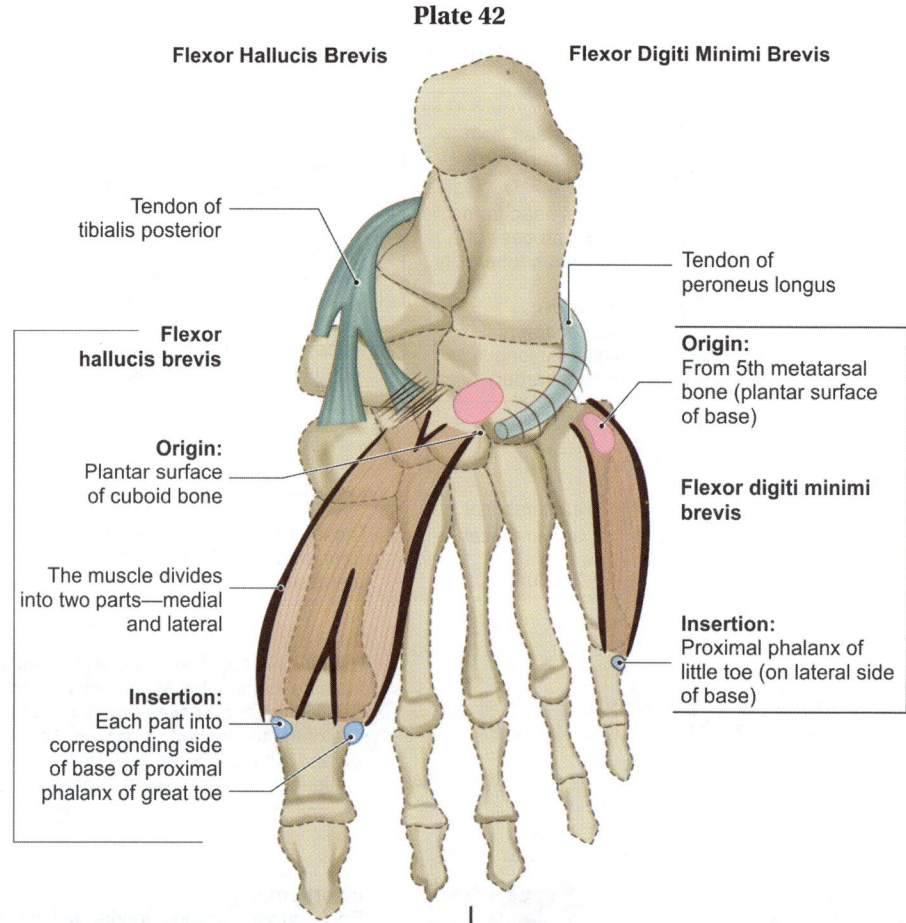

Flexor Hallucis Brevis

Tendon of tibialis posterior

Flexor hallucis brevis

Origin: Plantar surface of cuboid bone

The muscle divides into two parts—medial and lateral

Insertion: Each part into corresponding side of base of proximal phalanx of great toe

Flexor Digiti Minimi Brevis

Tendon of peroneus longus

Origin: From 5th metatarsal bone (plantar surface of base)

Flexor digiti minimi brevis

Insertion: Proximal phalanx of little toe (on lateral side of base)

Some fibers also arise from the lateral cuneiform bone, and from the tendons of insertion of the tibialis posterior.

Nerve supply:
From the medial plantar nerve (S2, S3).

Action:
See under flexor digiti minimi brevis.

Nerve supply:
From the lateral plantar nerve (S1, S2).

Actions of flexor hallucis brevis and flexor digiti minimi brevis: As indicated by their names, the flexor hallucis brevis and the flexor digiti minimi brevis flex the corresponding toes. However, their main function is to stabilize the toes (by preventing extension) while walking. This is necessary as the propulsive force is transmitted to the ground through the toes. These muscles also help in maintaining the arches of the foot.

Plate 43
Adductor Hallucis

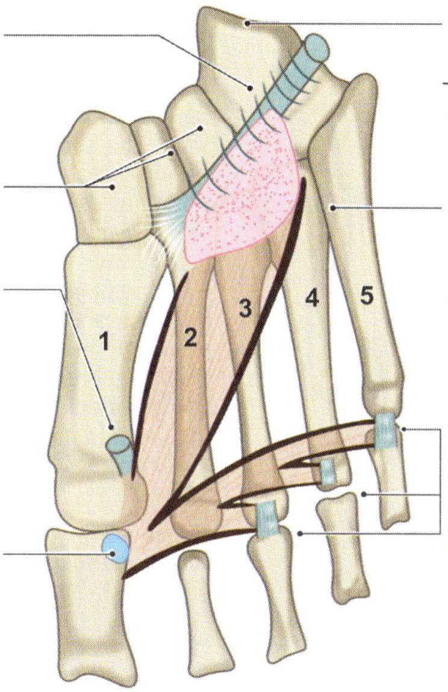

- Tendon of peroneus longus (covered by sheath)
- Cuboid bone
- Cuneiform bones
- Flexor hallucis brevis

Origin:
Oblique head from bases of 2nd, 3rd and 4th metatarsal bones. Some fibers from sheath of peroneus longus tendon.

Transverse head from plantar aspect of metacarpophalangeal joints of 3rd, 4th and 5th toes.

Nerve supply:
Lateral plantar nerve (S2, 3).

Insertion into:
Lateral side of base of proximal phalanx of great toe (in common with lateral part of flexor hallucis brevis)

Interosseous Muscles of the Foot
See next page also

Introductory remarks

These are small muscles placed between the metatarsal bones. There are three plantar, and four dorsal, interossei. They are numbered from medial to lateral side.

Each plantar interosseous muscle arises from one metatarsal bone (from the plantar aspect of the shaft). It is inserted into the base of the proximal phalanx, and into the dorsal digital expansion of the corresponding digit. Each dorsal interosseous muscle arises from the shafts of two adjoining metatarsal bones. The dorsal interossei are inserted into the bases of the proximal phalanges, and into the dorsal digital expansions.

Details of the attachments of individual interosseous muscles are easily remembered if their actions are first understood.

Actions of interossei

The interossei adduct or abduct the toes with reference to an axis passing through the second digit. The plantar interossei are adductors. They pull the 3rd, 4th and 5th toes toward the second toe. The dorsal interossei are abductors. To understand their action note that as the axis of the second digit is the line of reference for defining abduction: movement of this digit to either the medial or lateral side is described as abduction. The first dorsal interosseous muscle pulls the second toe medially; and the second dorsal interosseous muscle pulls the same (2nd) digit laterally. The 3rd muscle pull the 3rd digit, and the 4th muscle pulls the 4th digit laterally (i.e. away from the 2nd digit).

In addition to abduction and adduction, the interossei flex the metatarsophalangeal joints and extend the interphalangeal joints by virtue of their insertion into the dorsal digital expansions.

Plate 44
Plantar Interossei

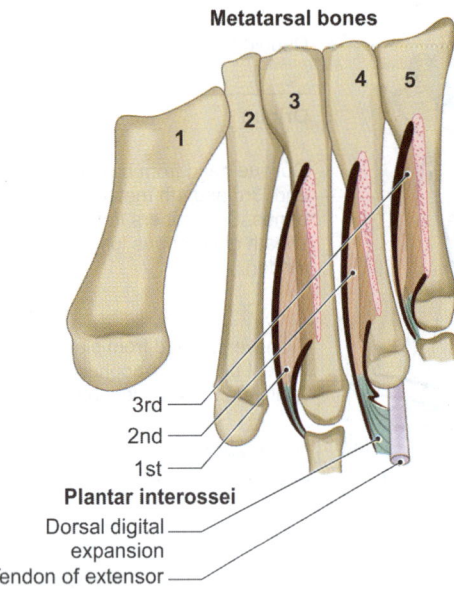

Origin:
The first plantar interosseous muscle arises from the plantar aspect of the shaft of the 3rd metatarsal bone. The second muscle has a similar origin from the 4th metatarsal bone, and the third muscle from the 5th metatarsal bone.

Insertions:
Each plantar interosseous muscle is inserted into the base of the proximal phalanx of one digit; and partly into the dorsal digital expansion of that digit. The 1st plantar interosseous muscle is inserted into the medial side of the 3rd digit; the second muscle into the medial side of the 4th digit; and the third muscle into the medial side of the 5th digit.

Nerve supply:
All the interossei are supplied by the lateral plantar nerve (S2, S3).

Dorsal Interossei of the Foot

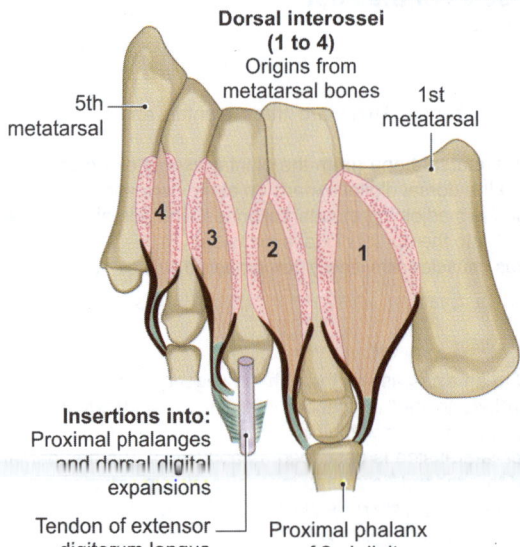

Origins:
Each dorsal interosseous muscle arises from the adjacent sides of the shafts of two metatarsal bones as follows: The first muscle arises from the 1st and 2nd metatarsal bones. The second muscle arises from the 2nd and 3rd metatarsal bones. The third muscle arises from the 3rd and 4th metatarsal bones; and the fourth muscle from the 4th and 5th metatarsal bones.

Insertions:
Each dorsal interosseous muscle ends in a tendon which is inserted on one side (medial or lateral) of the base of a proximal phalanx; and also into the corresponding dorsal digital expansion as follows: The first muscle is inserted on the medial side of 2nd digit. The second muscle is inserted on the lateral side of the 2nd digit. The third muscle is inserted on the lateral side of the 3rd digit. The fourth muscle is inserted on the lateral side of the 4th digit.

5 CHAPTER

Sternum and Ribs

THE STERNUM

AN 21.1 Identify and describe the salient features of sternum.

The vertically elongated sternum lies in the midline in the anterior wall of the thorax. This *flat bone* consists of three parts. From above downward these are manubrium, body and the xiphoid process.

The sternum presents anterior and posterior surfaces.

The body joins the manubrium at the *manubriosternal joint* and the xiphoid process at the *xiphisternal joint*. The anterior ends of the upper seven costal cartilages are attached to the margins of the sternum. The first costal cartilage is attached to the lateral margin of the manubrium. The second costal cartilage is attached partly to the manubrium, and partly to the upper end of the body. The third, fourth, fifth, and sixth cartilages are attached to the lateral margin of the body. The seventh costal cartilage is attached to the lateral side of the xiphisternal joint. The area of attachment of each cartilage is marked by a notch on the lateral margin of the sternum **(Fig. 5.1)**.

Manubrium: On either side, the upper border of the manubrium articulates with the medial end of the clavicle to form the *sternoclavicular joint* through *clavicular notches*. Between the right and left clavicular notches it presents the *jugular* (suprasternal) *notch*. The manubrium and the body of the sternum lie at a slight angle; the manubriosternal junction projects forward. This projection forms the *sternal angle*; guide to identify costal cartilages and ribs and intercostal spaces.

Body: It consists of four parts (*sternebrae*) united by cartilage till puberty; fuse thereafter to form a single bone. The lines of fusion are seen on the anterior aspect of the bone. The manubriosternal joint is a secondary cartilaginous joint (*symphysis*).

Xiphoid process: It is cartilaginous in children; undergoes ossification in the adults. The xiphisternal joint is a *symphysis*. However, unlike a typical symphysis, the joint disappears in old age.

Junction of the first costal cartilage with the manubrium is a *synchondrosis*. Other sternocostal joints are *synovial joints*.

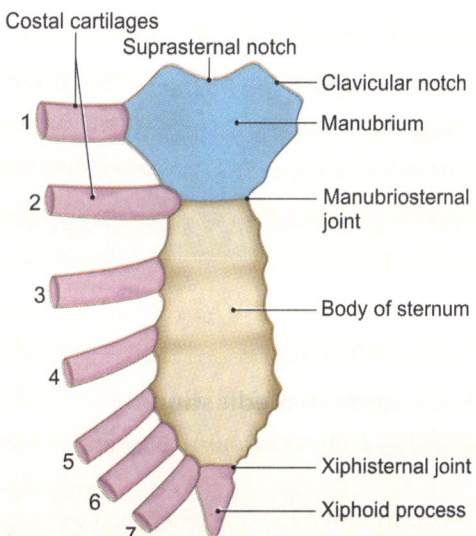

Fig. 5.1: Sternum and costal cartilages from the front.

Sternoclavicular Joint

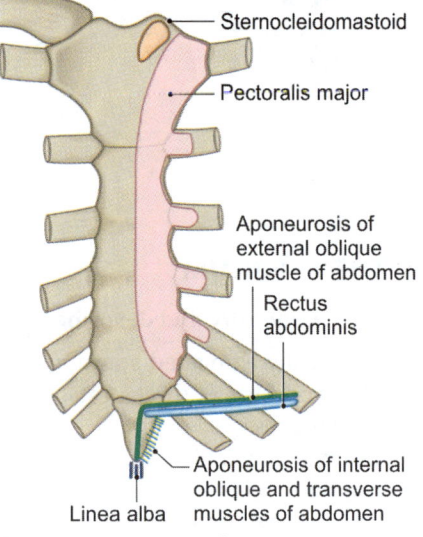

Fig. 5.2: Sternum: Attachments on anterior aspect.

AN 13.4 **Describe sternoclavicular joint.**

Sternoclavicular joint is a double synovial (*plane variety—gliding*) joint; united by the fibrous capsule. Its intracapsular articular disc separates joint cavity into two compartments. It provides the only bony attachment between the appendicular and axial skeletons. It is reinforced by the anterior and posterior sternoclavicular, interclavicular, and costoclavicular ligaments. It allows elevation and depression, protraction and retraction, and circumduction of the shoulder.

Sternoclavicular joint is rarely dislocated because its location protects it from most injury forces. A direct blow to medial end of clavicle may dislocate clavicle posteriorly. An indirect force on the lateral aspect of shoulder may rotate medial end of clavicle to either anterior or posterior to sternum.

Attachments

Attachments to the Anterior Aspect (Fig. 5.2)

Muscle/structure	Attachment
Sternocleidomastoid (sternal head)	Upper part of the manubrium (*origin*)
Pectoralis major	Corresponding half of manubrium and body of sternum; extends to costal cartilages (*origin*)
Rectus abdominis	Xiphoid process; extends to 7th, 6th, and 5th costal cartilages (*insertion*)
External oblique aponeurosis	(Covers rectus abdominis) beyond insertion of rectus abdominis (*origin*)
Internal oblique and transversus abdominis aponeuroses	Sides of xiphoid process
Linea alba	Lower end of xiphoid process

Attachments to the Posterior Aspect (Fig. 5.3)

Muscle	Origin
Sternohyoid	Upper part of posterior surface of manubrium; extends onto the back of clavicle (*origin*)
Sternothyroid	Posterior surface of manubrium (below origin of sternohyoid); extends onto first costal cartilage (*origin*)
Sternocostalis	Lower one-third of posterior surface of body and xiphoid process (also adjoining parts of costal cartilages) (*origin*)
Diaphragm (*sternal slips*)	Back of xiphoid process

Boundaries of Mediastinum

AN 21.11 Mention boundaries and contents of the superior, anterior, middle and posterior mediastinum.

Mediastinum is the space between two pleural cavities. It is divided into superior and inferior mediastinum by an imaginary line from the sternal angle called angle of Louis (*manubriosternal joint*) to T4/5 intervertebral disc.

Superior mediastinum: It is above the transverse thoracic plane passing through sternal angle and junction of T-4 and T-5 vertebrae. It communicates with the root of neck through the *thoracic inlet*; bounded anteriorly by manubrium, posteriorly by T-1 vertebra and laterally by 1st rib.

Contents (from anterior to posterior)
- Thymus, Trachea, Esophagus and Thoracic duct
- Great vessels related to heart and pericardium
   a. Brachiocephalic veins
   b. Superior part of SVC
   c. Arch of aorta and its branches (Brachiocephalic trunk, Left common carotid and Left subclavian arteries)
- *Nerves*: Vagus, phrenic nerves, Left recurrent laryngeal nerve and cardiac plexus of nerves.

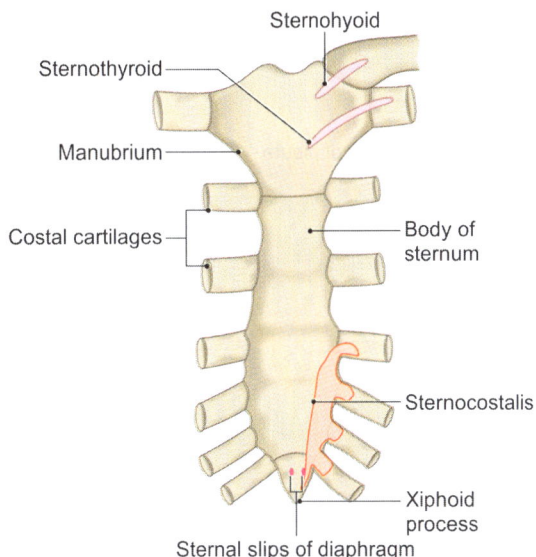

Fig. 5.3: Sternum: Attachments on posterior aspect.

Inferior mediastinum is divided into:
a. **Anterior mediastinum** (region in front of pericardium)
b. **Middle mediastinum** (consists of pericardium and heart)
c. **Posterior mediastinum** (region between pericardium and vertebrae).

Anterior mediastinum: Lies between the body of sternum and transversus thoracis muscles anteriorly and pericardium posteriorly. It continues with superior mediastinum at sternal angle, limited inferiorly by diaphragm. It contains sternopericardial ligaments, branches of internal thoracic vessels and few lymph nodes. In infants and children it also contains lower part of thymus.

Middle mediastinum: Contains pericardium, heart, ascending aorta, pulmonary trunk, SVC, arch of azygos vein and principal bronchi.

Posterior mediastinum: It is anterior to T-5 to T-12 vertebrae, posterior to pericardium and diaphragm and between parietal pleura of two lungs. It contains descending thoracic aorta, thoracic duct, azygos and hemiazygos veins, esophagus, thoracic sympathetic trunks and thoracic splanchnic nerves and posterior mediastinal lymph nodes.

Sternum: Relations

Posterior aspect of manubrium:
- Arch of aorta and its branches
   - Left brachiocephalic vein
- Lateral part: Lungs and pleura
- Body of the sternum:
   - Lungs and pleura **(Fig. 5.4)**
   - Pericardium
- Xiphoid process: Liver.

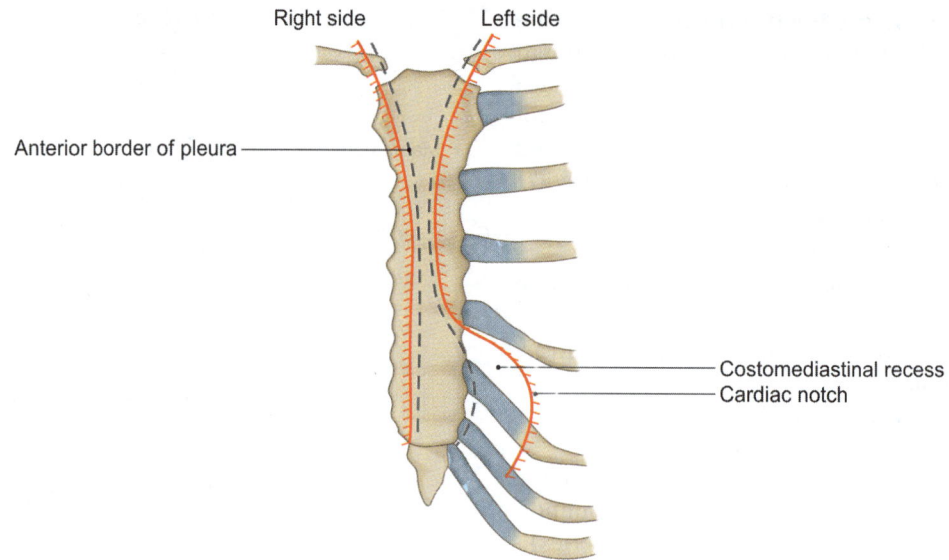

Fig. 5.4: Sternum: Pleural reflections.

Sexual Differences

Feature	Male	Female
Length	Longer (average: 7 inches)	Shorter (average: 6.5 inches)
Sternal angle	More pronounced	Less pronounced
Muscular impressions	More marked	Less marked

Sternal Angle: Anatomical Events
* Attachment of second costal cartilage; counting of ribs
* Trachea bifurcates into two principal bronchi
* Marks the plane separating superior and inferior mediastinum
* Termination of ascending aorta
* Arch of aorta begins and ends
* Descending thoracic aorta commences
* Marks upper limit of the base of the heart
* Azygos vein arches over root of right lung; opens into superior vena cava (SVC)
* Pulmonary trunk divides into two pulmonary arteries just below the sternal angle
* Cardiac plexuses are located at this level.

Ossification and Development (Figs. 5.5A and B)

Number of ossification centers in different sternal segments is variable:
* One to three in the manubrium
* One or two in each sternebra
* Centers appear around fifth month of fetal life
* Ossification in the xiphoid process begins around third year

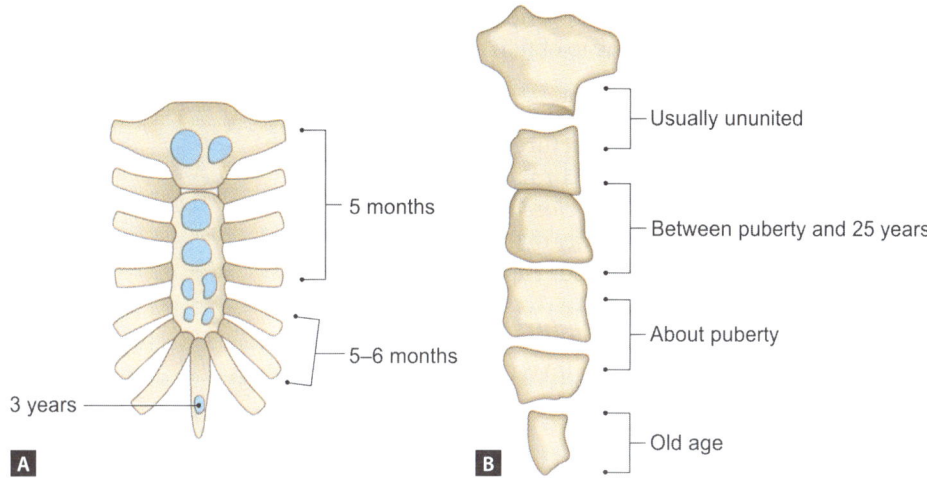

Figs. 5.5A and B: Sternum: ossification: (A) Time of appearance; (B) Time of fusion.

❖ Sternebrae unite with each other between puberty and 25 years; union starts inferiorly and proceed upward.

AN 21.8 Describe and demonstrate type, articular surfaces and movements of manubriosternal and xiphisternal joints.

Manubriosternal joint: It is a secondary cartilaginous joint (*symphysis*) between manubrium and the body of the sternum.

Xiphisternal joint: It is a secondary cartilaginous joint (*symphysis: disappears later*) between the xiphoid process and the body of the sternum.

Clinical Anatomy

Congenital Anomalies

Ectopia cordis: The sternum develops in two lateral halves, which unite from below upward. In ectopia cordis (heart is exposed), the two sternal halves remain nonunited **(Fig. 5.6)**.

Sternal foramen: Sometimes an opening may persist in the body of the sternum due to defective ossification.

Bifid sternum: Depending on the range of incomplete ossification, at times lower part of the sternum remains nonunited called bifid sternum (*cleft sternum*) **(Figs. 5.7A and B)**.

Certain congenital defects in the chest make sternum either projects anteriorly (*pigeon chest*) **(Fig. 5.8A)** or inferoposteriorly making the chest appears as funnel (*funnel chest*) **(Fig. 5.8B)**.

Sternal Puncture

Being radially accessible, the sternum is a common site for bone marrow aspiration. The sternum is covered by a thin plate

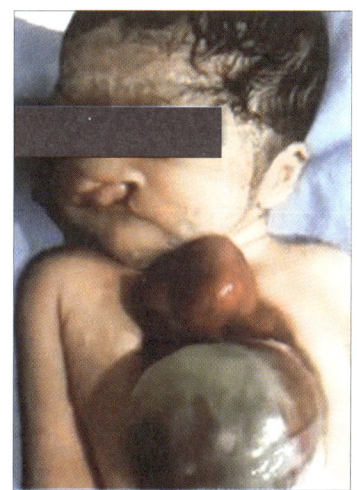

Fig. 5.6: Ectopia cordis.

of cortical bone through which a wide bore needle is pushed into the highly vascular spongy bone to obtain the sample.

Sternal Fracture

In automobile accidents, sternal fracture is commonly seen near the sternal angle. The broken fragments remain concealed under the skin (*closed comminuted fracture*). Depending upon the severity of the impact, the mediastinal structures may get injured/ruptured.

Sternal Division for Surgical Procedures

Complete vertical cutting of the sternum is required when operating on the heart or great vessels. Divided sternal parts are approximated and wired.

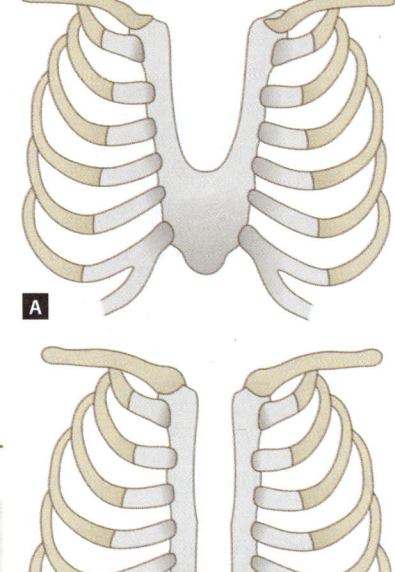

Figs. 5.7A and B: Bifid sternum: (A) Incomplete; (B) Complete.

> **QUESTIONNAIRE**
> - Classify the bone.
> - Name the parts of the sternum.
> - Enumerate the articulations of sternum. Classify these joints.
> - What type of joint is between first costal cartilage and the sternum?
> - Mark the posterior relations of the manubrium sterni.
> - Mark the pleural reflections on the right and left sides.
> - Mark the attachments of sternocleidomastoid and pectoralis major.
> - Mark the muscles attached to the posterior surface of the manubrium sterni.
> - Name the muscles attached to the xiphoid process.
> - What is the sternal angle? Enumerate the anatomical events at this level.
> - What is sternal foramen? How it is formed?
> - What is bifid sternum?
> - What is ectopia cordis?
> - What is the clinical importance of the sternum?
> - Comment on its ossification and development.

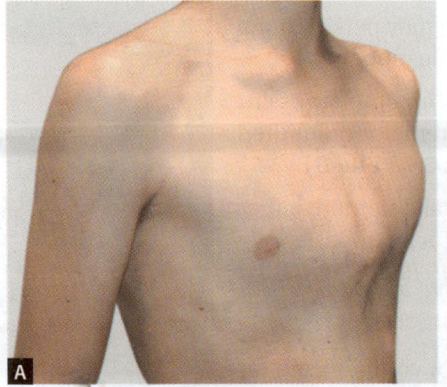
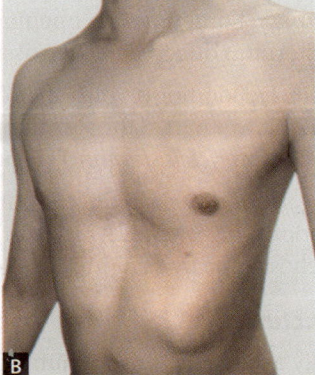

Figs. 5.8A and B: (A) Pigeon chest; (B) Funnel chest.

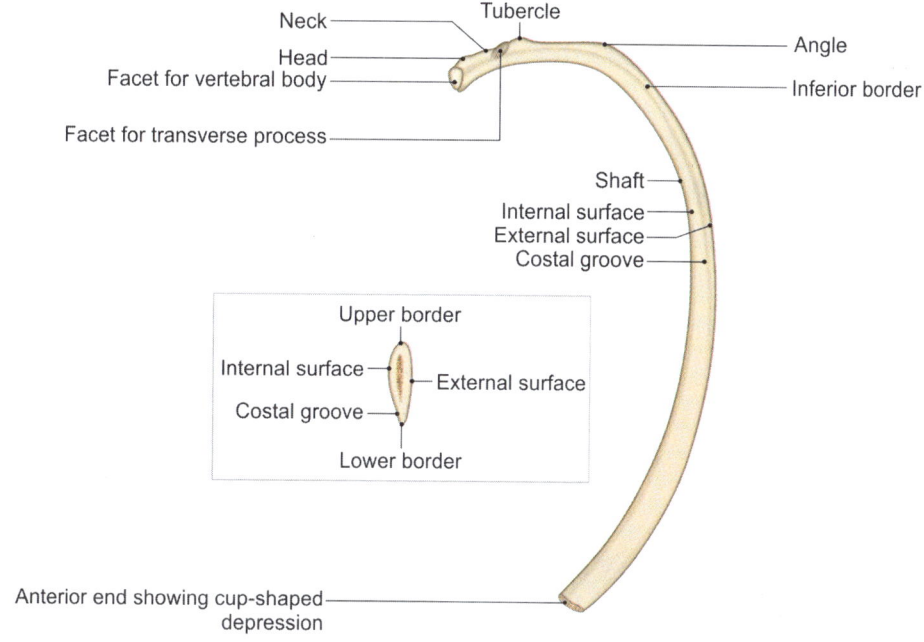

Fig. 5.9: Typical rib from below.

TYPICAL RIBS

AN 21.1 Identify and describe the salient features of typical rib.

General Features

The ribs are curved *flat bones* that form the side walls of the thorax (**Fig. 5.9**). There are 12 ribs on either side. They vary considerably in length; seventh rib is the longest, those above and below it become progressively shorter. Adjacent ribs are separated by *intercostal spaces*.

The ribs are attached behind to the thoracic vertebrae. The anterior ends of the upper seven ribs through their *costal cartilages* are attached to the sternum. These are *true ribs*.

The costal cartilages of the eighth, ninth, and 10th ribs do not reach the sternum directly, but end by gaining attachment to the next higher costal cartilage. These are *false ribs*.

The anterior ends of the 11th and 12th ribs have small pieces of cartilage. These ends are free; called *floating ribs*.

At the posterior end of a typical rib a *head*, a *neck*, and a *tubercle* are noted.

Head: It articulates partly with the superior costal facet on the body of the numerically corresponding vertebra; partly with the inferior costal facet on the next higher vertebra.

Neck: It is lateral to the head; in front of the transverse process of the numerically corresponding vertebra. It has a sharp upper border—the *crest* of the neck. Just lateral to the neck, the rib presents the *tubercle*. The tubercle has *medial articular part* which bears a facet that articulates with the costal facet on the transverse process of the corresponding vertebra and *lateral nonarticular part*—rough for attachment of ligaments.

Anterior end of rib: It shows a cup-shaped depression for the attachment of the costal cartilage.

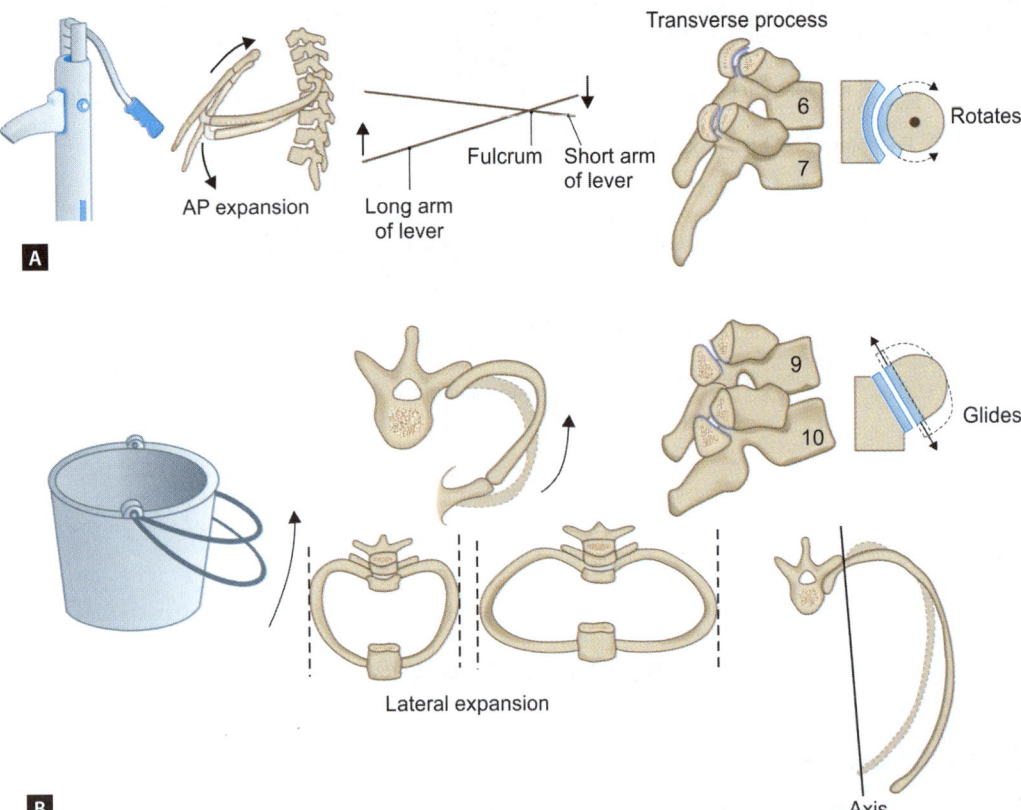

Figs. 5.10A and B: Movements of thoracic cage: (A) Pump handle movement; (B) Bucket handle movement.

Shaft: It is flat and curved. It has two surfaces (*inner and outer*) and two borders (*upper and lower*). The upper border is rounded; lower border is sharp. The inner surface is concave. Just above the lower border, the inner surface shows *costal groove*. The external surface is convex. A short distance lateral to the tubercle, it is marked by a rough line. At this point the rib appears bent; called the *angle*. The shaft is also twisted along its long axis. Thus, the external surface faces downward in the posterior part and upward in its anterior part.

Movements of Thoracic Cage

Movements of Rib (Figs. 5.10A and B)

Pump handle movement: It increases anteroposterior and transverse diameters (2nd–6th ribs).

Mechanism and demonstration of movement:
- Hold the rib at fulcrum (tubercle).
- Rotate the neck a little backwards and downwards.
- This rotation is possible because of the nature of facets. Facets on the tubercle of rib are convex but concave on transverse process. The movement is magnified at the anterior end which moves upwards and forwards because of the long segment (shaft) of the lever. Sternum is pushed forwards so that AP diameter is increased.

❖ Transverse diameter is also increased simultaneously as the middle part of the rib is elevated. The axis for increasing the AP diameter passes through the neck of the rib.

Bucket handle movement: It increases transverse diameter but anteroposterior diameter is reduced (7th–10th ribs).

Mechanism and demonstration of movement:
❖ Fix both the ends of the rib.
❖ Elevate the middle part of the rib.
❖ Elevation increases the transverse diameter like the handle of a bucket. The AP diameter is reduced as both the ends of the rib slide backwards. Slide occurs because of the nature of the facets. Facets on the tubercle of the rib and transverse process of thoracic vertebra are flat. The movement occurs at costovertebral and costotransverse joints (plane synovial).
❖ Elevation of the ribs makes the costal cartilages transverse which are otherwise obliquely placed, thus the infrasternal angle is increased.
❖ Axis for increase in transverse diameter passes through both ends of the rib.

Typical Ribs: Attachments

Part	Attached structure
Head	• Fibrous capsule Radiate ligament • Intra-articular ligament of costovertebral joint
Neck and tubercle give attachment to ligaments of costotransverse joint	
Crest of neck	Superior costotransverse ligament
Posterior surface of neck	Costotransverse ligament
Rough nonarticular part of the tubercle	Lateral costotransverse ligament

Muscle/structure	Attachment
Internal intercostal membrane	*Neck of rib:* Lower border and anterior surface
External intercostal muscle	• *Superiorly:* Lower border of shaft • *Inferiorly:* Outer lip of superior border (of next lower rib)
Internal intercostal muscle	• *Above:* Floor of costal groove • *Below:* Inner lip of superior border (of next lower rib)
Intercostalis intimus (innermost intercostal)	• *Above:* Upper border of costal groove • *Below:* Inner lip of superior border (of next lower rib, with internal intercostal)
Serratus anterior, pectoralis minor, latissimus dorsi, external oblique abdomen, levator costae, and iliocostalis cervicis (part of erector spinae)	External surfaces of typical ribs; attachments varying from rib to rib

Typical Ribs: Relations

❖ Intercostal vessels and nerve (*of intercostal space*) lie in relation to the costal groove; separated from the floor of the groove by internal intercostal muscle.
❖ Sympathetic trunk descends vertically across the anterior aspect of the heads of lower ribs.
❖ Internal surfaces of the ribs are covered by costal pleura.

Ribs: Ossification

Typical rib has one primary center; appears in shaft during second month of fetal life. Secondary centers appear around puberty:
- One for the head
- One each for articular and nonarticular parts of the tubercle.

Center for nonarticular part of the tubercle is absent in lower ribs. As 11th and 12th ribs have no tubercles, the relevant centers are absent in them.

AN 21.8 Describe and demonstrate type, articular surfaces and movements of costovertebral and costotransverse joints.

Costovertebral joints: These are synovial (*plane variety*) joints between heads of the ribs with corresponding and supra-adjacent vertebral bodies.

Costotransverse joints: These are synovial (*plane variety*) joint between tubercle of the rib with transverse process of the corresponding vertebra.

AN 21.10 Describe costochondral and interchondral joints.

Costochondral joints: These are the joints between anterior ends of the ribs and their costal cartilages.

Interchondral joints: These are synovial (*plane variety*) joints between 6th and 10th costal cartilages of ribs.

QUESTIONNAIRE

- What type of bone is rib? Why?
- Side determination of the typical rib.
- Demonstrate the articulations of a typical rib. Classify these joints.
- Which ligament connects head of the rib to the vertebra? How many slips does the ligament have? Mark their attachments.
- What are the contents of the subcostal groove?
- Mark the muscles attached to the upper border of the rib.
- Mark the attachments to lower border and the subcostal groove.
- What is the direction of the anterior angle? What are the muscles attached close to the angle?
- What is the direction of the posterior angle?
- Pump handle movement occurs in which ribs? What diameters are increased? Explain its mechanism.
- Bucket handle movement occurs in which ribs? What diameters are increased? Explain its mechanism.
- Name the accessory muscles of the respiration.
- What is the common site of rib fracture? Why?
- In which condition notching of the lower border of the ribs is seen? Why?
- Comment on the ossification of the rib.

ATYPICAL RIBS

AN 21.1 Identify and describe the features of 1st, 2nd, 11th and 12th ribs.

First Rib

This smallest rib with broad and flat shaft presents *upper* and *lower* surfaces with *inner* and *outer* borders. Its head has a single facet (first rib articulates only with first thoracic vertebra). The tubercle is prominent and coincides with the angle.

Shaft: The upper surface of the shaft presents two shallow grooves (for subclavian vessels). At the inner border these grooves are separated by the *scalene tubercle*. The lower surface is smooth without a costal groove **(Figs. 5.11 and 5.12)**.

Features

❖ Shortest and most curved
❖ Broad and flat
❖ Twist in the shaft is absent
❖ Costal groove is absent.

Side Determination

❖ *Posterior*: Vertebral end (head)
❖ *Superior*: Rough surface
❖ *Medial*: Inner border with scalene tubercle.

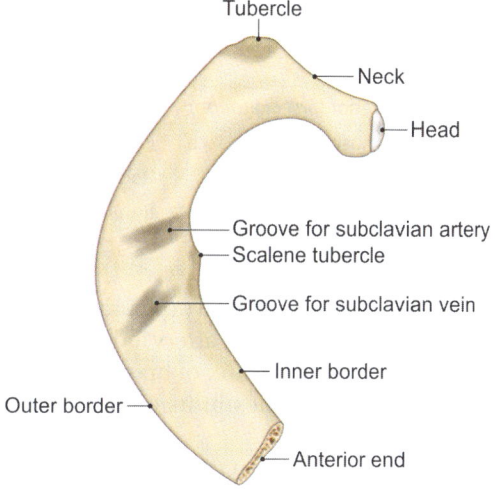

Fig. 5.11: First rib from above.

When the rib is placed on a horizontal plane (superior surface facing upward) both ends of the rib touch the surface.

Anatomical Position

Posterior vertebral end (head) is raised so that the shaft makes an angle of 45° with the horizontal.

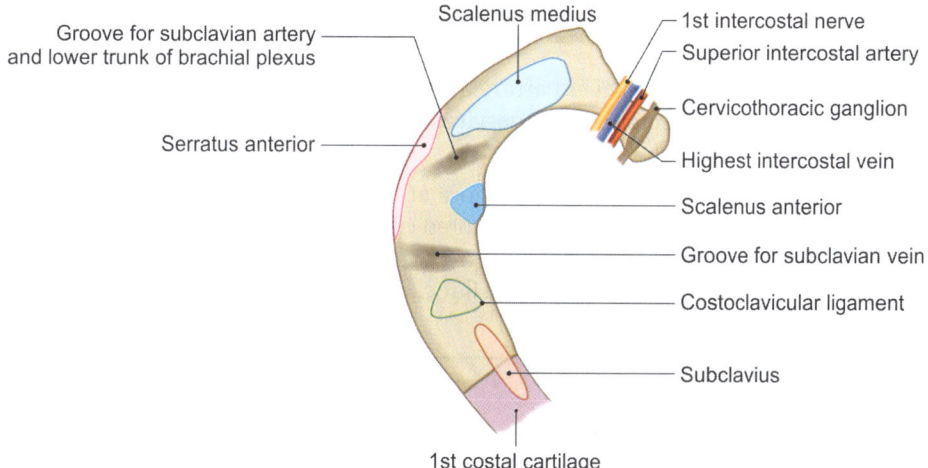

Fig. 5.12: First rib: Attachments and relations from above.

Attachments

Muscle/structure	Attachment
Scalenus anterior	Scalene tubercle; adjoining part of the upper surface (*insertion*)
Scalenus medius	Rough area on the superior surface, behind groove for subclavian artery (*insertion*)

(Contd...)

(Contd...)

Subclavius	Anterior end of the upper surface and adjoining part of first costal cartilage (*origin*)
Serratus anterior (*first digitation*)	Outer border near the groove for subclavian artery (*origin*)
Intercostal muscles of first space	Outer border
Costoclavicular ligament	Rough area in front of the groove for subclavian vein
Suprapleural membrane	Inner border

Relations

- Inferior surface is related to pleura and lung.
- Groove for subclavian artery lodges named artery and lower trunk of brachial plexus; subclavian vein lies in its own groove in front
- Structures related on the anterior aspect of the neck of first rib; from medial to lateral side:
  - Sympathetic trunk (*cervicothoracic ganglion*)
  - Superior intercostal artery
  - First posterior intercostal vein
  - Ventral ramus of first thoracic nerve (*ascends across first rib*).

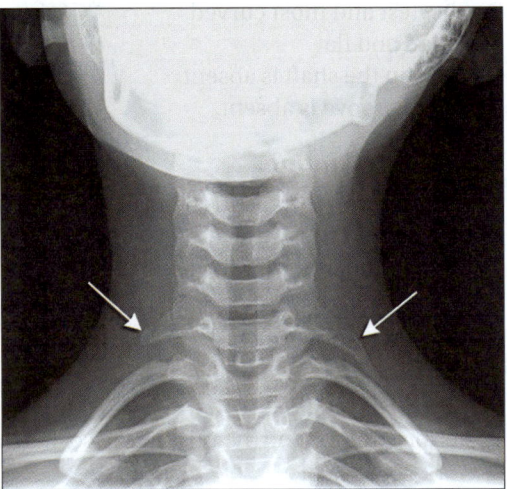

Fig. 5.13: Bilateral cervical ribs.

Clinical Anatomy

Thoracic inlet syndrome: Subclavian artery and first thoracic nerve arch over the first rib. These may be pressed or stretched by a cervical rib. This causes various vascular or neural symptoms.

Cervical rib: The costal element of C-7 vertebra at times enlarges to form various grades of cervical rib. A fully formed cervical rib is anchored close to anterior end of first rib (**Fig. 5.13**). In such situation, lower trunk of brachial plexus overrides cervical rib causing its stretching. This leads to various neurological symptoms. Subclavian artery is also likely to be compressed causing various vascular symptoms.

QUESTIONNAIRE

- Which are atypical ribs?
- Side determination and anatomical position of this bone.
- What is attached to the inner border of the first rib?
- Enumerate the structures related to the neck of the first rib.
- What is the function of the suprapleural membrane? What is it a remnant of?
- Identify the scalene tubercle. What is attached to it?
- Mark the attachments of scalenus medius, subclavius, and serratus anterior.
- Mark the attachment of the costoclavicular ligament.
- Identify the grooves for the subclavian vessels.
- What is a cervical rib? What are its symptoms?
- Comment on its ossification.

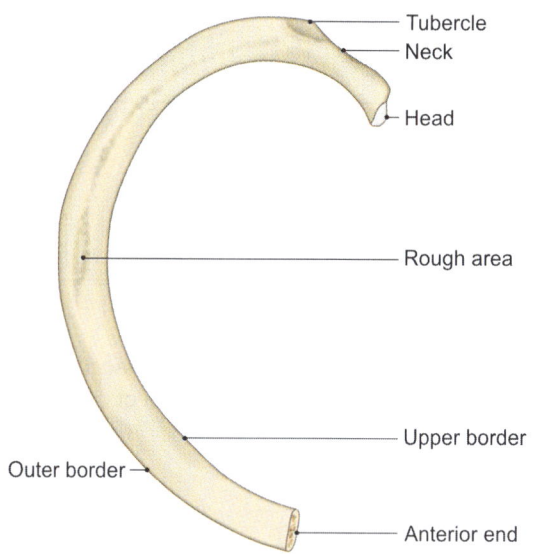

Fig. 5.14: Second rib (right) from above.

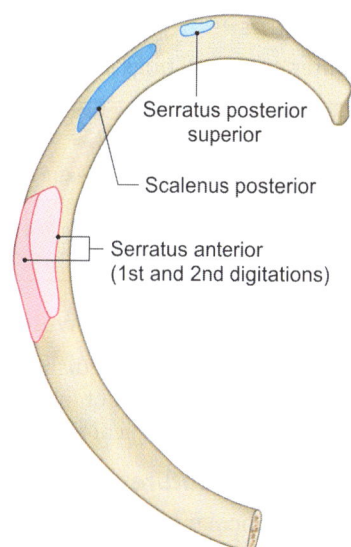

Fig. 5.15: Attachments on the superior aspect of the second rib.

Second Rib

The second rib when placed on a flat surface the entire rib touches the surface (in typical rib: posterior end is lifted off the surface). The external surface is directed outward and upward (*not directly upward as in first rib*). Near its middle, it has a prominent rough area. The inner surface points medially and downward. A short costal groove is present on its posterior part (**Figs. 5.14 and 5.15**).

Features
- Double the size of the first rib; bearing similar curvature
- Nonarticular part of the tubercle is small
- Angle is close to the tubercle
- Twist is absent in the shaft
- External surface of the shaft faces upward and outward
- Inner surface is smooth and concave; faces downward and inward.

Attachments

Muscle/structure	Attachment
Intercostal muscles	Upper and lower borders
Scalenus posterior	Posterior part of the outer surface (*insertion*)
Serratus anterior (first and second digitations)	Tubercle on the outer surface behind the middle of shaft (*origin*)
Serratus anterior (first digitation)	Outer border near the groove for subclavian artery (*origin*)
Serratus posterior superior (slip)	Just lateral to the tubercle (*insertion*)
Costoclavicular ligament	Rough area in front of the groove for subclavian vein

Relations

Inner surface: Lungs and pleura.

> **QUESTIONNAIRE**
> - What are the identifying features of the second rib?
> - Side determination and anatomical position.
> - Why is the costal groove shallow for the second rib?
> - Why is the rib thicker near the outer border in front of the posterior angle? Name the muscles attached.

Tenth, Eleventh, and Twelfth Ribs

These ribs can be distinguished from typical ribs they present only a single articular facet on the head because they articulate only with the corresponding vertebra. In other respects the 10th rib is similar to a typical rib (**Fig. 5.16**).

Tenth Rib: Feature

Single articular facet for T-10 vertebra.

Eleventh Rib: Features

- Relatively short
- Single articular facet on the head for T-11 vertebra
- No neck or tubercle
- Anterior end is pointed (in contrast to broad anterior ends of typical ribs)
- Angle is slight
- Costal groove is shallow.

Twelfth Rib: Features

- Single articular facet on the head for T-12 vertebra
- No neck or tubercle
- Anterior end is pointed; covered with cartilage

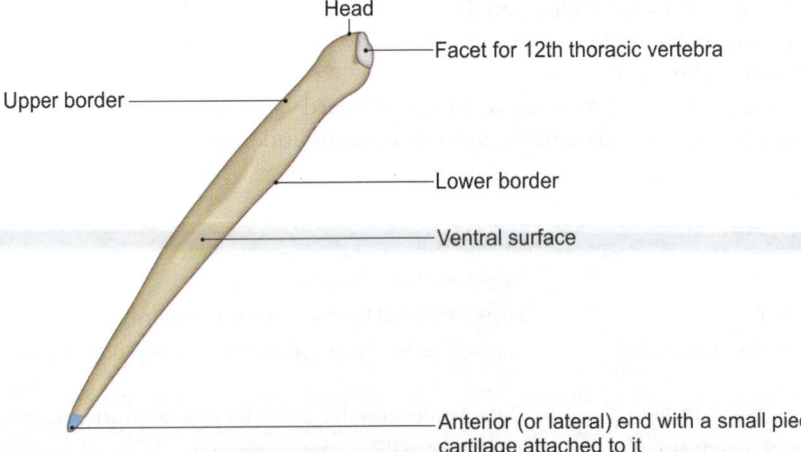

Fig. 5.16: Right 12th rib from the front (absence of neck, tubercle, angle, and costal groove).

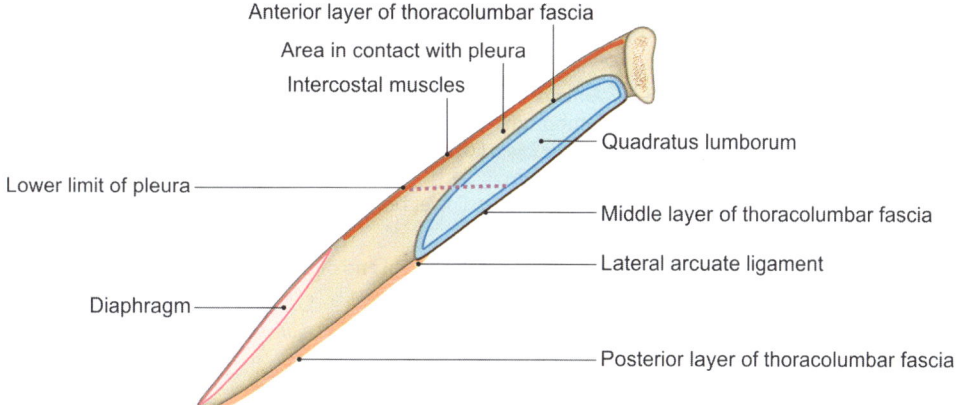

Fig. 5.17: 12th rib, anterior aspect: Attachments.

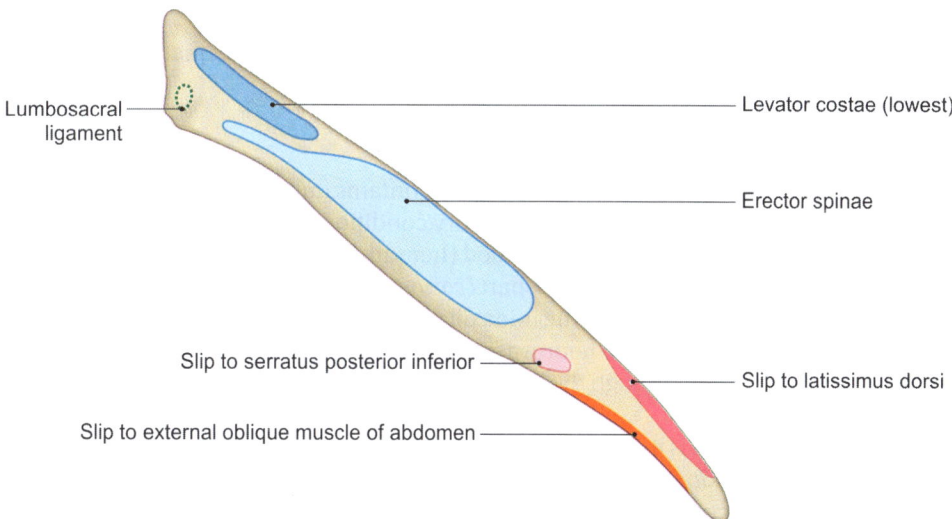

Fig. 5.18: 12th rib, posterior aspect: Attachments.

- No angle
- Costal groove is absent
- Vertebral end is directed slightly upwards.

Twelfth Rib: Attachments (Figs. 5.17 and 5.18)

Muscle/Structure	Attachment
Ligaments of costovertebral joint and lumbocostal ligament	Near the medial end
Intercostal muscles	Medial part of the upper border
Diaphragm	Lateral part of the upper border and adjoining part of the anterior surface (*origin*)

Muscle/Structure	Attachment
Quadratus lumborum	Lower part of the medial half of the anterior surface (*insertion*)
Thoracolumbar fascia	• *Anterior layer*: Anterior surface above the attachment of quadratus lumborum • *Middle layer*: Lower border below the attachment of quadratus lumborum • *Posterior layer*: Lower border, lateral to attachment of quadratus lumborum
Lateral arcuate ligament	Lower border at the lateral end of the area for attachment of quadratus lumborum
Levator costae (lowest) and part of erector spinae	Medial part of the posterior surface (*insertion*)
Latissimus dorsi (slips), external oblique abdomen and serratus posterior inferior	Lateral part of the posterior surface (*origin*)

Twelfth Rib: Pleural Relationship

The upper part of the medial half of the anterior surface (area above for quadratus lumborum) is in contact with pleura (*costodiaphragmatic recess*).

Clinical Anatomy

- ❖ ***Pleural tap:*** Pleural cavity is a potential space. It contains fluid that forms a firm to facilitate the movements of lung. In certain inflammatory conditions, the pleural cavity may contain excessive fluid (pleurisy with effusion), blood (hemothorax) or pus (pyothorax). By gravity, the fluid accumulates in the dependent part (*costodiaphragmatic recess*). To drain this fluid (*pleural tap*) a needle is inserted in the midaxillary line in the chosen intercostal space. Care has to be taken to avoid injury to neurovascular bundle in the intercostal space **(Fig. 5.19)**. For this needle is inserted through the lower part of intercostal space along the upper border of the rib below.
- ❖ ***Notching of the ribs***: This is the radiographic confirmation of blockade in the axillary/brachial artery and/or coarctation of aorta (localized narrowing of descending thoracic aorta distal to the attachment of ductus arteriosus). The radiological findings reveal irregular notching of the ribs **(Fig. 5.20)**. This is caused by posterior intercostal arteries, which become tortuous and dilated to erode the lower borders of the ribs.

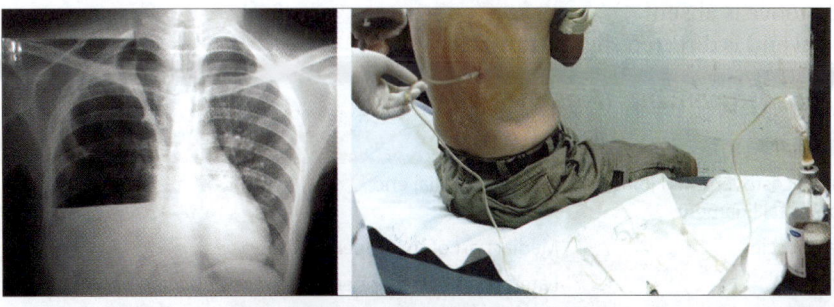

Fig. 5.19: Pleural effusion and tapping.

❖ ***Fracture of ribs***: Fracture of the ribs in children is rare due to highly elastic chest wall. In adults fracture of the ribs is seen due to direct violence or indirect compression. The most weak spot is the angle of the rib. The lower two ribs having no angles are least injured while the upper two ribs being protected by clavicle also escape fracture.

In severe compression injuries to the chest many vertebrosternal ribs may be fractured in front as well as behind. This makes a part of thoracic cage almost free (*stove-in chest/flail chest*). The affected side of the chest shows paradoxical respiratory movements (in inspiration the loose part of the chest wall is sucked in while in expiration it blows out).

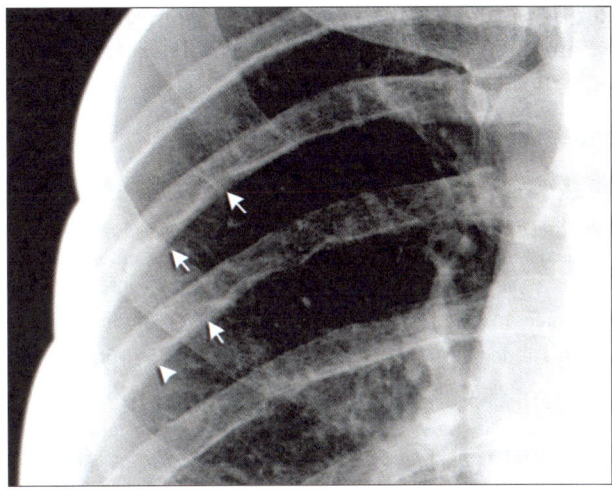

Fig. 5.20: Notching of ribs.

QUESTIONNAIRE

- What are the identifying features of the 12th rib?
- Side determination and anatomical position.
- Mark the attachment of the quadratus lumborum muscle.
- Mark the attachment of the thoracolumbar fascia.
- Mark the pleural reflections on this rib.
- What are the nonarticular parts of the tubercle not present for 11th and 12th ribs?

COSTAL CARTILAGES (HYALINE CARTILAGE)

A typical costal cartilage presents two ends (medial and lateral), two surfaces (anterior and posterior), and two borders (upper and lower).
❖ Lateral end of each costal cartilage is attached to the anterior end of the rib.
❖ Medial ends of the upper seven costal cartilages are attached to the lateral margin of the sternum.
   a. First costal cartilage is attached to the lateral margin of the manubrium sterni.
   b. Medial end of the second cartilage is attached partly to the manubrium and partly to the first sternebra.
   c. 3rd, 4th, and 5th cartilages are attached to the lateral edge of the sternum at the points of junction of sternebrae; 6th on the fourth sternebra; and 7th at the junction of fourth sternebra and xiphoid process.
❖ Medial ends of 8th, 9th, and 10th costal cartilages are connected to the next higher costal cartilage.
❖ Cartilages of 11th and 12th ribs are small; attached to the tips of the ribs. Their lateral ends are free.
❖ Joint between first costal cartilage and the manubrium sterni is a *synchondrosis*.

- 2nd to 7th costal cartilages join the sternum through *synovial joints*.
- Junctions of 8th, 9th, and 10th cartilages with the next higher cartilage are marked by the synovial joints.

Costal Cartilages: Attachments

Muscle/structure	Attachment
Internal intercostal muscles and external intercostal membranes	• Superior and inferior borders • Internal intercostal muscles (internally) and external intercostal membranes (externally)
Pectoralis major	Anterior surfaces of first 6th or 7th cartilage
Rectus abdominis	5th, 6th, and 7th cartilages
Internal oblique abdominis aponeurosis	7th, 8th, and 9th cartilages
Sternocostalis	Posterior surfaces of 2nd to 6th cartilages
Transversus abdominis	Posterior surfaces of 7th to 12th cartilages
Subclavius	First costal cartilage (anteriorly)
Sternothyroid (part)	First costal cartilage (posteriorly)
Costoclavicular ligament and articular disc of sternoclavicular joint	Upper surface of first costal cartilage

ATLAS OF MUSCLE ATTACHMENTS: THORAX AND ABDOMEN

Plate 1

Intercostal Muscles

The intercostal muscles fill the intervals between adjacent ribs. They are arranged in three layers: external, internal and innermost.

Attachments of intercostal muscles:

Each external intercostal muscle arises from the lower border of the rib above, and is inserted into the upper border of the rib below. The fibers of the muscle run obliquely from one rib to the other, the upper attachment being nearer the sternum. Therefore, on the back of the thorax the fibers run downward and laterally, and on the front of the thorax the fibers are directed downward and medially.

Each internal intercostal muscle arises from the costal groove of the rib above and is inserted into the upper border of the rib below. Its fibers run at right angles to those of the external intercostal: on the front of the thorax they pass downward and laterally. The innermost layer is made up of three distinct muscles as follows:
1. The intercostal is intimi (or *innermost intercostal muscle*) is seen only in the middle two-fourths of the intercostal space.
2. The subcostales are present only over the posterior part of the intercostal space (near the angles of the ribs).
3. In the anterior part of the thoracic wall the innermost layer is formed by a muscle called the sternocostalis. Some details of these are given on the next page.

Actions of intercostal muscles:

The external intercostal muscles are generally regarded as elevators of ribs, and the internal intercostal muscles as depressors. However, the role played by these muscles in respiratory movements is highly controversial. Their main importance seems to be to provide strong, but elastic, supports that prevent the thoracic wall from bulging inward or outward as a result of pressure changes associated with inspiration or expiration.

Nerve supply:

The intercostal and subcostal muscles are supplied by the intercostal nerves of the spaces concerned.

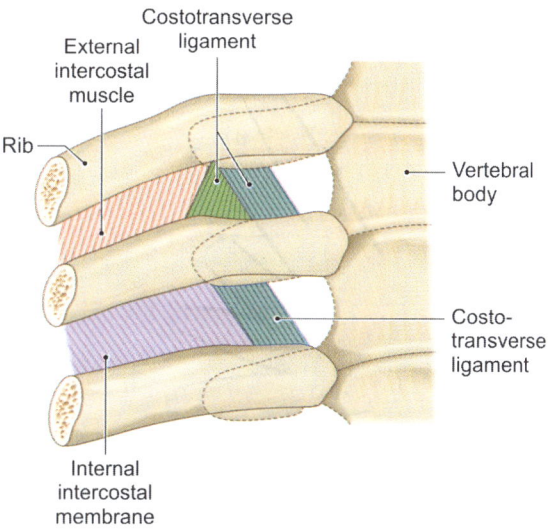

Posterior ends of two intercostal spaces viewed from within the thorax. The internal intercostal membrane has been removed in the upper space.

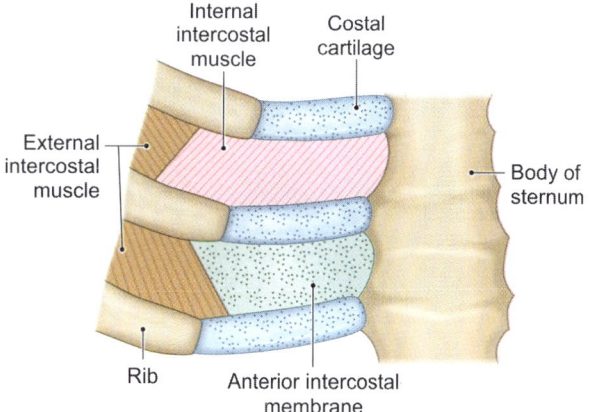

Anterior ends of two intercostal spaces viewed from the front. Some layers have been removed in the upper space.

Plate 2

Sternocostalis

The muscle is also called the transversus thoracis. The sternocostalis lies behind the sternum and costal cartilages.

It arises from the posterior aspect of (a) the lower one-third of the body of the sternum, (b) the xiphoid process, and (c) the adjoining parts of the costal cartilages (usually 4th to 7th).

From this origin (d) the fibers pass upward and laterally to be inserted into the 2nd, 3rd, 4th, 5th and 6th costal cartilages (lower borders and inner surfaces). The lowest fibers are horizontal and lie parallel with those of the transversus abdominis.

The intercostal vessels and nerves lie between the sternocostalis and the internal intercostal muscle.

Action:

The muscle depresses the costal cartilages into which it is inserted.

Nerve supply:

This is through the intercostal nerves.

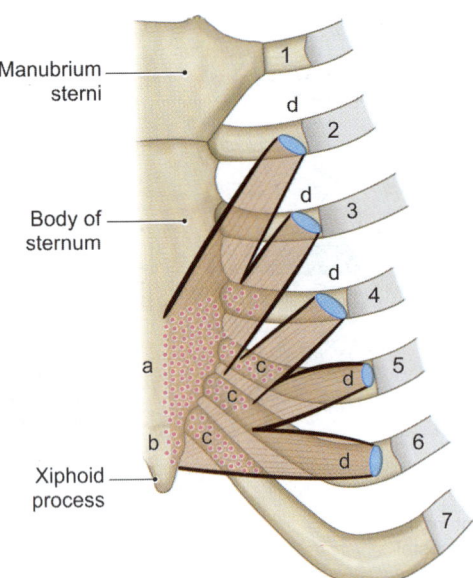

The innermost intercostal muscles are attached both above and below to the inner surfaces of adjoining ribs. The direction of their fibers is the same as that of the internal intercostal. They are separated from the internal intercostals by the intercostal nerves and vessels.

The subcostales are well developed only in the lower part of the thorax. Each muscle arises from the inner surface of a rib near its angle. It runs downward crossing two or three intercostal spaces before being attached to the surface of another rib. The direction of the fibers is the same as that of the internal intercostals.

Nerve supply is by intercostal nerves.

Actions are similar to intercostal muscles.

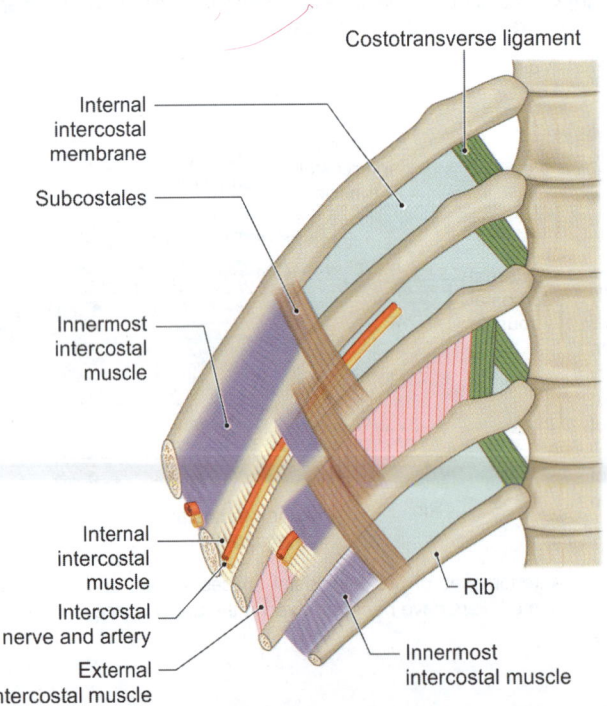

Atlas of Muscle Attachments: Thorax and Abdomen

Plate 3

The Diaphragm

This is the main muscle of respiration.

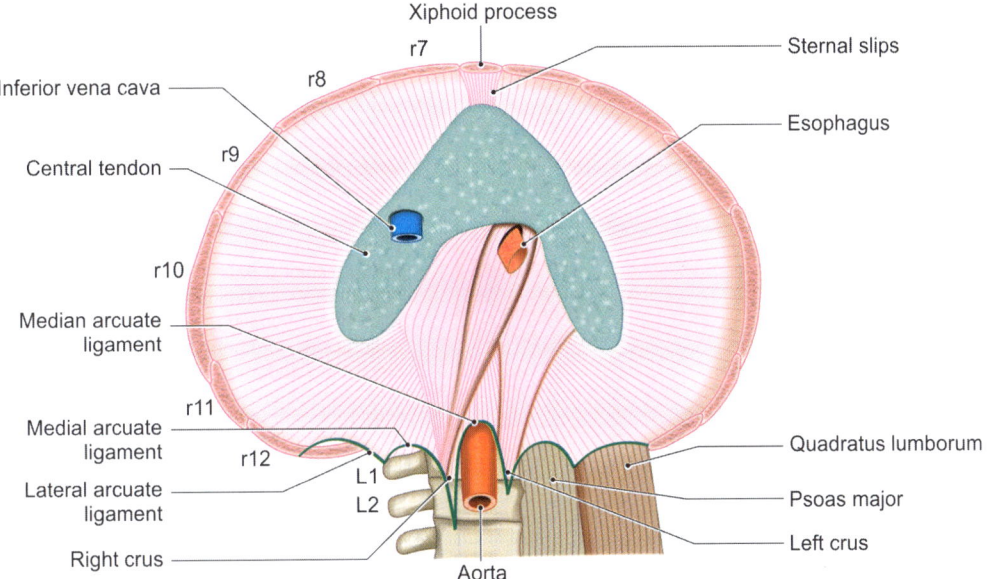

Attachments of the diaphragm:

The origin of the diaphragm can be divided into sternal, costal and vertebral parts. The *sternal part* consists of two slips, right and left, that arise from the back of the xiphoid process. The *costal part* consists of broad slips one from the inner surface of each of the lower six ribs (i.e. 7th to 12th) and their costal cartilages. The *lumbar part* consists of two crura (right and left) that arise from the anterolateral aspects of the bodies of lumbar vertebrae; and of fibers that arise (on either side) from two tendinous arches called the lateral and medial arcuate ligaments. The right crus is larger than the left: it arises from the bodies of vertebrae L1, L2, L3 and from the intervening intervertebral discs. The left crus arises similarly from vertebrae L1 and L2. The medial margins of the two crura are joined to each other (at the level of the lower border of vertebra T12) to form the median arcuate ligament.

From its extensive origin, described above, the muscular fibers of the diaphragm run upward and converge to be inserted on the margins of a large, flat, central tendon which is located just below the pericardium and heart. It is usually described as being made up of three leaf-like parts (or folia) that are fused together. There is an anterior (triangular) leaf: its apex is directed toward the xiphoid process and its base posteriorly, where it becomes continuous with two tongue shaped posterior leaves. The apex of the anterior leaf receives the sternal fibers, while the sides of the leaf receive the anterior costal fibers.

The posterior costal fibers reach the lateral sides of the posterior folia, while the fibers of the crura and those arising from the arcuate ligaments reach the apices and medial margins of the posterior folia.

The diaphragm receives a double nerve supply. Motor innervation is through the right and left phrenic nerves. The diaphragm is also supplied by the lower six intercostal nerves which provide a sensory supply.

228 Atlas of Muscle Attachments: Thorax and Abdomen

Plate 4

External Oblique Muscle of Abdomen

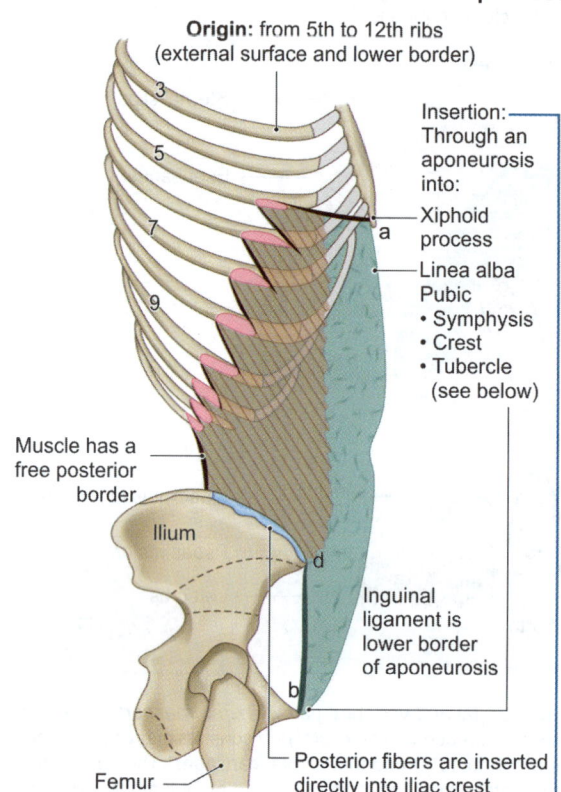

Origin: from 5th to 12th ribs (external surface and lower border)

Insertion: Through an aponeurosis into:
- Xiphoid process
- Linea alba
- Pubic
  - Symphysis
  - Crest
  - Tubercle (see below)

Muscle has a free posterior border

Ilium

Inguinal ligament is lower border of aponeurosis

Posterior fibers are inserted directly into iliac crest

Femur

The external oblique muscle is supplied by the lower six thoracic spinal nerves (i.e. 7th, 8th, 9th, 10th and 11th intercostal nerves and by the subcostal nerve).

Actions:
1. It supports the abdominal viscera, counteracting the effect of gravity especially in the sitting or standing position.
2. By active contraction it increases the intra-abdominal pressure which pushes up the diaphragm during expiration: and helps to expel contents of abdominal viscera in defecation, micturition, vomiting and in child-birth. These actions are common to all anterolateral muscles of the abdomen.

Between the anterior superior iliac spine and the pubic tubercle the aponeurosis of the external oblique has a free lower edge that is folded on itself to form the inguinal ligament. The aponeurosis bears an opening called the superficial inguinal ring. Some details of the ring are shown in the figure below.

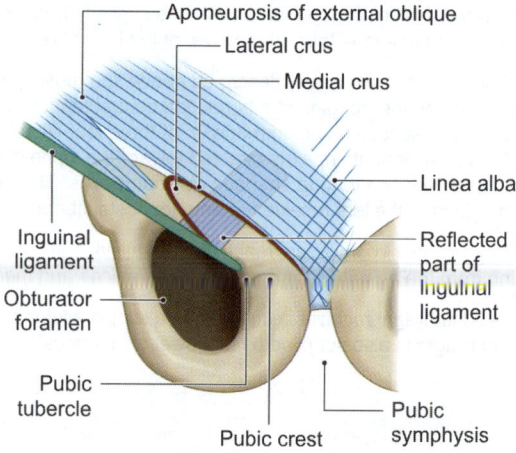

- Aponeurosis of external oblique
- Lateral crus
- Medial crus
- Linea alba
- Reflected part of Inguinal ligament
- Pubic symphysis
- Pubic crest
- Pubic tubercle
- Obturator foramen
- Inguinal ligament

Plate 5

Internal Oblique Muscle of Abdomen

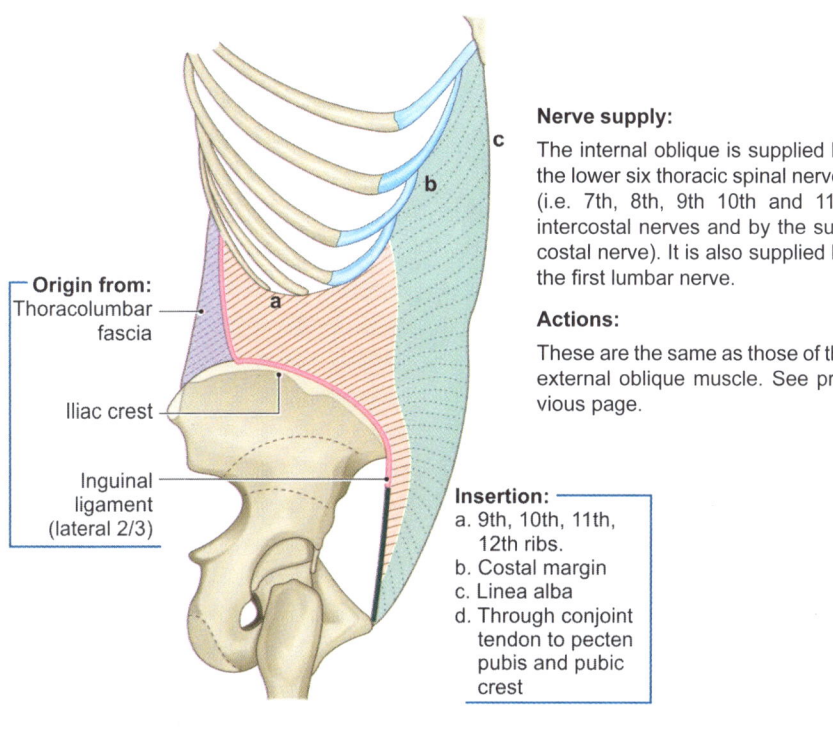

Origin from:
Thoracolumbar fascia
Iliac crest
Inguinal ligament (lateral 2/3)

Insertion:
a. 9th, 10th, 11th, 12th ribs.
b. Costal margin
c. Linea alba
d. Through conjoint tendon to pecten pubis and pubic crest

Nerve supply:
The internal oblique is supplied by the lower six thoracic spinal nerves (i.e. 7th, 8th, 9th 10th and 11th intercostal nerves and by the subcostal nerve). It is also supplied by the first lumbar nerve.

Actions:
These are the same as those of the external oblique muscle. See previous page.

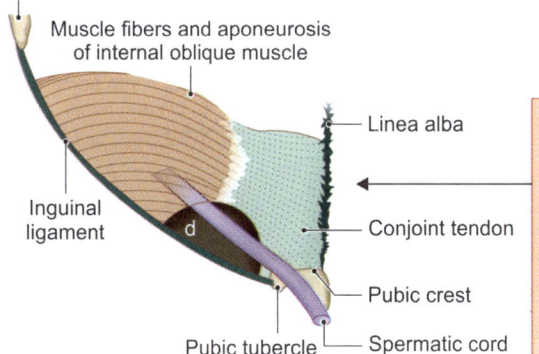

Relationship to inguinal canal:

The fibers of the internal oblique muscle take an important part in forming the walls of the inguinal canal. Fleshly fibers arising from the inguinal ligament from the anterior wall of the canal. They then form the roof of the canal (arching over the spermatic cord). They end in the conjoint tendon which forms the medial part of the posterior wall.

Atlas of Muscle Attachments: Thorax and Abdomen

Plate 6

Transversus Abdominis

The transversus abdominis is the deepest muscle of the anterolateral part of the abdominal wall. It has its origin posteriorly. From the origin the fibers run forward around the abdominal wall to their insertion in front.

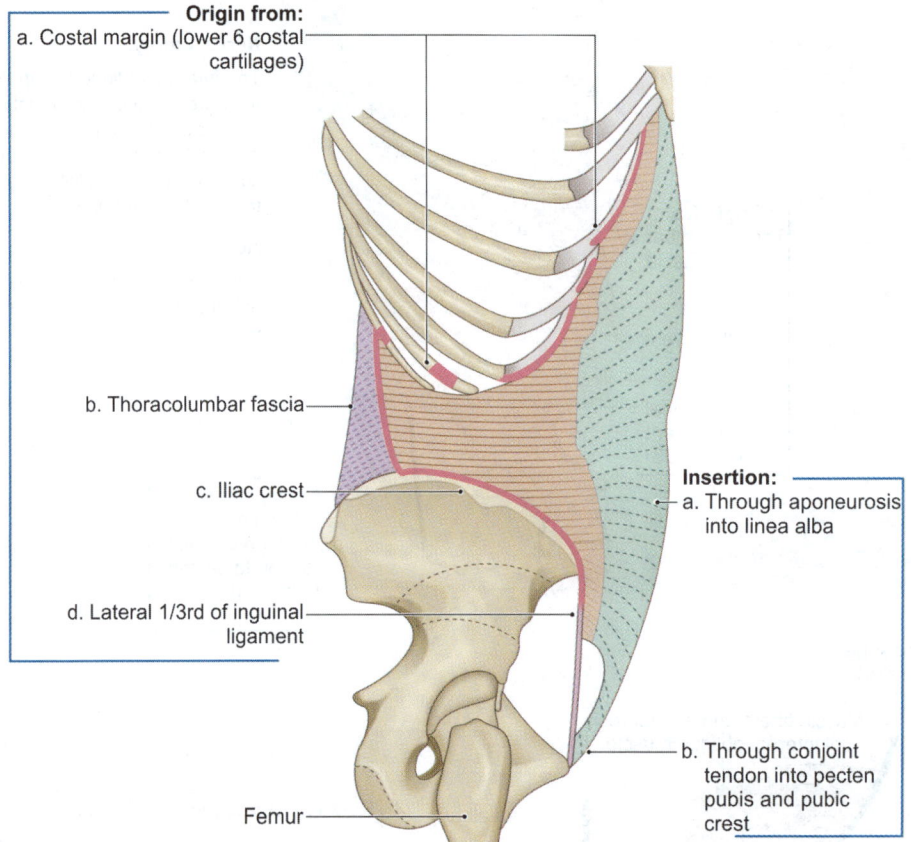

Origin from:
a. Costal margin (lower 6 costal cartilages)
b. Thoracolumbar fascia
c. Iliac crest
d. Lateral 1/3rd of inguinal ligament

Insertion:
a. Through aponeurosis into linea alba
b. Through conjoint tendon into pecten pubis and pubic crest

Femur

Nerve supply:

The transversus abdominis is supplied by the lower six thoracic spinal nerves (i.e. 7th, 8th, 9th, 10th and 11th intercostal nerves and by the subcostal nerve). It is also supplied by the first lumbar nerve. (The supply is the same as that of the internal oblique).

Actions of anterolateral muscles of abdomen

The actions of these muscles are as follows:
1. They support the abdominal viscera, counteracting the effect of gravity especially in the sitting or standing position.
2. By active contraction they increase the intra-abdominal pressure which pushes up the diaphragm during expiration and helps to expel contents of abdominal viscera in defecation, micturition, vomiting and in childbirth.
3. Theoretically, these muscles can bend the trunk forward or laterally, but their role in such movements is negligible.

Plate 7

Rectus Abdominis

The rectus abdominis runs vertically in the anterior abdominal wall next to the midline. The muscles of the two sides are separated by the linea alba. The origin of the muscle lies at its lower end, and the insertion at its upper end.

Note that the upper end of the muscle is the insertion.

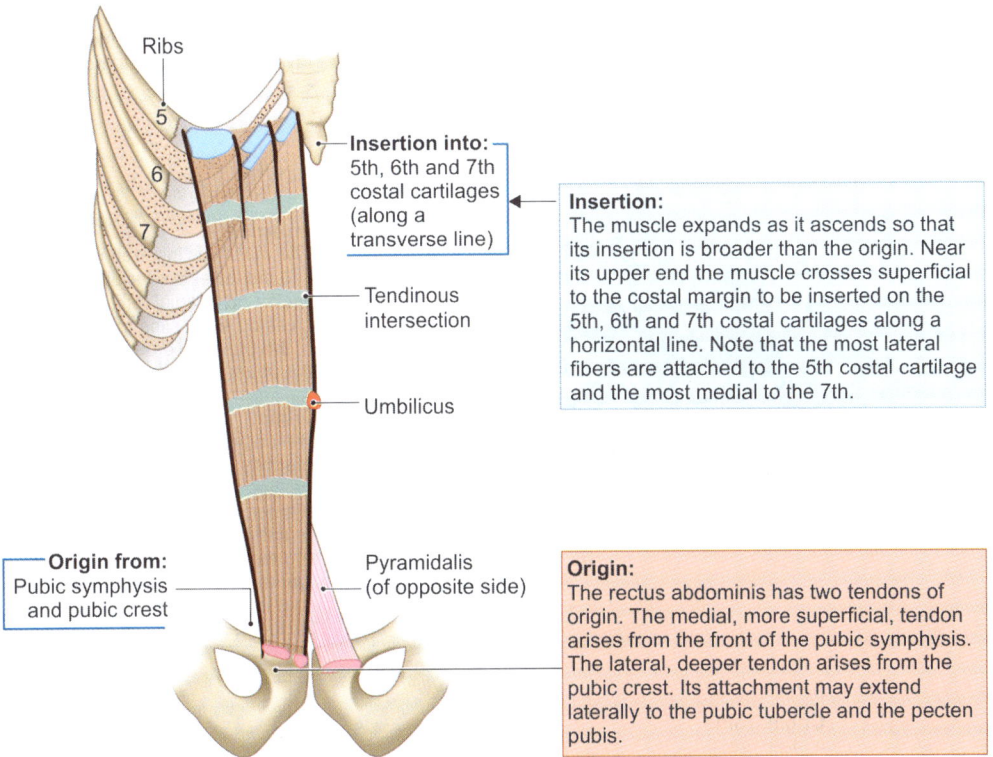

Insertion into: 5th, 6th and 7th costal cartilages (along a transverse line)

Tendinous intersection

Umbilicus

Origin from: Pubic symphysis and pubic crest

Pyramidalis (of opposite side)

Insertion:
The muscle expands as it ascends so that its insertion is broader than the origin. Near its upper end the muscle crosses superficial to the costal margin to be inserted on the 5th, 6th and 7th costal cartilages along a horizontal line. Note that the most lateral fibers are attached to the 5th costal cartilage and the most medial to the 7th.

Origin:
The rectus abdominis has two tendons of origin. The medial, more superficial, tendon arises from the front of the pubic symphysis. The lateral, deeper tendon arises from the pubic crest. Its attachment may extend laterally to the pubic tubercle and the pecten pubis.

Nerve supply:
The rectus abdominis is supplied by the lower six or seven thoracic nerves.

Action:
The rectus abdominis can bend the trunk forward. It assists the anterolateral muscles in supporting the abdominal viscera and in increasing intra-abdominal pressure.

The lateral border of the rectus abdominis can be made out on the surface of the living as a groove called the linea semilunaris.

A number of tendinous intersections (*usually three*) run transversely across the muscle; one at the level of the umbilicus, one at the level of the lower border of the xiphoid, and one midway between these two. An occasional intersection may be present below the umbilicus. The intersections have been regarded by some to represent embryonic septa between different myotomes, but this is uncertain. Their presence increases the number of muscle fibers present and hence increases the power of muscle.

Plate 8

Quadratus Lumborum

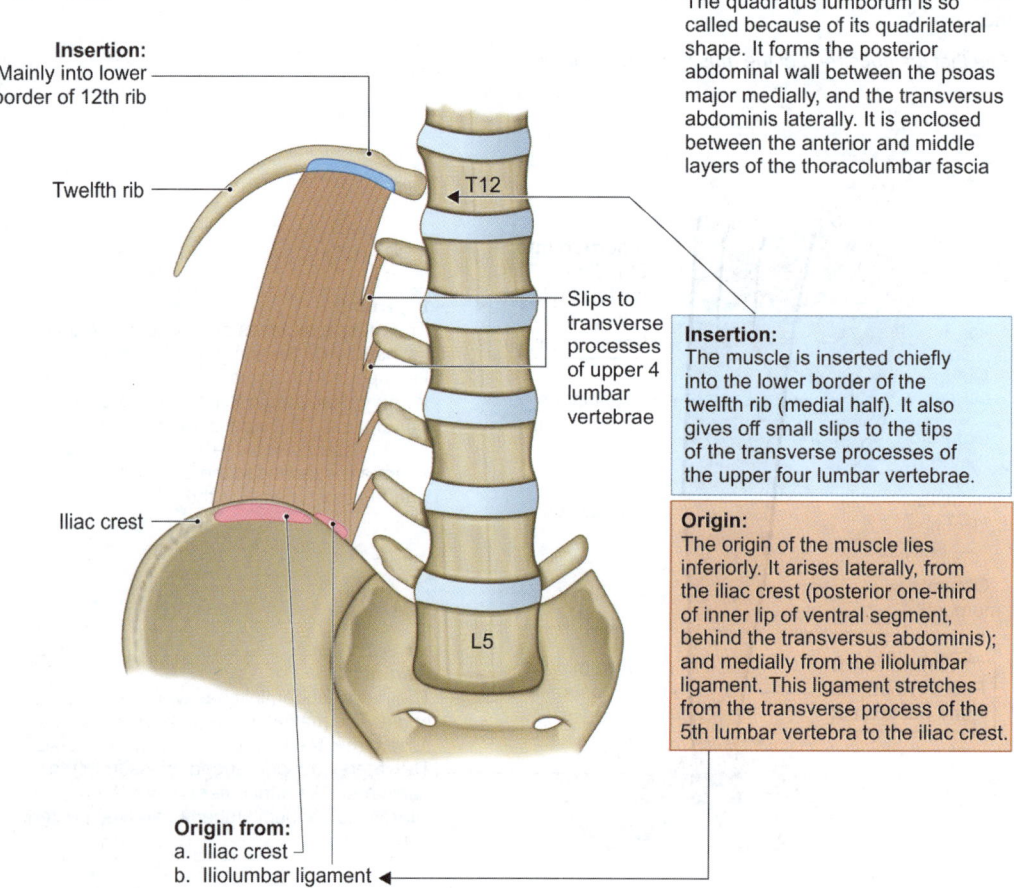

The quadratus lumborum is so called because of its quadrilateral shape. It forms the posterior abdominal wall between the psoas major medially, and the transversus abdominis laterally. It is enclosed between the anterior and middle layers of the thoracolumbar fascia

Insertion:
Mainly into lower border of 12th rib

Twelfth rib

Slips to transverse processes of upper 4 lumbar vertebrae

Iliac crest

T12

L5

Origin from:
a. Iliac crest
b. Iliolumbar ligament

Insertion:
The muscle is inserted chiefly into the lower border of the twelfth rib (medial half). It also gives off small slips to the tips of the transverse processes of the upper four lumbar vertebrae.

Origin:
The origin of the muscle lies inferiorly. It arises laterally, from the iliac crest (posterior one-third of inner lip of ventral segment, behind the transversus abdominis); and medially from the iliolumbar ligament. This ligament stretches from the transverse process of the 5th lumbar vertebra to the iliac crest.

Nerve supply:

It is supplied by the ventral rami of the twelfth thoracic and upper lumbar nerves.

Actions:

The muscle aids respiration by fixing the twelfth rib allowing the diaphragm to act to better advantage. It can cause lateral flexion of the vertebral column.

Plate 9

Levator Ani and Coccygeus

The levator ani is shown schematically in the upper figure in which the pelvis has been out transversely along a line passing through the upper part of the pubis (in front) and the ischial spine behind. The origin of the muscle from the pelvic aspect of the lower part of the hip bone is shown in the lower figure.

The levator ani and the coccygeus form a transverse partition across the pelvis which is called the pelvic diaphragm.

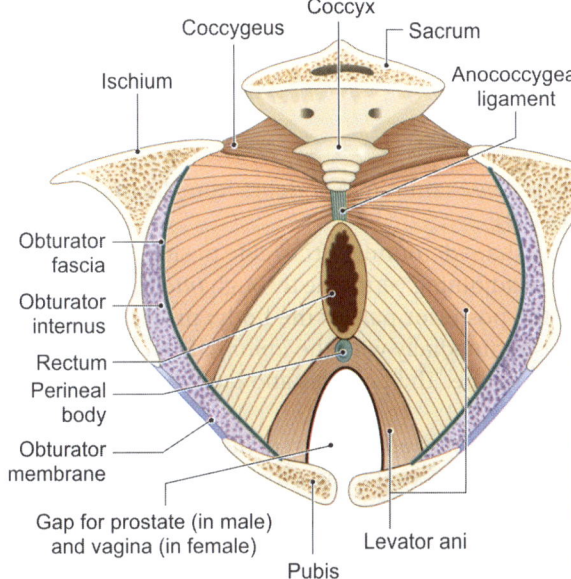

Origin:

The levator ani arises from the following (from front to back):
1. The pelvic surface of the body of the pubis (a)
2. The obturator fascia (b).
3. The spine of the ischium (c)

Insertion (See upper figure):

From the origin described about ethers of the leator ani arch backward and medial to be inserted as follows:

a. In the male the most anterior bers pass across the sides of the prostate to end in the leator prostate muscle. In the famale the corresponding bers pass across the sides of the agina to end in the perineal body. They are then called the pubo aninalis which acts as a sphincter for the agina.

b. The intermediate bers pass across the sides of the rectum and become continuous with those of the opposite side behind the anorectal junction. These bers constitute the puborectalis. They merge wtih the internal and external sphincters of the anal canal to form the anorectal right.: the ring can be felt by anger placed in the rectum.

c. The most posterior bers are attached to the coccyx, and to a brous band called the anococcygeal ligament. The posterior margin of the muscle is continuous with the coccygeus.

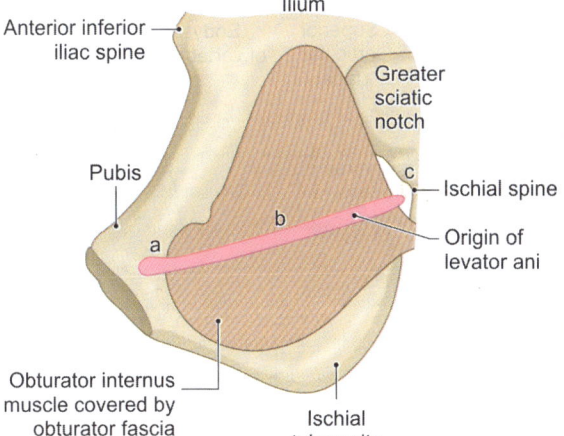

Nerve supply of levator ani and coccygeus

The levator ani is supplied by a branch from the 4th sacral nerve; and another branch from the inferior rectal nerve or from the perineal division of the pudendal nerve. The coccygeus is supplied by the 4th and 5th sacral nerves.

Vertebral Column

CHAPTER 6

AN 21.1 Identify and describe the salient features of typical vertebra.

TYPICAL VERTEBRA

General Considerations

The parts of a typical vertebra are best observed by examining a vertebra from the mid-thoracic region. The parts identified are (**Figs. 6.1 to 6.3**):

- **Body** lies anteriorly. It is short cylindrical shaped; rounded from side to side. Its flat upper and lower surfaces are attached to those of adjoining vertebrae through *intervertebral discs*.
- **Pedicles** are short rounded bars from the posterior part of the body; project backwards and laterally. Each pedicle continues posteromedially with the *lamina*. Both laminae pass backward and medially and meet in the midline. The pedicles and laminae constitute the *vertebral arch*.
- **Vertebral foramen** is bounded anteriorly by the posterior aspect of the body on the sides by the pedicles and behind by the laminae. Each vertebral foramen forms a short segment of the *vertebral canal* that runs through the whole length of the vertebral column and transmits the spinal cord.
- **Spine (spinous process)** passes backwards (and downwards) from the junction of the two laminae.

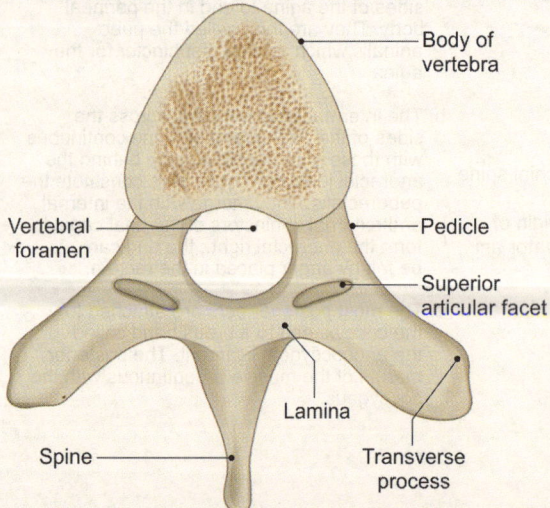

Fig. 6.1: Typical vertebra from above.

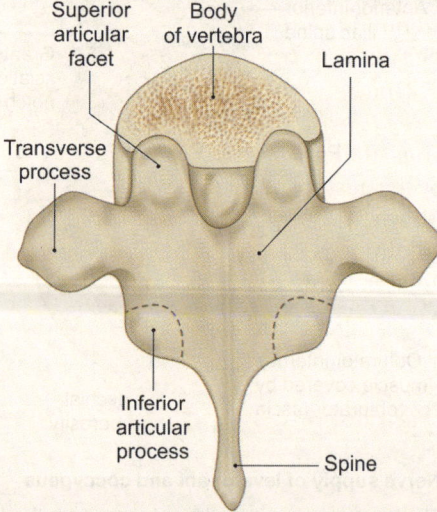

Fig. 6.2: Typical vertebra from behind.

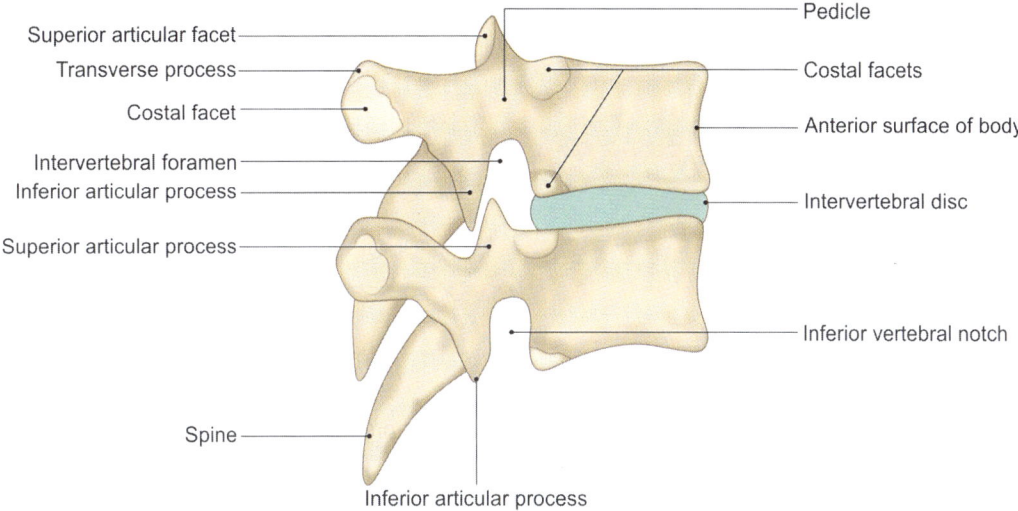

Fig. 6.3: Typical vertebrae from lateral side (costal facets for ribs, are shown on the bodies and transverse processes: Present only in the thoracic region).

❖ *Transverse process* passes laterally (and usually somewhat downwards) from the junction of each pedicle and the corresponding lamina. The spinous and transverse processes serve as levers for muscles acting on the vertebral column.

Vertebrae from the Lateral Side: Additional Features

Superior articular process projects upwards from the junction of the pedicle and the laminae and *inferior articular process* projects downward. Each process bears a smooth articular facet (directed posteriorly and laterally) and the *inferior facet* (directed forwards and medially). The superior facet of one vertebra articulates with the inferior facet of the vertebra above it. Two adjoining vertebrae articulate at three joints:
❖ Two between right and left articular processes
❖ One between bodies of the vertebrae (through intervertebral disc).

Pedicle is narrower than the body (in vertical diameter); attached nearer its upper border. Thus, there is a large *inferior vertebral notch* below the pedicle. The notch is bounded in front by the posterior surface of the body of the vertebra, and behind by the inferior articular process. Above the pedicle, there is a shallow *superior vertebral notch*. Superior and inferior notches of adjoining vertebrae join to form the *intervertebral foramina* for the passage of spinal nerves emerging from the spinal cord.

Cervical, Thoracic, and Lumbar Vertebrae

Cervical, thoracic, and lumbar vertebrae are identified on the basis of the following characteristics:
❖ Transverse process of a cervical vertebra is pierced by *foramen transversarium* **(Figs. 6.4 and 6.5)**
❖ Thoracic vertebrae present *costal facets* for articulation with ribs (present on the sides of vertebral bodies and transverse processes).

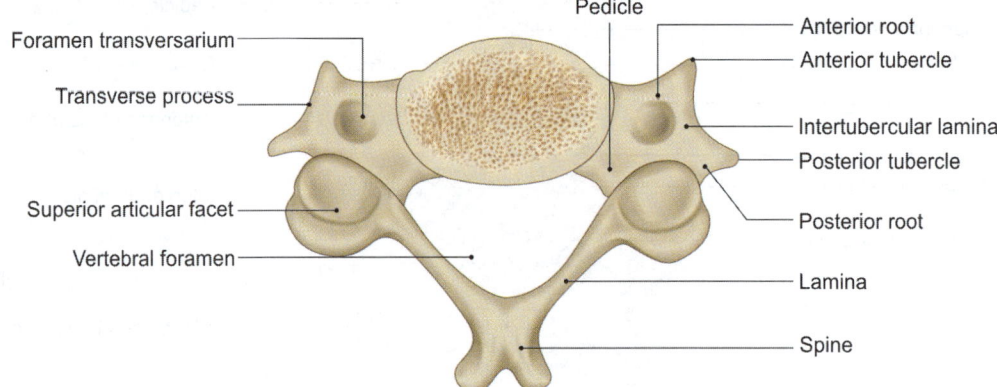

Fig. 6.4: Typical cervical vertebra from above.

- Lumbar vertebra is recognized by the large sized body; no foramina transversaria or facets for ribs.

Cervical, Thoracic, and Lumbar Vertebrae: Differences

Vertebral bodies: These progressively increase in size from above downward; smallest in cervical vertebrae and largest in lumbar vertebrae. The body is oval in the cervical and lumbar regions and triangular (heart shaped) in the thoracic region.

The upper and lower surfaces are flat in the thoracic and lumbar region. In cervical vertebrae, the upper surface is concave from side to side; the posterolateral parts of its edge are raised to form distinct lips. Thus, superior vertebral notch is prominent in cervical vertebrae; barely perceptible in thoracic vertebrae.

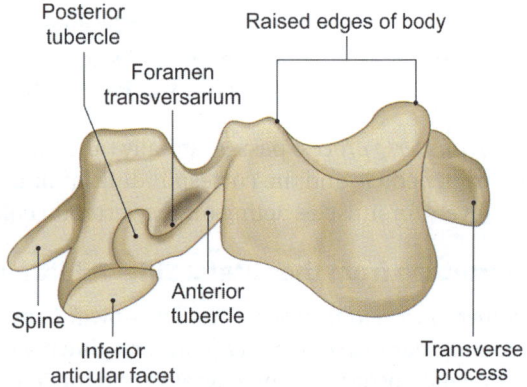

Fig. 6.5: Typical cervical vertebra from anterolateral side.

In thoracic region, the head of a typical rib articulates with the sides of the bodies of two vertebrae. For this, each side of the body of a typical thoracic vertebra presents two costal facets (upper and lower) adjoining upper and lower borders. Each of these is only half a facet (*demifacet*), the other half being on the adjoining vertebra. The upper facet is large and articulates with the numerically corresponding rib. The lower, smaller facet articulates with the next lower rib.

Vertebral foramen: It is triangular and large in cervical vertebrae. In lumbar vertebrae, it is also triangular **(Fig. 6.6)**. In thoracic vertebrae, it is small and circular (or oval). These variations in size correspond with those of the spinal cord which is largest (in diameter) in the cervical region **(Fig. 6.7)**.

Pedicles: They are long and directed backward and laterally in the cervical region. In the thoracic region, they pass almost directly backward. They are thick and short in the lumbar region; directed backward and laterally **(Fig. 6.8)**.

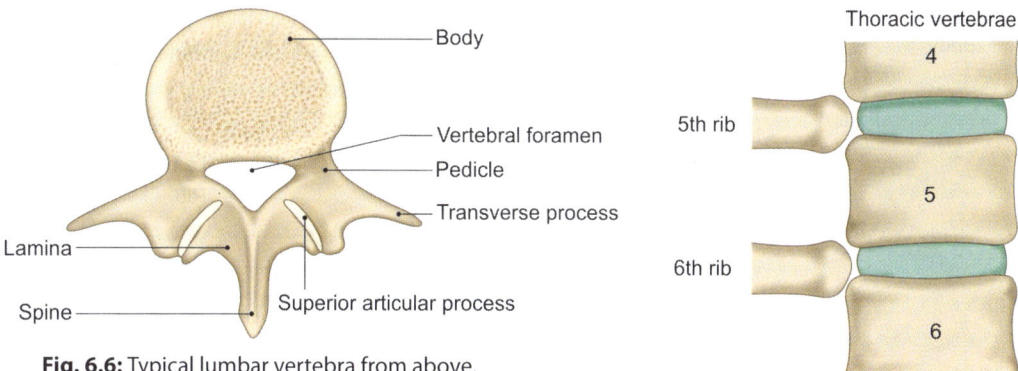

Fig. 6.6: Typical lumbar vertebra from above.

Fig. 6.7: Numerical relationship of thoracic vertebrae to ribs.

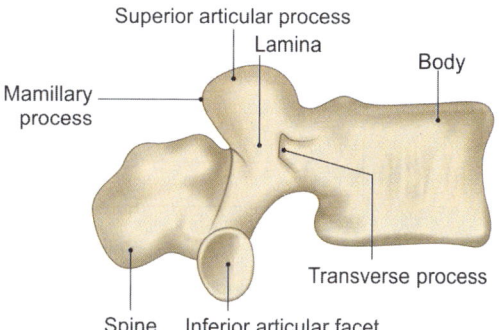

Fig. 6.8: Typical lumbar vertebra from the lateral side.

Laminae: Those of cervical vertebrae are long (transversely) and narrow (vertically). In the thoracic region, they are short (transversely) and so broad (vertically) that the laminae of adjacent vertebrae overlap. In the lumbar region, they are short and broad, but do not overlap.

Spinous processes: These are short and bifid in a typical cervical vertebra. They are long and project downward in the thoracic region. In lumbar vertebrae, they are large and quadrangular (horizontal) and have a thick posterior edge.

Transverse processes (Figs. 6.9 A to C): Those of typical cervical vertebrae are relatively short; pierced by foramina transversaria. The part of the process in front of the foramen is the *anterior root*; and the part behind, is the *posterior root*. The part lateral to the foramen is the *costotransverse bar*. The anterior and posterior roots end in the *anterior* and *posterior tubercles*. From the lateral side, the transverse process appeared grooved. The cervical nerves lie in these grooves after coming out of the intervertebral foramina.

The transverse processes of a typical thoracic vertebra are large with blunt ends. They are directed backward and laterally. Each process lies just behind the corresponding rib and bears prominent facet for the articulation with the rib.

The lumbar transverse processes are relatively small with tapering ends. The posteroinferior aspect of the root of each transverse process bears an elevation called the *accessory process*.

Proper ribs are formed only in the thoracic region; but rudimentary ribs are formed in the cervical and lumbar regions during fetal life. These become fused with the true transverse processes. The part of the transverse process derived from the rudimentary rib is called the *costal element*.

In Cervical Region, Costal Element Forms
a. Anterior root
b. Costotransverse bar
c. Both anterior and posterior tubercles.

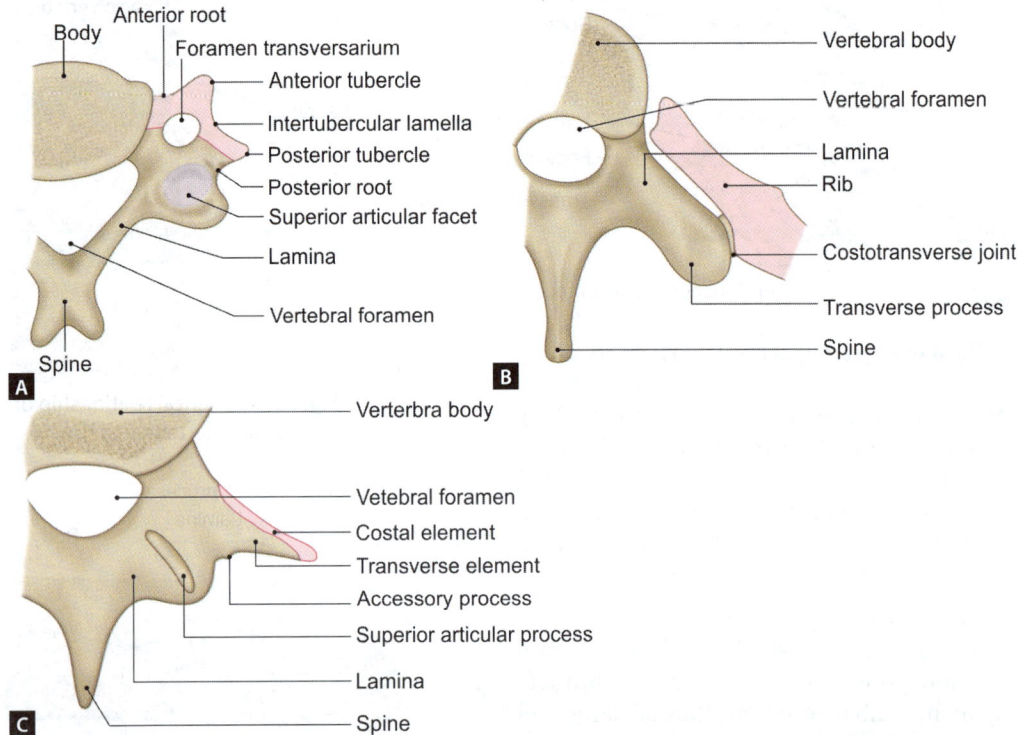

Figs. 6.9A to C: (A) Cervical; (B) Thoracic; (C) Lumbar. Transverse processes: Parts derived from costal elements (red shading).

In Lumbar Region, Costal Element Forms
❖ Strip along the anterior margin of transverse process.

Direction of Articular Facets (Figs. 6.10 to 6.13)

In cervical region, the facets are flat:
❖ Superior facets are directed equally backward and upward
❖ Inferior facets are directed forward and downward.

In thoracic region, the facets are flat and almost vertical.
❖ Superior facets face backward, slightly upward, and slightly laterally
❖ Inferior facets face forward, slightly downward, and slightly medially.

In lumbar region, the facets are vertical; curved from side to side.
❖ Superior facets are slightly concave; directed equally backward and medially
❖ Inferior facets are slightly convex; directed equally forward and laterally.
Each superior articular process of a lumbar vertebra shows a rough projection called the *mamillary process*, on its posterior border.

In the cervical region, superior and inferior articular processes form a solid *articular pillar* that helps to transmit some weight from one vertebra to the next lower one. This is not so in the thoracic and lumbar regions.

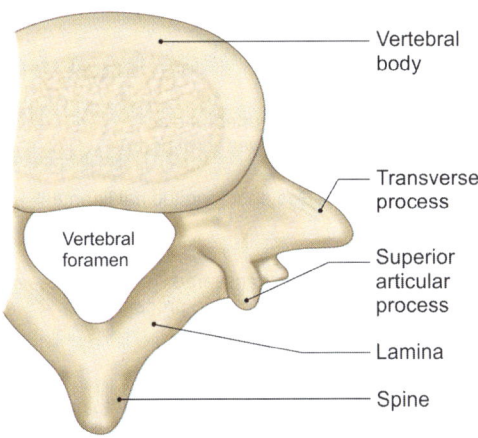

Fig. 6.10: L-5 vertebra from above.

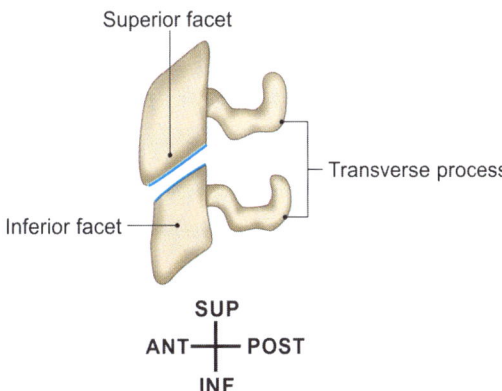

Fig. 6.11: Orientation of the articular facets of cervical vertebrae (lateral view).

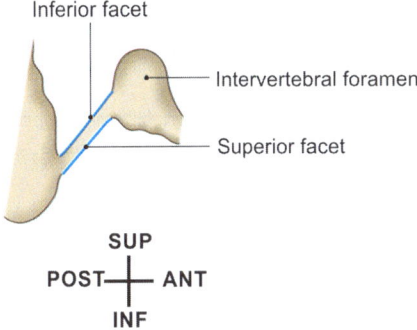

Fig. 6.12: Orientation of the articular facets of thoracic vertebrae (lateral view).

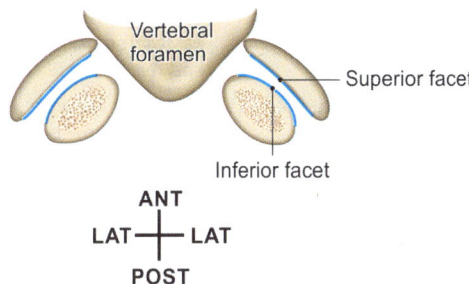

Fig. 6.13: Orientation of the articular facets of lumbar vertebrae (facets seen from above); inferior processes are cut across.

Vertebrae: Attachments

Vertebrae give attachment to many muscles and ligaments. The muscles attached to vertebrae vary from vertebra to vertebra **(Fig. 6.14)**.

Adjoining vertebrae are connected to each other at three joints. They are:
* One median joint between the vertebral bodies
* Two joints (right and left) between the articular processes.

Adjoining vertebral bodies are connected to each other by intervertebral discs (fibrocartilage). Each disc has an outer fibrous part (*annulus fibrosus*) and an inner soft part (*nucleus pulposus*).

Joints between the articular processes are *synovial joints*. The capsules of these joints are attached along the margins of articular facets.

Apart from intervertebral discs and the capsular ligaments, adjoining vertebrae are connected to one another by a series of ligaments. These include:

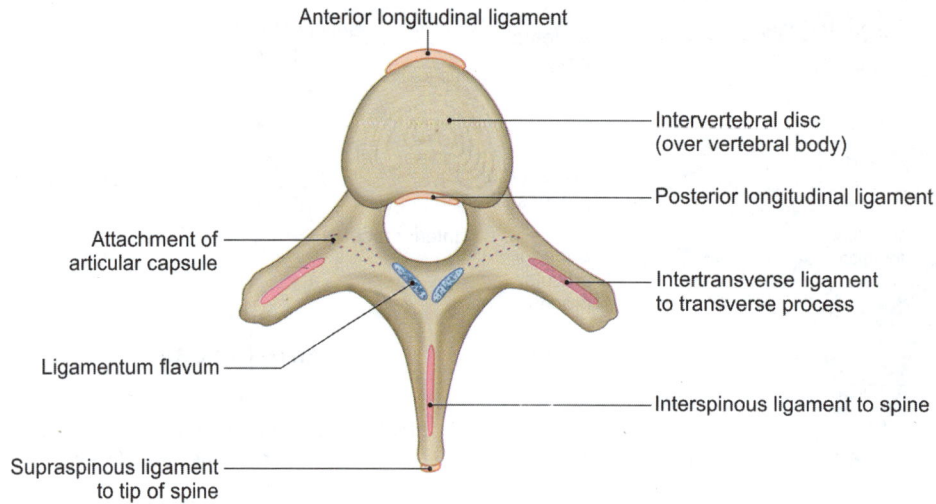

Fig. 6.14: Position of various ligaments interconnecting adjoining vertebrae.

Anterior longitudinal ligament	Passes from the anterior surface of the body of one vertebra to another; upper end reaches basilar part of occipital bone
Posterior longitudinal ligament	Present on the posterior surface of the vertebral bodies (*within vertebral canal*); upper end reaches the body of axis beyond which it continues with membrana tectoria
Intertransverse ligaments	Connect adjacent transverse processes
Interspinous ligaments	Connect adjacent spinous processes
Supraspinous ligaments	Connect tips of the spines of vertebrae from 7th cervical vertebra to sacrum (*in neck replaced by ligamentum nuchae*)
Ligamenta flava	Connect laminae of adjacent vertebrae; right and left ligaments meet in the middle line

Vertebral Column: Movements (Fig. 6.15)

Cervical region

Flexion and extension:
- At atlanto-occipital joint: Free
- At remaining joints (C-2 to C-7): Limited by:
  - Shape of the body
  - Intervertebral disc
  - Spinous processes

Rotation:
- At atlanto-axial joint: Free; rotates by almost 90°
- C-3 to C-7: Considerable freedom

Cervical articular facets are angled coronally by about 30°, permitting considerable freedom of movements in sagittal, coronal, and horizontal planes

Lumbar region

Plane of lumbar articular facets is more or less sagittal, thus they resist rotation

Since L-1 to S-1 articular facets joints are in more coronal plane, they permit rotation. L-4 and L-5 facets joints permit greatest degree of movements in all planes

CHAPTER 6 ✦ Vertebral Column

AN 50.2 Describe and demonstrate movements of intervertebral joints.

Vertebral Column: Intervertebral Movements (Fig. 6.15)

Region	Movements		
	Flexion and extension	Lateral flexion	Rotation
Cervical	+++ More	++ Possible	+ Very little
Reasons			Superior and inferior facets of adjacent vertebrae do not lie in the arc in which rotation occurs
Thoracic	Very little	Very little	More
Reasons			Superior and inferior facets of adjacent vertebrae lie in the arc in which rotation occurs
Lumbar	++ More	Possible	Very little
Reasons			Superior and inferior facets of adjacent vertebrae do not lie in the arc in which rotation occurs

Vertebral Column: Curvatures

AN 50.1 Describe the curvatures of the vertebral column.

Vertebral column presents four anteroposterior curvatures (**Fig. 6.16**):
- Thoracic and sacral curvature: Concave anteriorly
- Cervical and lumbar curvature: Concave posteriorly.

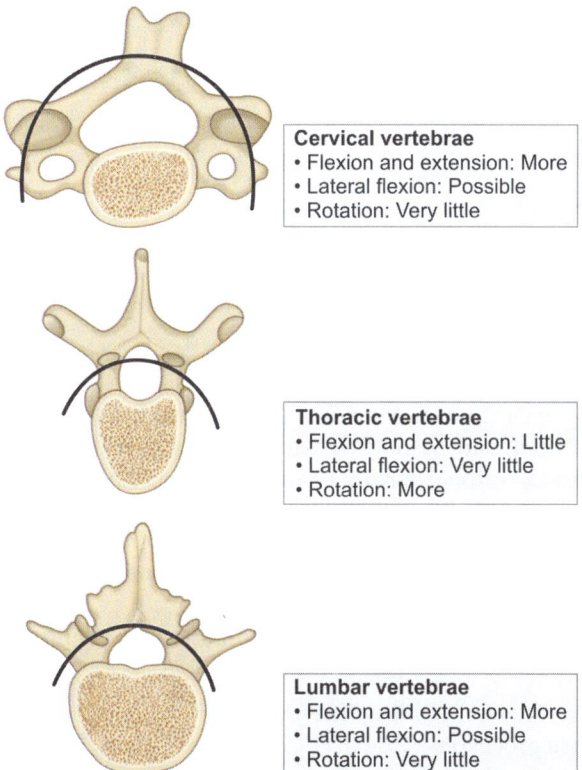

Fig. 6.15: Vertebral column: Movements.

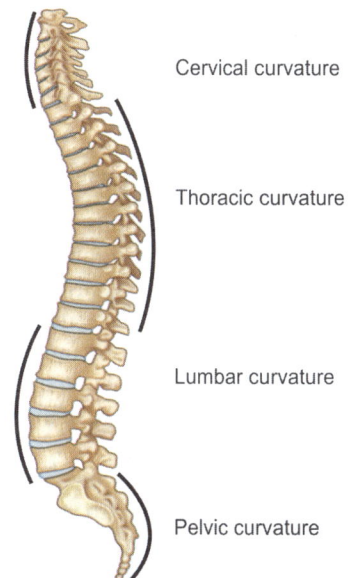

Fig. 6.16: Vertebral column: Curvatures.

Primary curvatures: Thoracic and sacral curvatures are primary; appear before birth.
Secondary curvatures: Cervical and lumbar curvatures are secondary; appear after birth.
- Cervical curvature develops when child starts holding his head (3–6 months).
- Lumbar curvature develops when child adopts upright posture (18 months).

Differences Between Vertebrae

Feature	Cervical	Thoracic	Lumbar
Body			
Shape	Transversely oval	Heart shaped	Kidney shaped
Cupping of body	Present	Absent	Absent
Facet on the body	Absent	Present	Absent
Transverse process	Short, thin, horizontal	Long, thick, directed downward	Thin, intermediate sized, horizontal
Foramen transversarium	Present	Absent	Absent
Facet	Absent	Present	Absent
Spinous process	Short, bifid, horizontally backward	Long, triangular, obliquely downward	Intermediate sized, quadrangular, horizontally backward
Vertebral foramen	Large, triangular	Small, round	Intermediate, triangular
Facet on superior articular process	Upward and backward	Backward	Backward and medially
Facet on inferior articular process	Downward and forward	Forward	Forward and laterally
Superior vertebral notch	Deep	Shallow	Shallow
Inferior vertebral notch	Deep	Deep	Deep
Movements			
Flexion and extension	More	Little	More
Lateral flexion	Possible	Very little	Possible
Rotation	Very little	More	Very little

AN 51.1 Describe and identify the cross-section at the level of T-8, T-10 and L-1 (transpyloric plane).

Vertebral Column: Ossification and Development

Typical vertebra: It has three primary ossification centers. One center appears in the body and one in each half of neural arch; centers appear between 9 weeks and 12 weeks of fetal life.

The posterolateral parts of the vertebral bodies are ossified by extension from the centers for the neural arches. Remaining part of the body is the *centrum*. For some time, the centrum is connected to the neural arches by the cartilage forming the *neurocentral joints*.

Sometimes, the vertebral body may ossify from two primary centers. If one of these centers fails to develop one half of the body may be missing. This condition is *hemivertebra* (cuneiform vertebra).

Two neural arches fuse (posteriorly) after birth during first year. They unite with the centrum between third and sixth years.

Five secondary centers appear in each vertebra after puberty. These are:
- Second and third at the tips of transverse processes
- Fourth and fifth centers that form ring-shaped epiphyses over upper and lower surfaces of the vertebral body

Epiphyses derived from the secondary centers fuse with the rest of the vertebra at about 25 years.
- *Atlas:* It ossifies from three centers, one appearing in each lateral mass and one in the anterior arch. The posterior arch is formed by extension from the center for the lateral masses.
- *Axis:* It has five primary centers: one for each half of the vertebral arch, one for the centrum, and two for the dens.

Lumbar vertebrae: They ossify like typical vertebrae; additional secondary centers for the mamillary processes are present.

> **QUESTIONNAIRE**
> - Classify vertebrae.
> - How will you differentiate cervical, thoracic, and lumbar vertebrae?
> - What type of joint is present between the bodies of the vertebrae?
> - Enumerate the functions of the intervertebral disc.
> - What type of cartilage is intervertebral disc? What is its structure?
> - What are the types of joints between articular processes?
> - Name the ligaments connecting the two vertebrae.
> - What is ligamentum flavum? What does it connects?
> - Where is foramen for basivertebral vein? Comment on its clinical importance.
> - Are the body and the centrum of a vertebra same?
> - Are the vertebral arch and the neural arch of a vertebra same?
> - What are the costal and the transverse elements?

ATYPICAL CERVICAL VERTEBRAE

AN 26.5 Describe features of atypical cervical vertebrae (Atlas and Axis).

First Cervical Vertebra (Atlas)

The first cervical vertebra is the atlas.

Identifying Features

- Body is absent
- No spinous process
- Two lateral masses connected by anterior and posterior arches

Atlas (ring like) consists of two *lateral masses* joined anteriorly by a short *anterior arch*, and posteriorly by a longer *posterior arch*. A large transverse process (*with foramen transversarium*) projects laterally from the lateral mass. The superior aspect of each lateral mass shows an elongated concave facet which articulates with the corresponding condyle of the occipital bone to form *atlanto-occipital joint*. The long axis of the facet runs forward and medially. Nodding and lateral movements of the head take place at these atlanto-occipital joints. The inferior aspect of each lateral mass shows a large almost circular facet for articulation with the superior articular facet of the second cervical vertebra (*axis*) to form *lateral atlantoaxial joint*. The facet is flat; directed downward and medially and backward. The medial side of the lateral mass shows a tubercle which gives attachment to the *transverse ligament of atlas*. This ligament divides large foramen (bounded by lateral masses and arches) into anterior and posterior parts. The posterior part corresponds to the vertebral foramen; spinal cord passes through it. The anterior part is occupied by the *dens* (upward projection from the body of axis). The dens articulates with the

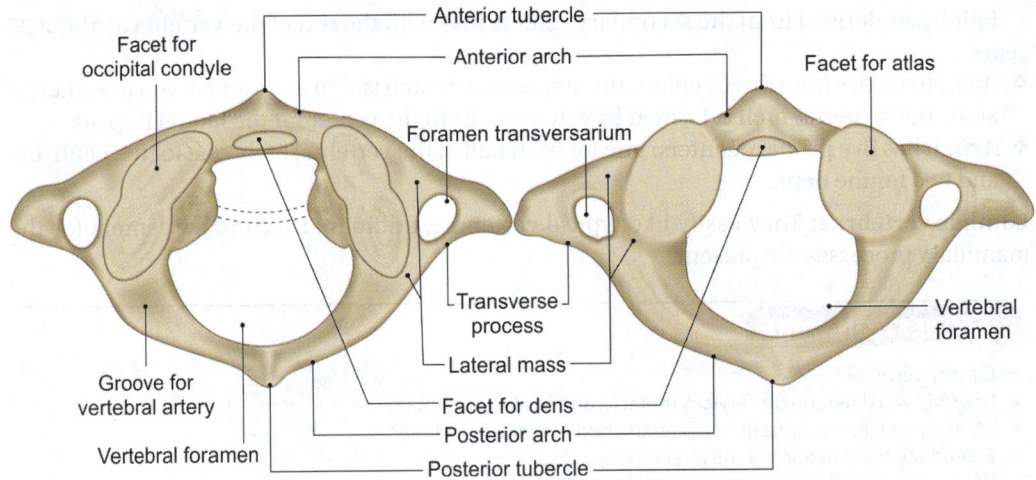

Fig. 6.17: Atlas (C-1 vertebra) from above and atlas (C-1 vertebra) from below.

posterior aspect of the anterior arch. It also articulates with the transverse ligament. These two articulations collectively form *median atlanto-occipital joint*. In side-to-side movement of the head, the atlas moves with the skull around the pivot formed by the dens **(Fig. 6.17)**.

The anterior arch presents a small midline projection called the *anterior tubercle*. The posterior arch bears the *posterior tubercle* (*rudimentary spine*). The upper surface of the posterior arch is grooved by the vertebral artery.

The transverse processes are large. Their tips correspond to the posterior tubercles of the transverse processes of a typical cervical vertebra.

Attachments and Relations

Vertebral artery passes upward through the foramen transversarium. It then runs medially on the groove over the posterior arch. It is accompanied by the vertebral vein and a plexus of sympathetic nerve fibers.

First cervical nerve crosses the posterior arch deep to the vertebral artery; divides here into anterior and posterior primary rami.

Structures passing through the vertebral canal **(Fig. 6.18)**:
a. Spinal cord
b. Meninges
c. Spinal part of accessory nerve
d. Anterior and posterior spinal arteries.

Atlas: Attachments

Ligament	Attachment
Capsules of atlanto-occipital joints and atlanto axial joints	Margins of the corresponding facets
Anterior and posterior atlanto-occipital membranes	Upper margins of the corresponding arches of atlas
Transverse ligament	Medial side of lateral mass
Ligamentum nuchae	Tip of posterior tubercle

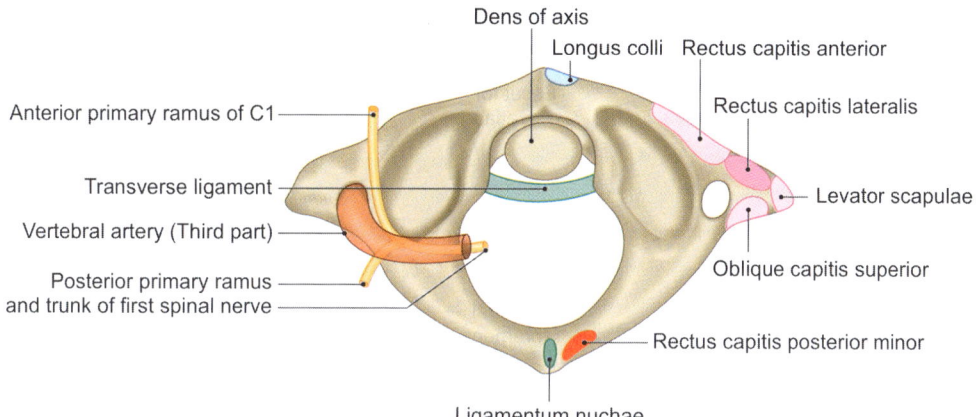

Fig. 6.18: Atlas: Structures attached/related.

Atlas is attached to axis by ligaments; similar as seen between typical cervical vertebrae.

Muscle	Attachment
Rectus capitis anterior	Front of lateral mass and root of transverse process (*origin*)
Rectus capitis lateralis	Anterior part of the upper surface of transverse process (*origin*)
Rectus capitis posterior minor	Posterior tubercle (*origin*)
Superior oblique capitis	Posterior part of the upper surface of transverse process (*origin*)
Inferior oblique capitis and splenius cervicis	Inferior aspect of transverse process (*insertion*)
Levator scapulae	Lateral margin of transverse process (*origin*)
Longus colli (*some fibers of upper oblique part*)	Anterior tubercle (*insertion*)

Second Cervical Vertebra (Axis)

The second cervical vertebra is the axis.

Identifying Features

- Presence of tooth like projection (*dens*)
- Very small transverse process.

The axis presents a thick tooth-like projection from the upper part of the body called the *dens* (*odontoid process*). It fits into the space between the anterior arch of the atlas and its transverse ligament to form the *median atlanto-occipital joint* (pivot joint). The anterior aspect of the dens bears a convex oval facet for articulation with the anterior arch. Its posterior aspect shows a transverse groove for the transverse ligament.

On either side of the dens, the axis shows an oval facet for articulation with the corresponding facet on the inferior aspect of the atlas. The transverse process of the axis lies lateral to this facet. It is small and ends in a single tubercle corresponding to the posterior tubercle of a typical cervical vertebra. The transverse process is pierced by foramen transversarium.

The pedicles, laminae, and spine are thick and strong. The inferior articular facets (below the junction of pedicles and laminae) are orientated as in a typical cervical vertebra.

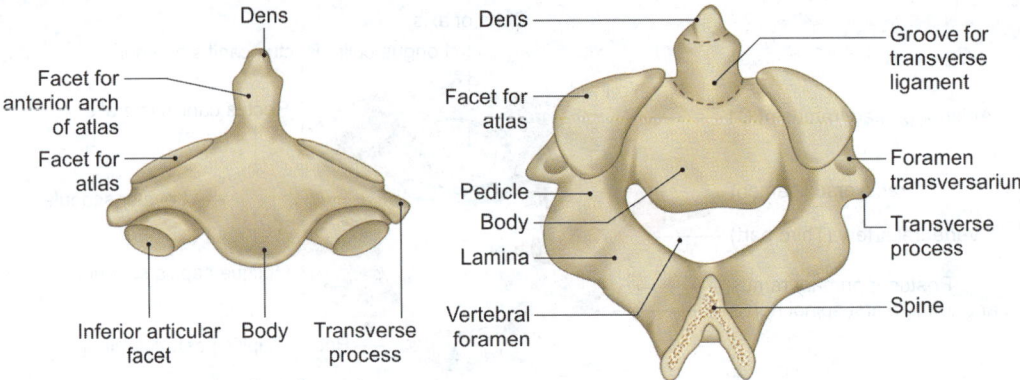

Fig. 6.19: Atlas (C-1 vertebra) from above.

Fig. 6.20: Atlas (C-1 vertebra) from below.

Attachments (Figs. 6.19 and 6.20)

Ligament	Attachment
Apical ligament	Apex of the dens
Right and left alar ligaments	Dens on depressions below and lateral to the apex
Membrana tectoria (lower end)	Posterior surface of the body
Ligamentum nuchae	Tip of the spine

Axis is connected to the atlas and to the third cervical vertebra through ligaments similar to those between typical vertebrae **(Fig. 6.21)**.

Muscle	Attachment
Rectus capitis posterior major	Posterior edge of the spine (origin)
Inferior oblique capitis	Side of the spine (origin)
Scalenus medius	Anterior aspect of the transverse process (origin)
Levator scapulae	Lateral aspect of the transverse process (origin)
Splenius cervicis	Posterior aspect of the transverse process (insertion)
Semispinalis cervicis	Lower part of the spine and lamina (insertion)
Longus colli (vertical part)	Attached to anterior aspect of the body
Multifidus, spinalis cervicis, and interspinalis	Attached to the spine

AN 43.1 Describe and demonstrate the movements with muscles producing the movements of atlanto-occipital and atlantoaxial joints.

Atlanto-occipital and Atlantoaxial Joints

Atlanto-occipital joint is a synovial joint (*condylar variety*) between the superior articular facets of the atlas and the occipital condyles. It permits flexion, extension, and lateral flexion of the head.

Atlantoaxial joints are synovial joints consisting of two lateral plane joints between the articular facets of the atlas and the axis. The median atlantoaxial joint is a pivot joint between the dens of the axis and the anterior arch of the atlas. These joints are involved in rotation of the atlas and head on the axis.

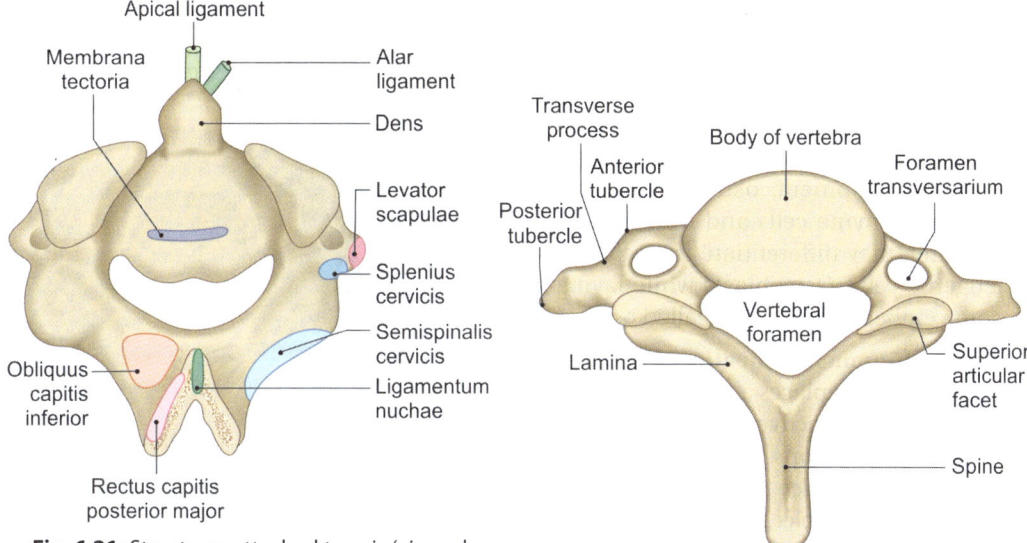

Fig. 6.21: Structures attached to axis (viewed from above and behind).

Fig. 6.22: C-7 vertebra seen from above.

AN 26.7 Describe the features of the 7th cervical vertebra.

Seventh Cervical Vertebra

The seventh cervical vertebra is also called vertebra prominens.

Identifying Features

- Presence of a long, thick and nearly horizontal spinous process
- Spine is not bifid
- Transverse processes are large; posterior root is larger than anterior root
- Foramen transversarium is relatively small; may be absent or doubled.

Long and thick spinous process of C-7 vertebra ends in a single tubercle. The tip of the process forms a prominent surface landmark. The transverse processes are also large with prominent posterior tubercles.

The vertebral artery and vein do not traverse the foramen transversarium of C-7 vertebra. An accessory vertebral vein passes through the foramen (**Fig. 6.22**).

Cervical Vertebrae: Movements

Movement	
Flexion and extension	These movements are more when • Intervertebral discs are thicker • Articular facets are on an inclined plane • Spines are directed horizontally
Lateral flexion	Possible
Rotation	Very little *except* between C-1 and C-2 (*pivot joint*). Plane of articular facets are not in the line of a circle whose center is in the body of the vertebra (axis of movement)

Intramembranous Ossification

AN 26.6 Explain the concept of bones that ossify in membrane.

Ossification consists of deposition of organic matrix by osteoblasts with its subsequent mineralization. In early development, osteoblasts differentiate from mesenchyme cells and from fibroblast like cells. Later, they differentiate from fibroblast like osteogenic cells. Osteoblasts while laying matrix become embedded in it; and called osteocytes.

Intramembranous ossification: Here the bone is formed where it replaces a pre-existing membrane of embryonic connective tissue. An outer covering (*periosteum*) develops this newly formed bone, and osteoblasts (*which differentiate in it*) continue osteogenesis. Example: Bones of skull and clavicle.

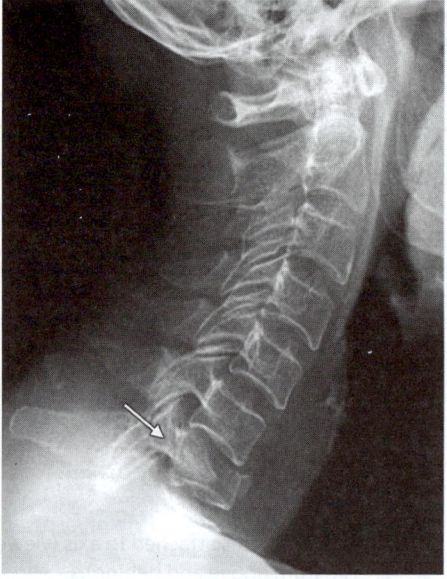

Fig. 6.23: Fracture cervical vertebra.

Clinical Anatomy

Fracture of cervical vertebrae: This may results from a fall on the head with flexed neck. Dislocation results from automobile accidents. The dislocation results as the intervertebral facets are in a horizontal plane **(Fig. 6.23)**.

Prolapsed intervertebral disc (Fig. 6.24): The relatively thin posterior part of the nucleus pulposus ruptures (trauma/degenerative changes). The nucleus pulposus protrudes posteriorly into the vertebral canal. The common sites are C-5 and C-6 and C-6 and C-7.

Klippel–Feil syndrome: Congenital fusion of the cervical vertebrae is one of the features of this syndrome. Fusion of cervical vertebrae results in grossly restricted movements of the neck.

Cervical spondylosis: This degenerative condition of cervical vertebrae may be seen after 50 years of age. This is fairly common in people who are susceptible to neck strain (keeping the neck in one position for long time), e.g., reading and writing.

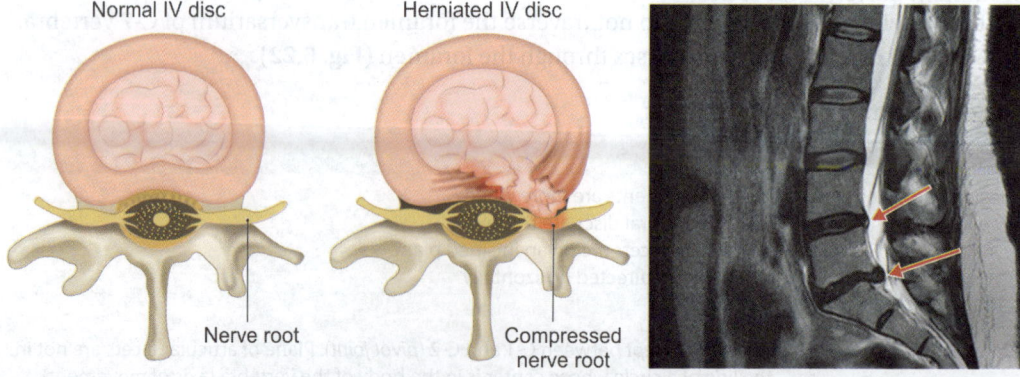

Fig. 6.24: Prolapsed intervertebral disc.

AN 21.2 Identify and describe the features of 1st, 11th and 12th thoracic vertebrae.

ATYPICAL THORACIC VERTEBRAE

First Thoracic Vertebra

This can be distinguished from a typical thoracic vertebra **(Figs. 6.25 and 6.26)**.

Identifying Features
- Small body similar in shape to that of a cervical vertebra
- Posterolateral parts of the body are raised (as in cervical vertebrae)
- Definite superior vertebral notch (absent in other thoracic vertebrae)
- Superior costal facets (on the body) are complete; first rib articulates wholly with T-1 vertebra
- Spine is long and horizontal.

Tenth, Eleventh, and Twelfth Thoracic Vertebrae

These vertebrae resemble lumbar vertebrae in shape and size of their bodies, of the vertebral foramina and of the spines **(Fig. 6.27)**.

These vertebrae can be distinguished from typical thoracic vertebrae because they have only one costal facet on each side of the body.
- T-10 vertebra has a costal facet on each transverse process (*transverse process is large as in typical thoracic vertebrae*)
- Facets on transverse processes are absent in T-11 and T-12 vertebrae which have small transverse processes.
- T-11 and T-12 vertebrae are distinguished from each other by inferior articular facets:
  - Thoracic type in T-11 vertebra
  - Lumbar type in T-12 vertebra.

Transverse Processes
- Transverse processes of T-12 vertebra show superior, inferior, and lateral tubercles
- Transverse processes are absent or rudimentary on T-11 vertebra.

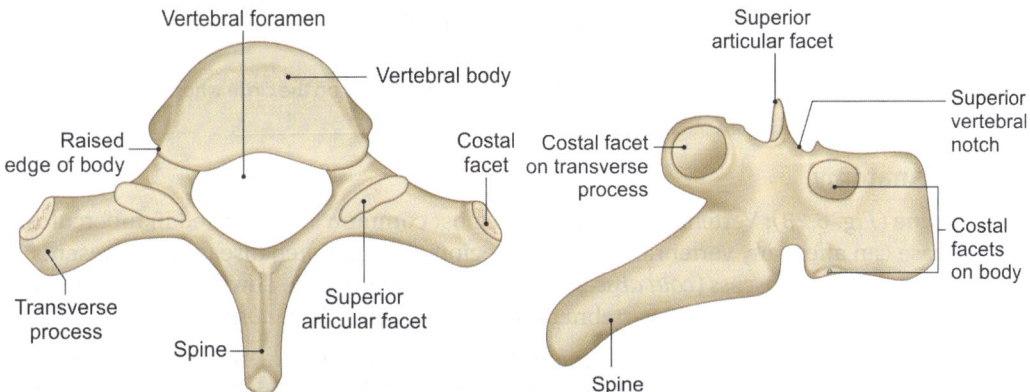

Fig. 6.25: First thoracic vertebra from above. **Fig. 6.26:** First thoracic vertebra from the lateral side.

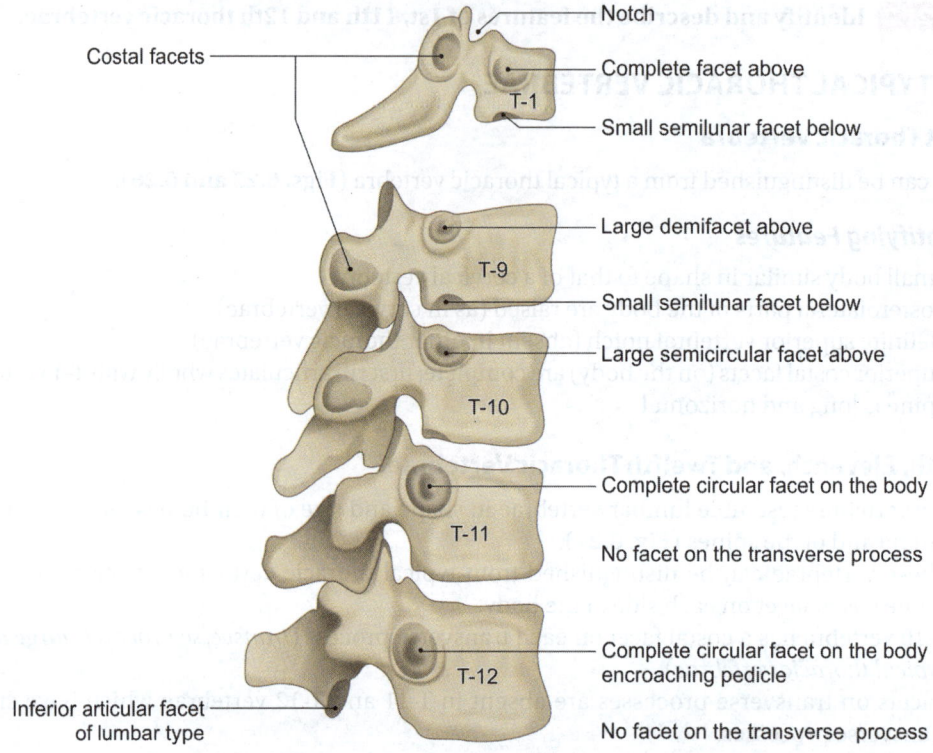

Fig. 6.27: Atypical thoracic vertebrae from the lateral side.

Thoracic Vertebrae: Movements

Movement	
Flexion and extension	These movements are little when • Intervertebral discs are thinner • Articular facets are in a vertical plane • Spines are long and directed downward
Lateral flexion	Very little due to presence of ribs
Rotation	More as the plane of the articular facets lies on the circle whose center is in the body of the vertebra (axis of movement)

Clinical Anatomy

Pott's spine (Fig. 6.28): Vertebrae are one of the most common sites affected in tuberculosis. The disease can affect any vertebra. In thoracic region, the untreated disease may presents as pre- or paravertebral abscess (*cold abscess*). This abscess may trickle down into the upper part of the front of the thigh from T-12 vertebra under psoas fascia (*psoas abscess*).

Kyphosis/scoliosis: It may cause collapse of the vertebrae resulting in the spine deformity (*kyphosis/scoliosis*) **(Figs. 6.29A to D)**. In severe cases, neurological involvement may manifest as paraplegia.

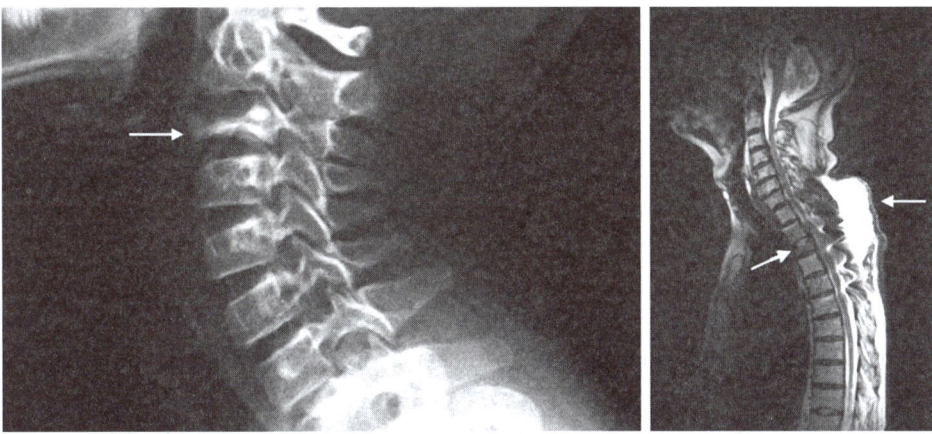

Fig. 6.28: Pott's spine.

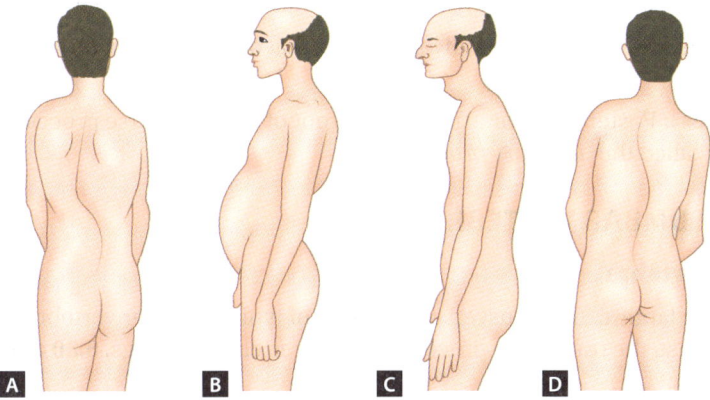

Figs. 6.29A to D: Spine deformities: (A) Lumbar scoliosis; (B) Lordosis; (C) Kyphosis; (D) Dorsal scoliosis.

Fracture of the vertebrae: Fracture of the vertebral column may involve the body of the vertebral arch. Associated with automobile accidents sudden forceful flexion can cause compression fracture of the body. It can also cause dislocation of the vertebral arch.

Compression of spinal cord in thoracic region: Vertebral canal in the thoracic region is the narrowest. Hence, any intrusion into the vertebral canal is bound to cause neurological symptoms (paraplegia, paresthesia).

QUESTIONNAIRE

- What are the differences between C-7 and T-1 vertebrae?
- Why is the body of the first, second, and the third thoracic vertebrae grooved on either side of the midline?
- Enumerate the characteristic features to identify T-12 vertebra.
- What do the tubercle of the T-12 vertebra correspond into the lumbar vertebra?
- Is psoas major attached to the T-12 vertebra? Where?
- Which movements are possible in the thoracic part of the vertebral column?
- Which spinal nerve passes through the inferior vertebral notch at T-1? Why?

LUMBAR VERTEBRAE

There are five lumbar vertebrae. The fifth lumbar vertebra is atypical in nature.

Features of Lumbar Vertebrae

Body: Large and wide transversely. Its vertical extent is more on the anterior aspect than on the posterior aspect. This accounts for the ventral convexity of the lumbar part of the vertebral column.

Pedicle: Short and the laminae are directed backwards so that vertebral foramen is triangular shaped which is not so marked in the thoracic and cervical regions.

Spinous process: Quadrangular shaped with thickened posterior and inferior borders; projects almost horizontally.

Superior articular processes: Gently concave and face medially and backwards. Posterior border of each process presents roughened elevation called the *mamillary process*.

Inferior articular process: Has slightly convex articular facet that faces laterally and forwards.

Transverse process: Relatively thin and long except that of fifth lumbar vertebra which is thick and stout.

Accessory process: Posteroinferior aspect of the root of the transverse process shows a small rough elevation called the *accessory process*.

ATYPICAL LUMBAR VERTEBRA

Fifth Lumbar Vertebra

L-5 vertebra is the largest. The transverse processes of typical lumbar vertebrae are small and tapering. In contrast, the transverse processes of L-5 vertebra are **(Figs. 6.30 and 6.31)**:
a. Very large
b. Encroaches on the body
c. Short and thick
d. Blunt tipped.

AN 53.4 Explain and demonstrate clinical importance sacralization of lumbar vertebra and lumbarization of 1st sacral vertebra.

Clinical Anatomy

Sacralization of L-5 vertebra (Fig. 6.32): The fusion of the L-5 vertebra completely or in part with the sacrum is termed as sacralization of L-5 vertebra.

Lumbarization of S-1 vertebra: When S-1 vertebra is no longer joined with the rest of the sacrum and instead it is partly or completely fused with L-5 vertebra **(Fig. 6.33)**. Painful symptoms like backache are generally presenting complaints.

In both sacralization and lumbarization conditions the normal spine curvature is altered thus it is natural that weight transmission would be affected resulting in degenerative changes in the vertebrae involved.

Spina bifida (Fig. 6.34): The failure of fusion of two halves of the vertebral arches posteriorly results in spina bifida. It affects lumbar region usually. When not associated with neurological

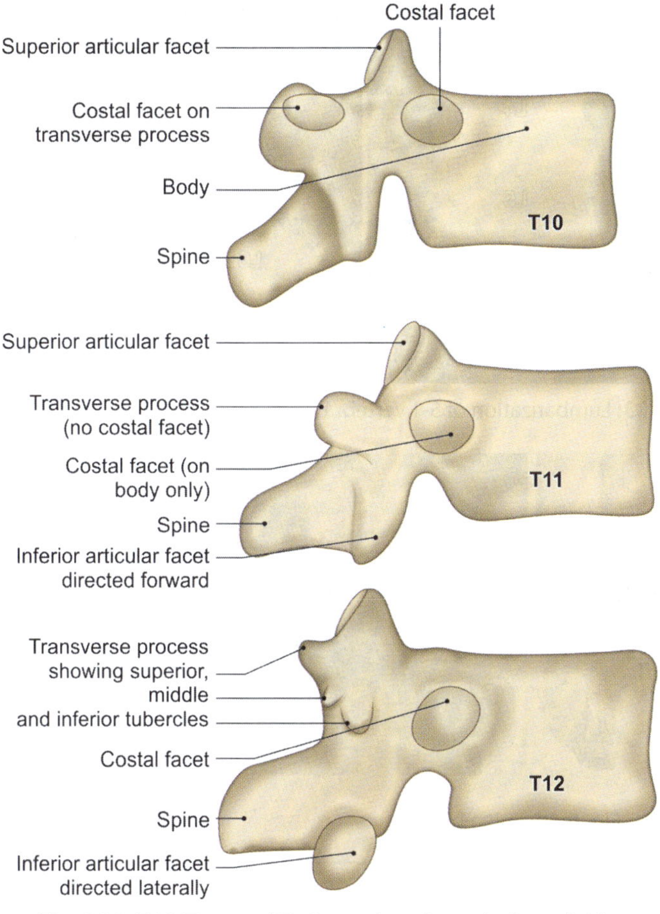

Fig. 6.30: T-10, T-11, and T-12 vertebrae from the lateral side.

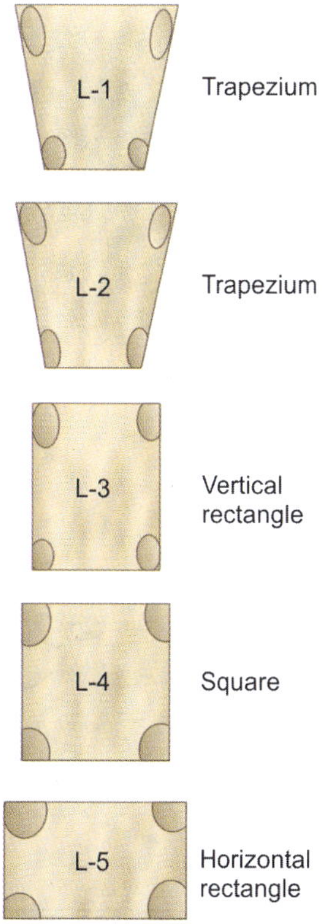

Fig. 6.31: Identification of lumbar vertebrae: Fawcett's method.

abnormalities the condition is termed as *spina bifida occulta*. It is marked on the surface by a dimple.

Spondylolysis: It is a stress fracture through the pars interarticularis (thin bone segment joining two vertebrae) of the lumbar vertebrae. This fairly common condition can present at birth or occur after injury. Repeated stress fractures caused by hyperextension of the back (in gymnastics and football players) and traumatic fractures result in this condition. The most common cause in adults is degenerative arthritis.

Spondylolisthesis: In this condition, there is anterior displacement of the centrum. In this, there is pressure on the spinal nerves causing backache.

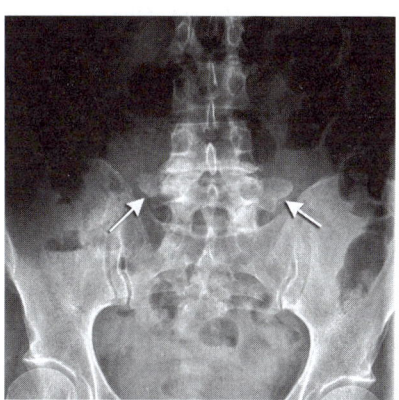

Fig. 6.32: Bilateral sacralization of L-5.

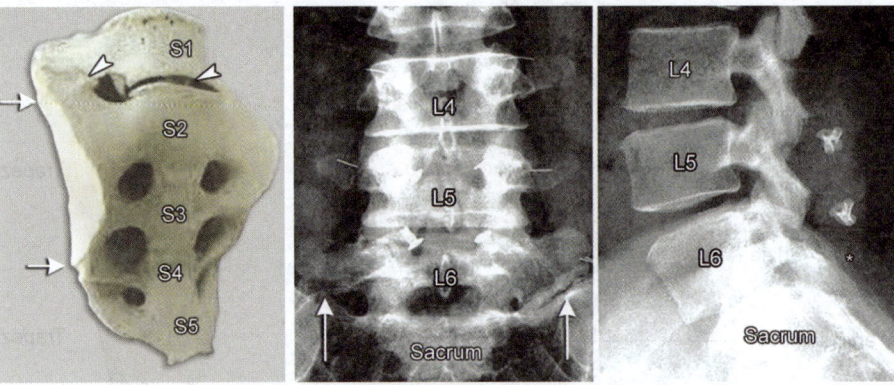

Fig. 6.33: Lumbarization of S-1 vertebra.

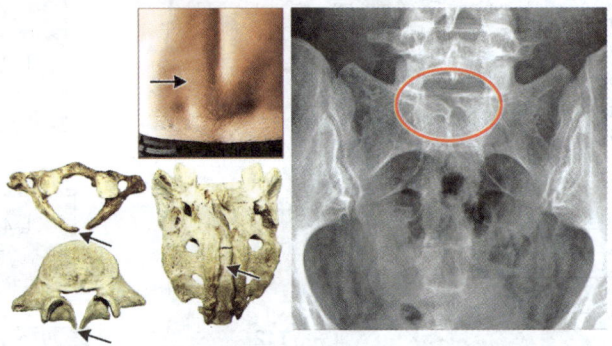

Fig. 6.34: Spina bifida.

QUESTIONNAIRE

- Classify lumbar vertebrae.
- Which is the atypical lumbar vertebra?
- Enumerate the characteristic features of L-5 vertebra.
- Is psoas major attached to L-5 vertebra? Where it is attached?
- Mark the attachment of the crus of diaphragm to the L-3 vertebra.
- What are the muscles attached to the transverse process of the lumbar vertebra.
- What are the structures passing through the vertebral foramen? Which lumbar nerve passes through the inferior vertebral notch of L-3 vertebra?
- What are the costal and transverse elements of the lumbar vertebra?
- What are the attachments of the median, medial and lateral arcuate ligaments? Enumerate the structures passing underneath these ligaments.
- What are the mamillary and accessory processes? What is attached there?
- What are the developmental anomalies of the lumbar vertebrae?
- What is lumbarization and sacralization of the vertebrae?
- What movements are possible in the lumbar part of the vertebral column?
- At what level is lumbar puncture is done? Why?
- At what level the spinal cord ends?
- What is cauda equina?
- What is spina bifida?
- What is spondylolisthesis?

SACRUM

The sacrum lies below the L-5 vertebra. It is made up of five fused sacral vertebrae. It is wedged between the two hip bones and takes part in forming the pelvis. It is triangular shaped. It presents:
* *Upper end (base)*: Articulates with L-5 vertebra
* *Lower end (apex)*: Articulates with the coccyx
* Concave anterior *(pelvic)* surface
* Convex posterior *(dorsal)* surface
* *Right and left lateral surfaces*: Articulate with ilium of the corresponding side.
* *Sacrum from front*: When viewed from the front, pelvic sacral surface shows four pairs of *anterior sacral foramina* (first foramen is largest; fourth is smallest) **(Fig. 6.35)**. The foramina separate the *medial part* of the sacrum from its *lateral part*.
* Medial part is formed by fused bodies of sacral vertebrae
* Lateral part represents fused transverse processes, including costal elements.

The anterior sacral foramina (on pelvic surface) continue posteriorly with the *posterior sacral foramina* which open on to the dorsal surface. The canals connecting the anterior and posterior foramina open into the *sacral canal*. It is the downward continuation of the vertebral canal.

Sacrum from above: Viewed from above, the base is formed by the first sacral vertebra with a large oval body that articulates with the body of the L-5 vertebra. The body has a projecting anterior margin called the *sacral promontory*. Behind the body, there is a triangular vertebral (sacral) canal bounded by thick pedicles and laminae. Where the laminae meet, there is a small tubercle representing the *spine*. The superior articular facets arise from the junction of the pedicles and laminae that articulate with the inferior articular facets of the L-5 vertebra. Lateral to the body, the superior surface of the lateral part (*ala*) is seen **(Fig. 6.36)**.

Sacrum from behind: When viewed from behind, the medial and lateral parts of sacrum are distinguished; separated by four pairs of posterior sacral foramina. These foramina give passage to the dorsal rami of sacral nerves. The medial part of the dorsum of the sacrum is formed by the fused laminae of sacral vertebrae **(Fig. 6.37)**.

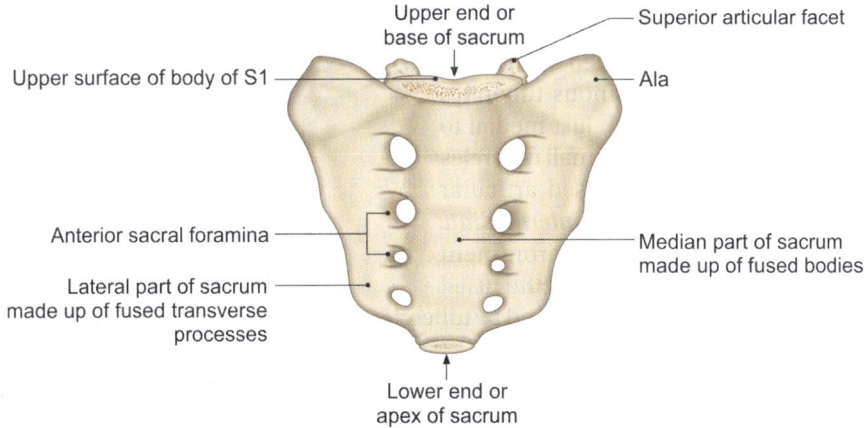

Fig. 6.35: Sacrum from the front.

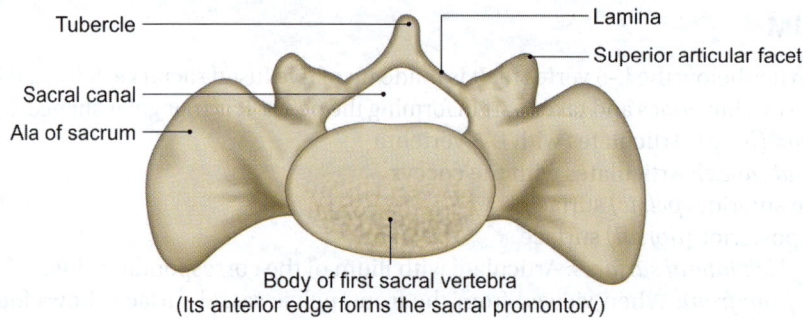

Fig. 6.36: Sacrum from above.

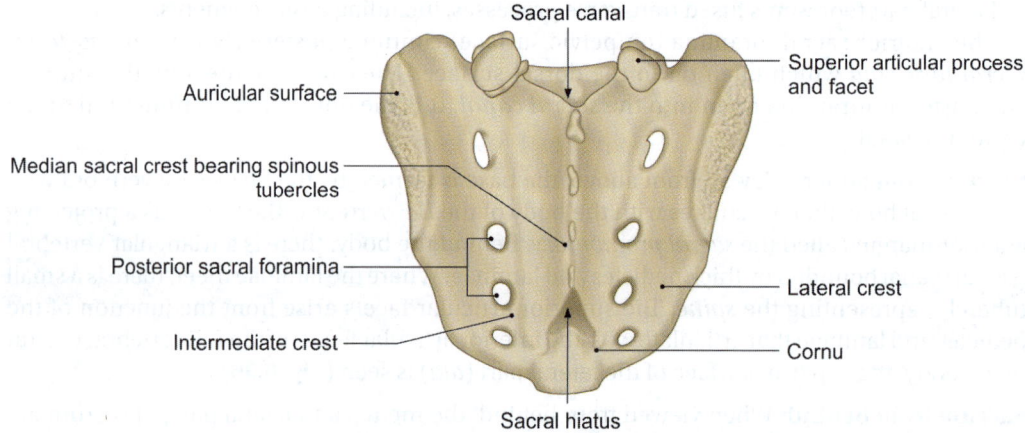

Fig. 6.37: Sacrum from behind.

The laminae of the S-5 vertebra (*sometimes also of fourth*) are deficient leaving an inverted U-shaped gap called the *sacral hiatus*. The midline is marked by a ridge called the *median sacral crest* on which four spinous tubercles (*representing spines*) are noted. Just medial to the dorsal sacral foramina, four small tubercles are identified that represent fused articular processes; collectively form the *intermediate crest*. Lateral to the foramina, a prominent lateral sacral crest is seen formed by the fused transverse processes. The crest is marked by tubercles which represent the tips of the transverse processes **(Fig. 6.38)**.

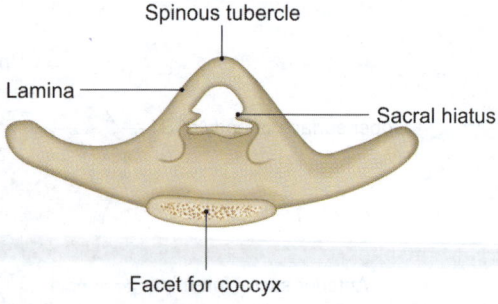

Fig. 6.38: Sacrum from below.

The lower end (apex) bears an oval facet for the articulation with the coccyx. At the sides of the sacral hiatus, two small downward projections (*sacral cornua*) are seen. They represent inferior articular processes of S-5 vertebra; connected to the coccyx by ligaments.

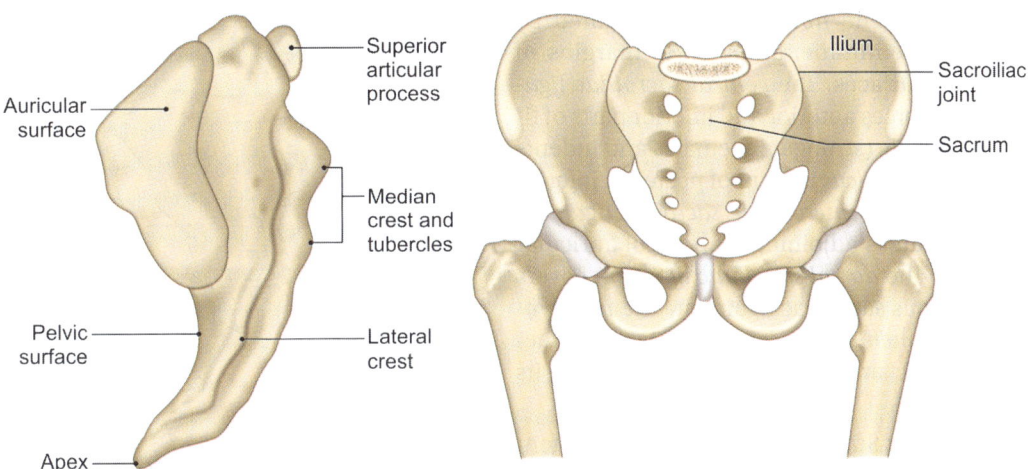

Fig. 6.39: Sacrum from the lateral side.

Fig. 6.40: Sacroiliac joint.

Sacrum from the side: The lateral surface bears a large L-shaped *auricular area* (articulates with ilium). It consists of a superior limb present on the S-1 vertebra, and an inferior limb that lies on the S-2 and S-3 vertebrae. The area behind the auricular surface is rough; gives attachment to ligaments that connect the sacrum to the ilium **(Fig. 6.39)**.

Sex Differences

Feature	Male	Female
Ala—body relation	Breadth of body of S-1 vertebra is more than of ala	Breadth of body of S-1 vertebra is less than of ala
Sacroiliac articulation (auricular surface)	Extends up to 3rd segment	Extends up to 2.5 to 3rd segment
Pelvic curvature	Uniformly curved anteriorly	Abruptly curved at last two segments
Dorsal convexity	Less marked	More marked
Sacral promontory	More projected	Less prominent and less projected
Sacral index	Less than 114 (usually 105)	More than 114 (usually 115)

Sacral Index

$$\frac{\text{Transverse diameter of sacrum}}{\text{Anterior length of sacrum}} \times 100$$

❖ Males: Less than 114 (usually 105)
❖ Females: More than 114 (usually 115).

AN 50.2 Describe and demonstrate the type, articular ends, ligaments and movements of sacroiliac joint.

Sacroiliac Joint

Sacroiliac joint is a synovial joint (*plane variety*). The articular surfaces are auricular surface of sacrum and auricular surface of ilium **(Fig. 6.40)**.

Ligaments: The *fibrous capsule* is lined by synovial membrane; attached to margins of articular surfaces. The *ventral sacroiliac ligament* reinforces anterior and inferior parts of fibrous capsule (stronger in females and indents *preauricular sulcus* in front of posterior inferior iliac spine). The *interosseous sacroiliac ligament* connects areas adjoining margins of auricular surfaces. The *dorsal sacroiliac ligament* covers interosseous sacroiliac ligament. The *vertebropelvic ligaments* (accessory ligaments to sacroiliac joint) are important in maintaining its stability.

Movements: Stability is primary requirement of joint because it transmits body weight from vertebral column to lower limbs. It is maintained by interlocking device of articular surfaces, sacroiliac ligaments and vertebropelvic ligaments (iliolumbar, sacrotuberous and sacrospinous). During flexion and extension of trunk (*stooping & straightening*) sacroiliac joint permits some anteroposterior rotatory movement around a transverse axis.

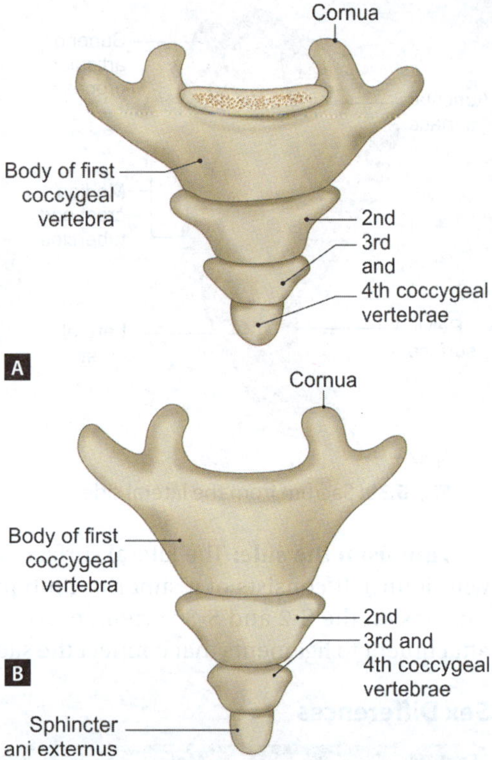

Figs. 6.41A and B: (A) Coccyx from front; (B) Coccyx from behind.

Ossification

- Ossification of sacrum is complicated
- Each sacral piece ossifies like a typical vertebra
- Upper pieces have additional centers for the parts derived from costal elements
- Sacral pieces are united by cartilage till 20 years of age after which they fuse with each other.

COCCYX

The coccyx consists of four rudimentary vertebrae fused together.

It has pelvic and dorsal surfaces. The base (upper end) has an oval facet for articulation with the apex of the sacrum. Lateral to the facet, there are two cornua that project upward; connected to the sacral cornua by ligaments.

First coccygeal vertebra has rudimentary transverse processes.
Remaining vertebrae are represented by nodules of bone **(Figs. 6.41A and B)**.

Ossification

- Each coccyx segment has one primary center
- Centers for most segments appear after birth
- Segments unite with each other by about the 20th year.

Attachments on the sacrum and coccyx **(Figs. 6.42 and 6.43)**.

CHAPTER 6 ✦ Vertebral Column

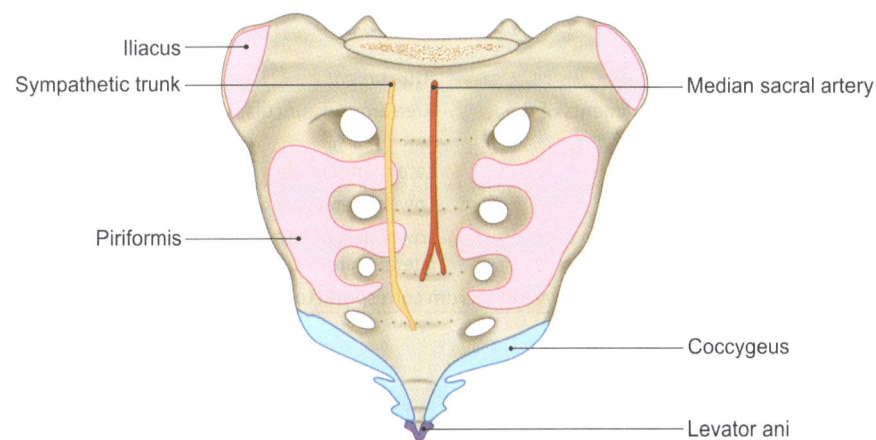

Fig. 6.42: Pelvic aspect of sacrum and coccyx: Attachments.

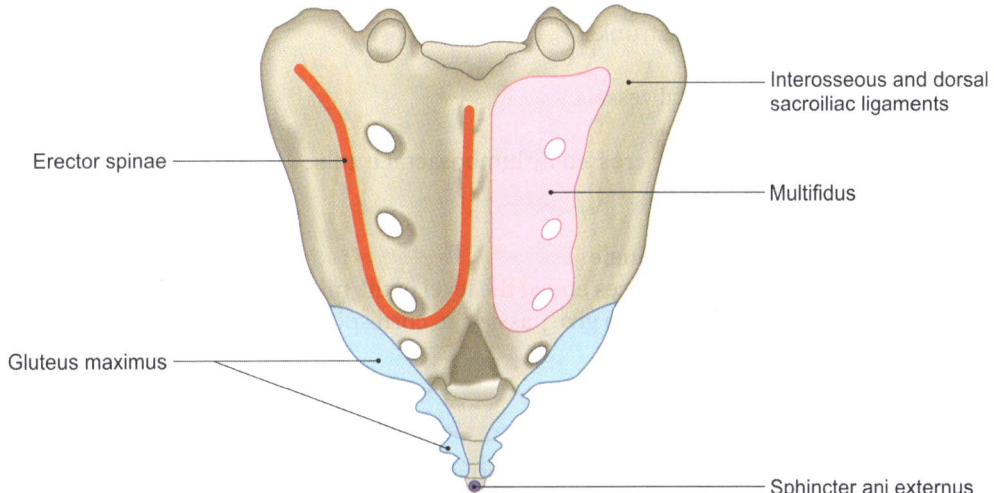

Fig. 6.43: Dorsal aspect of sacrum and coccyx: Attachments.

Muscles

Muscle	Attachment
Iliacus	Pelvic surface; anterolateral part of ala (*origin*)
Piriformis	Pelvic surface; in the form of three digitations from the areas between sacral foramina (*origin*)
Coccygeus	Lateral side of pelvic aspect of the last piece of sacrum and coccyx (*insertion*)
Levator ani	Sides of lower two segments of the coccyx (*insertion*)
Gluteus maximus	Lateral margin of the lowest part of sacrum and coccyx (*origin*)
Erector spinae	U-shaped; dorsal aspect of sacrum; medial limb of "U" to spinous tubercles and lateral limb to transverse tubercles (*origin*)
Multifidus	Area within U-shaped origin of erector spinae (*origin*)

Ligaments

Ligament	Attachment
Ventral, dorsal and interosseous ligaments of the sacroiliac joint	Area around auricular surface
Iliolumbar ligament	Lateral part of ala
Sacrotuberous ligament	Lower lateral part of the dorsal surface of sacrum
Sacrospinous ligament	Lower part of lateral margin of sacrum and adjoining lateral margin of coccyx
Ligaments of the joints between L-5 vertebra and sacrum correspond to those of other intervertebral joints	

Sacrum: Relations

- Rectum is in contact with the ventral surfaces of 3rd, 4th, and 5th sacral pieces
- Ventral surfaces of first three sacral pieces are covered by peritoneum; give attachment to sigmoid mesocolon
- Deep to rectum, ventral surface is crossed by:
  a. Right and left sympathetic trunks
  b. Median sacral vessels
  c. Right and left lateral sacral vessels
  d. Superior rectal vessels
- Ala is covered by psoas major; crossed by lumbosacral trunk
- Sacral canal contains:
  a. Cauda equina
  b. Spinal meninges filum terminale
- Subarachnoid and subdural spaces end at the level of the middle of sacrum
- Ventral and dorsal sacral foramina give passage to corresponding rami of sacral nerves.

QUESTIONNAIRE

- What is the anatomical position of the sacrum?
- How do you differentiate male sacrum from female sacrum? Mention three important points.
- What are the structures passing through the sacral canal?
- Enumerate the structures emerging through the sacral hiatus.
- What are the structures passing through pelvic sacral foramina? Do they pierce the piriformis muscle?
- What are the structures passing through dorsal sacral foramina? Do they pierce multifidus and erector spinae?
- Which are the transverse elements of the sacrum?
- Show the costal elements of the sacrum.
- Mark the relation of sympathetic trunk and the sacrum. How many ganglia are there in the sympathetic trunk in the cervical, thoracic, lumbar, and sacral parts?
- Mark the relation of the root of the sigmoid mesocolon. What is the shape of the sigmoid mesocolon? Where is its apex related?
- Mark the attachments of:

Ligaments	Muscles
Ventral and dorsal sacroiliac ligaments	Iliacus
Uterosacral ligament	Piriformis
	Multifidus and erector spinae

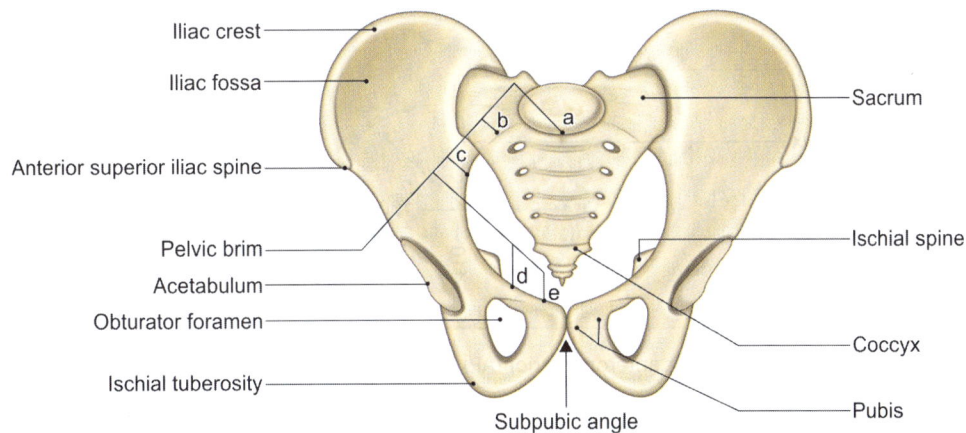

Fig. 6.44: Pelvis from the front.

AN 53.2 Demonstrate the anatomical position of bony pelvis and show boundaries of pelvic inlet, pelvic cavity and pelvic outlet.

BONY PELVIS

Bony pelvis is made up of two hip bones, sacrum, and the coccyx. It is subdivided into:
- Greater (false) pelvis
- Lesser (true) pelvis.

The walls of the *greater pelvis* are formed by the broad upper parts of the two iliac bones *(iliac fossae)*, and posteriorly by the base of the sacrum. The greater pelvis has no bony anterior wall; it is merely the lower part of the abdomen. The communication between the greater and lesser pelvis is the superior pelvic aperture (pelvic inlet). The margins of the aperture constitute the pelvic brim **(Fig. 6.44)**.

Pelvic Brim

It is formed by:
- *Behind*: Sacral promontory and ridge separating superior and anterior surfaces of sacrum
- *On either side*: Arcuate line of ilium
- *Anteriorly*: Pecten pubis and pubic crest
- Arcuate line, pecten pubis, and pubic crest constitute the *linea terminalis*.

Cavity of Lesser Pelvis

It is bounded by:
- *In front*: Body and pubic rami
- *On either side*: Pelvic surfaces of ilium and ischium below the arcuate line
- *Behind*: Anterior surfaces of the sacrum and coccyx.

Inferior Pelvic Aperture

It is bounded by:
- *Anteriorly*: Pubic arch.
- *Laterally*: Ischial tuberosity, lesser sciatic notch, ischial spine and greater sciatic notch.
- *Posteriorly*: Lateral margin of sacrum and coccyx.

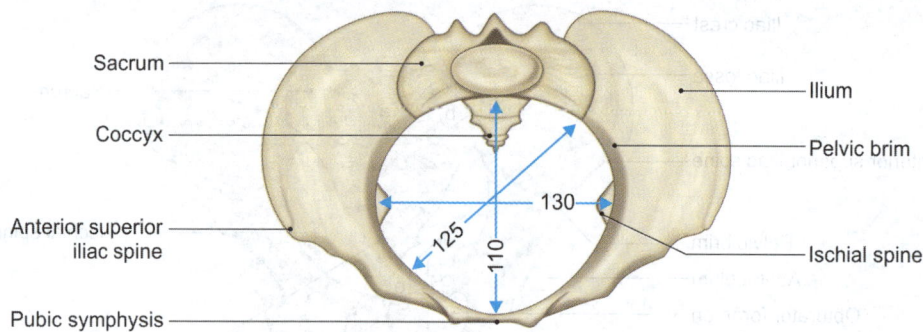

Fig. 6.45: Pelvis anteroposterior (AP) view: Diameters of pelvic inlet.

When ligaments are intact, lateral margins are formed by sacrotuberous ligaments (from side of sacrum and coccyx to ischial tuberosity). Inferior aperture appears rhomboidal.

Pelvis Orientation
- Anterior superior iliac spines and the upper margin of pubic symphysis are in same vertical plane
- Pelvic inlet faces forward and upward, its plane at an angle of 50-60° with the horizontal plane
- Pelvic outlet faces downward and slightly backward at an angle of 15° with the horizontal plane.

Axis of the pelvic passage is curved; corresponding to the sacral curvature.

Pelvis Diameters
These diameters are important in obstetrics. Dimensions given below are those in the females.

Pelvic Inlet (Fig. 6.45)

Diameter	Landmarks	Value
Anteroposterior	Upper border of pubic symphysis to sacral promontory	110 mm
Transverse	Measured across the widest part of pelvic brim	130 mm
Oblique diameter	One iliopubic eminence to opposite sacroiliac joint	125 mm

Pelvic Outlet (Figs. 6.46 and 6.47)

Diameter	Landmarks	Value
Anteroposterior	Apex of coccyx to the lower border of pubic symphysis	125 mm
Transverse	Measured between two ischial tuberosities	110 mm
Oblique diameter	Midpoint of sacrotuberous ligament of one side to the junction of ischiopubic rami on the other side	118 mm

AN 53.3 Define true pelvis and false pelvis and demonstrate sex determination in male and female bony pelvis.

Sex Differences in the Pelvis

The sexual differences are most marked in the pelvis.
- *Male pelvis*: It is more strongly built, with more prominent muscular markings. All articular areas (including acetabulum) are larger in males, for transmission of greater body weight.

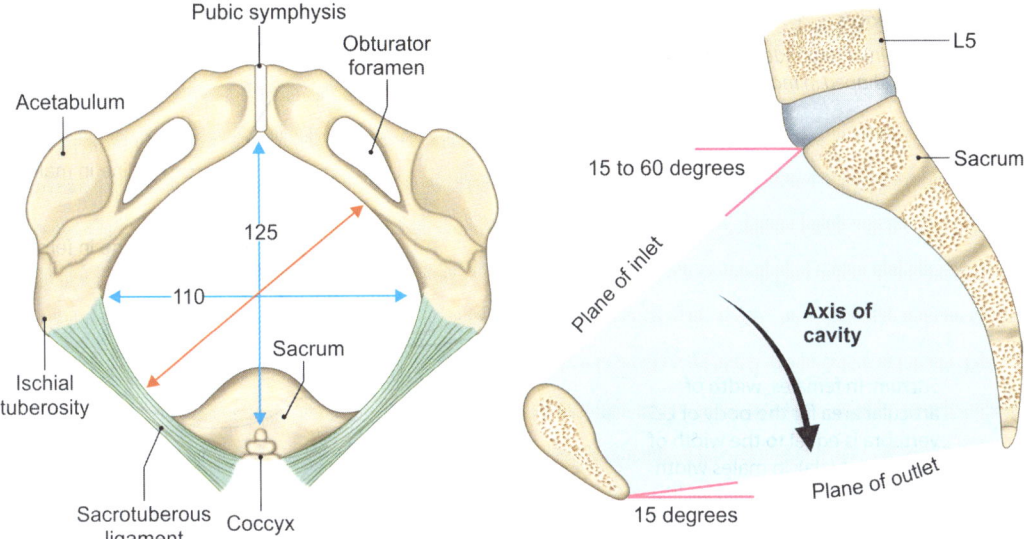

Fig. 6.46: Pelvic outlet from below.

Fig. 6.47: Schematic sagittal section of the pelvis to show orientation of pelvic inlet and outlet.

❖ *Female pelvis*: It is adapted for child-bearing function. Thus, female pelvis is broader and shallower.

The points used in deciding the sexing of a given pelvis are given below. However, all the features have to be taken together as no singular feature being decisive.

Sl. No.	Differences	Illustration
1.	Subpubic angle (angle between right and left ischiopubic rami) is almost 90° in female; 50–60° in male ("a"). Angle is sharp in male; rounded in female	
2.	Medial edges of ischiopubic rami are markedly everted in male ("b" in Figure) for attachment of crura of penis	
3.	In **Figures A and B** lines xy represent distance from pubic symphysis to anterior margin of acetabulum. Lines yz represent total width of acetabulum. In male (**Fig. A**) xy = yz; in female (**Fig. B**) xy is more than yz	
4.	Pubis, ischium and ilium meet at a point in the floor of acetabulum ("m" in Figure B). Line mn represents height of ischium, and xm is the length of pubis. Puboischial index: xm/mn × 100 is less than 90 in male and more than 90 in female	

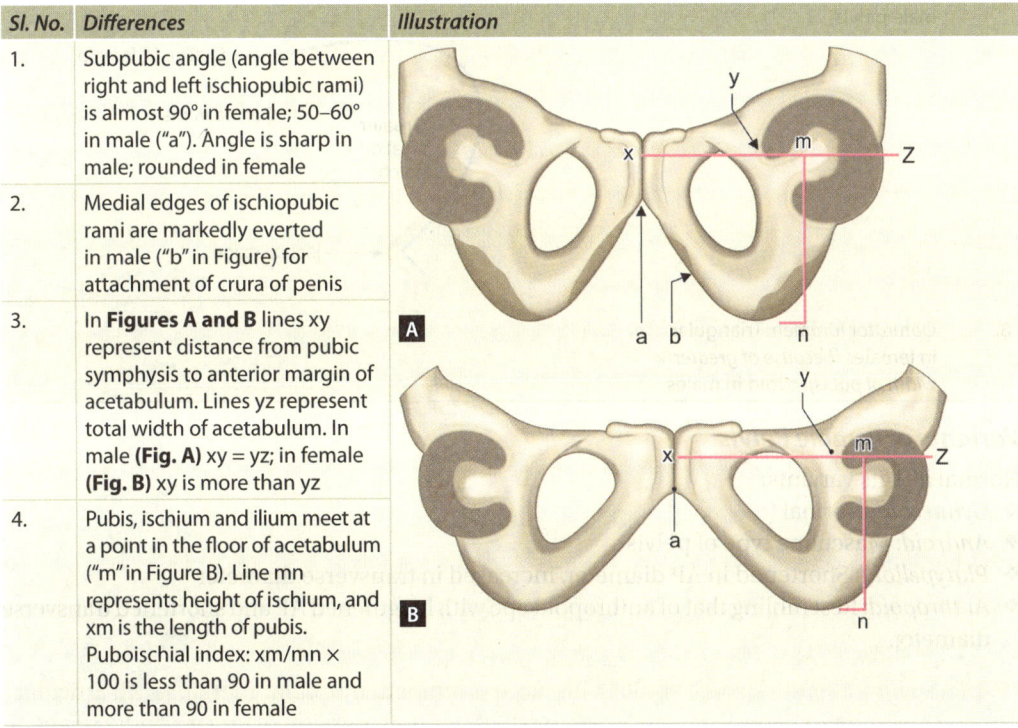

Sl. No.	Differences	Illustration
5.	Pelvic inlet is rounded in female; heart shaped in male	
6.	Sacrum: In females, width of articular area for the body of L-5 vertebra is equal to the width of lateral part (ala); in males width of the body is more than width of the lateral part	
7.	Greater sciatic notch is wide and deep in female pelvis; narrow in male pelvis	
8.	Obturator foramen: Triangular in females (because of greater width of pubis); ovoid in males	

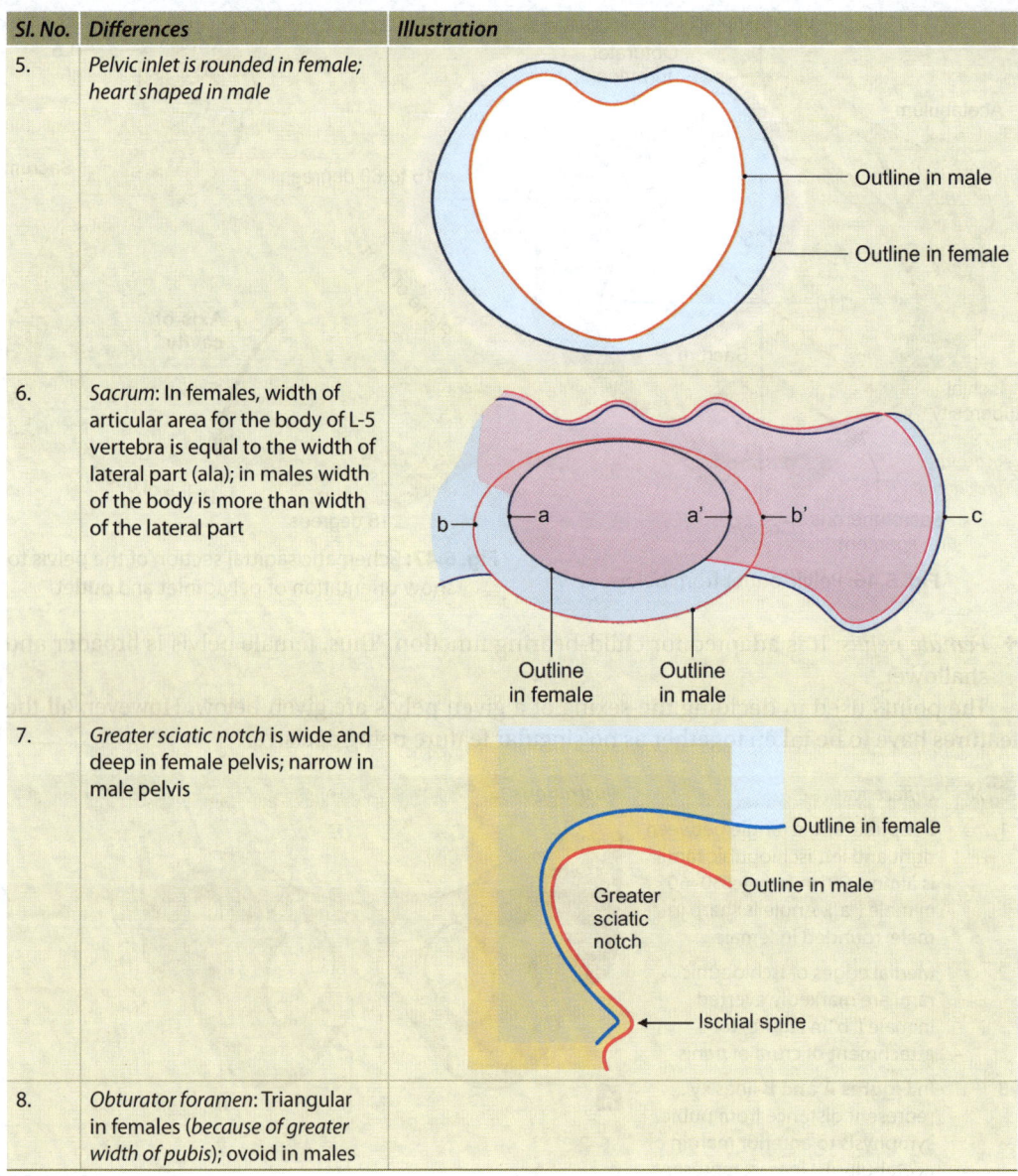

Variants of Female Pelvis

Normal and its variants:
- *Gynaecoid*: Normal
- *Android*: Masculine type of pelvis
- *Platypelloid*: Shortened in AP diameter, increased in transverse diameter
- *Anthropoid*: Resembling that of anthropoid ape with lengthened AP and shortened transverse diameter.

AN 53.4 Explain and demonstrate types of bony pelvis.

Pelvis: Types

Pelvis	Features	Illustration
Gynaecoid (mesatipellic)	• Inlet is round • Transverse diameter of inlet is greatest • Most female pelvis of this type • No difficulty in parturition	
Android (brachypellic)	• Inlet is heart shaped • Posterior segment of inlet is wider • Fair number of females possess android pelvis • Parturition is difficult	
Anthropoid (dolichopellic)	• Inlet is oval anteroposteriorly • AP diameter of inlet is more than transverse diameter • Difficulty in parturition	
Platypelloid (platypellic)	• Flat type • Inlet is transversely oval • Transverse diameter is disproportionately greater than AP diameter of inlet • Vitamin D deficiency (rickets/osteomalacia) results in this type pelvis	

Clinical Anatomy

Fractures of pelvis (Fig. 6.48): These may be isolated lesions due to localized blow or displacements of part of pelvic ring due to compression injuries. Associated with pelvic fractures might be soft tissue injuries to bladder, urethra, and rectum; penetrated by spicules of bone or torn by wide displacements of pelvic fragments.

Positive Trendelenburg's sign: It is seen in:
* Fracture of femoral neck
* Dislocated hip joint
* Paralysis of gluteus medius and minimus

If the right gluteus medius and minimus muscles are paralyzed, the unsupported left side of the pelvis falls instead of rising.

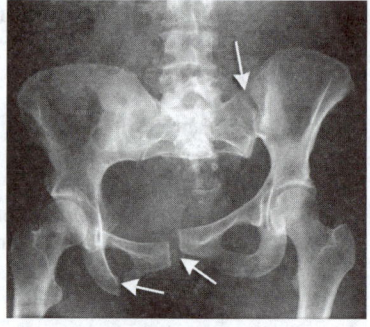

Fig. 6.48: Fracture pelvis.

Contracted pelvis: The variations in the pelvic cavity account for change in the dimensions of the pelvic cavity.

Symmetrically contracted pelvis: It is associated with small stature women.

Asymmetrically contracted pelvis: It is due to scoliosis, poliomyelitis, pelvis fractures, congenital dislocation of hip and Naegele's pelvis (*degenerative/absence of one ala of sacrum*).

Rachitic flat pelvis: The sacrum is rotated; thus sacral promontory projects forward and coccyx tips backward **(Fig. 6.49)**. AP diameter of inlet is narrowed but outlet is increased. This deformity is typical of rickets.

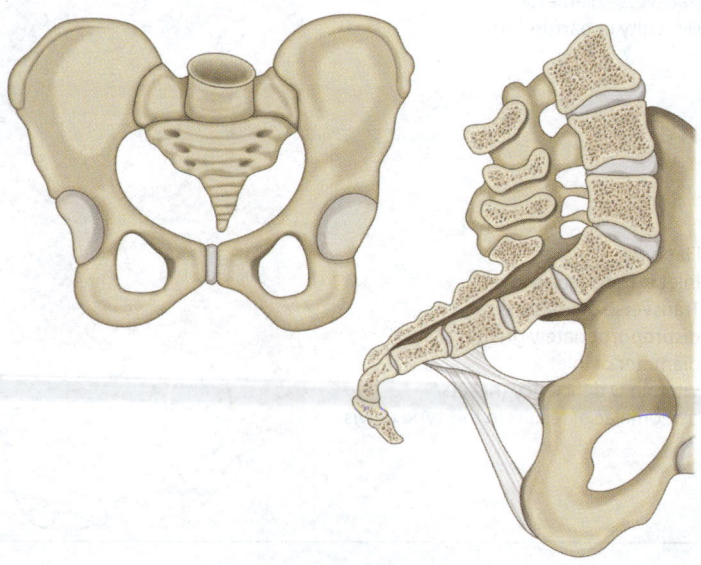

Fig. 6.49: Rachitic flat pelvis.

CHAPTER 6 ✦ Vertebral Column

QUESTIONNAIRE

- What is the meaning of the word pelvis?
- Hold the pelvis in the anatomical position. How much is the angle of inclination at the inlet and the outlet?
- Enumerate important points to differentiate male pelvis from the female pelvis.
- What is puboischial index? What are its value in male and female?
- What parts of the sacrum and the hip bone form pelvic brim?
- What is linea terminalis?
- Enumerate the structures which are in direct contact with the pelvic brim.
- Does psoas major pass through the true pelvis?
- What are the structures that pass through the pelvis but not necessarily in contact with the pelvic brim?
- What is greater or false pelvis and lesser or true pelvis?
- How do you measure the diameters at pelvic brim, cavity, and outlet?
- What is the plane of the least pelvic dimensions?
- What is pelvic brim index?
- Mark the attachment of the levator ani muscle.
- Where is the pudendal block given?
- How many lumbar arteries are there? What are they branches of?
- What is preauricular sulcus? How it is produced?

Bones of Head and Neck

CHAPTER 7

THE SKULL

General Considerations

The skull consists of many bones. Students should be familiar with their names as a preliminary to further study.

The skull bones collectively form the cranium (*cranium = skull minus mandible*). The upper part of the cranium is the skull vault. The remainder of the skull constitutes the *facial skeleton* including the mandible. Lower part of the facial skeleton is freely movable at the *temporomandibular joints*.

The mandible forms the lower jaw. Other skull bones are firmly united to one another at joints called *sutures*.

The cranium consists of two main parts. Its upper and posterior part contains a large cranial cavity which contains the brain. Anteriorly and inferiorly the cranium forms:
❖ Facial skeleton including orbital walls
❖ Cavity of the nose
❖ Upper part of the cavity of the mouth.

The upper dome-like part of the skull is the vault (*calvaria*). It forms the upper, lateral, anterior, and posterior walls of the cranial cavity. Its anterior wall forms the forehead. The part of the skull forming the floor of the cranial cavity is the base.

AN 26.1 Demonstrate anatomical position of skull.

Skull: Anatomical Position

Frankfort plane: This horizontal plane passes along the inferior margin of the bony orbit to the upper margin of the external acoustic meatus.

Reid's base line: This horizontal line passes through the lower margin of the bony orbit and the middle of the external acoustic meatus.

AN 26.2 Describe the features of norma frontalis, verticalis, occipitalis, lateralis and basalis.

Methods of Study of the Skull

Skull can be studied in the following manner:
❖ Study of exterior (outer aspect)
  - Norma verticalis: From above
  - Norma frontalis: From front
  - Norma lateralis: From the side

- Norma occipitalis: From behind
- Norma basalis: From below.
❖ Study of interior (inner aspect)
  - On removing the skull cap, the interior (base of skull) is seen. It shows three depressions (cranial fossae). From before backward these are called anterior, middle, and posterior cranial fossae.
❖ Individual skull bones.

Skull Bones (22)

❖ *Cranium bones* (8): Frontal, occipital, parietal (2), temporal (2), sphenoid, and ethmoid
❖ *Facial bones* (14): Nasal (2), maxilla (2), lacrimal (2), zygomatic (2), palatine (2), inferior nasal concha (2), vomer, and mandible.

When the skull is viewed from above (*norma verticalis*) four bones are seen. The bone forming the anterior part of the vault is the frontal bone. The greater part of the roof and side walls of the cranial cavity are formed by the right and left parietal bones. The two parietal bones meet in the midline at the *sagittal suture*. Their anterior margins join the frontal bone at the *coronal suture*. The posterior part of the vault is formed by the occipital bone. The suture joining the occipital bone to the parietal bones is the *lambdoid suture* (**Fig. 7.1**).

When the skull is viewed from the front (*norma frontalis*), the most conspicuous features are the jaws which bear the teeth. The mandible forms the lower jaw. The upper jaw is formed by the right and left maxillae (**Fig. 7.2**).

The forehead region is formed by the frontal bone. The prominence of the cheek is formed by the zygomatic bone. A median nasal aperture is present between the two maxillae; leads into the nasal cavities. In the aperture depth, bones seen are:
❖ Ethmoid
❖ Inferior nasal concha
❖ Vomer

Above and lateral to the nasal aperture, right and left orbits cavities are noted which contain eyeballs. Orbital walls receive contributions from following bones:
❖ Frontal
❖ Zygomatic

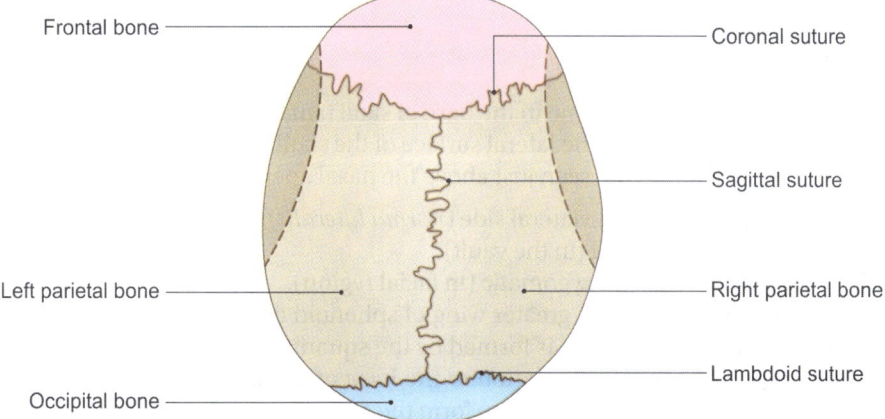

Fig. 7.1: Skull from above.

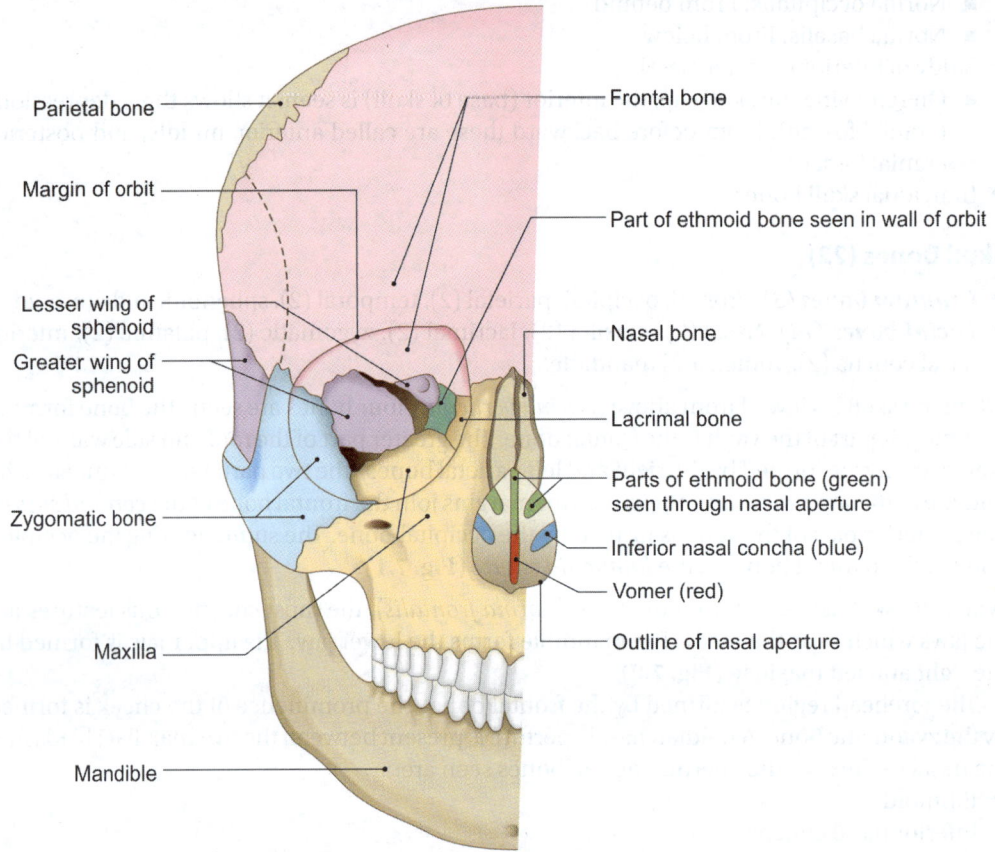

Fig. 7.2: Skull from the front.

- Ethmoid
- Maxilla
- Lacrimal
- Sphenoid

Sphenoid is a large unpaired bone in the base of skull (small part seen in orbit). The greater wing of sphenoid is also seen on the lateral surface of the skull. In the area between two orbits, the right and left nasal bones are seen just above the nasal aperture.

When the skull is viewed from the lateral side (*norma lateralis*), bones noted are **(Fig. 7.3)**:
- Frontal, parietal, and occipital (in the vault)
- Ethmoid, lacrimal, nasal, and zygomatic (in facial region).

The maxilla, mandible, and the greater wing of sphenoid are also seen. Below the parietal bone the lateral wall of the cranium is formed by the squamous temporal bone. Lower down, the mastoid temporal bone lies in relation to the base of skull. The temporal bone gives off zygomatic process; joins zygomatic bone to form the *zygomatic arch*.

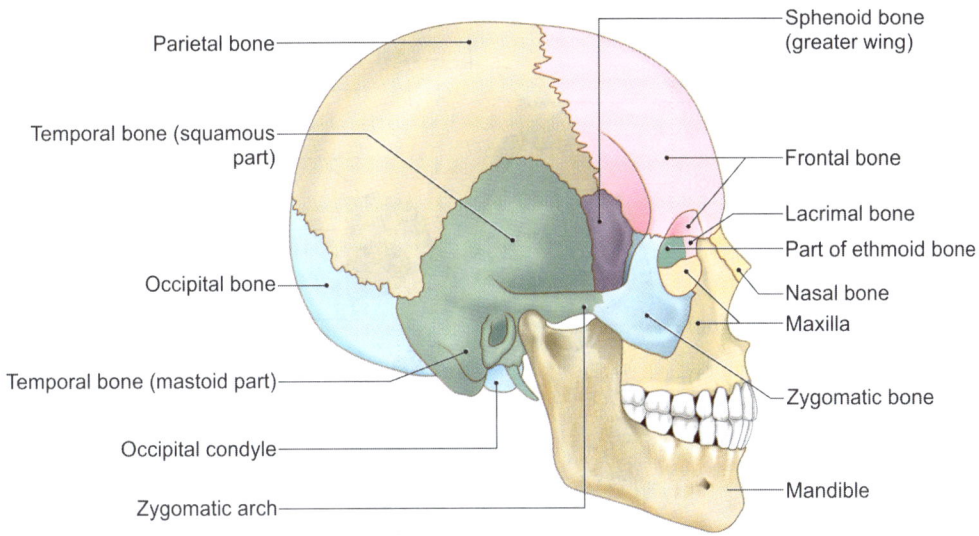

Fig. 7.3: Skull from the lateral side.

When the skull is viewed from below (*norma basalis*), bones identified are **(Fig. 7.4)**:
- Maxilla
- Sphenoid
- Temporal
- Occipital
- Parts of zygomatic
- Vomer
- Palatine.

The maxillae bear the upper teeth. Lateral to the teeth, the maxilla articulates with the zygomatic bone. Medial to the teeth, the maxilla forms the anterior part of the *bony palate*. The posterior part of the palate is formed by the right and left palatine bones. Above the posterior edge of the palate, the posterior openings of the right and left nasal cavities are seen; separated by the vomer. Part of the vomer is seen on the front of the skull through the anterior nasal aperture. Behind the vomer, the sphenoid presents the body. On either side of the body, the greater wing is noted. Posteriorly, the body of the sphenoid continues with the basilar part of the occipital bone. Just behind the basilar part, the occipital bone has a large *foramen magnum* through which the cranial cavity communicates with the vertebral canal. Posterior to the foramen magnum, the occipital bone forms significant part of the base of the skull.

The lateral part of the base of the skull is formed by the temporal bone (wedged between sphenoid and occipital bones). It consists of medial petrous part, posterolateral mastoid part and the anterolateral squamous part.

Temporal bone gives off zygomatic process that joins the zygomatic bone to form the *zygomatic arch*.

Skull: Functions

The primary function is to protect the brain. Parts of the skull most exposed to external violence are thicker than those which are shielded by overlying muscles. Thus, the skull cap is thick and

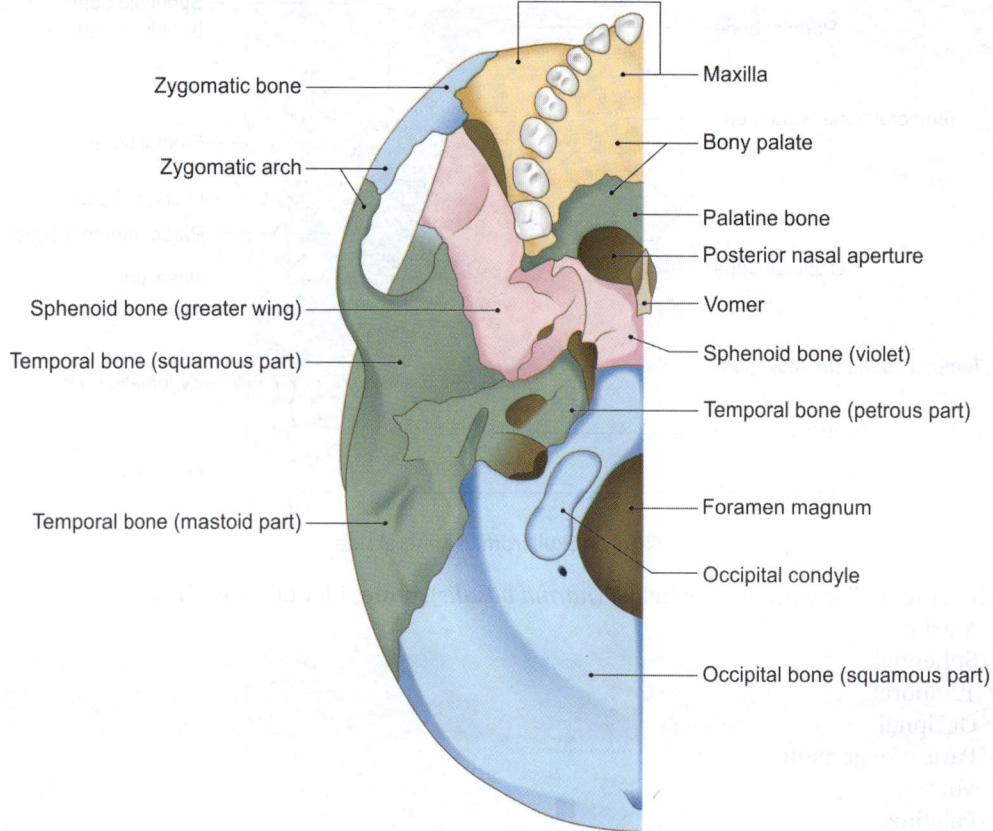

Fig. 7.4: Skull from below.

dense; squamous temporal are protected by temporalis muscles, and thin and fragile inferior part of occipital bone is shielded by the muscles at the back of the neck. Skull fracture is further prevented by its elasticity and its rounded shape.

AN 26.3 Describe cranial cavity, its subdivisions, foramina and structures passing through them.

Cranial Fossae

When the skull cap (*calvaria*) is removed, the floor of the cranial cavity is noted. It is divided into three depressions called the anterior, middle, and posterior cranial fossae **(Fig. 7.5)**.

Anterior cranial fossa: The floor of the anterior cranial fossa is formed mainly by the frontal bone; anteriorly near the midline a small part is formed by the ethmoid. Posteriorly, the median part of the floor is formed by the body of the sphenoid; and the lateral parts by the lesser wings of sphenoid. The floor has a sharp posterior margin that separates it from the middle cranial fossa. The medial part of the margin is formed by the lesser wing of sphenoid and its lateral part by the frontal bone.

Middle cranial fossa: The floor of middle cranial fossa is narrow (anteroposteriorly) in its median part and broad laterally. The narrow median part is formed by the body of the sphenoid.

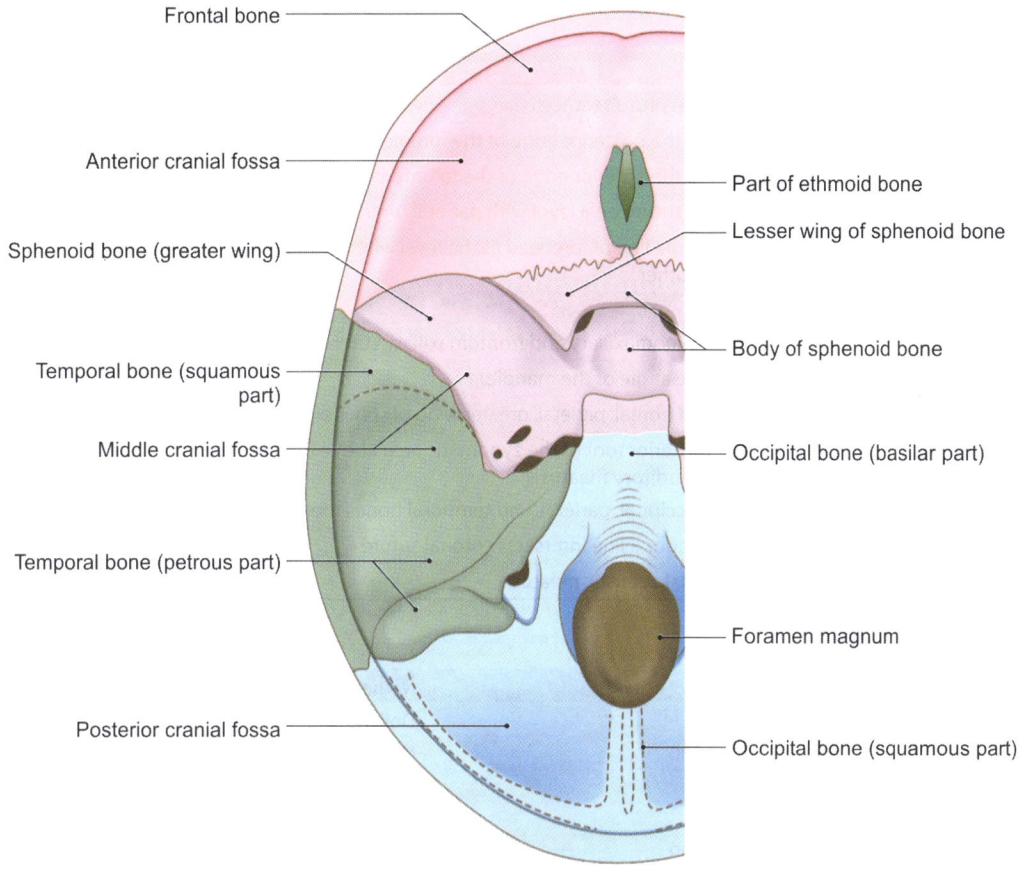

Fig. 7.5: Floor of the cranial cavity.

The broad lateral part is formed by the greater wing of the sphenoid, the squamous temporal, and the anterior surface of the petrous temporal bone.

Posterior cranial fossa: The greater part of the floor of the posterior cranial fossa is formed by the occipital bone. The foramen magnum is seen. The anterolateral part of the floor is formed by the posterior surface of the petrous temporal bone.

Cranial Points

In the midline	
Gnathion	Point of the chin
Prosthion	Lowest point on the upper jaw between the central incisors
Acanthion	Anterior nasal spine
Nasion	Junction of frontal and nasal bones
Glabella	Midpoint at the level of superciliary arches
Bregma	Junction of coronal and sagittal sutures
Lambda	Junction of coronal and lambdoid sutures
Opisthocranion	Most posteriorly projecting point on the occipital bone

(Contd...)

(Contd...)

In the midline	
Inion	External occipital protuberance
Opisthion	Central point of the posterior edge of the foramen magnum
Basion	Central point of the anterior edge of the foramen magnum
Obelion	Point in sagittal suture on a level with parietal foramina
Ophryon	Point in the middle line of forehead at the level where temporal lines most nearly approach each other
At the side of the skull	
Dacryon	Junction of lacrimomaxillary and frontomaxillary sutures
Gonion	Outer side of the angle of the mandible
Pterion	Meeting point of frontal, parietal, greater wing of sphenoid, and squamous temporal bones
Porion	Point on the posterior root of the zygomatic arch above the middle of the upper border of the external auditory meatus
Asterion	Region where occipital, parietal, and temporal bones meet
Stephanion	Point where temporal line intersects coronal suture
Auricular point	Center of external acoustic meatus

Skull: Classification

Index	Classification	Nomenclature
Cephalic	Below 75	Dolichocephalic
	Between 75 and 80	Mesaticephalic
	Above 80	Brachycephalic
Orbital	Below 84	Microseme
	Between 84 and 89	Mesoseme
	Above 89	Megaseme
Nasal	Below 48	Leptorrhine
	Between 48 and 53	Mesorrhine
	Above 53	Platyrrhine
Gnathic	Below 98	Orthognathous
	Between 98 and 103	Mesognathous
	Above 103	Prognathous

Skull: Measurements

❖ *Length*: It is measured from glabella to occipital point, while *breadth* or greatest transverse diameter is found near external acoustic meatus.
   Proportion of breadth to length (breadth × 100)/length is called *cephalic index*.
❖ *Height*: It is measured from basion to bregma.
   Proportion of height to length (height × 100)/length is called *vertical (height) index*.
❖ *Length of face*: It is measured from nasion to chin; its *width* is the distance between the zygomatic arches.

By comparing facial length with width; skulls are divided into two groups:
❖ *Dolichofacial*: Long faced
❖ *Brachyfacial*: Short faced.

Skull: Ossification

Development and ossification of the skull is complex.

Relevant features: Skull develops from mesenchyme surrounding the developing brain. The mesoderm of the occipital myotomes, otic capsule, nasal capsule, and the first branchial arch also contributes to the formation of the skull.

The mesenchyme shows condensations in the regions where the skull bones develop. A number of chondrification centers appear in relation to the base of the skull. The cartilages formed do not correspond to individual bones. The base of the skull is formed by ossification in relation to these cartilages.

The mesenchyme that is to form the sides and vault of the skull, and also the facial skeleton is not chondrified, but converted into bone by *intramembranous ossification*. Thus, some skull bones are formed in membrane, some in cartilage, and some in both.

- *Bones formed in membrane*: Frontal, parietal, zygomatic, palatine, nasal, lacrimal, maxilla, and vomer.
- *Bones formed in cartilage*: Ethmoid and inferior nasal concha.
- *Bones formed in cartilage and membrane*: Occipital, sphenoid, temporal, and mandible.

Time at which skull bones begin to ossify is variable. Ossification centers appear in many bones in 7th or 8th prenatal week; but in some ossification begin after birth. Number of ossification centers is variable.

- *Bones developing from one center*: Zygomatic, palatine, lacrimal, nasal, vomer, and inferior nasal concha.
- *Parietal bone* ossifies from two centers that appear in the region of the future tuberosity.
- *Frontal bone* has two centers on each side. At birth, the bone is in two halves; two halves occasionally remain separate and united by a midline suture—*metopic suture*.
- *Ethmoid bone* has three ossification centers one for perpendicular plate and one for each labyrinth.
- *Maxilla* has one main center, but additional centers appear in its anterior part.
- *Occipital bone* ossifies from several centers. In newborn, bone consists of separate squamous, condylar and basilar parts that are united by cartilage. These parts fuse with each another by sixth year. The basilar part fuses with the corresponding part of the sphenoid between 18 years and 25 years.
- *Sphenoid bone* ossifies from several centers. At birth, the bone is in three parts. The central part consists of the body and lesser wings; each lateral part consists of greater wing and pterygoid process. The parts unite during the first year of life. The sphenoid body fuses with the basilar part of occipital bone between 18 years and 25 years.
- *Temporal bone* ossifies from several centers. The squamous, tympanic, and styloid parts ossify independently. Petrous and mastoid parts constitute *petromastoid element* that has several ossification centers. The squamous part ossifies first.

Clinical Anatomy

Fracture of orbital plate of frontal bone: It causes trickling of blood under conjunctiva—*subconjunctival hemorrhage* (**Fig. 7.6**). Other fractures in the anterior cranial fossa may present with bleeding into nose or mouth. Tearing of meninges leads to cerebrospinal fluid (CSF) leakage from the nose. Meningitis may result due to communication with the exterior through the nasal cavity.

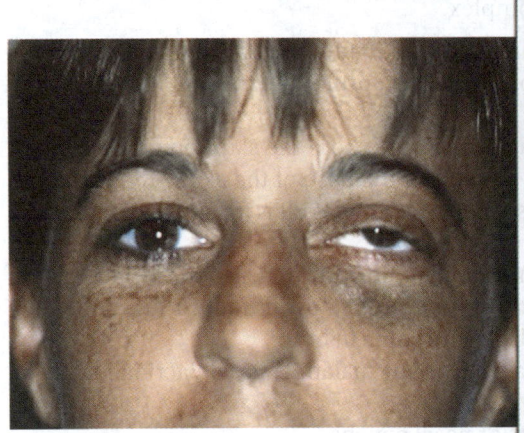
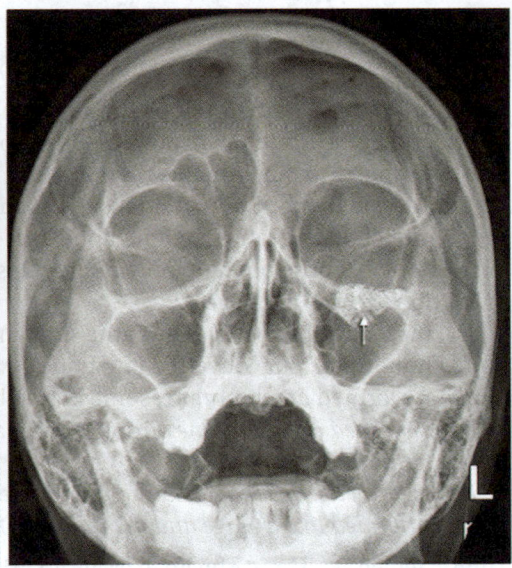

Fig. 7.6: Fracture orbital plate with subconjunctival hemorrhage.

Foramen cecum: When patent, it transmits a vein from nasal mucosa to superior sagittal sinus. It is a potential site for transmission of infection from nasal cavity to the cranium.

Fracture of middle cranial fossa: It is characterized by bleeding and CSF leakage from ear, bleeding into mouth and involvement of abducens nerve (*squint and diplopia*). Facial nerve may be involved.

Fracture of posterior cranial fossa: It can cause extravasation of blood in the suboccipital region. Ninth, tenth and eleventh cranial nerves may get injured in the jugular foramen.

SKULL FROM ABOVE (NORMA VERTICALIS)

The meeting point of the coronal and sagittal sutures is the *bregma*. The sagittal suture meets the lambdoid suture at the *lambda*. In the fetal skull (and few months after birth), there are gaps in the skull bones at these points; filled by membranes. These gaps are the *anterior and posterior fontanels*. The parietal bone posterolaterally is more convex; called the parietal tuber (eminence). Near the posterior part of the sagittal suture, each parietal bone presents a parietal foramen (may be absent) for the parietal emissary vein. The temporal lines are seen on the lateral parts of the parietal and frontal bones **(Fig. 7.7)**.

Clinical Anatomy

Emissary Veins

These connect intracranial dural venous sinuses to subcutaneous veins of scalp **(Fig. 7.8)**. These are valveless and blood can flow in either direction. Infection of scalp can spread via these veins to cause:
❖ Meningitis
❖ Dural venous sinus thrombosis.

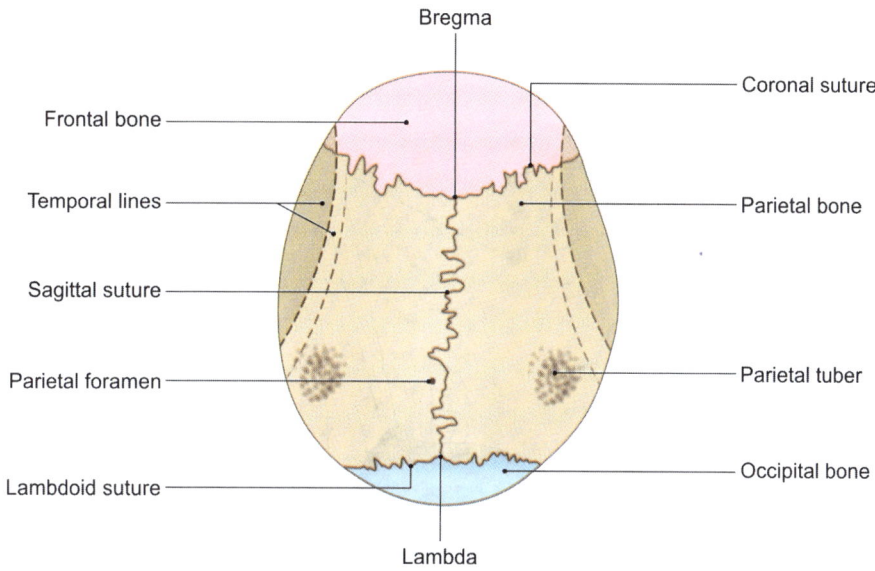

Fig. 7.7: Skull viewed from above.

Safety Valve Hematoma

The fracture of vault may tear dura and pericranium. This results in collection of intracranial hemorrhage in subaponeurotic layer of skull through fracture line. No signs of brain compression develop until subaponeurotic space is filled with blood. After this signs of cerebral compression develop rapidly. This collection of blood is termed safety valve hematoma.

SKULL FROM THE FRONT (NORMA FRONTALIS)

When the skull is viewed from the front, the bones seen have been identified; the orbits and the anterior nasal aperture have been noted. We shall now consider further details (**Fig. 7.9**).

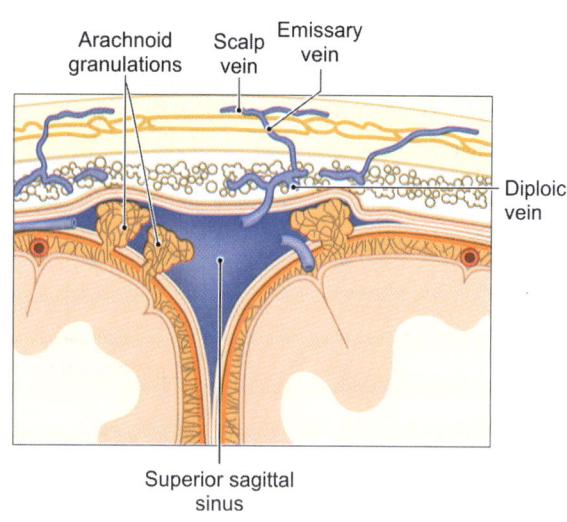

Fig. 7.8: Emissary vein.

Articulations: Lateral to the orbit, the frontal bone gives off zygomatic process which joins the frontal process of the zygomatic bone at the *frontozygomatic suture*. The nasal part of the frontal bone projects downward. On either side of the midline, it joins the frontal process of the maxilla at the *frontomaxillary suture* and the nasal bone at the *frontonasal suture*. Two nasal bones join at the *internasal suture* and the frontal process of the maxilla at the *nasomaxillary suture*. Below the nasal aperture, the right and left maxillae meet at the *intermaxillary suture*. Laterally, the zygomatic process of maxilla articulates with the maxillary process of the zygomatic bone at the *zygomaticomaxillary suture*.

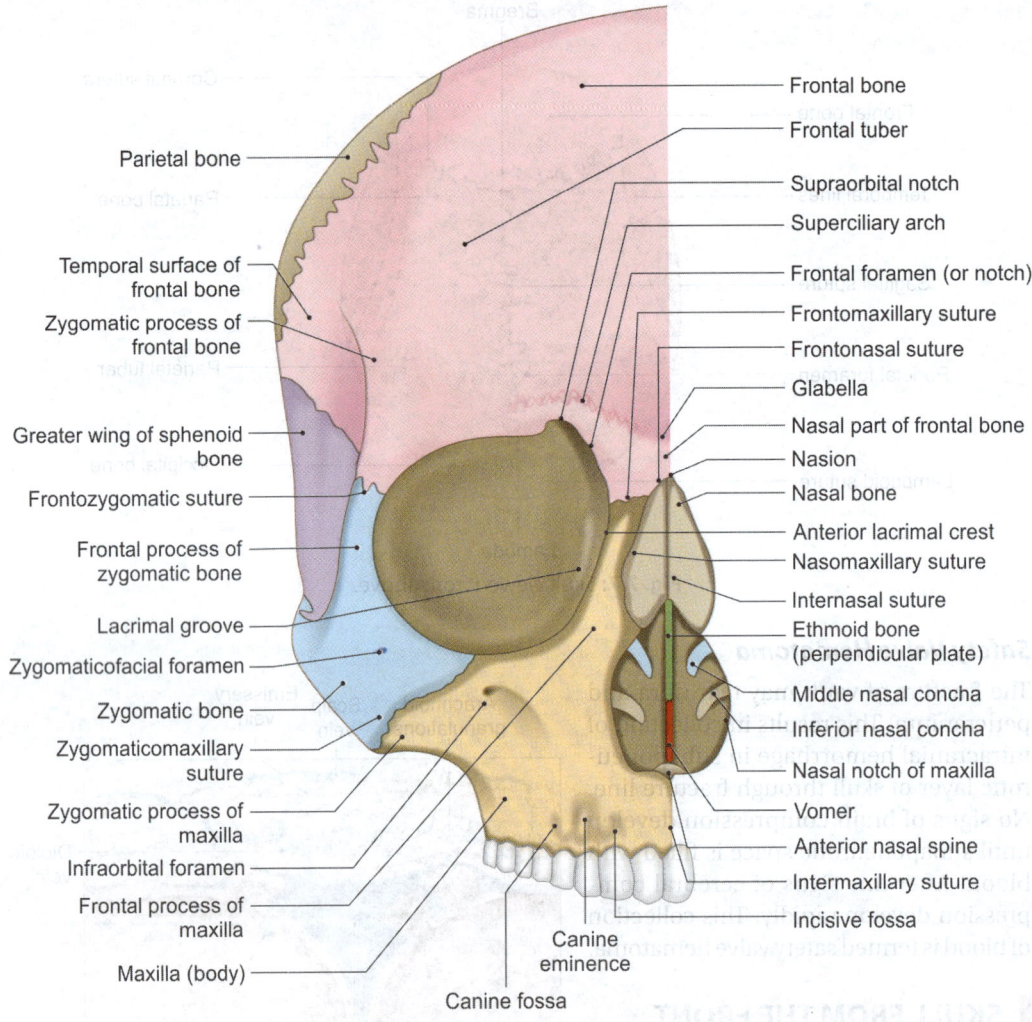

Fig. 7.9: Skull from the front.

Other Features

Frontal Bone

The external surface of the frontal bone about 3 cm above the orbit is the *frontal eminence* (frontal tuber). Just above the medial part of the orbit a raised ridge called the *superciliary arch* is noted. The two arches meet in the midline at the *glabella*. The meeting point of the frontonasal and internasal sutures is the *nasion*. When traced upward, the zygomatic process of the frontal bone runs as a ridge which continues posteriorly with the temporal lines. The ridge separates the external surface of the frontal bone from the temporal surface.

Maxilla

The frontal process is marked by a sharp vertical ridge called the *anterior lacrimal crest*; forms part of the medial orbital margin. The part of the frontal process behind the crest forms the lacrimal groove. In the lower part of the nasal aperture, the maxillae show a sharp forward projection called the *anterior nasal spine*. The maxilla presents sockets (*alveolar process*) for the eight teeth. From the midline, there are two incisors, one canine, two premolars, and three molars. Just above the canine tooth the maxilla shows a vertical elevation produced by the root of this tooth called the *canine eminence*. Medial to this eminence and above the incisor teeth, there is a depression—the *incisive fossa* and laterally, there is another depression called the *canine fossa*.

Foramina

At the junction of medial one-third and lateral two-thirds of the upper orbital margin, the supraorbital notch is noted (may be converted into a foramen). Medial to it a smaller frontal notch (or foramen) is seen. On the lateral surface of the zygomatic bone, the *zygomaticofacial foramen* is noted (sometimes double). About one centimeter below the inferior margin of the orbit *infraorbital foramen* is seen.

Anterior Nasal Aperture

It is a pear-shaped opening. On either side, its margin is formed mainly by the nasal notch of the maxilla. Its upper part is bounded by the lower borders of the nasal bones. In the depth of aperture, the nasal septum separates the right and left nasal cavities. Its upper part is formed by the perpendicular plate of ethmoid and lower part by the vomer.

Lateral to the septum, two curved bony plates project into nasal cavity from the lateral side. These are the *middle* and *inferior nasal conchae*. The middle concha is a part of the ethmoid bone; inferior concha is an independent bone attached to the maxilla.

Some features mentioned above can be visualized better in a coronal section through the nasal cavity and the orbit. Note the orientation of the ethmoid bone in relation to these cavities and to the floor of the anterior cranial fossa (**Fig. 7.10**).

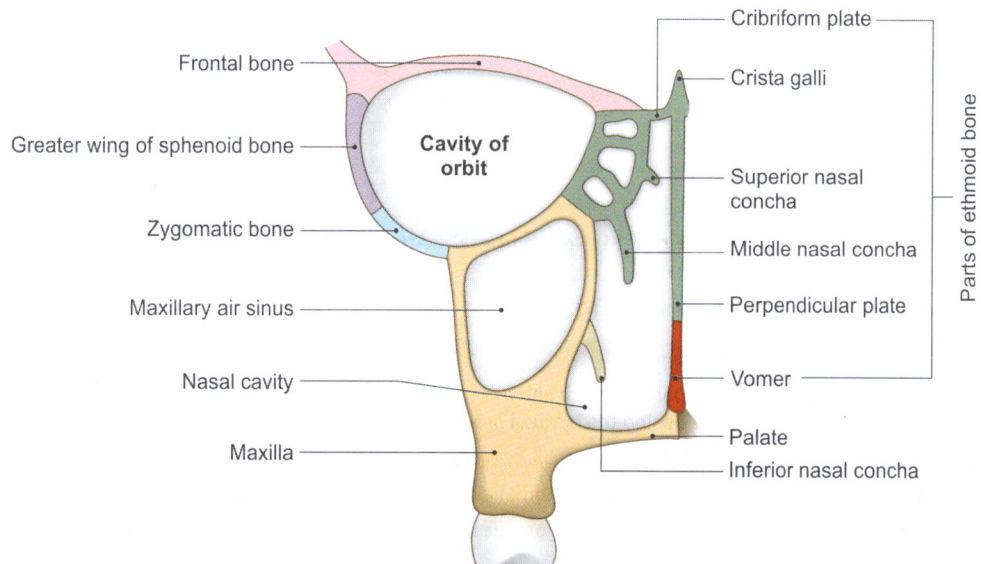

Fig. 7.10: Coronal section through the orbit and nasal cavity to show the bones related.

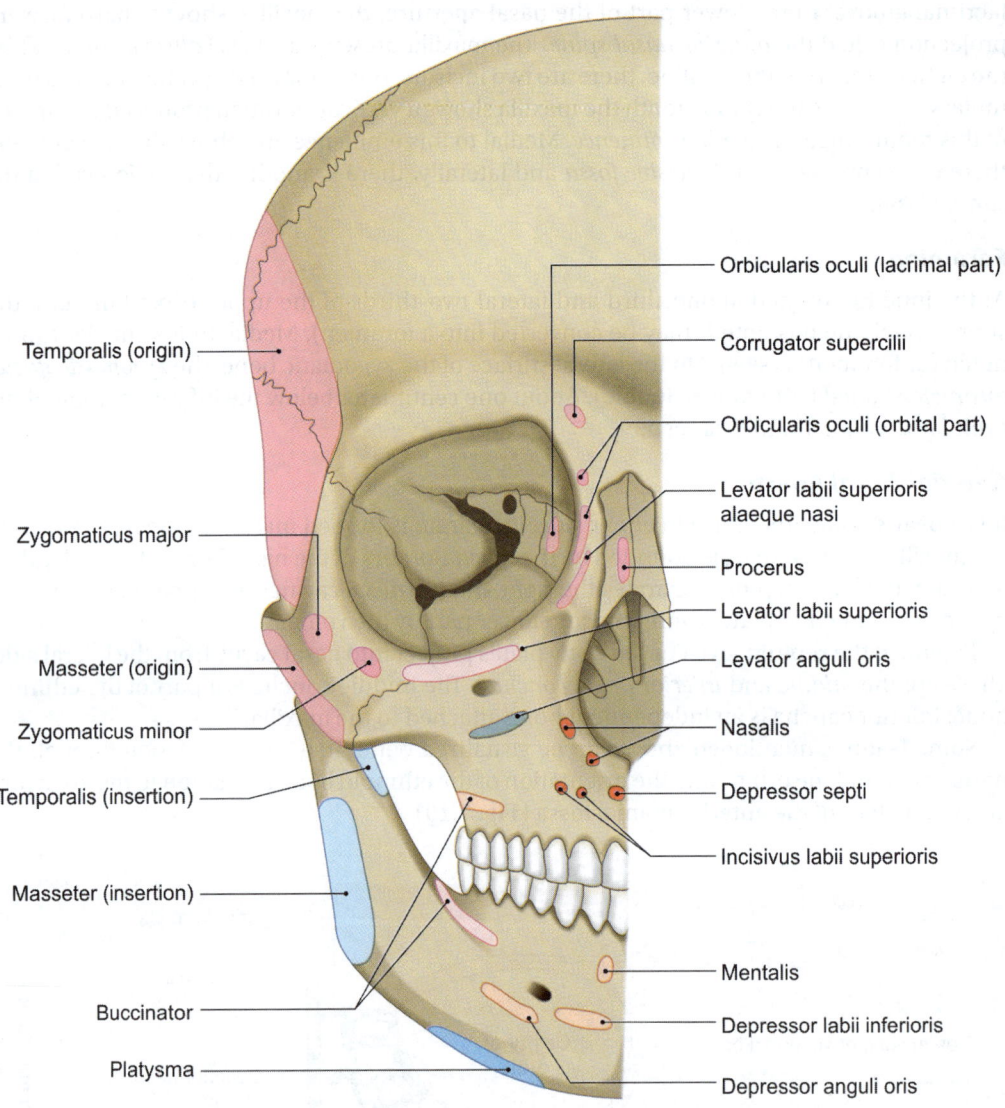

Fig. 7.11: Norma frontalis: Attachments.

Norma Frontalis: Attachments (Fig. 7.11)

Muscle	Attachment
Orbicularis oculi (*orbital part*)	Nasal part of frontal and frontal process of maxilla; *lacrimal part* from the lacrimal bone behind the lacrimal groove
Corrugator supercilii	Medial end of superciliary arch
Zygomaticus major	Lateral surface of zygomatic bone in front of zygomaticotemporal suture
Zygomaticus minor	Lateral surface of zygomatic bone behind zygomaticomaxillary suture

(Contd...)

(Contd...)

Muscle	Attachment
Levator labii superioris	Lower margin of orbit: Partly from maxilla, partly from zygomatic bone
Levator anguli oris	Canine fossa of maxilla below infraorbital foramen
Levator labii superioris alaeque nasi	Frontal process of maxilla
Procerus	Lower part of nasal bone
Nasalis	*Transverse part*: Maxilla just lateral to nasal notch *Alar part*: Maxilla below and medial to transverse part
Depressor septi	Maxilla just above central incisor tooth
Incisivus labii superioris	Maxilla above lateral incisor tooth

BONY ORBIT

Orbital Margins

It is formed by bones as under:
- *Upper margin*: Frontal bone
- *Lateral margin*: Mainly by zygomatic; upper part by zygomatic process of frontal
- *Inferior margin*: Zygomatic bone (lateral part) and maxilla (medial part)
- *Medial margin*: Mainly by frontal process of maxilla; upper part by nasal part of frontal bone.

Structures Attached to Whitnall Tubercle

- Check ligament of lateral rectus
- Lateral end of LPS aponeurosis
- Suspensory ligament of Lockwood
- Lateral end of superior and inferior tarsus.

Orbital Walls

The orbit is pyramid shaped. The orbital opening represents the base with the apex at the posterior end. The orbit presents roof, floor, medial, and lateral walls **(Fig. 7.12)**.
- *Roof* is formed mainly by the orbital plate of frontal bone. Posteriorly, it is completed by the lesser wing of sphenoid. The anterolateral part of the roof has a depression called the *lacrimal fossa*. Close to the orbital margin, at the junction of the roof and medial wall, there is a small depression called the *trochlear fossa*.
- *Floor* is mainly formed by the orbital surface of maxilla. The anterolateral part of the floor is formed by the zygomatic bone. Posteromedially, a small part is formed by the palatine bone (orbital process).
- *Lateral* wall is formed by the zygomatic bone anteriorly and completed by the greater wing of sphenoid posteriorly.
- *Medial* wall is formed mainly by the orbital plate of ethmoid. Posterior to ethmoid, a small part is formed by the body of the sphenoid. Anterior to ethmoid, the wall is formed by the lacrimal bone, and still anteriorly by the frontal process of maxilla. The maxilla shows a deep lacrimal groove (*for lacrimal sac*). The groove is bounded by:
  - *Anteriorly*: Anterior lacrimal crest of the frontal process of maxilla
  - *Posteriorly*: Crest of the lacrimal bone.

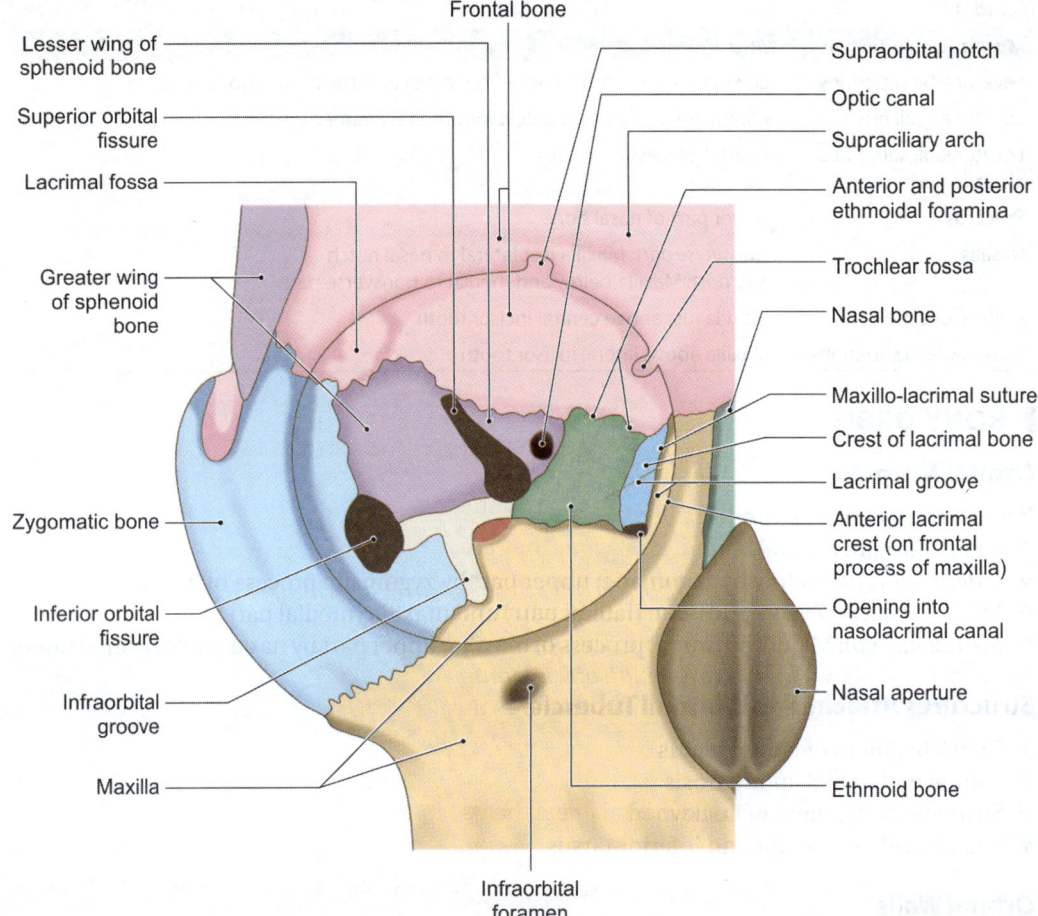

Fig. 7.12: Orbit and surrounding structures.

Orbit: Apertures

Superior orbital fissure: It separates roof and lateral wall posteriorly. It is bounded by (**Fig. 7.13**):
- *Above and medially*: Lesser wing of sphenoid
- *Below and laterally*: Greater wing of sphenoid.

Inferior orbital fissure: It is seen between the floor and lateral wall posteriorly. It is bounded by:
- *Above and laterally*: Greater wing of sphenoid
- *Below and medially*: Orbital surface of maxilla.

This fissure continues anteriorly with the infraorbital groove on the maxilla. Anteriorly, the groove ends in a canal which passes through the maxilla to open on the surface through the *infraorbital foramen*.

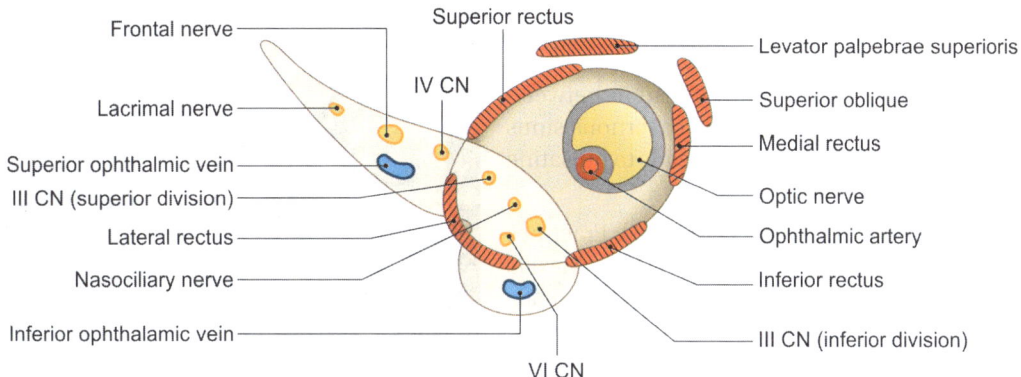

Fig. 7.13: Superior orbital fissure and optic canal: Structures passing.

Optic canal: It is at the junction of the medial wall and the roof posteriorly. It transmits optic nerve surrounded by three meninges and the ophthalmic artery.

Anterior and posterior ethmoidal foramina: They are at the junction of the roof and the medial wall on the suture separating the orbital plate of ethmoid from the frontal bone.

On the lateral wall, there are two small foramina on the orbital surface of the zygomatic bone: both open into canals within the bone. The other end of one canal opens on the external surface of the zygomatic bone as the *zygomaticofacial foramen*. The other end of second canal opens on the temporal surface of the zygomatic bone as the *zygomaticotemporal foramen*.

Orbital Index

It signifies proportion which the orbital height bears to the orbital width

$$\frac{\text{Orbital height}}{\text{Orbital width}} \times 100$$

Clinical Anatomy

Black eye: It is the blackish discoloration of the eyelids **(Fig. 7.14)**.

Direct black eye is due to local blow to the eye causing blackish discolorations of both eyelids simultaneously within 2 hours due to subcutaneous hemorrhage.

Indirect black eye is due to injury causing hemorrhage in subaponeurotic layer. The hemorrhage fills subaponeurotic space up to highest nuchal liner posteriorly; superior temporal line laterally and slowly gravitates

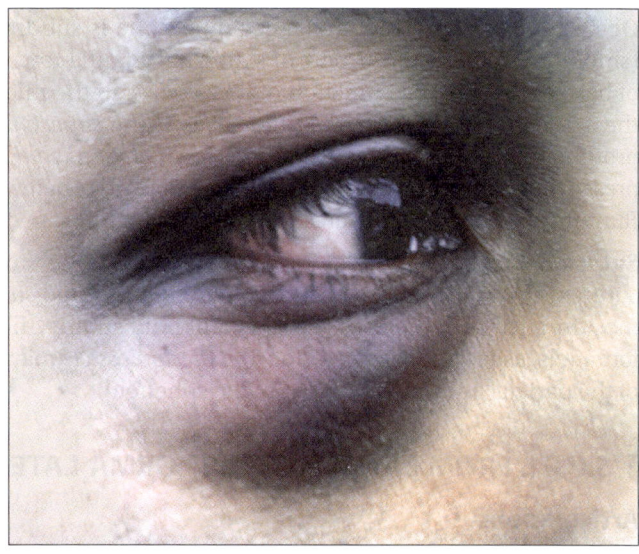

Fig. 7.14: Black eye.

under frontalis to upper eyelid followed by lower eyelid. This takes 1–2 days to appear.

Pulsating eyeball: A communication between the internal carotid artery and cavernous sinus (*carotid cavernous aneurysm*) leads to pulsating and bulging eyeball.

Fractures of facial bones (Fig. 7.15): Fractures of nasal bones are due to direct violence. Maxilla fractures are seen in road traffic injuries. Zygomatic arch may be fractured by violence to the side of skull. Fractures of mandible are most common fractures of facial bones; usually bilateral.

Compression of supraorbital nerve: This nerve emerges from the supraorbital foramen/ notch. Compression of nerve here causes considerable pain. This is used by anesthetists to determine depth of anesthesia/consciousness.

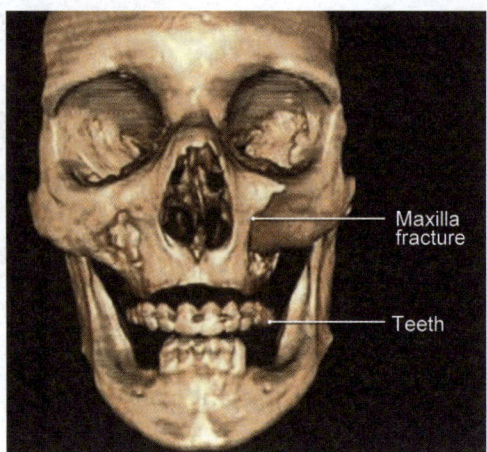

Fig. 7.15: Fracture of facial bones.

SKULL FROM BEHIND (NORMA OCCIPITALIS)

When skull is viewed from behind, the parietal tuber, the parietal foramina, the temporal lines, the sagittal suture, the lambdoid suture, and the lambda are noted.

Sutures: The outline of the lambdoid suture at times is complicated. Sometimes small bony pieces are surrounded by parts of the suture called the *sutural bones.* Below the lambdoid suture, the *occipitomastoid suture* unites the lower part of the lateral border of the occipital bone to the mastoid temporal bone. The *parietomastoid suture* joins the posterior part of the parietal bone to the mastoid temporal bone.

Occipital bone: The squamous occipital bone is subdivided into an upper triangular part (smooth: forms posterior part of skull vault) and a lower part (rough: forms posterior part of base of skull). At the junction of these parts, in the midline, a prominent projection called the *external occipital protuberance* is seen. The *superior nuchal lines* run laterally from the protuberance. A little above these lines the *highest nuchal lines* may be noted (faint, not always present). The *external occipital crest* is a median ridge below the external occipital protuberance. Running laterally from the crest, *inferior nuchal lines* are noted **(Fig. 7.16)**.

Sutural (Wormian) bones: Some ossification centers others may occur in relation to the sutures, giving rise to irregular, isolated bones, called *sutural (Wormian) bones.* They occur most frequently in the course of the lambdoid suture. These may be occasionally seen at the fontanels, especially the posterior. The *pterion ossicle* may exist between the sphenoidal angle of the parietal and the great wing of the sphenoid.

SKULL FROM LATERAL SIDE (NORMA LATERALIS)

Articulations

Frontal bone: The lower margin of the frontal bone articulates with several bones. It forms *frontonasal, frontomaxillary, frontolacrimal, frontoethmoid,* and *frontozygomatic* sutures.

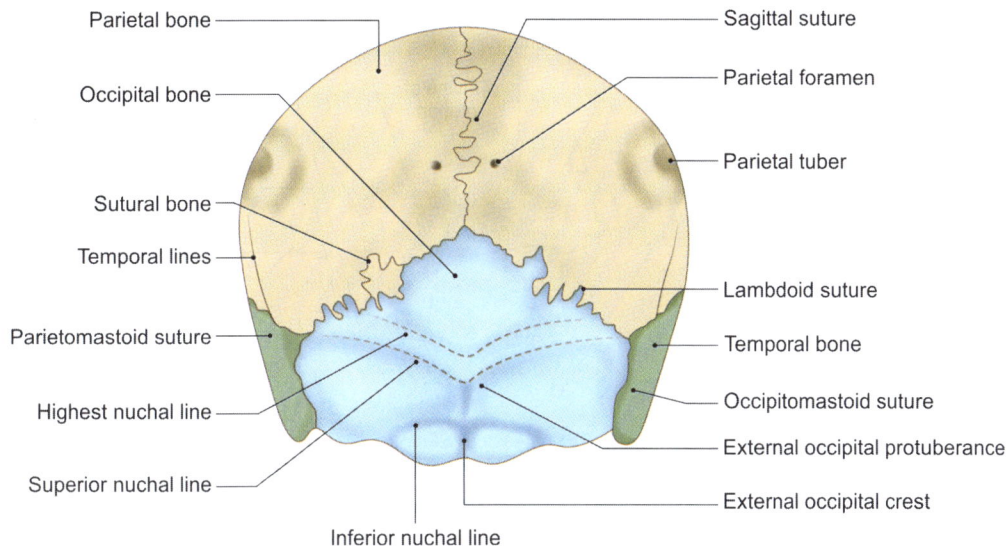

Fig. 7.16: Skull from behind.

Behind the frontozygomatic suture the frontal bone articulates with upper border of the greater wing of sphenoid at the *frontosphenoid* suture. The posterior end of this suture meets the coronal suture.

Parietal bone: Anterior end of the parietal bone meets the posterior border of the frontal bone at the *coronal suture*. The anteroinferior angle of parietal bone joins greater wing of sphenoid at the *parietosphenoid* suture. Further back, the inferior border articulates with the squamous and mastoid temporal bone at the *parietosquamous* and *parietomastoid* sutures **(Figs. 7.17 to 7.19)**.

The posterior border of the parietal bone joins occipital bone at the *lambdoid suture*. Each parietal bone articulates with opposite parietal bone at the *sagittal suture*. Near the anteroinferior angle of the parietal bone the sutures form H-shaped arrangement. Four bones, the parietal, frontal, sphenoid (greater wing) and temporal (squamous part) meet; meeting point is the pterion. The center of pterion lies 4 cm above the zygomatic arch and 3.5 cm behind the frontozygomatic suture.

Zygomatic bone: Frontal process of zygomatic bone joins frontal bone and its maxillary process articulates with the maxilla. Its temporal process runs backward and joins zygomatic process of the temporal bone to form the *zygomatic arch*. Posteriorly, frontal process of the zygomatic bone articulates with the anterior margin of the greater wing of sphenoid.

Temporal bone: It articulates with the parietal bone above, in front with greater wing of sphenoid, and with zygomatic bone (by zygomatic process), and behind with the occipital bone (through mastoid part). Inferiorly, it shows mandibular fossa that articulates with the head of the mandible to form the temporomandibular joint.

Occipital bone: It articulates with two parietal bones at the *lambdoid suture*. Lower down, it articulates with the mastoid temporal bone.

Maxilla: Posterior border of the maxilla joins *pterygoid process* of the sphenoid bone and the *pyramidal process* of the palatine bone.

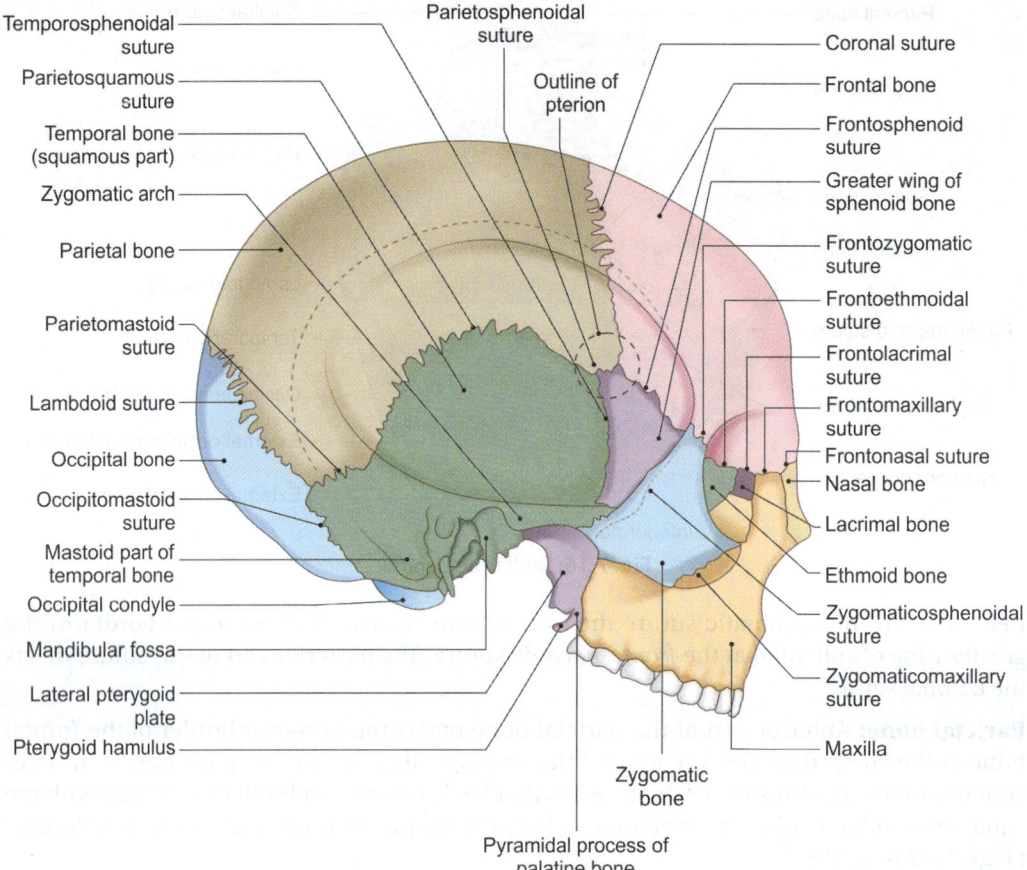

Fig. 7.17: Sutures on the lateral aspect of the skull.

Foramina

- *Zygomaticotemporal foramen*: On the temporal surface of zygomatic bone
- *Mastoid foramen*: On or near occipitomastoid suture.

Other Features

The lateral side of the skull vault is marked by a prominent curved ridge called the *temporal line*. This line starts anteriorly as a continuation of the sharp lateral edge of the zygomatic process of the frontal bone. It curves backward as it crosses the coronal suture. It then runs backward across the parietal bone. Anteriorly a single ridge is seen but posteriorly two lines are made out (superior and inferior).

Superior temporal line fades away on the posteroinferior part of the parietal bone.

Inferior temporal line curves forward on to the temporal bone to continue with a ridge called the *supramastoid crest*.

Supramastoid crest separates squamous and mastoid parts of the temporal bone and continues anteriorly with the posterior root of the zygomatic process. Just below this root the *external acoustic meatus* is seen.

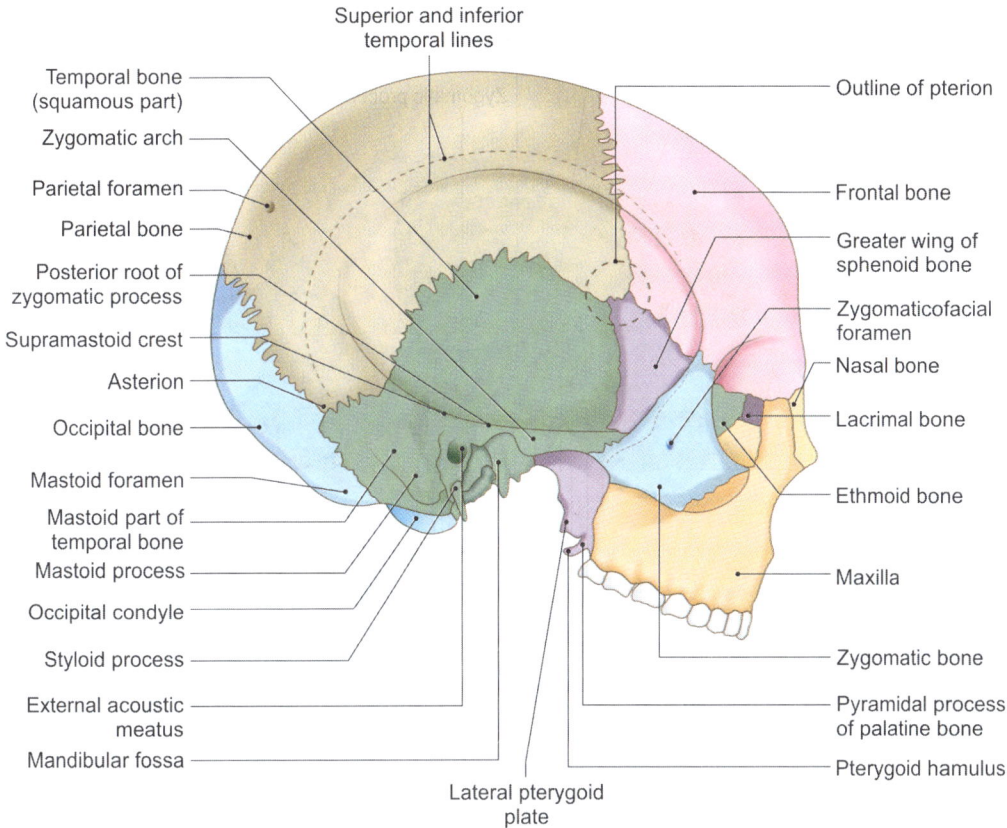

Fig. 7.18: Skull from lateral side.

Temporal Fossa

The region between the temporal lines (above) and the zygomatic arch (below) is the temporal fossa. In its floor bones seen are:
❖ Parts of frontal and parietal
❖ Squamous temporal
❖ Greater wing of sphenoid.

The anterior wall of the fossa is formed mainly by the temporal surface of the zygomatic bone. It also receives contributions from the greater wing of sphenoid and the frontal bone.

The mastoid temporal bone in the young is separated from the squamous part by the *squamomastoid suture*. The mastoid part articulates with the parietal bone at the *parietomastoid suture* and with the occipital bone at the *occipitomastoid suture*. The point at which these two sutures meet is the *asterion*. Just behind the external acoustic meatus the mastoid part shows a large downward projection—the *mastoid process* (*mastoid = like breast*). The styloid process (*styloid = needle like*) projects downward and forward from the inferior aspect of the bone.

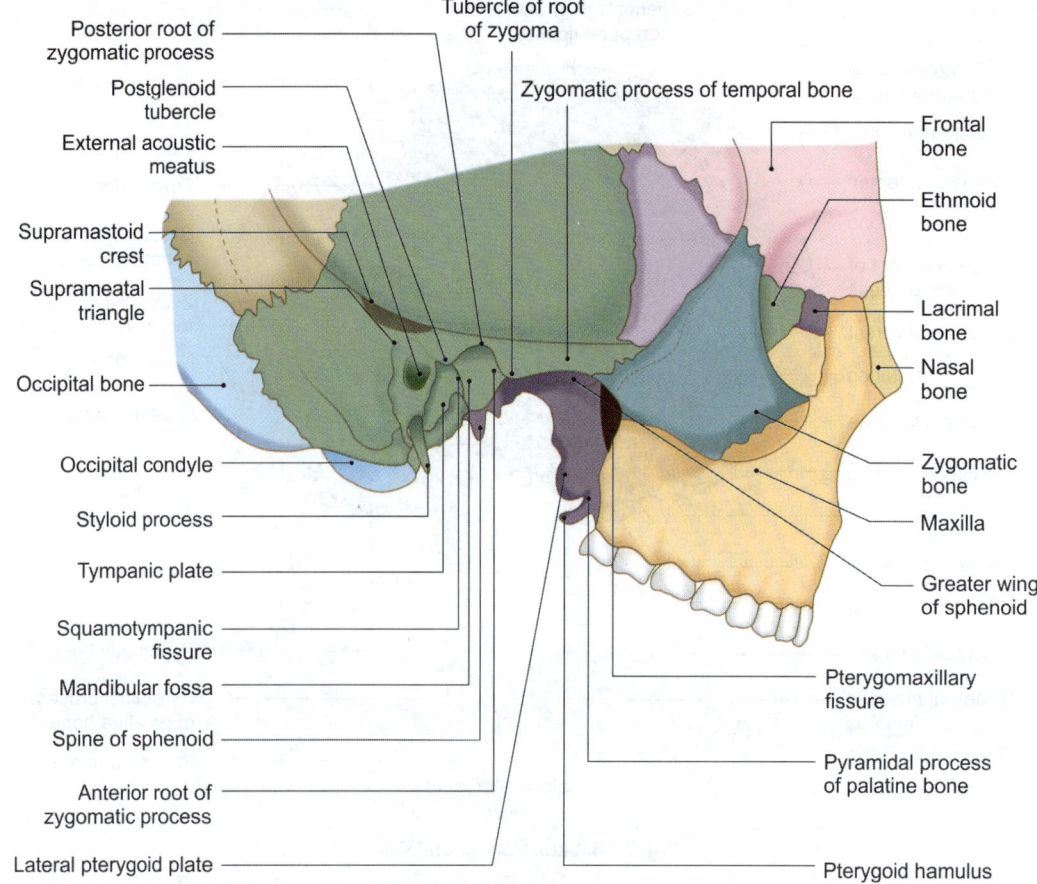

Fig. 7.19: Norma lateralis: Features.

Zygomatic Arch Region: Features

Formation of zygomatic arch is as under:
* *Anterior part*: Temporal process of zygomatic bone
* *Posterior part*: Zygomatic process of temporal bone.

At its posterior end, zygomatic process of temporal bone divides into anterior and posterior roots:
* Posterior root passes backward along the lateral margin of mandibular fossa, then above the external acoustic meatus to continue with supramastoid crest
* Anterior root passes medially in front of the mandibular fossa.

Two projections are noted in relation to the roots of the zygomatic process. At the junction of the anterior root with the process (in front of mandibular fossa), there is the tubercle of the root of zygoma. Other projection behind the mandibular fossa is the *postglenoid tubercle*.

Bone around the opening of the external acoustic meatus is rough; gives attachment to the cartilaginous part of the meatus.

Tympanic plate forms the anterior margin, inferior margin, and the lower part of posterior margin of the meatus. Posteriorly, the tympanic part joins the mastoid part of the bone. The tympanic plate has a broad anterior surface which lies behind the mandibular fossa (formed by squamous temporal); two being separated by the *squamotympanic fissure*.

Just above and behind the external acoustic meatus, there is an area called the *suprameatal triangle*. Its boundaries are:
❖ *Upper border:* Supramastoid crest
❖ *Anteroinferior border:* Posterosuperior part of external acoustic meatus
❖ *Posterior border:* Imaginary vertical line touching posterior margin of the meatus.

Importance of triangle: Mastoid antrum (important cavity) lies deep to it in the petrous temporal bone.

Some features are obscured from view by the zygomatic arch are seen when the arch is cut away. The temporal surface of the greater wing of sphenoid is seen in the floor of temporal fossa. Inferiorly, this surface ends in a sharp ridge called the *infratemporal crest*. Medial to the crest, the infratemporal surface of the greater wing is seen **(Fig. 7.20)**.

Further medially, the pterygoid process (of sphenoid) is seen. It projects downward from the junction of the body and the greater wing. It consists of medial and lateral pterygoid plates.

These are free posteriorly, but meet anteriorly to enclose the pterygoid fossa. Below and medial to the mandibular fossa, the *spine* of sphenoid is observed.

Infratemporal Fossa

It is the space lateral to the pterygoid process. It communicates with temporal fossa through the gap between zygomatic arch and the side of skull **(Fig. 7.21)**.

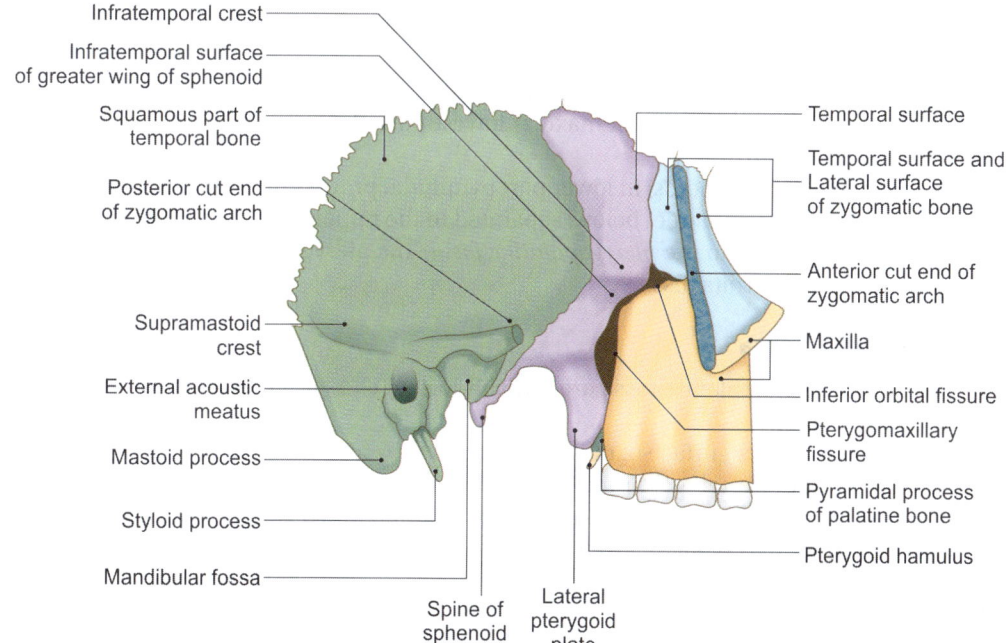

Fig. 7.20: Lateral aspect of the skull after removal of zygomatic arch.

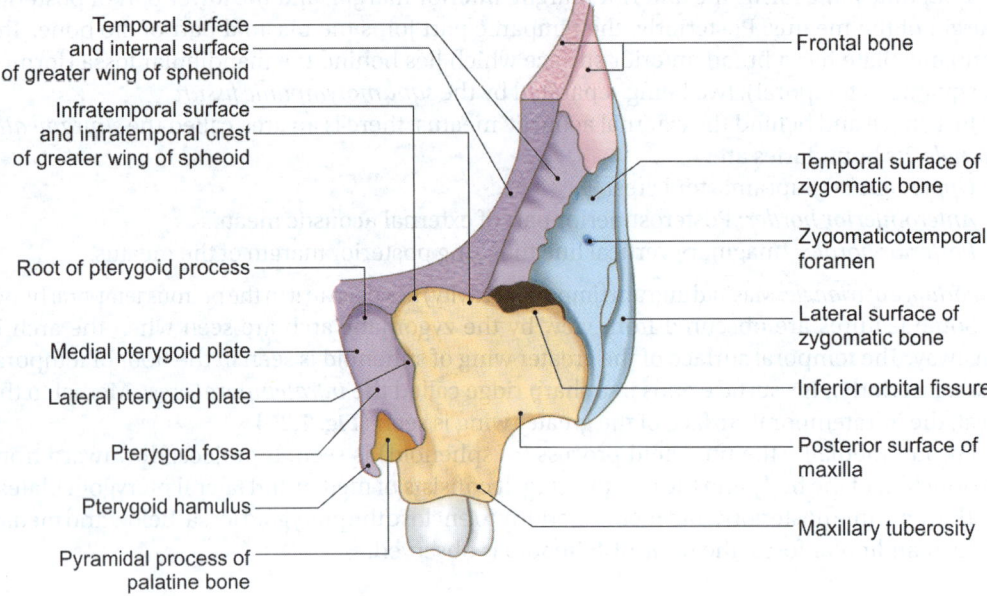

Fig. 7.21: Anterior wall of temporal and infratemporal fossae seen from behind (zygomatic process of temporal bone removed; coronal section cut through middle cranial fossa).

Formation

* *Roof*: Infratemporal surface of the greater wing of sphenoid and squamous temporal.
* *Anterior wall*: Posterior surface of maxilla; lowest part of this surface forms a projection called *maxillary tuberosity*.
* *Medial wall*: Pterygoid process; in lower part pyramidal process of the palatine bone.

Anterior and medial walls meet below; separated in the upper part by the *pterygomaxillary fissure*. This fissure leads into the *pterygopalatine fossa*. The pterygomaxillary fissure continues above with the inferior orbital fissure.

Pterygopalatine Fossa

The walls of the pterygopalatine fossa are difficult to see (shown schematically in **Fig. 7.22**). Walls and their formation:

* *Anterior wall*: Posterior surface of maxilla
* *Posterior wall*: Root of pterygoid process
* *Medial wall*: Mainly by perpendicular plate of palatine bone; separates fossa from nasal cavity. Uppermost part of medial wall is formed by body of sphenoid.

Communications

* *Laterally*: Opens into infratemporal fossa through pterygomaxillary fissure
* *Above*: Communicates with the orbit through inferior orbital fissure.

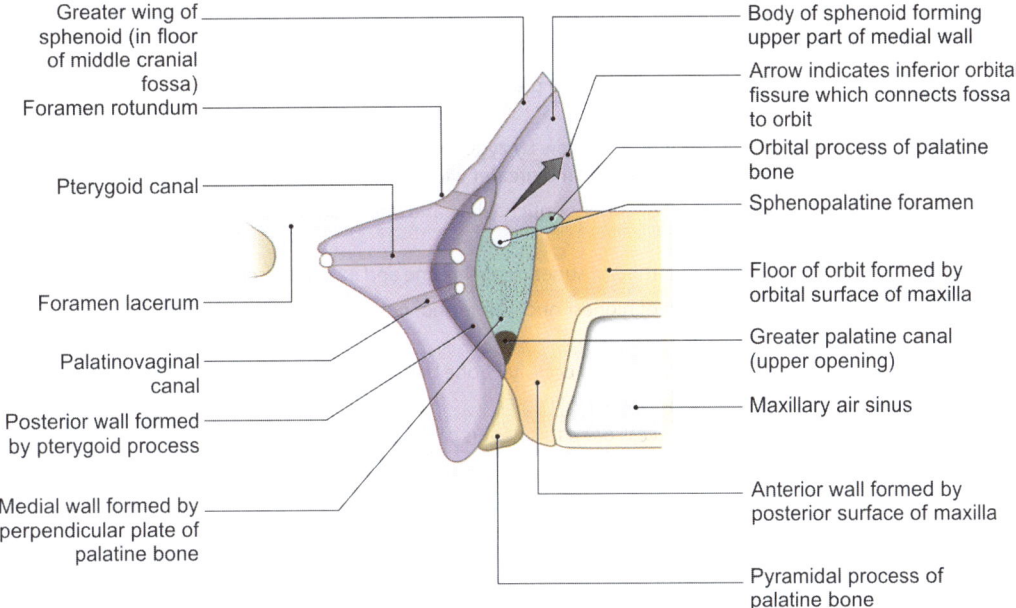

Fig. 7.22: Scheme to show the walls of the pterygopalatine fossa.

Openings

Posterior wall of the fossa presents three openings:
1. *Upper and largest*: Anterior end of foramen rotundum (other end opens into middle cranial fossa).
2. Below this is the opening of pterygoid canal (posterior end of canal opens on the anterior wall of foramen lacerum).
3. *Lower down on the posterior wall*: Opening of palatinovaginal canal.

Medial wall of the fossa shows *sphenopalatine foramen* through which the fossa communicates with the nasal cavity.

Inferiorly, the fossa is closed on the surface by meeting of the maxilla and the pterygoid process; but at a deeper plane, there is an opening in the floor of the fossa which leads into the greater palatine canal (opens inferiorly on the posterior part of the palate).

Norma Lateralis: Attachments (Fig. 7.23)

Muscle	Attachment
Masseter	Zygomatic arch (lower border and deep surface) (*origin*)
Buccinator	Lateral aspect of maxilla (above three molar teeth); also from mandible (*origin*)
Lateral pterygoid	Lower head: Lateral surface of lateral pterygoid plate Upper head: Infratemporal surface and crest of greater wing of the sphenoid (*origin*)
Medial pterygoid (superficial head)	Lateral aspect of pyramidal process of palatine bone and maxillary tuberosity (*origin*)

(Contd...)

(Contd...)

Muscle	Attachment
Medial pterygoid (deep head)	Medial surface of lateral pterygoid plate (*origin*)
Temporalis	Temporal line and below by zygomatic arch; includes parts of frontal, parietal, squamous temporal and greater wing of sphenoid (*origin*)
Sternocleidomastoid	Lateral half of superior nuchal line and lateral surface of mastoid process (*insertion*)
Trapezius	Medial one-third of superior nuchal line and external occipital protuberance
Occipitalis (occipital belly of occipitofrontalis)	Lateral part of highest nuchal line and mastoid process (*origin*)
Splenius capitis	Mastoid process and occipital bone below lateral one-third of superior nuchal line (deep to SCM) (*insertion*)
Longissimus capitis	Mastoid process deep to splenius capitis (*insertion*)

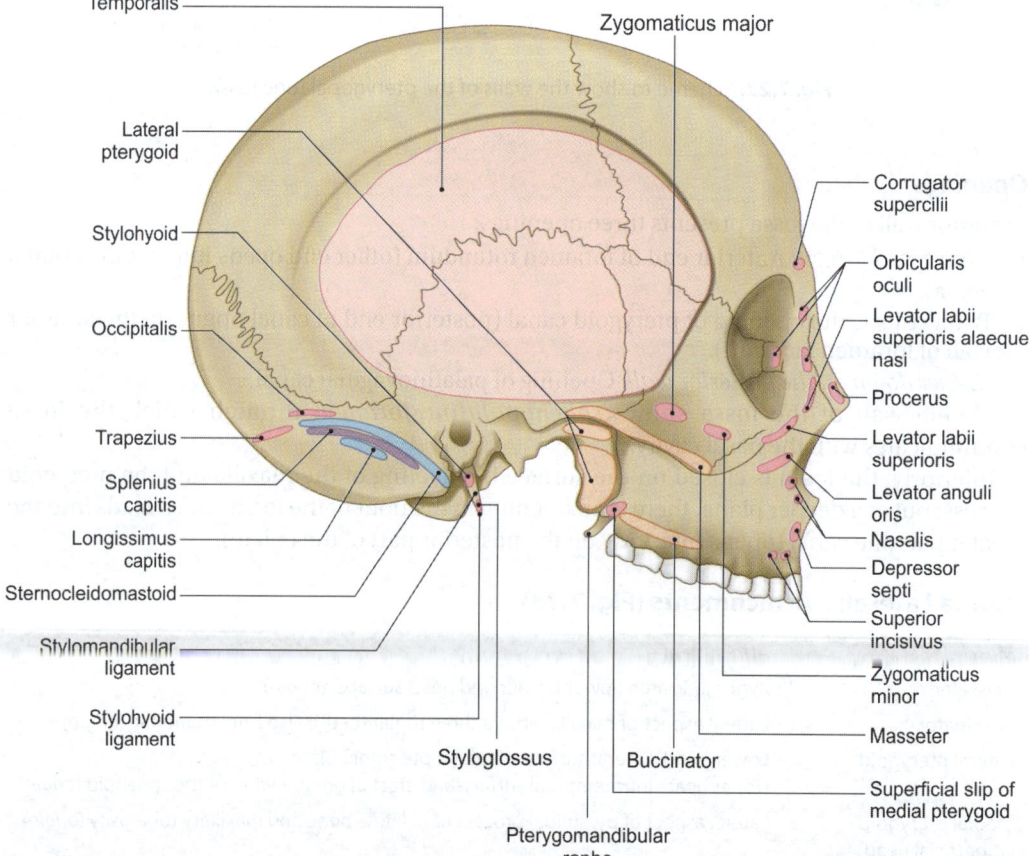

Fig. 7.23: Norma lateralis: Attachments.

Styloid Process: Attachments

Structure	Attachment
Stylohyoid muscle	Posterior aspect (*origin*)
Styloglossus muscle	Anterior aspect (*origin*)
Stylopharyngeus muscle	Medial aspect (*origin*)
Stylohyoid ligament	Attached to tip
Stylomandibular ligament	Attached to lateral side

SKULL FROM BELOW (NORMA BASALIS)

In the anterior part, the inferior aspect of the maxillae are seen. The alveolar process of the maxilla provides attachment to the upper teeth. The posterior end of alveolar process forms a backward projection called the *maxillary tuberosity*. Within the concavity of the alveolar arch (formed by alveolar process) the bony palate is noted; separates the nasal cavities (above) from the mouth cavity (below) **(Fig. 7.24)**.

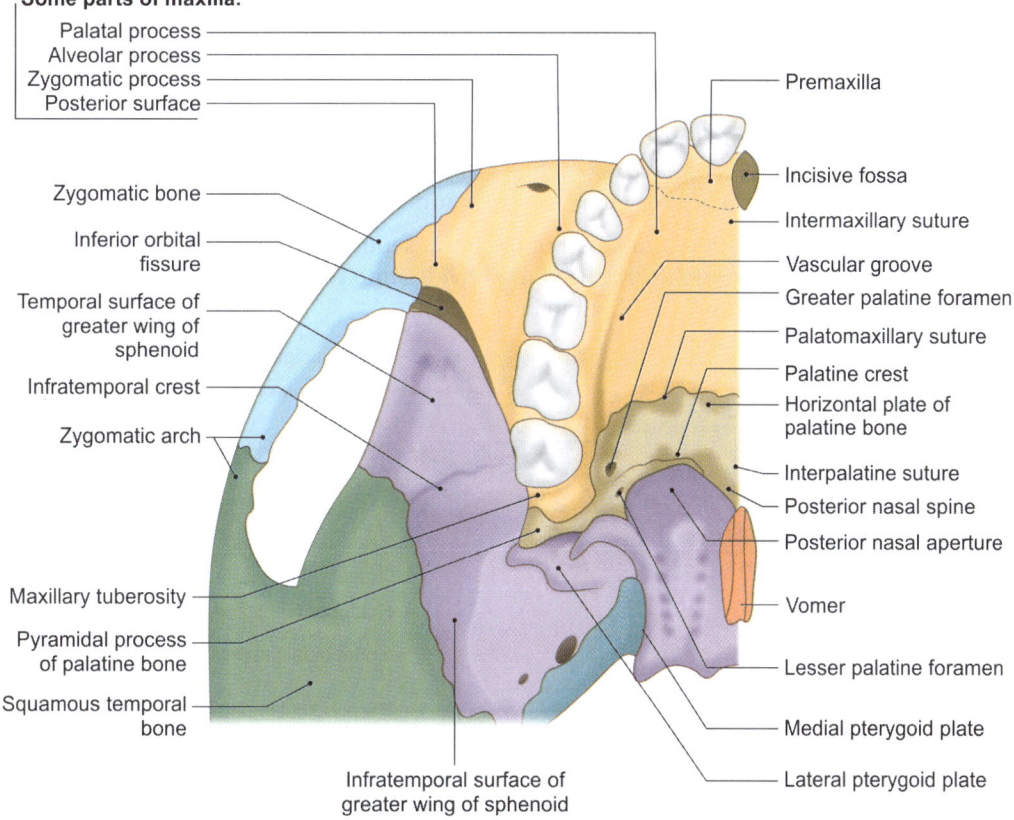

Fig. 7.24: Norma basalis: Anterior part.

Hard palate: Anterior part of the palate is formed by the palatal processes of the maxillae. Both processes meet in the midline at the *intermaxillary suture*. Overlying the anterior part of this suture, the *incisive fossa* is seen. On the side walls of this fossa, the *lateral incisive foramina* are noted (in place of lateral incisive foramina, there may be anterior and posterior median incisive foramina). The part of the alveolar process bearing incisor teeth including the adjoining part of the palate is the *premaxilla*. Lateral to the alveolar arch, the inferior aspect of the zygomatic process of the maxilla passes laterally to meet the zygomatic bone. The posterior surface of the maxilla is noted; separated (posterolaterally) from the greater wing of sphenoid by the inferior orbital fissure.

The posterior part of the hard palate is formed by the horizontal plate of palatine bones. Both bones articulate at the *interpalatine suture*. They also articulate with the posterior margins of the palatal processes of the maxillae at the *palatomaxillary sutures*. The posterior borders of the horizontal plates of the palatine bones are free; from the posterior margin of the hard palate. In the midline, the margin projects backward and forms the *posterior nasal spine*. Just in front of the posterior border, a curved ridge called *palatine crest* is seen. The posterolateral part of the horizontal plate gives a projection called the *pyramidal process*. It projects backward and laterally; between the lower ends of the medial and lateral pterygoid plates.

Greater and lesser palatine foramina: The greater palatine foramen is on the horizontal plate, medial to last molar tooth. It is the lower opening of the canal of the same name present in relation to the floor of the pterygopalatine fossa. The lesser palatine foramina (usually two) are on the pyramidal process just behind the greater palatine foramen.

Posterior nasal apertures: Just above the posterior margin of the hard palate, these are seen. Each aperture is bounded below by the posterior edge of the horizontal plate of the palatine bone. Its lateral wall is formed by the perpendicular plate the palatine bone. The posterior edge of the perpendicular plate is fused to the medial pterygoid plate of the sphenoid. Perpendicular plate separates the nasal cavity from the pterygopalatine fossa.

Vomer: This flat plate of bone forms part of the nasal septum. It separates the right and left posterior nasal apertures. Superiorly, the vomer divides into two alae that articulate with the inferior surface of the body of the sphenoid **(Fig. 7.25)**.

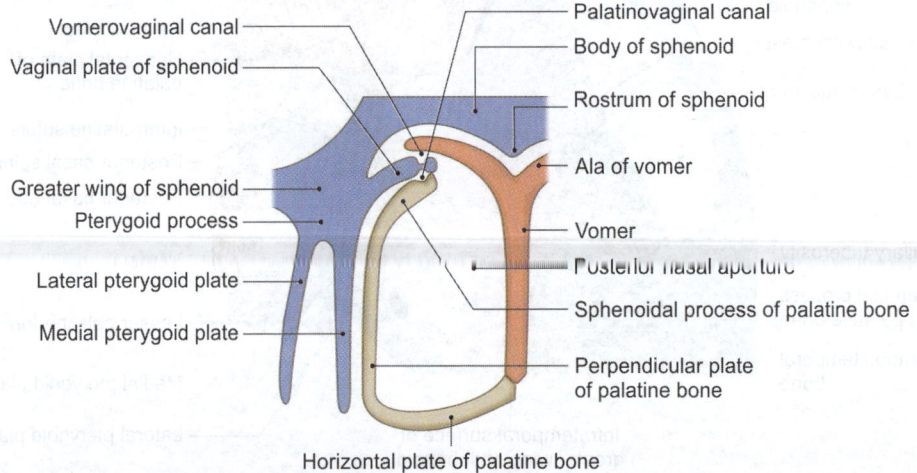

Fig. 7.25: Scheme to show the bones around the posterior nasal aperture.

Sphenoid: Additional Features

It extends across the entire width of the base of the skull and also onto the side wall of the vault. It is made up of body, right and left greater and lesser wings and the right and left pterygoid processes.

When viewed from below, the body of the sphenoid is seen in the roof of the posterior part of the nasal cavity and adjoining nasopharynx.

A median ridge called the *rostrum* projects downward from the body of the sphenoid. The rostrum fits into the gap between the alae of the vomer.

From the root of the pterygoid process, a horizontal *vaginal plate* projecting medially which overlaps the lateral part of the ala.

From the upper part of the perpendicular plate of the palatine bone, its *sphenoidal process* projects medially which overlaps anterior part of vaginal plate. The *palatovaginal canal* is placed between these two plates. It runs forward to open on the posterior wall of the pterygopalatine fossa.

The *vomerovaginal canal* (not always present) when present, lies between the vaginal plate of the sphenoid and the ala of vomer. It runs forward to join the palatinovaginal canal. Posteriorly, the body of the sphenoid continues with the basilar part (body) of the occipital bone.

Pterygoid process (consisting medial and lateral pterygoid plates) projects downward from the junction of the body of the sphenoid with the greater wing. These plates meet anteriorly; free posteriorly. The space between them is the *pterygoid fossa*. Anteriorly, the pterygoid process is fused to the posterior aspect of the maxilla in its middle part. Higher up, it is separated from the maxilla by the *pterygomaxillary fissure*. The perpendicular plate of the palatine bone closes the pterygopalatine fossa medially and at the same time meets the anterior margin of the medial pterygoid plate. In their lowest parts, the pterygoid plates are separated by a gap; filled by pyramidal process of the palatine bone. This process can be seen from behind and from the lateral side in the medial wall of the infratemporal fossa **(Figs. 7.26 and 7.27)**.

Medial pterygoid plate is directed backward. It has medial and lateral surfaces, and a free posterior border. The upper end of posterior border divides to enclose a triangular depression—the *scaphoid fossa*. Medial to this fossa, there is a small tubercle which projects into the *foramen lacerum*. It hides from view the posterior opening of the pterygoid canal;

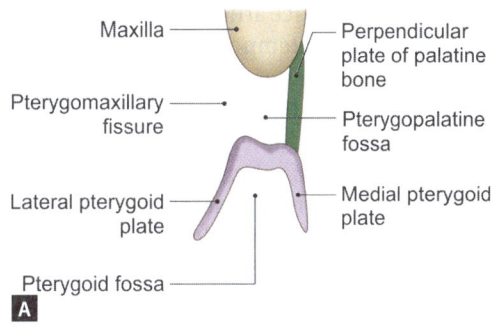
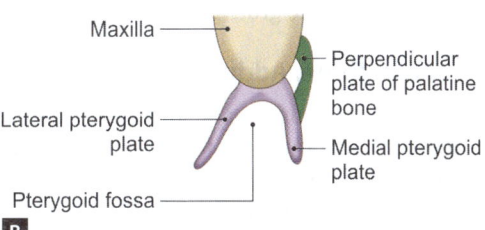
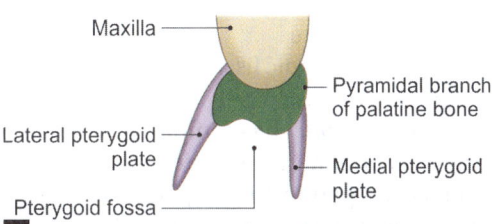

Figs. 7.26A to C: Schematic TS to show the arrangement of medial and lateral pterygoid plates.

anterior end of this canal opens on the posterior wall of the pterygopalatine fossa. The lower end of the posterior border is prolonged downward and laterally to form the *pterygoid hamulus* (**Fig. 7.28**).

Lateral pterygoid plate projects backward and laterally. It has medial and lateral surfaces. At its upper end its lateral surface continues with the infratemporal surface of the greater wing.

Greater wing of sphenoid has infratemporal and temporal surfaces (seen from below) and orbital surface (seen in lateral orbital wall). The anterior margin of the infratemporal surface is separated from the maxilla by the inferior orbital fissure. Laterally, it is separated from the temporal surface by the infratemporal crest. The posterior margin of the lateral part of the infratemporal surface articulates with the infratemporal surface of the squamous temporal bone. Medially, the infratemporal surface of the greater wing continues with the body of sphenoid. Posteriorly, the greater wing meets the anterior margin of the petrous temporal bone.

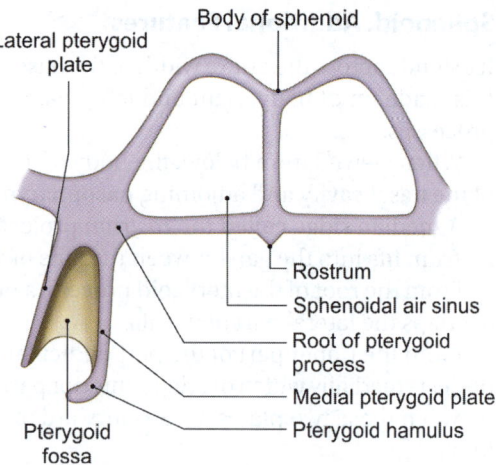

Fig. 7.27: Schematic CS to show relationship of pterygoid process to the rest of sphenoid bone.

Foramina near the posterior border of greater wing: The foramen ovale lies posterolateral to the upper end of the lateral pterygoid plate. Posterolateral to foramen ovale, foramen spinosum (in front of spine of sphenoid) is noted. A third foramen (sometimes medial to foramen ovale) is the emissary sphenoidal foramen. Between the foramen ovale and the foramen spinosum, small foramen called canaliculus innominatus is present. Posteromedial to these foramina and to the spine of sphenoid, the posterior margin of the greater wing forms the anterior wall of a prominent groove. The posterior wall of this groove is formed by the petrous temporal bone. The two bones meet in the floor of the groove which lodges the cartilaginous part of the auditory tube. Laterally, the groove ends in relation to the opening of the bony part of auditory tube.

Temporal Bone: Additional Features

Temporal bone consists of squamous, petrous, mastoid, and tympanic parts, with the styloid process. Important landmarks include (**Fig. 7.29**):
- Zygomatic process
- Tubercle of the root of zygoma
- Postglenoid tubercle
- Mastoid process
- Tympanic plate
- Squamotympanic fissure
- Styloid process.

Squamous part has temporal surface seen from the lateral aspect; part of it seen from below. Inferior and medial to temporal surface, the squamous part has infratemporal surface which takes part in forming the roof of the infratemporal fossa (with infratemporal surface of greater wing of sphenoid). Behind its infratemporal surface, the squamous part presents the *mandibular fossa.* This fossa is bounded anteriorly by the *articular tubercle.* The articular area for the mandible extends on to the tubercle.

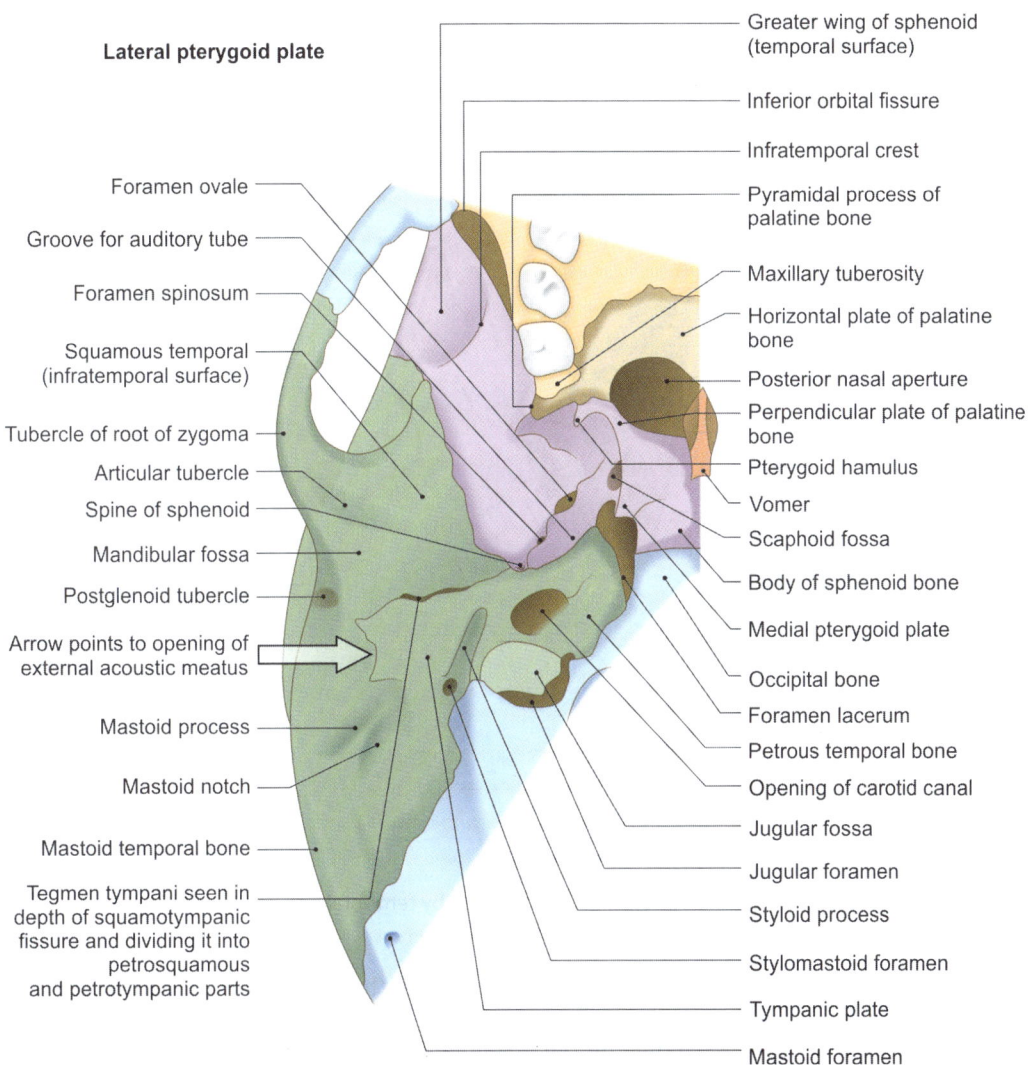

Fig. 7.28: Part of the base of skull formed by temporal and sphenoid bones.

Tympanic plate separates the mandibular fossa from the external acoustic meatus. The junction of the fossa (squamous part) with the tympanic plate is marked by the *squamotympanic fissure*. The lower edge of a plate of bone called the *tegmen tympani* (part of petrous temporal) projects through the fissure. It divides *squamotympanic fissure* into:
❖ Petrosquamous fissure (anteriorly)
❖ Petrotympanic fissure (posteriorly).

The posterior part of the tympanic plate partially surrounds the base of the styloid process and fuse with the mastoid temporal bone.

Petrous part runs forward and medially between the greater wing of sphenoid (anterolaterally), and the occipital bone (posteromedially). Its apex is separated from the body of the sphenoid,

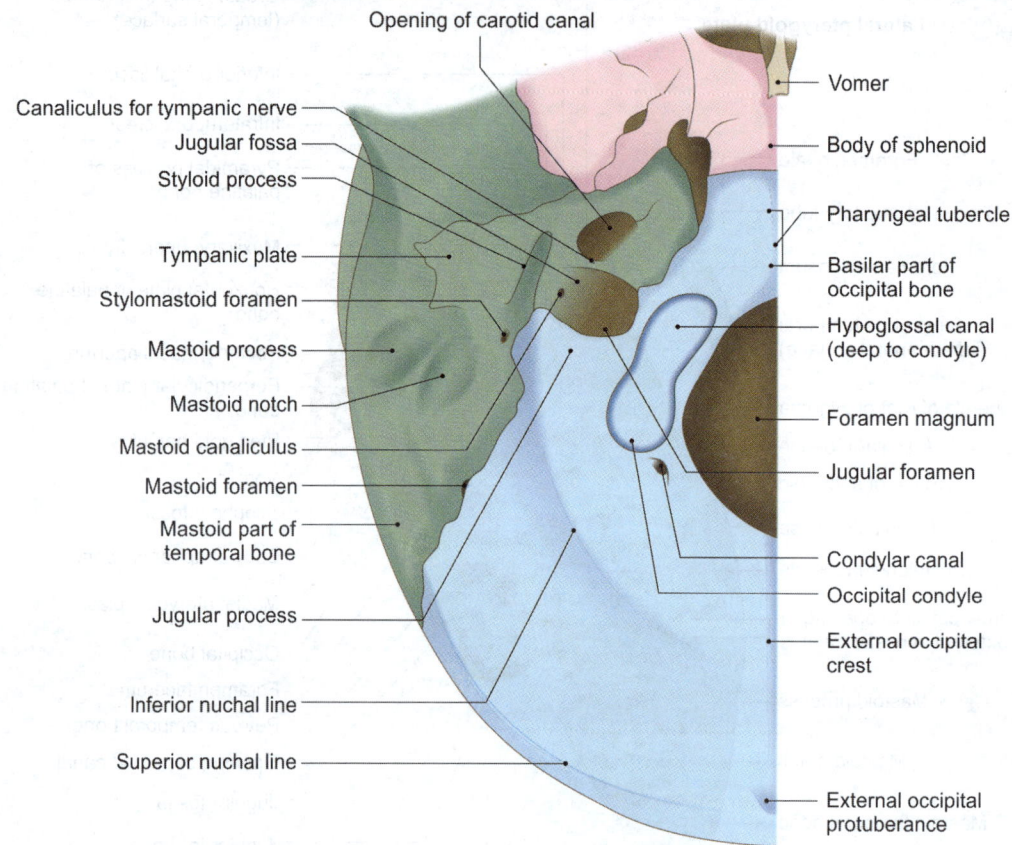

Fig. 7.29: Posterior part of base of skull (formed by temporal and occipital bones).

the root of the pterygoid process, and the basilar part of the occipital bone by the *foramen lacerum*. The inferior surface of the petrous temporal bone is marked by the lower opening of the *carotid canal* through which the internal carotid artery enters the cranial cavity. The canal passes medially, through the petrous temporal bone and opens into the posterior wall of the foramen lacerum. Behind the opening of the carotid canal, there is a large depression called the *jugular fossa*. This fossa leads posteriorly into the *jugular foramen* that opens into the posterior cranial fossa.

In the *mastoid part*, the mastoid process and the mastoid foramen are noted. Medial to the mastoid process, there is a deep *mastoid notch*. Near the anterior end of the notch, and just behind the styloid process the *stylomastoid foramen* is seen. Medial to the mastoid notch the bone is grooved by the occipital artery.

Occipital Bone: Additional Features

The greater part of the occipital bone is seen in the norma basalis. The most conspicuous feature is the large *foramen magnum* through which the cranial cavity communicates with the vertebral canal. The part of the bone anterior to the foramen magnum is the *basilar part*. Anteriorly, the basilar part continues with the body of the sphenoid. Both bones are separated by a plate of cartilage in the young, but fuse with each other in the adult. A short distance in front of the foramen magnum of the basilar part shows a small elevation in the midline called the *pharyngeal tubercle*.

The parts of the occipital bone lateral to the foramen magnum are the *occipital condyles*. Each condyle articulates with the corresponding superior articular facet on the C-1 vertebra (*atlas*) to form *atlanto-occipital joint*. The *hypoglossal* (anterior condylar) *canal* opens on the norma basalis above the lateral border of the anterior part of the condyle. The canal runs backward to open into the posterior cranial fossa. The opening of the *posterior condylar canal* is seen on the *condylar fossa* (depression behind the condyle).

Jugular process is lateral to occipital condyle. It forms posterior (and inferior) wall of the jugular fossa and foramen. The *jugular foramen* passes backward and medially from the fossa. Two small foramina in relation to the jugular fossa are noted:
* *Mastoid canaliculus* on the lateral wall of the fossa
* *Tympanic canaliculus* on the bony ridge that separates jugular fossa from the opening of the carotid canal.

The squamous part is behind the foramen magnum; articulates with mastoid temporal bone at the *occipitomastoid suture*. On or near this suture mastoid foramen is seen. Posteriorly, the squamous part forms the posterior part of the skull vault and joins the right and left parietal bones at the lambdoid suture. Its external surface is marked by:
* External occipital protuberance
* External occipital crest
* Inferior, superior and highest nuchal lines
* Many ridges; rough surface for muscular attachments.

Norma Basalis: Attachments (Fig. 7.30)

Muscle/structure	Attachment
Masseter	Lower border of zygomatic arch (*origin*)
Lateral pterygoid (upper head)	Infratemporal surface and infratemporal crest of greater wing of sphenoid (*origin*)
Lateral pterygoid (lower head)	Lateral surface of lateral pterygoid plate (*origin*)
Medial pterygoid	Medial surface of lateral pterygoid plate and pyramidal process of palatine bone (*origin*)
Tensor palati	Scaphoid fossa, medial side of spine of sphenoid and posterior margin of greater wing of sphenoid (*origin*) Posterior edge of palatine bone (*insertion*)
Tensor tympani	Greater wing of sphenoid (and adjoining part of wall of auditory tube) (*origin*)
Levator palati	Inferior surface of petrous temporal bone (*origin*)
Musculus uvulae	Posterior edge of hard palate near the midline from posterior nasal spine (*origin*)
Digastric (posterior belly)	Mastoid notch on the temporal bone (*origin*)
Longus capitis	Inferior surface of the basilar part of occipital bone (*insertion*)
Rectus capitis anterior	Occipital bone just in front of the condyle (*insertion*)

(Contd...)

(Contd...)

Muscle/structure	Attachment
Rectus capitis lateralis	Inferior surface of jugular process of occipital bone (*insertion*)
Rectus capitis posterior major	Lateral part of the area between inferior nuchal line and foramen magnum (*insertion*)
Rectus capitis posterior minor	Medial part of the area between inferior nuchal line and foramen magnum (*insertion*)
Semispinalis capitis	Medial part of the area between superior and inferior nuchal lines (*insertion*)
Superior oblique capitis	Lateral part of the area between superior and inferior nuchal lines (*insertion*)
Trapezius	Medial one-third of superior nuchal line and external occipital protuberance (*origin*)
Superior constrictor of pharynx (uppermost fibers)	Pharyngeal tubercle on basilar part of occipital bone (*origin*)
Pterygomandibular ligament	Tip of pterygoid hamulus
Pterygospinous ligament	Extends between spine of sphenoid and upper part of lateral pterygoid plate
Sphenomandibular ligament	Spine of sphenoid
Ligamentum nuchae (upper end)	External occipital protuberance and external occipital crest
Alar ligaments (of dens)	Occipital bone just medial to condyles
Anterior and posterior atlanto-occipital membranes	Corresponding margins of foramen magnum

AN 30.1 Describe the cranial fossae and identify related structures.

CRANIAL FOSSAE

When the upper part of the skull vault is removed the floor of the cranial cavity is seen. The floor is subdivided into three depressions called the anterior, middle, and posterior *cranial fossae*.

Anterior Cranial Fossa

The floor of the anterior cranial fossa is formed mainly by the orbital plates of the frontal bone. Anteriorly, the right and left halves of the frontal bone are separated by a median projection called the *frontal crest*. Just behind the crest, there is a depression called the *foramen cecum*.

Between the right and left orbital plates of the frontal bone, there is a notch occupied by the *cribriform plate* of the ethmoid bone. This plate presents numerous foramina for the olfactory nerve fibers. It also shows a median vertical projection called the *crista galli* which lies behind the foramen cecum.

The anterior and posterior ethmoidal canals open into the anterior cranial fossa near the lateral edge of the cribriform plate. The posterior part of the floor of the anterior cranial fossa is formed by the sphenoid bone. In the median part, it is formed by the anterior part of the superior surface of the body of sphenoid. This region is the *jugum sphenoidale*. Lateral to the jugum sphenoidale, the floor is formed by the lesser wing of sphenoid. The lesser wing also forms the posterior edge of the floor of the anterior cranial fossa. The medial edge of each lesser wing projects backward as the *anterior clinoid process* (**Fig. 7.31**).

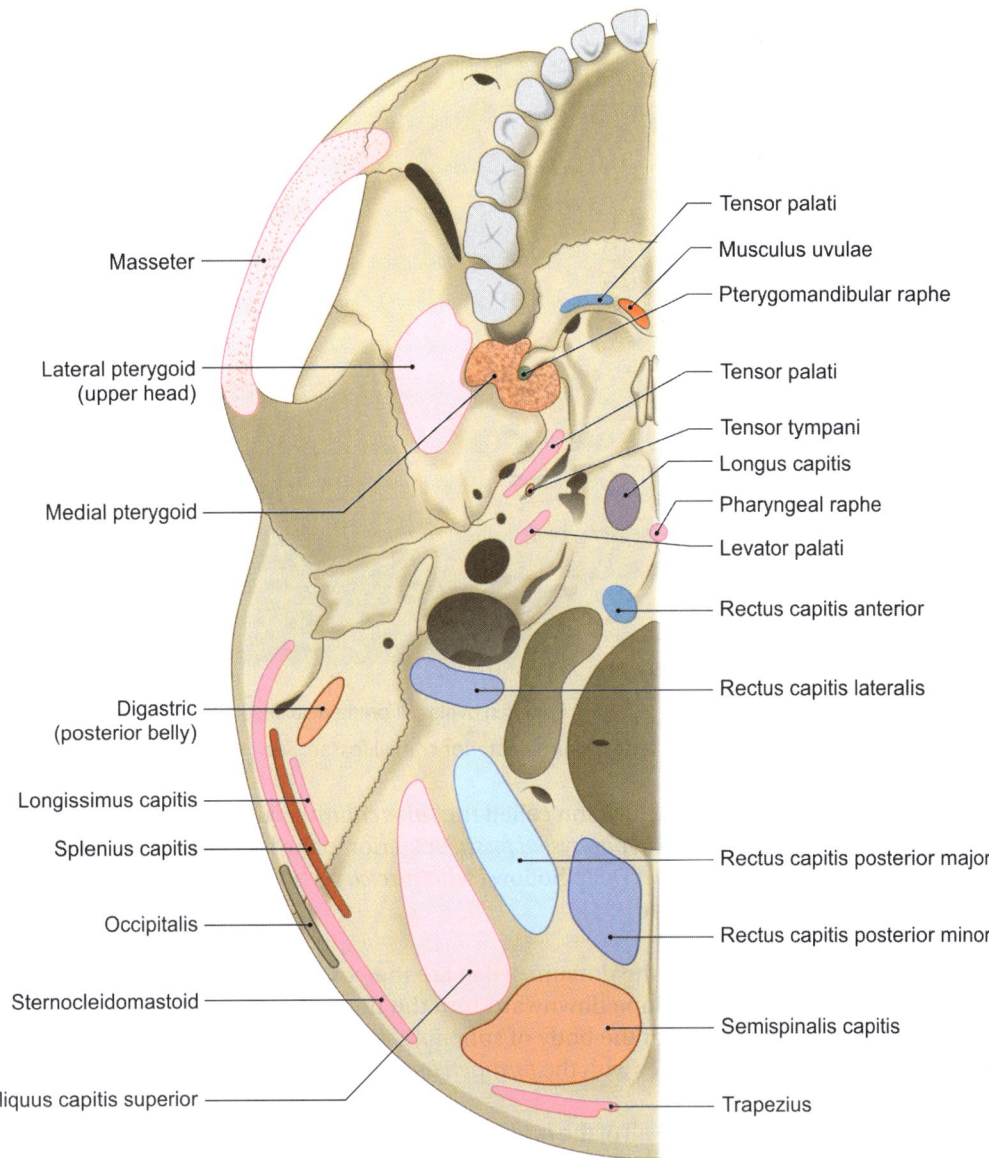

Fig. 7.30: Norma basalis: Attachments.

Middle Cranial Fossa

It has a raised median part (formed by the sphenoid body) and two large deep hollow areas on either side. Immediately behind the jugum sphenoidale, the body of the sphenoid is crossed by a transverse shallow groove that connects the two optic canals called the *sulcus chiasmaticus* (optic chiasma does not lie over sulcus). Behind the sulcus, the superior surface of the body of

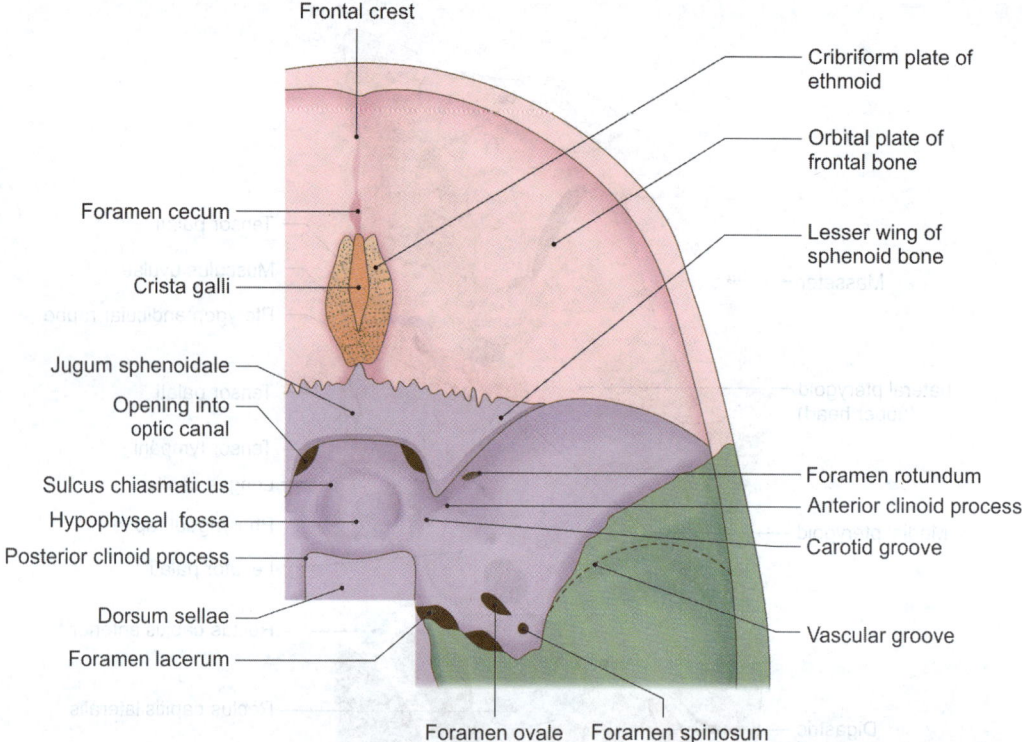

Fig. 7.31: Parts of anterior and posterior cranial fossae: Seen from above.

the sphenoid shows a median elevation called the *tuberculum sellae*. Behind the tuberculum, there is a depression called the *hypophyseal fossa*. Posterior to the fossa, there is a vertical plate of bone called the *dorsum sellae*. Deep hollow (*sella turcica*) is bounded by:

❖ *Anteriorly*: Tuberculum sellae
❖ *Posteriorly*: Dorsum sellae.

The superolateral angles of the dorsum sellae are the *posterior clinoid processes*. The sides of the body of the sphenoid slope downward into the floor of the lateral part of the middle cranial fossa. Here, each side of the body of sphenoid is marked by a shallow *carotid groove*. Posteriorly, the groove continues with the *foramen lacerum*. Anteriorly, it turns upward medial to the anterior clinoid process.

On either side, the anterior wall of the *middle cranial fossa* is formed by the greater and lesser wings of sphenoid. The lesser wings are attached to the sides of the body by two roots: anterior (upper) and posterior (lower).

Optic canal passes forward and laterally between the body of sphenoid and two roots of the lesser wing.

The greater and lesser wings are separated by the *superior orbital fissure* which leads into the orbit. Just below the medial end of the fissure and just lateral to the carotid groove is the *foramen rotundum;* opens anteriorly into the pterygopalatine fossa.

On either side, posterior wall of the middle cranial fossa is formed by the anterior sloping surface of the petrous temporal bone. The apex of the bone is separated from the body of

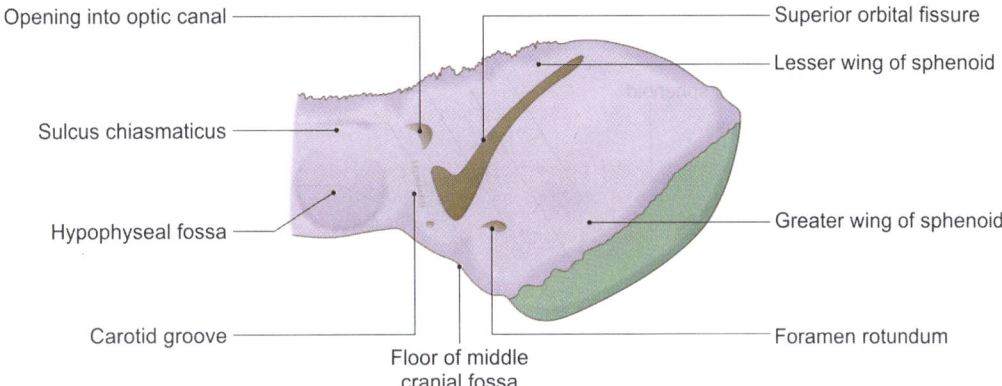

Fig. 7.32: Features in the anterior wall of middle cranial fossa: Schematic diagram.

the sphenoid by the foramen lacerum. A little above and lateral to the foramen, the petrous temporal bone shows a shallow depression called the *cavum trigeminale*. Lateral to this, two grooves run downward and medially. The upper and more prominent groove begins at a minute aperture called the *hiatus for greater petrosal nerve*. Below and lateral to it another groove is at the *hiatus for lesser petrosal nerve*. More laterally, the anterior surface is marked by an elevation called the *arcuate eminence*.

Lateral to arcuate eminence, the anterior surface of petrous temporal bone is formed by a thin plate of bone called the *tegmen tympani*. It separates middle cranial fossa from the cavities of the middle ear, auditory tube, and the mastoid antrum. Lower end of tegmen tympani projects in the squamotympanic fissure **(Fig. 7.32)**.

The floor of the lateral part of middle cranial fossa is medially formed by the greater wing of sphenoid and laterally by squamous temporal bone. Near the posterior margin of the greater wing, the *foramen ovale*, the *foramen spinosum*, and sometimes the *emissary sphenoidal foramen* are seen. Anteriorly, the lateral wall of the middle cranial fossa is formed by the greater wing of sphenoid and posteriorly by the squamous temporal bone. The anteroinferior angle of the parietal bone contributes to the most anterior part of the lateral wall (*at pterion*). A vascular groove (for middle meningeal vessels) starts at the foramen spinosum and runs forward on the floor. It divides into an anterior (*frontal*) and posterior (*parietal*) branches. The frontal branch runs upward and forward to the region of the inner surface of the pterion. The parietal branch runs backward first on the squamous temporal and then on the parietal bone.

Posterior Cranial Fossa (Fig. 7.33)

Here the most prominent landmark is the *foramen magnum*. Anterior to the foramen magnum, the wall of the fossa is formed by the basioccipital bone which continues above with the body of the sphenoid; area called the clivus. The lateral margin of the basiocciptal bone is separated from the petrous temporal bone by the petro-occipital fissure.

Between the jugular foramen (laterally) and the anterior part of foramen magnum (medially), there is a rounded elevation called the *jugular tubercle*. In the interval between the jugular tubercle and the foramen magnum, there is a fossa where the *hypoglossal canal* opens. The *posterior condylar canal* opens just lateral to the jugular tubercle immediately behind the jugular foramen. The lateral part of the anterior wall of the posterior cranial fossa is formed by

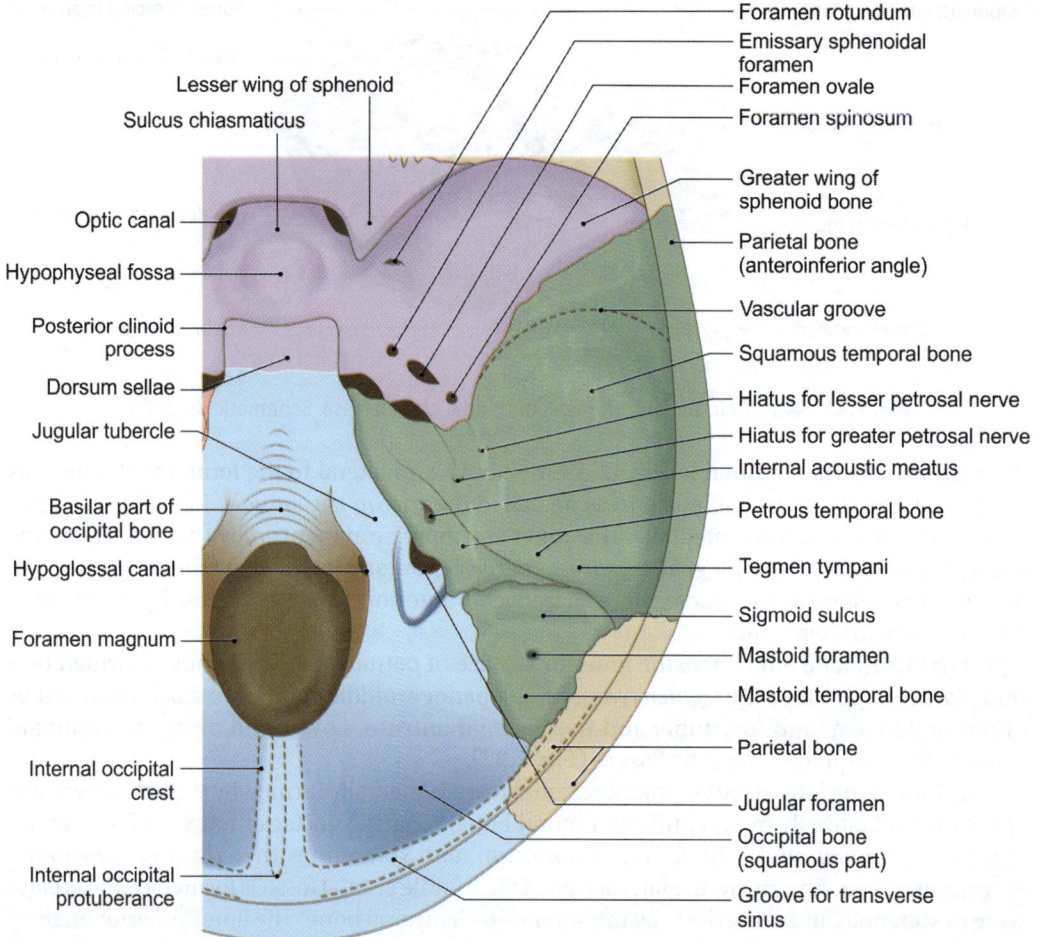

Fig. 7.33: Floor of the middle and posterior cranial fossae: Features.

the posterior surface of the petrous temporal bone. Just above the jugular foramen, this surface presents the opening of the *internal acoustic meatus*. Posterolateral to this opening, a slit in the bone leads into a canal called the *aqueduct of vestibule*. Posteriorly, the floor and lateral walls of the posterior cranial fossa are formed by the squamous occipital bone in anterolateral part by the mastoid temporal bone. The posteroinferior angle of the parietal bone makes small contribution to the anterior part of the lateral wall. Behind the foramen magnum, the two halves of the fossa are separated by the *internal occipital crest*. Posteriorly, the crest ends in the *internal occipital protuberance*. In the transverse plane, a prominent wide groove called the *transverse sulcus* runs laterally from the protuberance; lodges the transverse sinus (groove more prominent on the right). The groove first lies on the occipital bone and near its lateral (or anterior) end it crosses the posteroinferior angle of the parietal bone. It then runs downward and medially with an S-shaped curve. It deeply grooves petrous and mastoid parts of the temporal bone to reach the jugular foramen. This S-shaped groove is the *sigmoid sulcus*. The terminal part of the groove lies on the occipital bone just behind the jugular foramen. The mastoid foramen opens into the sigmoid sulcus formed by the mastoid temporal bone.

AN 30.2 Describe and identify major foramina with structures passing through them.

Foramina of the Skull (Fig. 7.34)

Structure passing	Foramen/openings
Medulla oblongata (lower end)	Foramen magnum
Internal carotid artery	Carotid canal
IJV sigmoid sinus	Jugular foramen
Olfactory nerve (I CN)	Cribriform plate of ethmoid
Optic nerve (II CN)	Optic canal
III, IV, and VI CNs	Superior orbital fissure
Ophthalmic division of V CN	Superior orbital fissure
Maxillary division of V CN	Foramen rotundum
Mandibular division of V CN	Foramen ovale
Facial nerve (VII CN)	Enters internal acoustic meatus; exit through stylomastoid foramen
Vestibulocochlear nerve (VIII CN)	Enters internal acoustic meatus to reach internal ear (*within petrous temporal bone*)
Glossopharyngeal, vagus, and accessory nerves (IX, X, and XI CNs)	Jugular foramen
Hypoglossal nerve (XII CN)	Hypoglossal canal

Skull Foramina and Structures Passing

On the anterior aspect of the skull: Supraorbital notch (or foramen), infraorbital foramen, and zygomaticofacial foramen transmit nerves, and vessels of the same names.

Foramina in the Orbit

Optic canal	Superior orbital fissure	Inferior orbital fissure	Infraorbital groove and canal	Nasolacrimal canal
• Optic nerve (surrounded by meninges) • Ophthalmic artery	*Upper lateral part*: • Trochlear nerve (IV CN) • Frontal and lacrimal branches of ophthalmic division of V CN • Recurrent branch of ophthalmic artery • Superior ophthalmic vein *Middle part (within tendinous ring)*: • Superior and inferior divisions of III CN • Nasociliary branch of ophthalmic division of V CN • Abducent nerve (VI CN) *Lower medial part*: • Inferior ophthalmic vein	• Maxillary nerve • Zygomatic nerve • Infraorbital vessels • Emissary vein connecting inferior ophthalmic veins to pterygoid venous plexus	• Infraorbital nerve (continuation of maxillary nerve) • Infraorbital vessels	Nasolacrimal duct

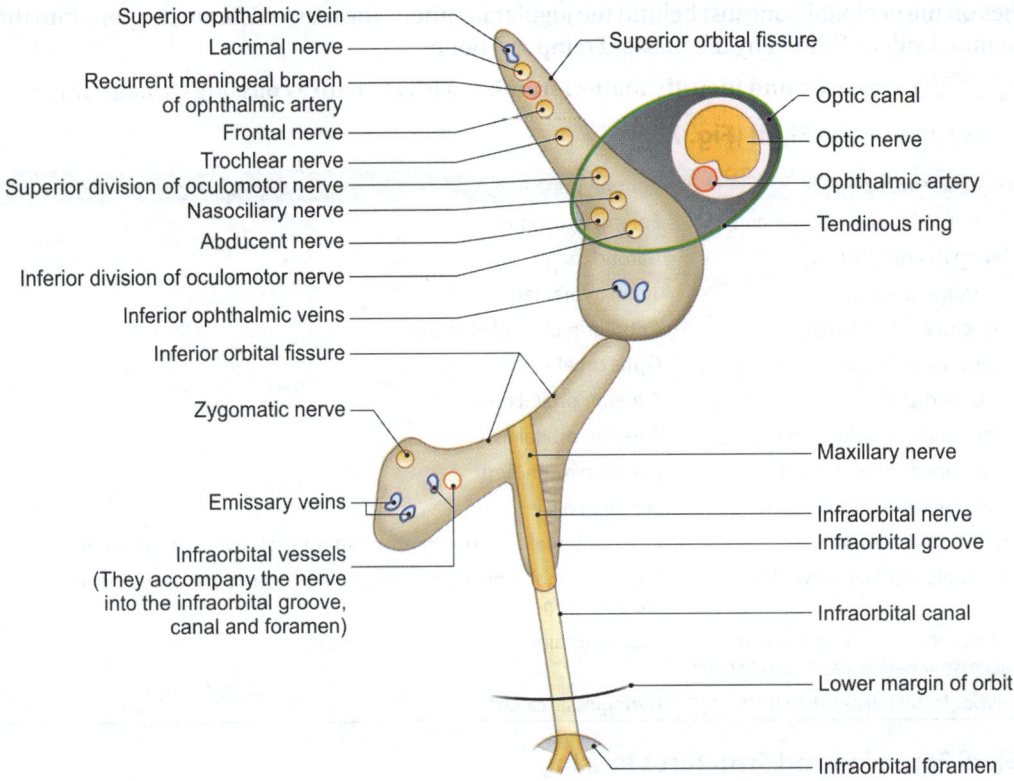

Fig. 7.34: Optic canal, superior, and inferior orbital fissures: Structures passing.

Walls of Orbit

Lateral wall of orbit	Medial wall of orbit
Zygomaticofacial foramen: Zygomaticofacial nerves and vessels	*Anterior ethmoidal canal*: Anterior ethmoidal nerves and vessels
Zygomaticotemporal foramen: Zygomaticotemporal nerves and vessels	*Posterior ethmoidal canal*: Posterior ethmoidal nerves and vessels

These openings are on the suture between the frontal and ethmoid bones.

Canals pass through the interval between these bones to reach the floor of the anterior cranial fossa at the lateral edge of the cribriform plate.

On the Lateral Side of the Skull

- *Zygomaticotemporal foramen*: Zygomaticotemporal nerves and vessels
- *Pterygomaxillary fissure*
    - Maxillary artery
    - Maxillary nerve
    - Sphenopalatine foramen: Nasopalatine nerve and vessels

- *Mastoid foramen*: Emissary vein connecting sigmoid sinus to occipital veins
- *Parietal foramen*: Emissary vein connecting superior sagittal sinus to the scalp veins.

On the Base of the Skull

- *Lateral incisive foramina*:
  - Terminal branches of greater palatine vessels (*from palate to floor of nose*)
  - Nasopalatine nerves (*from nose to palate*)

  Right and left incisive foramina may be replaced by anterior and posterior foramina; left nasopalatine nerve passes through the anterior foramen; right through the posterior foramen.
- *Greater and lesser palatine foramina*: Greater and lesser palatine nerves and vessels.
- *Foramen ovale* (**Fig. 7.35**):
  - Mandibular division of trigeminal nerve (V CN)
  - Lesser petrosal nerve
  - Accessory meningeal artery
  - Emissary veins connecting cavernous sinus to pterygoid venous plexus.
- *Foramen spinosum*:
  - Middle meningeal artery
  - Meningeal branch of mandibular nerve
  - Emissary vein.
- *Canalis innominatus (not always present)*: Lesser petrosal nerve.
- *Emissary sphenoidal foramen (present occasionally)*: Veins connecting cavernous sinus to pterygoid venous plexus.

Carotid Canal and Foramen Lacerum

The lower opening of the carotid canal is on the inferior aspect of the petrous temporal bone. The canal passes forward and medially through the petrous temporal bone and opens on the

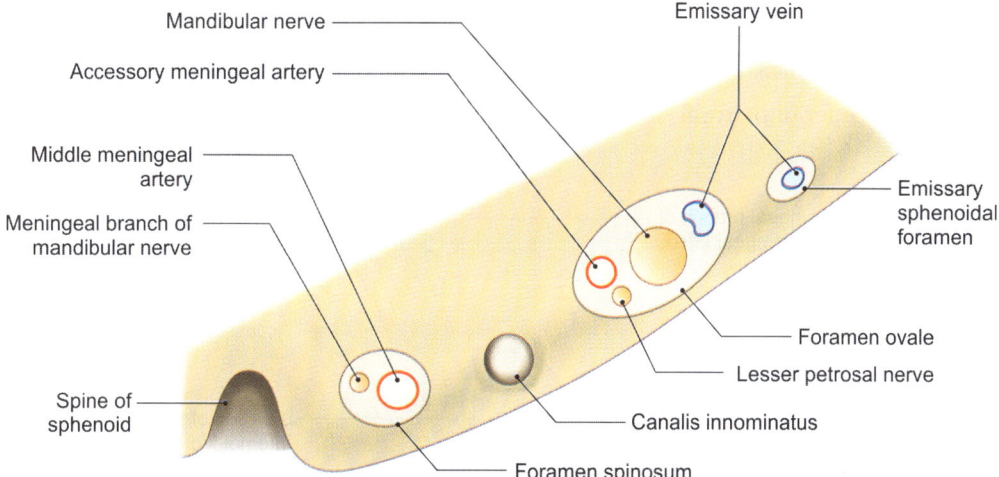

Fig. 7.35: Structures passing through foramen ovale and smaller foramina near it. Lesser petrosal nerve sometimes passes through canalis innominatus.

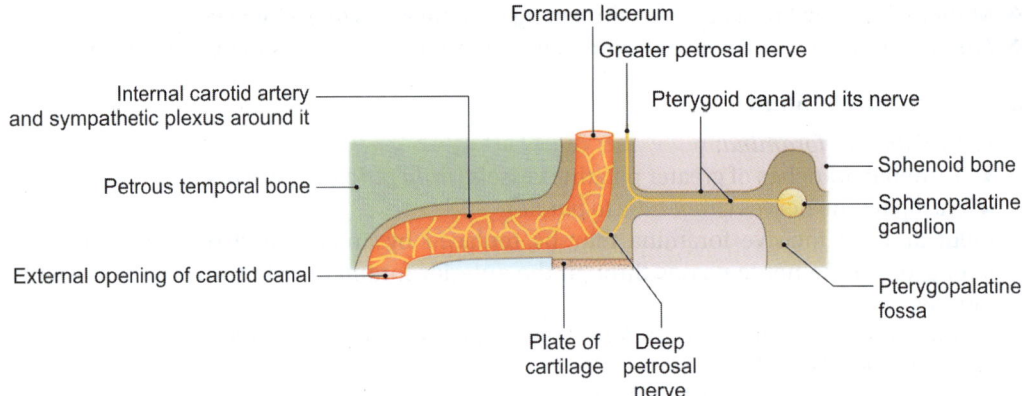

Fig. 7.36: Structures passing through carotid canal and foramen lacerum: Schematic.

posterior wall of the foramen lacerum. The internal carotid artery enters the skull through the carotid canal and the upper part of the foramen lacerum. Inferiorly, the foramen lacerum is closed by a plate of cartilage **(Fig. 7.36)**.

Other structures passing through the carotid canal and foramen lacerum:
- Sympathetic plexus on the internal carotid artery
- Venous plexus connecting cavernous sinus with pharyngeal venous plexus.

In addition, the foramen contains:
- *Deep petrosal nerve* arising from the sympathetic plexus in the foramen
- *Greater petrosal nerve* entering the foramen from above
- *Nerve of pterygoid canal* formed by the union of deep and greater petrosal nerves.

Structures passing through the whole length of foramen lacerum:
- Meningeal branch of ascending pharyngeal artery
- Emissary veins piercing cartilage closing lower end of the foramen.

Jugular foramen (consisting anterior, middle and posterior parts) **(Fig. 7.37)**.

Anterior part: Inferior petrosal sinus.

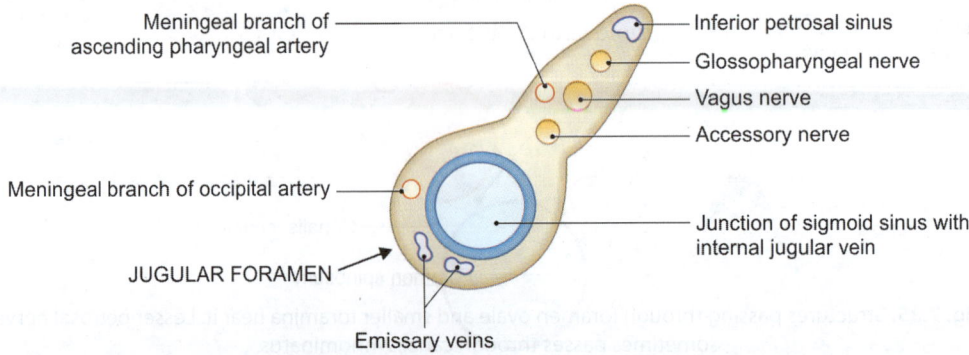

Fig. 7.37: Structures passing through jugular foramen: Schematic.

Middle part:
- Glossopharyngeal nerve (IX CN)
- Vagus nerve (X CN)
- Accessory nerve (XI CN)
- Meningeal branch of ascending pharyngeal artery.

Posterior part:
- Lower end of sigmoid sinus
- Emissary veins connecting sigmoid sinus to occipital veins
- Meningeal branch of occipital artery.

Two foramina are closely associated with the jugular foramen:

Tympanic canaliculus: Glossopharyngeal nerve (IX CN) carries secretomotor fibers for the parotid gland. These fibers leave IX CN through its tympanic branch. This nerve enters a small foramen on the ridge separating the jugular foramen from the carotid canal. This opening leads into the *tympanic canaliculus*. It passes through the petrous temporal bone to reach the middle ear. Here, these nerve fibers pass through the tympanic plexus into the *lesser petrosal nerve*. Lesser petrosal nerve emerges from the petrous temporal bone through the hiatus for lesser petrosal nerve. It then passes through the foramen ovale to reach the infratemporal fossa.

Mastoid canaliculus: Auricular branch of vagus (X CN) traverses petrous temporal bone. It enters through the mastoid canaliculus that opens on the lateral wall of the jugular fossa. It emerges through the *tympanomastoid fissure* **(Fig. 7.38)**.

Foramen magnum (largest foramen in the skull) **(Fig. 7.39)**:
- Lower end of medulla surrounded by meninges
- Anterior and posterior spinal arteries
- Lower end of the tonsil of cerebellum
- Vertebral artery
- Spinal root of accessory nerve (XI CN)
- Apical ligament of dens
- Superior band of cruciform ligament
- Membrana tectoria
- Alar ligaments of dens.

Hypoglossal canal:
- Hypoglossal nerve
- Meningeal branch of ascending pharyngeal artery
- Emissary vein connecting sigmoid sinus to internal jugular vein.

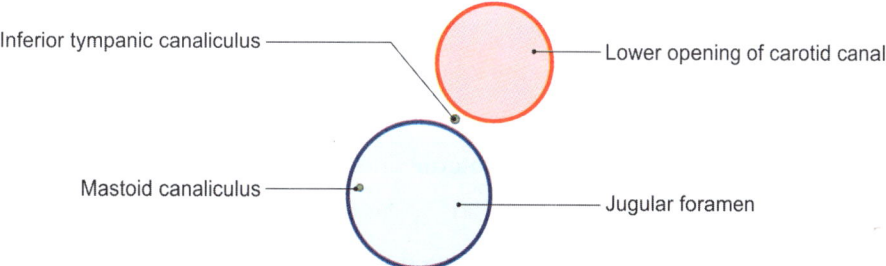

Fig. 7.38: Opening of the inferior tympanic canaliculus and mastoid canaliculus: Schematic.

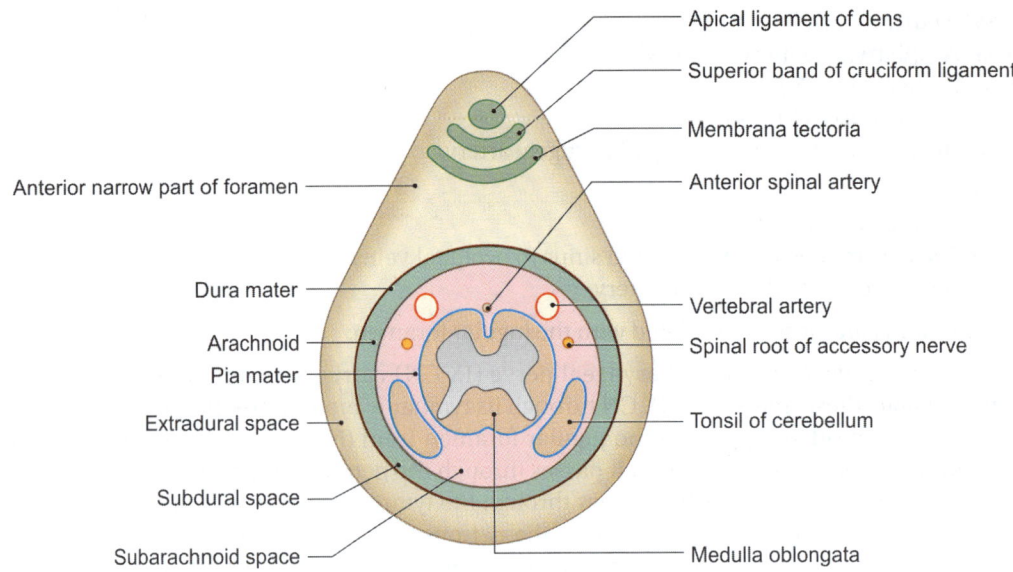

Fig. 7.39: Structures passing through foramen magnum: Schematic.

Posterior condylar canal: Emissary vein connecting lower end of sigmoid sinus to occipital veins.

Stylomastoid foramen:
- Facial nerve
- Stylomastoid branch of posterior auricular artery.

Floor of the Cranial Fossae: Foramina

Foramina already seen on the base of the skull are not included.
- *Apertures in cribriform plate of ethmoid*: Bundles of the olfactory nerves.
- *Foramen cecum* (blind) sometimes patent: Vein connecting the veins of the nose to the superior sagittal sinus.
- *Anterior ethmoidal canals*: Anterior ethmoidal nerves and vessels.
- *Posterior ethmoidal canals*: Posterior ethmoidal nerves and vessels.
- *Foramen rotundum*: Maxillary division of the trigeminal nerve.

Maxillary nerve then passes through the pterygopalatine fossa and finally through the inferior orbital fissure to reach the orbit.
- *Hiatuses for greater and lesser petrosal nerves*: Greater and lesser petrosal nerves.
  Greater petrosal nerve descends to the foramen lacerum and lesser petrosal nerve leaves the skull through the foramen ovale.
- *Internal acoustic meatus*:
  a. Facial nerve (motor root and nervus intermedius)
  b. Vestibulocochlear nerve
  c. Labyrinthine vessels.

Vestibulocochlear nerve terminates within petrous temporal bone by supplying membranous labyrinth.

Facial nerve emerges through the stylomastoid foramen. A little above its exit from stylomastoid foramen, the facial nerve gives chorda tympani nerve. This nerve passes through the posterior canaliculus to enter the middle ear cavity. It leaves middle ear cavity through *anterior canaliculus* that opens through the medial end of *petrotympanic fissure*. Here the nerve is medial to the spine of the sphenoid. The spine is also related to the auriculotemporal nerve on its lateral side.

NASAL CAVITY

The nasal cavity (consisting right and left halves) is separated by the nasal septum. Anteriorly, the cavity opens on the front through the *anterior nasal aperture* and posteriorly it opens on the base of the skull just above the posterior edge of the bony palate, through right and left *posterior nasal apertures*. Each half of the cavity presents lateral wall, medial wall (formed by septum), floor, and roof.

Lateral Wall

The medial surface of the maxilla forms the base of the lateral wall over which other bones are attached. Its features are:
- Large opening of maxillary air sinus—*maxillary hiatus*
- Nasolacrimal groove behind the lower part of frontal process
- Groove for greater palatine canal in the posteroinferior part.

Palatine bone (perpendicular plate) overlaps the posterior part of the maxilla. By this overlapping the greater palatine groove is converted into a canal, its medial wall being formed by the palatine bone. The palatine bone overlaps the posterior part of the maxillary hiatus reducing its size.

Lacrimal bone is behind the frontal process of maxilla. With its lower border the inferior nasal concha articulates. The lower part of the lacrimal bone and the upper part of the inferior nasal concha (*lacrimal process*) convert nasolacrimal groove into a canal and form its medial wall.

Inferior nasal concha is attached anteriorly to the conchal crest of the maxilla and posteriorly to the conchal crest of the palatine bone. Its upper margin overlaps the lower part of the maxillary hiatus. Here, a downward projection of the concha—*maxillary process* descends to articulate with the lower edge of the hiatus. Its *ethmoidal process* just upward into the hiatus. The space between the concha (medially) and the maxilla and palatine bones (laterally) is the *inferior meatus* (**Figs. 7.40 and 7.41**).

Part of the ethmoid bone overlaps the lacrimal bone and the upper parts of the maxilla and palatine bones. The relationship of the ethmoid to the nasal cavity is visualized by the coronal section through the region.

Ethmoid bone consists of a labyrinth closed medially by vertical medial plate is seen in the lateral wall of the nasal cavity. The plate descends vertically from the cribriform plate; its free lower part forms the middle nasal concha. Above the middle concha, a smaller projection, the superior nasal concha, arises from the medial plate. The spaces deep to these conchae are the *middle* and *superior meatuses*, respectively. The middle concha almost completely hides the maxillary hiatus from view. Deep to the concha, a rounded prominence called the *bulla ethmoidale* is seen in relation to the upper part of the hiatus. A little below the bulla a curved plate of bone runs downward and backward called the *uncinate process*. Its posterior end joins the ethmoidal process of the inferior concha. The curved gap between the bulla ethmoidale and the uncinate process is the *hiatus semilunaris* (**Fig. 7.42**).

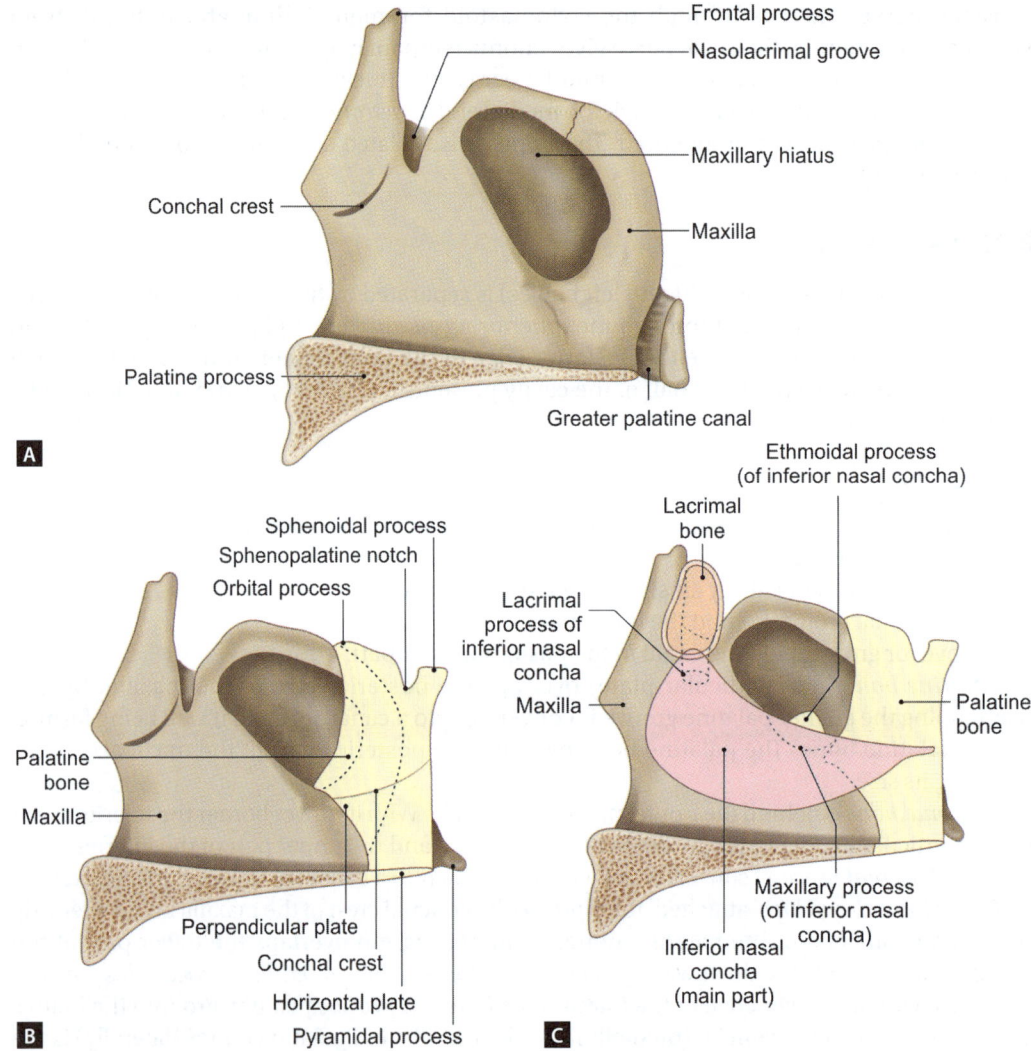

Figs. 7.40A to C: Lateral wall of the nose: bones. (A) Medial aspect of maxilla; (B) Palatine bone overlapping maxilla; (C) Lacrimal bone and inferior nasal concha overlapping maxilla and palatine bone.

Floor

It is formed by the upper surface of the bony palate. Each half of the palate is formed anteriorly by the palatine process of maxilla and posteriorly by the horizontal plate of palatine bone.

Roof

It is formed by many bones. From before backward these are:
❖ Parts of nasal bone
❖ Frontal bone
❖ Cribriform plate of ethmoid
❖ Anterior surface of the body of sphenoid.

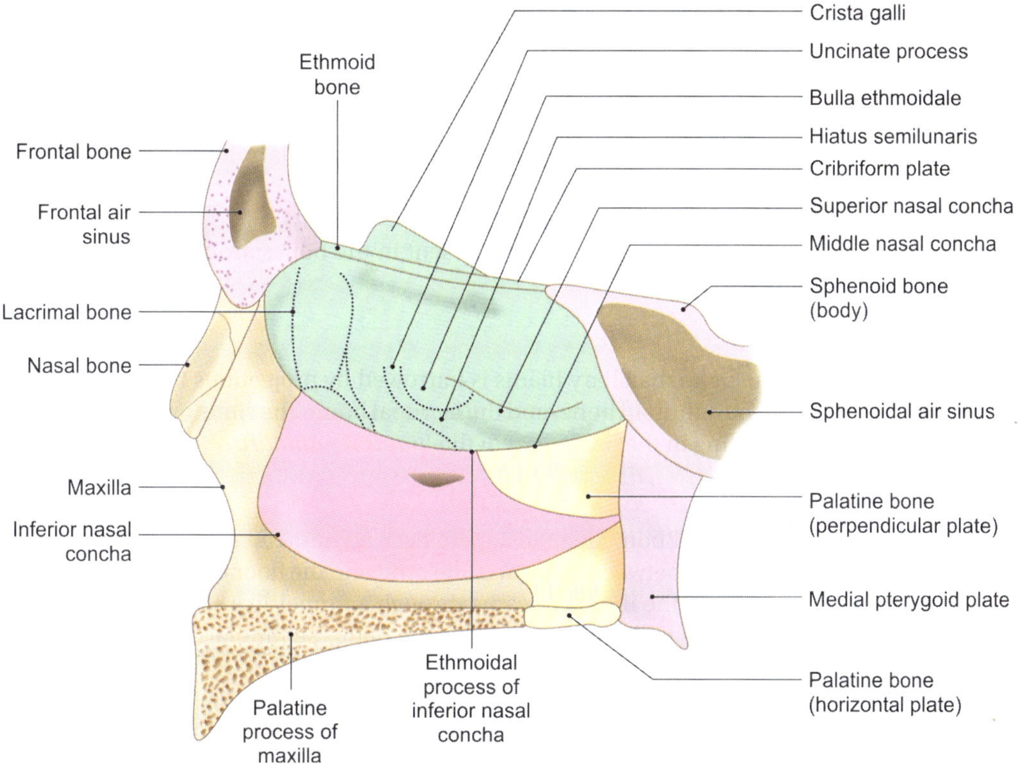

Fig. 7.41: Lateral wall of the nasal cavity with ethmoid. Parts shown in dotted line seen only when the middle concha is lifted off.

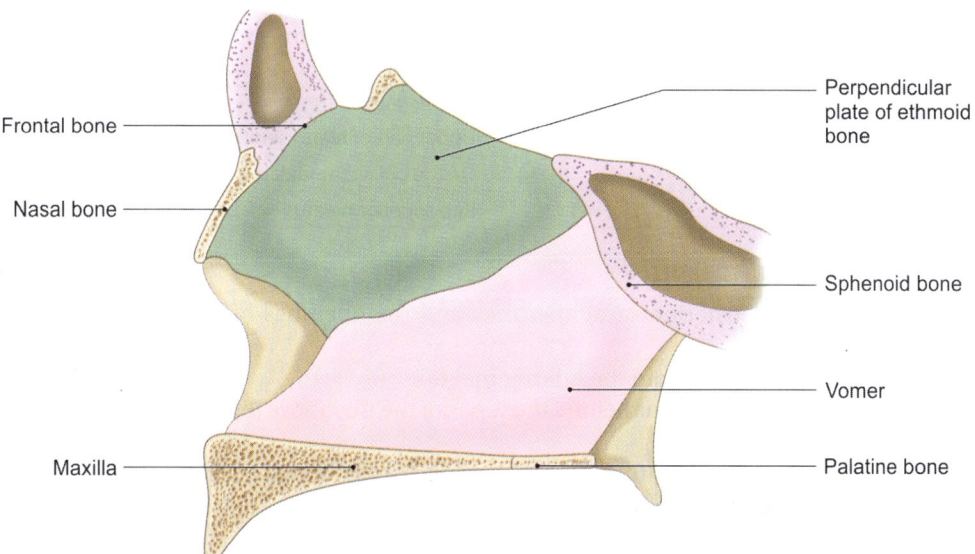

Fig. 7.42: Main bones forming the nasal septum.

Medial Wall

Also called the nasal septum; is formed by the plate of ethmoid (in upper part) and the vomer (in lower part).

Anteriorly, there is a gap in the septum; filled in by the cartilage. Around the edges of the septum, there are contributions from nasal, frontal, sphenoid, maxillary, and palatine bones.

Paranasal Air Sinuses

The paranasal sinuses (bilateral) are the spaces present in the bones around the nasal cavity and into which they open.

Maxillary Air Sinus

It lies within the maxilla. Large maxillary hiatus is narrowed by projections from the palatine bone, inferior nasal concha, ethmoid bone, and the lacrimal bone. The sinus opens into middle meatus of nose by an opening in the lower part of the *hiatus semilunaris*.

Frontal Air Sinuses

These are present in the frontal bone deep to superciliary arches. The sinus extends into the orbital plate of the frontal bone between the roof of the orbit and the floor of the anterior cranial fossa. Frontal sinus opens into the middle meatus through a funnel-like space, the *ethmoidal infundibulum* which continues with the upper end of the hiatus semilunaris.

Sphenoidal Air Sinuses

These are present in the body of sphenoid. Each sinus opens into the nasal cavity above the superior nasal concha. Their opening is the *sphenoethmoidal recess*.

Ethmoidal Air Sinuses

These are present within the labyrinth of the ethmoid bone. They are divided into anterior, middle, and posterior groups. The walls of some sinuses are incomplete. In intact skull, they are completed by frontal, maxillary, lacrimal, sphenoidal, and palatine bones **(Figs. 7.43 to 7.45)**.

Ethmoidal sinus	Opening
Anterior ethmoidal sinus	Upper part of hiatus semilunaris
Middle ethmoidal sinus	On the bulla ethmoidale
Posterior ethmoidal sinus	Into superior meatus

Nasal Cavity: Other Apertures

Besides anterior and posterior nasal apertures and the openings of the paranasal sinuses, following openings are noted:
- *Nasolacrimal canal* opens into the inferior meatus.
- *Sphenopalatine foramen* opens behind the superior meatus above the posterior end of middle concha.
- *Nasal cavity communicates* with the anterior cranial fossa through apertures in the cribriform plate of ethmoid and anterior ethmoidal canals.

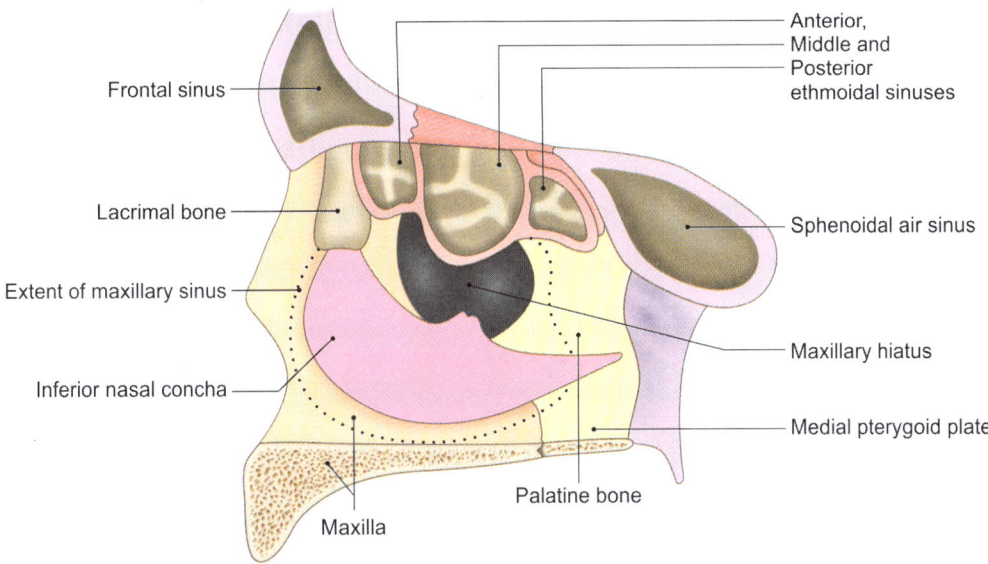

Fig. 7.43: Lateral wall of nasal cavity after removal of medial plate of ethmoid to expose ethmoidal air sinuses.

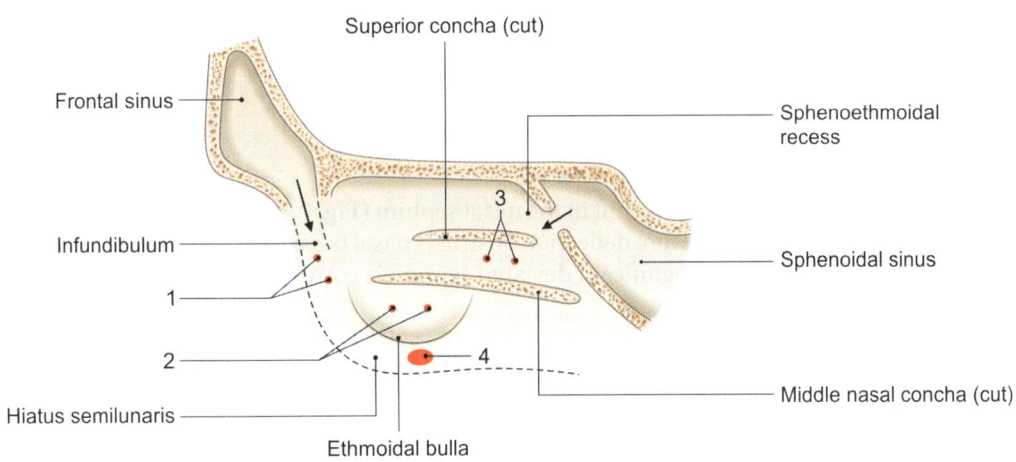

1 = Openings of anterior ethmoidal sinuses
2 = Openings of middle ethmoidal sinuses
3 = Openings of posterior ethmoidal sinuses
4 = Opening of maxillary sinus

Fig. 7.44: Openings of paranasal sinuses into the nasal cavity: Schematic.

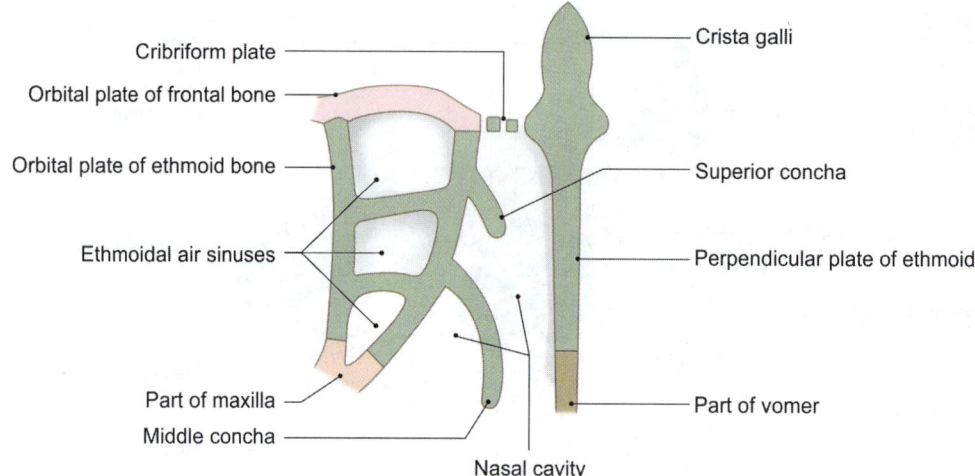

Fig. 7.45: Parts of ethmoid bone: Schematic.

❖ **Funnel-shaped opening** in the anterior part of the floor of the nasal cavity leads into the incisive canals which open on the lower surface of the palate.

Nasal Index

It is the proportion which the width of anterior nasal aperture bears to height of nose; latter being measured from nasion to lower margin of nasal aperture.

$$\frac{\text{Nasal width}}{\text{Nasal height}} \times 100$$

Clinical Anatomy

Deviated nasal septum: There is a shift in the nasal septum **(Fig. 7.46)**; more commonly shifts to left during normal growth. Severe deflection obstructs nasal passage. It may result in sinusitis and breathlessness. Clinically significant deviated septum is corrected by septoplasty.

FETAL SKULL

Features

Frontal Bone

It develops in two halves joined by *metopic suture*. The suture disappears subsequently. Most of the frontal bone develops in membrane except the orbital plates that develop in cartilage **(Figs. 7.47A to C)**.

Parietal Bone

It develops in membrane only. The parietal eminences are well marked in the fetal life. This is utilizing for relating fetal growth by measuring biparietal diameter using ultrasonography.

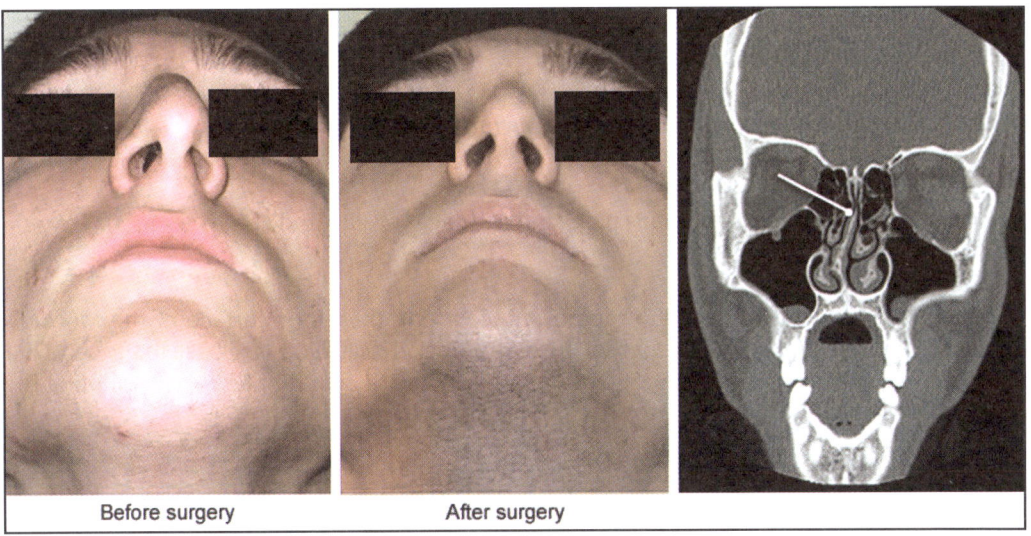

Fig. 7.46: Deviated nasal septum.

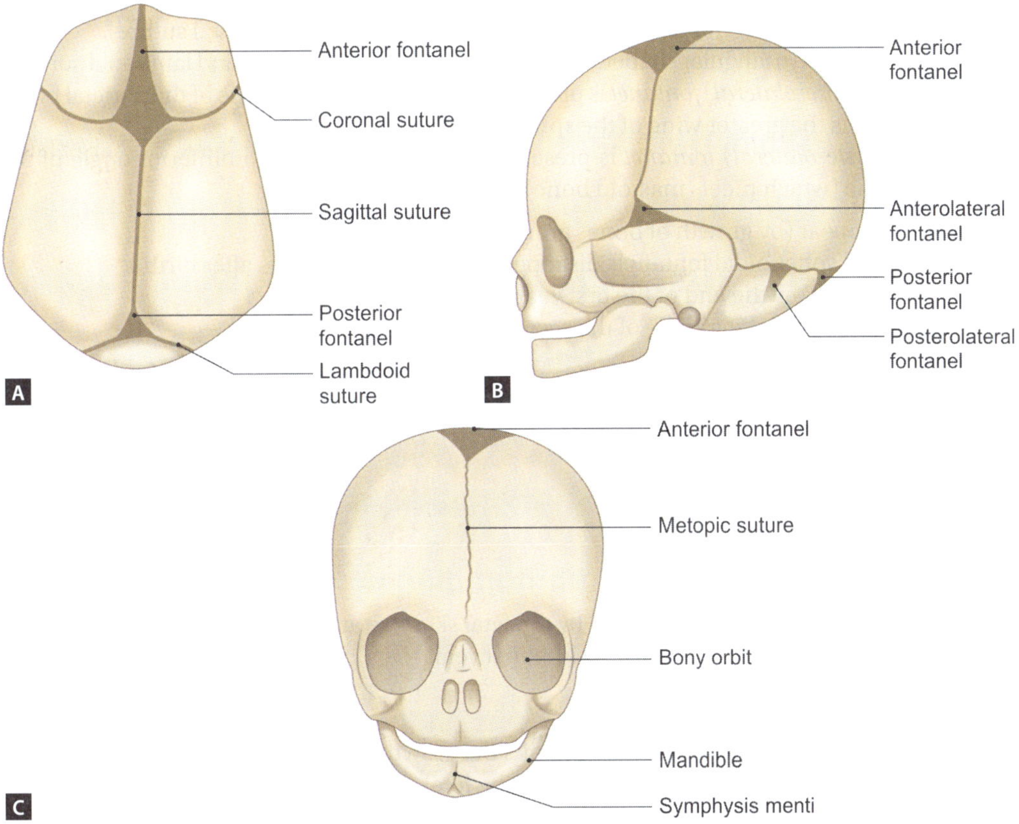

Figs. 7.47A to C: Fetal skull.

Temporal Bone

It ossifies by two processes:
- *Ossified in membrane:* Squamous part.
- *Ossified in cartilage:* Petromastoid, tympanic plate, and styloid process.

Occipital Bone

It develops in membrane (squamous part) and cartilage (basilar and condylar parts).

Mandible

It develops from two sources. The membrane covering the outer surface of the Meckel's cartilage forms the ramus and the part of the body. Meckel's cartilage gives rise to the condylar and coronoid processes and the part of the ramus above the mandibular canal including the lingula.

Fontanels

In newborn, there are some gaps in the vault of the skull that are filled by membrane. These gaps are fontanels (*fonticuli*). They are located in relation to the angles of the parietal bone. These include:
- *Anterior fontanel* (large and rhomboid shaped) lies at the junction of the sagittal, coronal and frontal sutures (at birth frontal bone is in two halves; separated by frontal suture).
- *Posterior fontanel* (triangular shaped) lies at the junction of the sagittal and lambdoid sutures.
- *Sphenoidal (anterolateral) fontanel* is present at the anteroinferior angle of the parietal bone, where it meets the greater wing of the sphenoid.
- *Mastoid (posterolateral) fontanel* is present in relation to the posteroinferior angle of the parietal bone (which meets mastoid bone).

Fontanels disappear (by growth of bones around them) after birth:
- Posterior and sphenoidal fontanels disappear within 2 or 3 months after birth
- Mastoid fontanel by the end of the first year
- Anterior fontanel by the middle of the second year.

Growth of Skull to Adult Size

Head circumference:
- In newborn: 14 inches
- At 4 months: 16 inches
- At 1 year: 18 inches
- At 5 years: 20 inches
- 7–10 years: 21 inches

Length and other dimensions gained by the fetal skull are attributed to the bone deposition and other factors. The maximum growth is in first year.

Mechanism of Growth

- *Sutural growth*: Mesenchymal tissue permits the growth at the sutures.
- *Endochondral growth*: Cartilaginous part of the fetal skull grows in all directions.
- *Surface accretion and resorption*: To meet the requirement of the growing structures, the capacity of the skull has to increase steadily and gradually. This is possible by deposition (accretion) of bone on the outer surface and resorption on the inner surface.

CHAPTER 7 ✦ Bones of Head and Neck

Features Influencing Skull Growth
- Appearance of dentition—growth of lower face
- Appearance of the paranasal sinuses
- General growth of the brain and the eyes
- Growth of upper face and nasal cavity due to increased respiratory need
- Development of the muscles of mastication
- Gender also influences the growth of the skull.

Growth in anteroposterior length: This takes place at the cartilaginous joints:
- Body of the sphenoid and the ethmoid
- Basiocciput with basisphenoid.

Growth in width: This takes place in:
- Sagittal suture
- Occipitomastoid suture
- Sutures around greater wing of sphenoid (sphenofrontal and sphenoparietal).

Growth in width: It is attained at:
- Frontozygomatic suture
- Pterion
- Asterion
- Squamosal suture (by temporal bone to parietal and sphenoid).

Closure of Sutures

It begins on the inner surface at around 30–40 years of age. At the outer surface, the process begins at about 40–50 years. There is a sequence of sutural obliteration beginning with the bregma and successively including sagittal, coronal, and the lambdoid sutures.

Craniometry

Anthropologists make use of measurements of indices of skull to compare them. Anthropometry is a wide technique which deals with the measurements of the entire body. Hence, craniometry is a part of the anthropometry. For this, certain bony land marks are used.

$$\text{Cephalic index} = \frac{\text{Breath}}{\text{Length}} \times 100$$

On the basis of cephalic index, the skull is classified as:
- Brachycephalic: 80.0–84.9
- Mesaticephalic: 75.0–79.9
- Dolichocephalic: 70–74.9.

Cranial Capacity

A reasonable estimate of the volume of the brain is 150–200 cc less than the cranial capacity. In male, the skull capacity on an average is 1,200–1,800 cc. In female, the capacity is 10% less.

Clinical Anatomy

Biparietal diameter: It is the maximum distance between the two parietal eminences **(Fig. 7.48)**. It is an important and reliable indicator of fetal growth—measured by

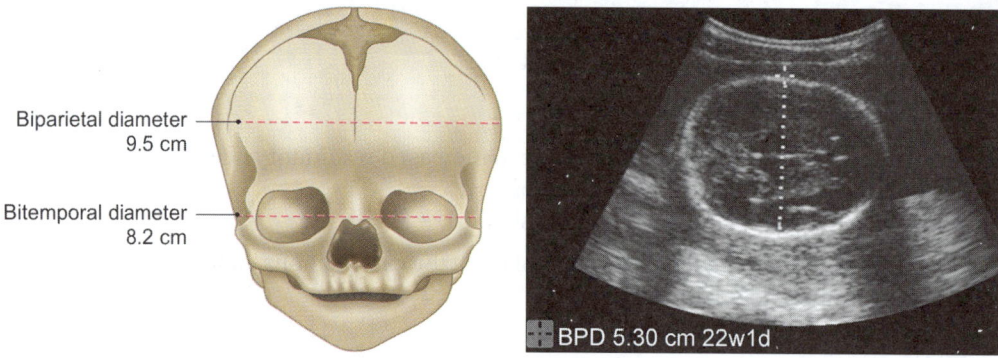

Fig. 7.48: Biparietal diameter.

ultrasonography. This distance increases with gestational age. In adults, this parameter is used in craniometry.

Anterior fontanel in infants (Fig. 7.49): In clinical practice, it is of invaluable help:
- Before its obliteration (18 months) abnormal bulging or depressed fontanel indicates increases or decreased intracranial tension and dehydration, respectively.
- Sample of CSF from the lateral ventricle can be obtained through it. The needle is passed downward and laterally through its lateral angle
- Superior sagittal sinus is accessed through it for intravenous injections
- By PV examination during delivery, anterior fontanel helps in determining presentation, position and attitude of the fetal head.

Fractures: The skull bones in a child are highly elastic. Their fracture is thus quite uncommon. However, in a localized blow depressed fracture may be seen, termed as *pond fracture* **(Fig. 7.50).**

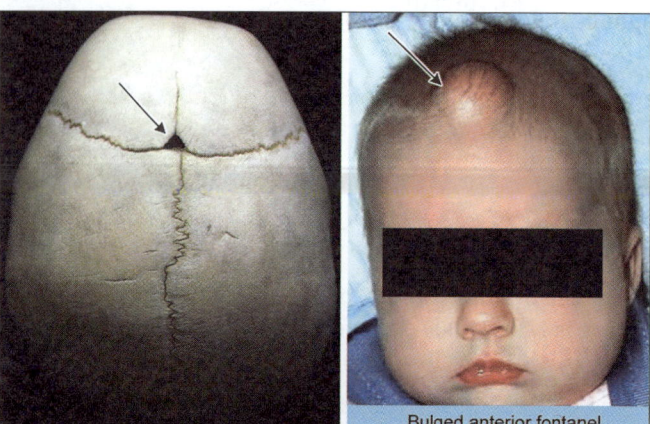
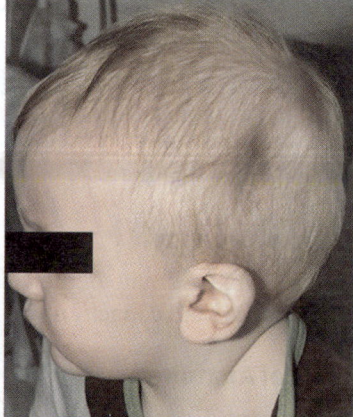

Fig. 7.49: Anterior fontanel. **Fig. 7.50:** Pond fracture.

CHAPTER 7 ✦ Bones of Head and Neck

QUESTIONNAIRE

- What is skull, cranium and the calvaria?
- Identify the sutures: Coronal, sagittal, and lambdoid.
- Identify the positions of various fontanels.
- Show these points and their importance: Bregma, lambda, pterion, asterion, glabella, suprameatal triangle, parietal eminence, and external occipital protuberance.
- Identify various fontanels in the adult skull.
- Show the attachments of the falx cerebri, falx cerebelli, tentorium cerebelli, and diaphragm sellae.
- Identify structures in the skull: Optic canal, foramen rotundum, foramen ovale, foramen spinosum, carotid canal, internal acoustic meatus, jugular foramen, hypoglossal canal, foramen magnum, foramen lacerum, supra and infraorbital foramina.
- Identify the fissures and enumerate the structures passing: Superior and inferior orbital fissures, pterygomaxillary fissure, and petrotympanic fissure.
- Identify crista galli. What is attached to it?
- What is a suture? Identify each type of suture in the skull.
- Identify clinoid processes. Name the structures attached to them.
- Identify the position of dural venous sinuses: Superior sagittal, cavernous, transverse, sigmoid, superior and inferior petrosal, sigmoid, and occipital.
- What is confluence of sinuses? Where it is present?
- Show clivus. Name the structures related to it.
- Show the course and relation with bone: Middle meningeal and internal carotid arteries.
- Show the course and relation with bone: Greater and lesser petrosal nerves.
- Identify cavum trigeminale. Name the structure located there.
- Identify styloid process. Enumerate the structures attached to it.
- Identify the various fontanels in the fetal skull.
- Enumerate various factors contributing to the growth of the fetal skull.

Individual Bones of Skull

CHAPTER 8

AN 26.4 Describe morphological features of mandible

MANDIBLE

The mandible consists of a U-shaped body, and two *rami* that project upward from the posterior part of the body. It has internal (medial) and external (lateral) surfaces. The body has an upper part that bears the teeth (*alveolar process*) and a lower border called the *base* **(Fig. 8.1)**.

Features

Ramus: It presents posterior border, a sharp anterior border, and a lower border that continues with the base of the body. The posterior and inferior borders of the ramus meet at the angle of the mandible. The anterior border of the ramus continues downward and forward on the lateral surface of the body as the *oblique line*. This line ends anteriorly near the *mental tubercle*. A little above the anterior part of the oblique line the *mental foramen* is seen that lies vertically below the second premolar tooth. Just below the incisor teeth the external surface of the ramus shows shallow *incisive fossa*.

Processes: Two processes arise from the upper part of the ramus. The anterior *coronoid process* is flat from side to side. The posterior *condylar process* is separated from the coronoid process by the *mandibular notch*. The upper end of the condylar process is expanded to form the head of the mandible.

Head: It is elongated transversely. Its smooth articular surface articulates with the mandibular fossa of the temporal bone to form the temporomandibular joint. The constricted part below the head is the *neck*. Its anterior surface has a rough depression called the *pterygoid fovea*.

Mandibular foramen: It is present a little above the center of the medial surface of the ramus foramen. It leads into the *mandibular canal* which runs forward within the bone. The medial margin of the foramen is formed by a projection called the *lingula*.

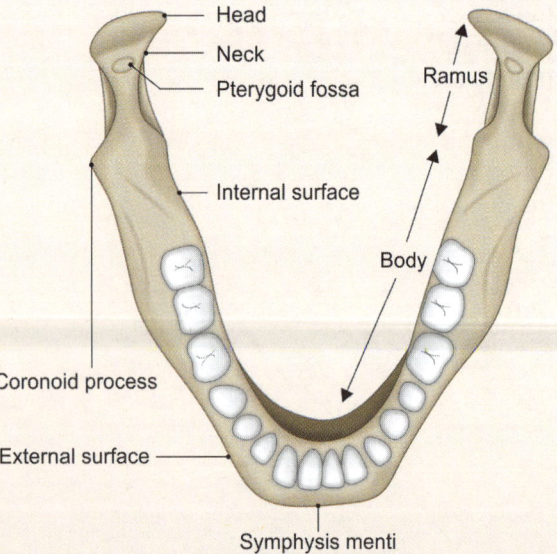

Fig. 8.1: Mandible seen from above.

Just behind the lingula, running downward and forward the *mylohyoid groove* is seen. A little above and anterior to the mylohyoid groove, the inner surface of the body of the mandible is marked by a ridge—the mylohyoid line. The posterior end of this line is just below and behind the third molar tooth. From here the line runs downward and forward to reach the symphysis menti. The mylohyoid line divides the inner surface of the body into a *sublingual fossa* (above mylohyoid line) and a *submandibular fossa* (below mylohyoid line).

Just below the anterior end of the mylohyoid line, the base of the mandible is marked by *digastric fossa*. In newborn, the mandible consists of right and left halves joined together at the *symphysis menti*; in later life two halves fuse to form one bone (**Figs. 8.2 and 8.3**).

When viewed from the front, the symphysis menti is marked by a slight ridge. Inferiorly, the ridge expands to form a triangular raised area called the *mental protuberance*. The lateral angles of the protuberance are prominent *mental tubercles*.

The posterior aspect of the symphysis menti also shows a median ridge the lower part of which is enlarged and may be divided into upper and lower parts called the mental spines (*genial tubercles*).

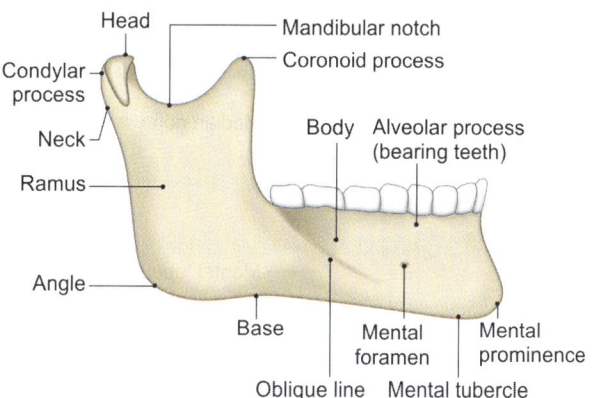

Fig. 8.2: Right half of mandible from the lateral side.

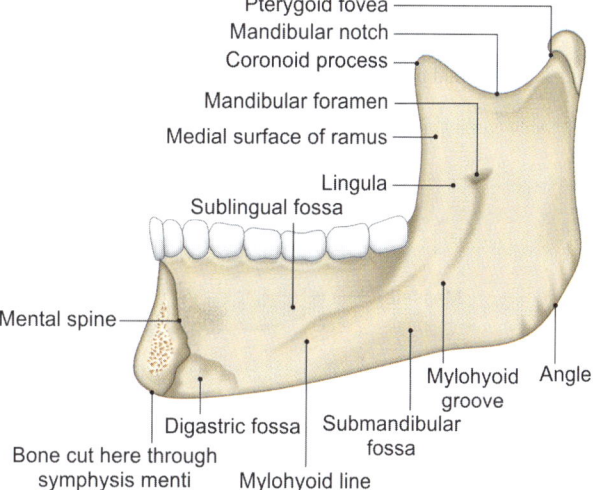

Fig. 8.3: Right half of the mandible from the medial side.

Attachments

Muscles on the External Aspect (Figs. 8.4 to 8.6)

Muscle	Attachment
Masseter	Lateral surface of the ramus and angle (*insertion*)
Buccinator	Outer surface of the body below molar teeth (*origin*)
Depressor labii inferioris	Anterior part of oblique line (*origin*)
Depressor anguli oris	Oblique line behind and below origin of depressor labii inferioris (*origin*)
Mentalis	Incisive fossa just below incisor teeth (*origin*)
Platysma (some fibers)	Lower border of the body (*insertion*)

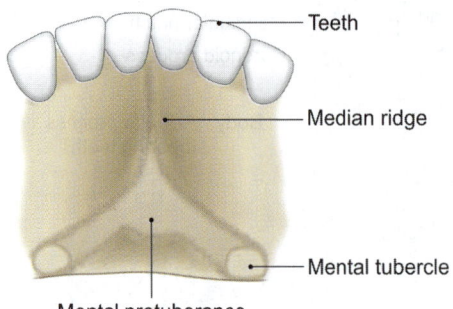

Fig. 8.4: Median part of the mandible: Anterior aspect.

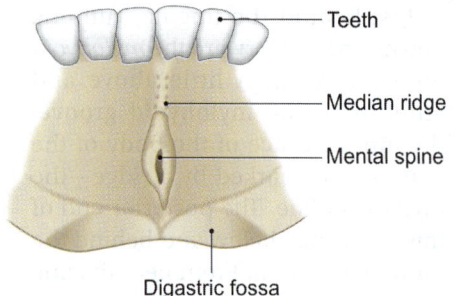

Fig. 8.5: Median part of mandible: Posterior aspect.

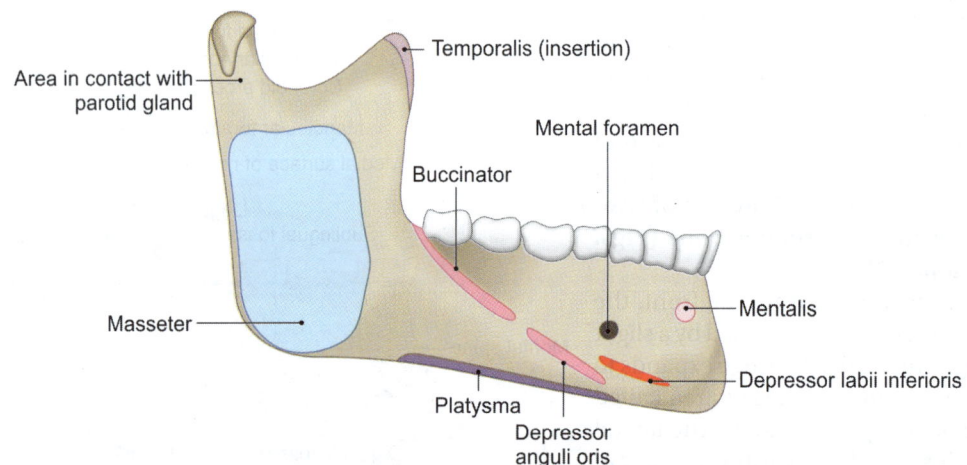

Fig. 8.6: Attachments on the mandible seen from the lateral side.

Muscles on the Internal Surface (Figs. 8.7 and 8.8)

Muscle	Attachment
Temporalis	Medial surface of coronoid process including its anterior and posterior borders; extends along anterior border of the ramus (*insertion*)
Lateral pterygoid	Fovea on the anterior aspect of neck (*insertion*)
Medial pterygoid	Medial surface of the angle and adjoining part of ramus (*insertion*)
Digastric (*anterior belly*)	Digastric fossa (*origin*)
Genioglossus	Upper mental spine (*origin*)
Geniohyoid	Lower mental spine (*origin*)
Mylohyoid	Mylohyoid line (*origin*)
Superior constrictor of pharynx	Posterior end of mylohyoid line near attachment of pterygomandibular raphe (*origin*)

CHAPTER 8 ✦ Individual Bones of Skull

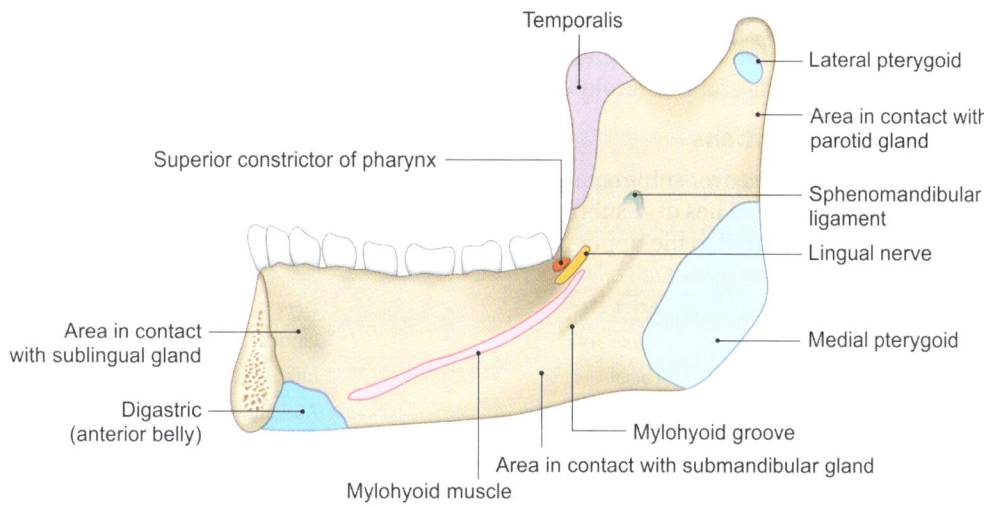

Fig. 8.7: Attachments on the mandible seen from the medial side.

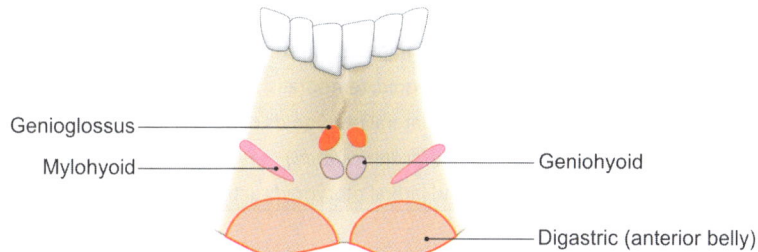

Fig. 8.8: Symphysis menti showing attachments, seen from behind.

Ligaments

Ligament	Attachment
Capsule of temporomandibular joint	Along the margins of the articular surface
Lateral temporomandibular ligament	Lateral aspect of the neck of the mandible
Sphenomandibular ligament	Lingula of the mandible
Stylomandibular ligament	Angle and posterior border of the ramus
Pterygomandibular raphe	Posterior end of the mylohyoid line

Mandible: Relations

Relations to Nerves and Vessels

- Masseteric nerve and vessels pass through the mandibular notch.
- Inferior alveolar nerve and vessels enter mandibular canal (*within bone*) through the mandibular foramen.
- Mylohyoid nerve and vessels run forward in the mylohyoid groove.
- Mental nerve and vessels emerge through the mental foramen.
- Lingual nerve is related above the posterior end of the mylohyoid line.

- Facial artery lies deep to ramus, near the angle. It then runs downwards and forwards; separated from the bone by the medial pterygoid muscle. It reaches lower border of the body of the mandible at the anteroinferior angle of masseter.

Salivary Glands: Relations
- **Sublingual gland** lies over sublingual fossa
- **Submandibular gland** lies over submandibular fossa
- **Parotid gland** is related to the upper part of the posterior border of the ramus.

Salivary glands	Arteries	Nerves
Parotid	Maxillary	Lingual
Submandibular	Facial	Inferior alveolar
Sublingual	Inferior alveolar	Auriculotemporal
	Masseteric	Masseteric
	Submental	Submental

Movements at Temporomandibular Joint (Fig. 8.9)

Movement	Muscles responsible
Depression (*opening of mouth*)	Lateral pterygoid and digastric
Elevation (*closing of mouth*)	Medial pterygoid, temporalis, and masseter
Protraction	Medial and lateral pterygoids of both sides
Retraction	Temporalis (*posterior fibers*)
Side to side movement	Medial and lateral pterygoids acting alternately

Mandible: Age Changes
Apart from fusion of the two halves of the bone and the progressive increase in size, the following points are noteworthy:
- *Prominence of chin* is absent at birth; forms during first and second year.
- *Direction of mental foramen* changes with age. In young it opens forwards; in the adult it opens backwards.

	Mental foramen	Opens below the sockets for deciduous molar teeth
	Mandibular canal	Runs near the lower border
	Angle of mandible	Obtuse (>140°)
At birth	Other features	Coronoid process is large; projects above the level of condyle
	Mental foramen	Opens midway between upper and lower borders
	Mandibular canal	Runs parallel with mylohyoid line
	Angle of mandible	110–120°
Adult	Other features	• Coronoid process is more or less at the same level as the condyle • Dentition/sockets for teeth are seen. Last molar appear 18–25 years
	Mental foramen	Opens close to alveolar border
	Mandibular canal	Runs close to alveolar border
	Angle of mandible	Obtuse (>140°)
Old age	Other features	Coronoid process projects above the level of condyle

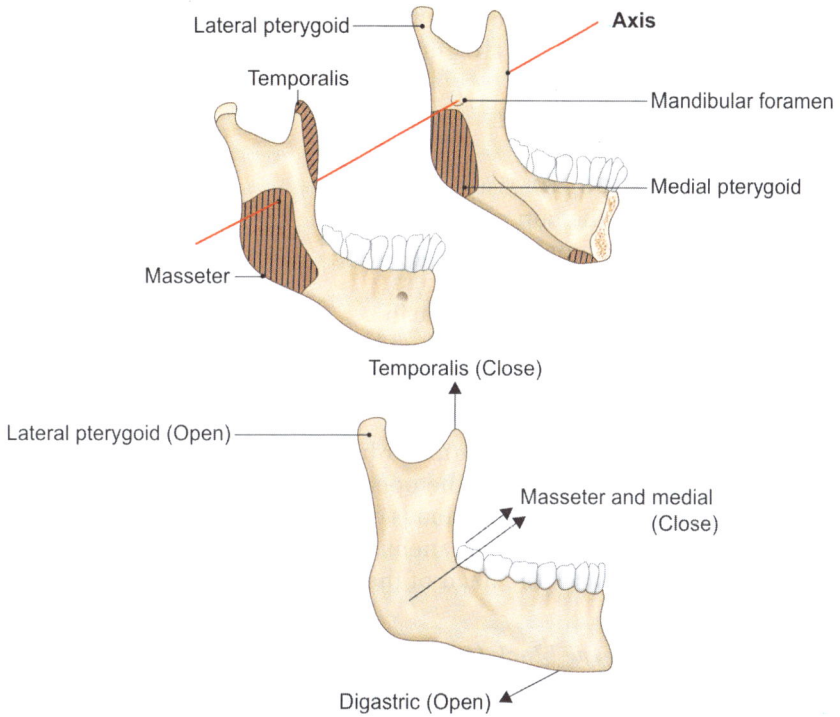

Fig. 8.9: Movements at temporomandibular joint.

Teeth Eruption

Teeth	LCI	UCI	ULI	LLI	Canines	1st PM	2nd PM	1st Molar	2nd Molar	3rd Molar
Temporary	5 months	6 months	7 months	8 months	18 months	X	X	1 year	2 years	X
Permanent	7 years	7 years	8 years	8 years	11 years	9 years	10 years	6 years	12 years	17–25 years

Gnathic (Alveolar) Index

Degree of projection of jaws is determined by this index. This represents proportion between basialveolar and basinasal lengths.

$$\frac{\text{Basialveolar length}}{\text{Basinasal Length}} \times 100$$

Development and Ossification

Greater part of mandible ossifies in the membrane in the mesenchyme of the mandibular process. Ossification of coronoid and condyloid processes is preceded by the formation of secondary cartilage.

Mandible is one of the first bones to start ossifying (*next to clavicle*). Each half is formed from one ossification center that appears (near mental foramen) during sixth week of fetal life. Small secondary centers may appear for genial tubercles.

At birth, the bone is in two halves—united at a fibrous joint (*symphysis menti*). Two halves unite between the first and third years of age.

Clinical Anatomy

Fractures of mandible (Fig. 8.10): Usually the mandible fractures occur on the opposite side of the blow. Frequently these fractures are bilateral. Commonly affected sites are coronoid process, mandibular neck, angle, and body of mandible in front of the mandibular foramen.

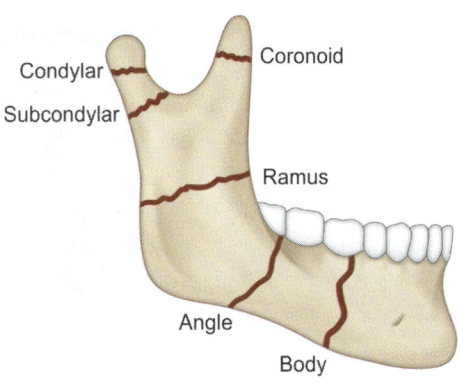

Fig. 8.10: Fracture of mandible.

Dislocation of temporomandibular joint (Figs. 8.11A and B): This may happen even without trauma. The forward dislocation of mandibular head is possible when the mouth is wide open (excessive yawning or a blow on the open mouth). The dislocated head comes to lie in the infratemporal region. The reduction is done by pressing the mandible down with the thumbs on the last molar teeth. Simultaneously upward pressure is applied at the chin (closure of mouth) which causes the head of the mandible to glide into the mandibular fossa.

Inferior alveolar/lingual nerve block (Fig. 8.12): To anesthetize the lower teeth, floor of the mouth and anterior two-thirds of the tongue adequately (for tooth extraction and root canal treatment), the inferior alveolar/lingual nerve is anesthetized. About half an inch above the crown of last molar tooth and just medial to the ramus of mandible, the needle is passed backwards and slightly outwards to infiltrate the nerve.

Referred pain from diseased tooth: Teeth of lower jaw are supplied by inferior alveolar nerve (branch of mandibular nerve). Thus, it is common to have pain from diseased tooth referred to external acoustic meatus—innervated by auriculotemporal nerve (branch of mandibular nerve).

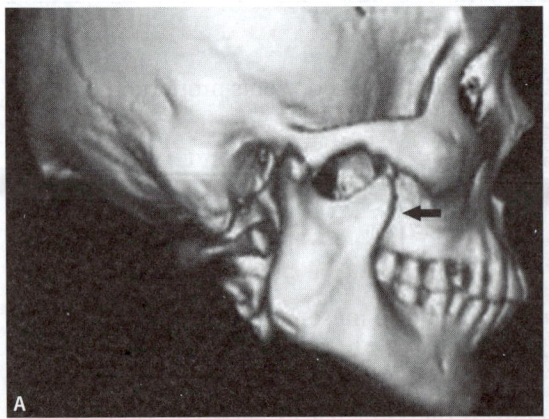 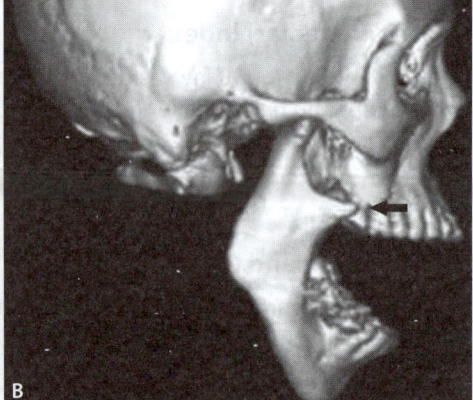

TMJ: Normal — TMJ: Dislocated

Figs. 8.11A and B: Dislocation of temporomandibular joint: (A) Normal; (B) Dislocated.

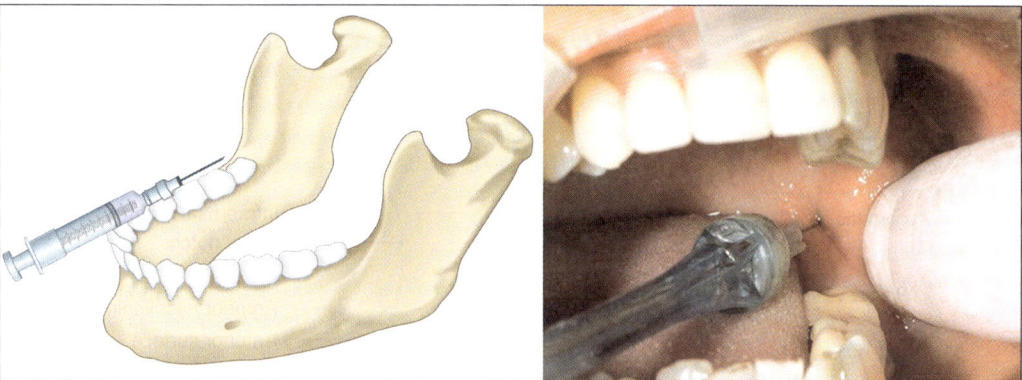

Fig. 8.12: Mandibular nerve block.

QUESTIONNAIRE

- Hold the bone in anatomical position and name its parts.
- Mark the nerves closely related to this bone.
- Mark the salivary glands related to the mandible.
- Mark the attachments of:

Ligaments	Muscles
Capsule of temporomandibular (TM) joint	Lateral pterygoid
Lateral ligament of TM joint	On the external aspect
Sphenomandibular	On the internal aspect
Stylomandibular	

- Comment on its ossification.
- Demonstrate the movements of the temporomandibular (TM) joint.
- What are the age changes in the mandible?
- What are the dental formulae for the temporary and permanent teeth?
- Show the arteries related to this bone.

MAXILLA

The right and left maxillae bear the upper teeth. Each maxilla takes part in forming (**Figs. 8.13 and 8.14**):
❖ Palate
❖ Floor and lateral wall of the nasal cavity
❖ Floor of the orbit.

Side Determination and Orientation

It is by examining the alveolar process. The alveolar process bearing teeth (or sockets for teeth) lies inferiorly and laterally. Sockets for the teeth reach the midline anteriorly. The maxilla presents:
❖ Body
❖ Alveolar process

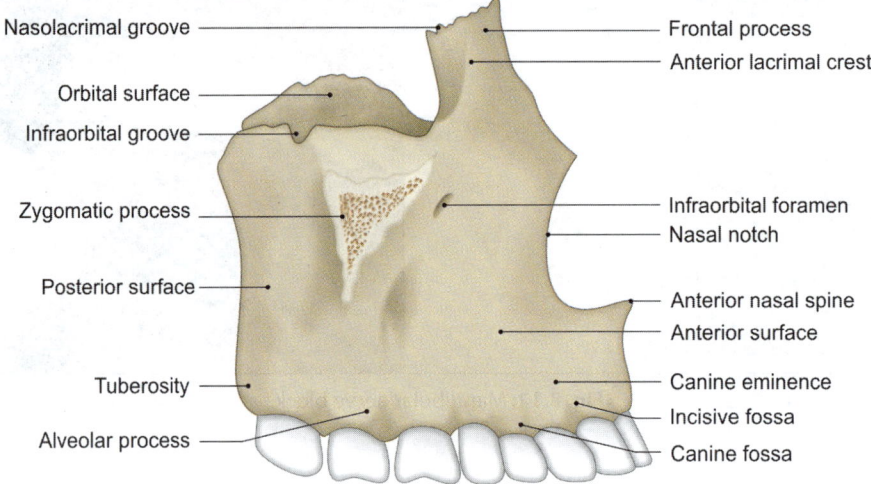

Fig. 8.13: Right maxilla: Lateral aspect.

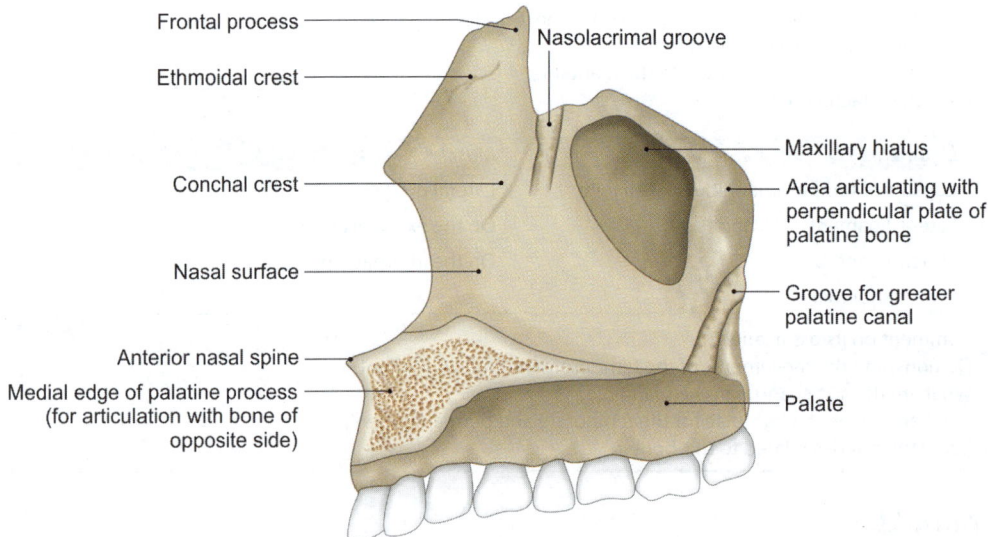

Fig. 8.14: Right maxilla: Medial aspect.

- Zygomatic process
- Frontal process
- Palatine process.

Features

Body

The body has anterior (anterolateral), posterior, medial, and superior surfaces. Inferiorly, it continues with the alveolar process. The body encloses the maxillary air sinus.

The upper margin of the *anterior surface* continues forms the inferior margin of the orbit. Medially, the anterior surface ends at the nasal notch which bounds the anterior nasal aperture.

Features seen include the infraorbital foramen, incisive and canine fossae, canine eminence, and the anterior nasal spine.

Superior (orbital) *surface* forms the floor of the orbit. Posterolaterally, it forms the lower margin of the inferior orbital fissure. The infraorbital groove runs forward over the orbital surface. This groove continues with the infraorbital canal; opens on the anterior surface at infraorbital foramen. Anteromedially, the orbital surface has a notch; forms the lateral margin of the upper opening of the nasolacrimal canal. The margins of the orbital surface articulate with the zygomatic, ethmoid, lacrimal, and the orbital process of the palatine bone.

Medial (nasal) *surface* takes part in forming the lateral wall of the nose. Its features include the maxillary hiatus, nasolacrimal groove, groove for greater palatine canal, and the conchal crest. This comes in contact with the palatine, ethmoid, and lacrimal bones, and the inferior nasal concha.

Posterior (infratemporal) *surface* forms the anterior wall of the infratemporal fossa and the pterygopalatine fossa. Inferiorly, it shows the maxillary tuberosity; posterior end of the alveolar process. The upper margin of this surface continues with the orbital surface at the inferior orbital fissure. Here, the surface is grooved by the maxillary nerve. Lower down, the infratemporal surface bears small openings for the posterior superior alveolar nerves and vessels. The infratemporal surface meets the pterygoid process of the sphenoid bone at the lower end of the pterygomaxillary fissure.

Zygomatic Process

This thick and strong process projects laterally from the junction of the anterior and infratemporal surfaces. It articulates with the zygomatic bone.

Palatine Process

It passes medially and forms the greater part of the hard palate. The features include intermaxillary suture, incisive fossa and incisive foramina. Posteriorly, it meets horizontal plate of the palatine bone at the *palatomaxillary suture*.

The upper surface of the palatine process forms the floor of the nasal cavity. On this surface, bone is thickened along the intermaxillary suture to form *nasal crest* which articulates with the vomer. The crest is more pronounced at its anterior end; seen in the floor of the anterior nasal aperture as the *anterior nasal spine*.

Frontal Process

This extends upward and medially from the body. Its upper edge meets the nasal part of the frontal bone. Medially (and anteriorly) it articulates with the nasal bone; and posteriorly it articulates with the lacrimal bone. The frontal process has external and internal surfaces. The external surface shows a vertical ridge called the anterior lacrimal crest. This crest continues with the inferior orbital margin. Behind this crest there is a vertical groove which forms the lacrimal groove along with the groove on the lacrimal bone.

Maxilla: Age Changes

- ❖ *At birth*: Transverse and anteroposterior diameters are greater than vertical diameter. Frontal process is well-marked. Body consists of little more than alveolar process; teeth sockets up to the orbital floor. Maxillary sinus is just a furrow on the lateral wall of nose.

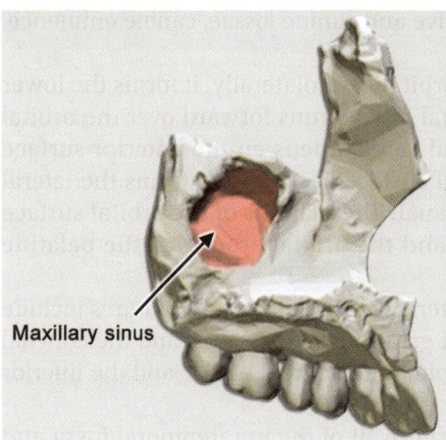
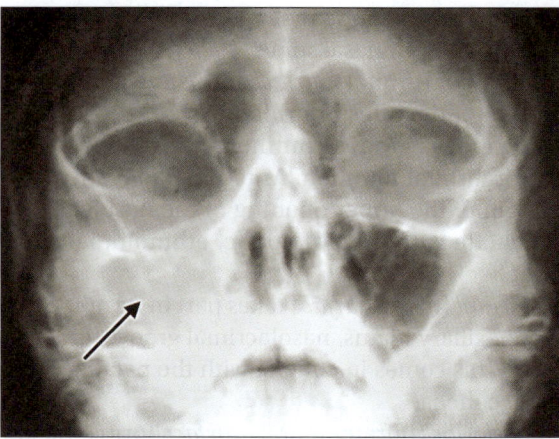

Fig. 8.15: Maxillary sinusitis.

❖ *In adult:* Vertical diameter is greatest; due to development of alveolar process and increase in sinus size.
❖ *In old age:* Bone height is diminished. After loss of teeth, alveolar process is absorbed. Lower part of the bone contracted and reduced in thickness.

Development and Ossification

The maxilla ossifies in membrane from two centers (one for maxilla proper; one for premaxilla). These centers appear during sixth week of fetal life; unite in the beginning of the third month.

Suture between two portions persists on the palate until nearly middle life. The frontal process develops from both centers.

Maxillary air sinus appears as a shallow groove on the nasal surface at the fourth month of fetal life. It develops fully after the second dentition.

Clinical Anatomy

Maxillary sinusitis (Fig. 8.15): It requires surgical intervention to drain stagnated inflammatory exudates by making an opening through incisive fossa called *Caldwell-Luc operation*. It is carried out when drainage of maxillary sinus fails.

Cleft lip (Harelip): This congenital anomaly consists of one or more clefts in upper lip **(Fig. 8.16)**. This results from failure of fusion of maxillary and median nasal processes in embryonic life.

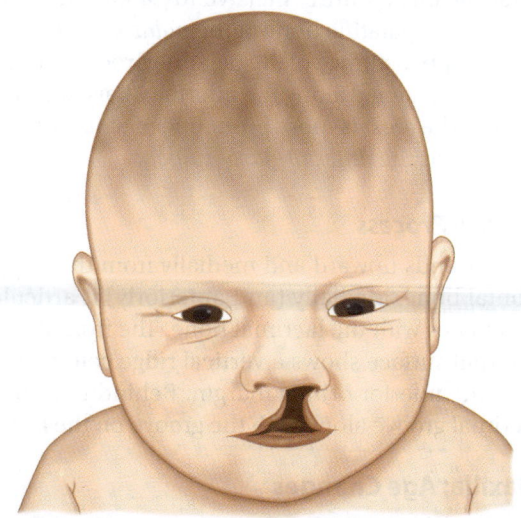

Fig. 8.16: Cleft lip.

CHAPTER 8 ✦ Individual Bones of Skull

📋 QUESTIONNAIRE

- Hold the bone in anatomical position and identify the side it belongs.
- Classify the bone and identify its parts.
- Enumerate the articulations of maxilla.
- Mark the attachments on the maxillary tuberosity.
- Identify the maxillary hiatus. What structures reduce it in the living?
- Show the orbital surface and name the groove on the orbital surface.
- Enumerate the structures passing through the orbital groove.
- Show the infratemporal surface. Name the nerves and vessels related here.
- Comment on its ossification.

ZYGOMATIC BONE

The zygomatic bone forms the prominence of the cheek. Parts of it are seen in the orbit and the anterior walls of the temporal and infratemporal fossae (**Figs. 8.17 and 8.18**).

Side Determination

The bone is orientated and its side determined by looking at the orbital margin. The orbital margin lies at the upper end of the anterior aspect. This margin contributes to the inferior and lateral margins of the orbit.

Articulations

- Body (anteromedially) with maxilla
- Frontal process with zygomatic process of frontal bone
- Temporal process with zygomatic process of temporal bone.

Zygomatic bone consists of:
- Body
- Frontal process
- Temporal process.

Features

Body and surfaces: It presents lateral, temporal, and orbital surfaces.

Lateral surface forms the prominence of cheek; perforated by the zygomaticofacial foramen (*or foramina*).

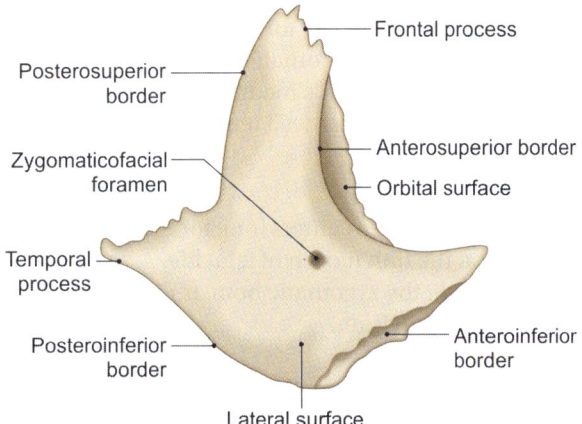

Fig. 8.17: Right zygomatic bone: Lateral aspect.

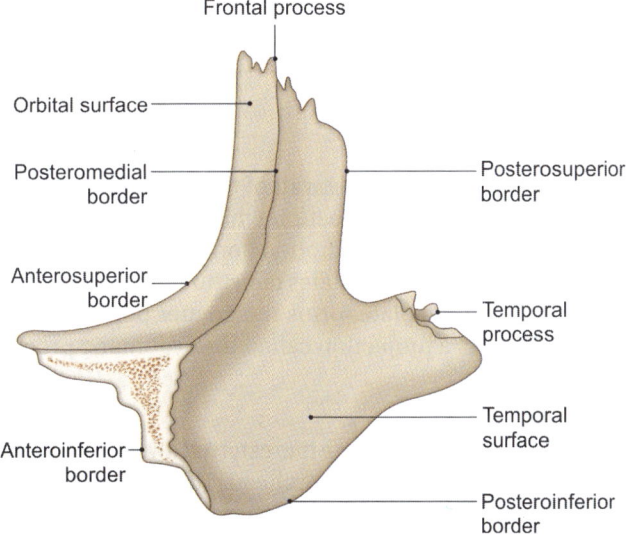

Fig. 8.18: Right zygomatic bone: Medial aspect.

Temporal surface (directed medially and posteriorly) forms anterior wall of the temporal fossa; also contributes to the anterior wall of infratemporal fossa. It is pierced by the zygomaticotemporal foramen.

Orbital surface forms part of the lateral wall of the orbit. Posteriorly, it meets the greater wing of sphenoid from which it is partially separated by the inferior orbital fissure. Medially it meets orbital surface of the maxilla.

Lateral surface is demarcated by four borders: (a) anterosuperior (orbital), (b) anteroinferior (maxillary), (c) posterosuperior (temporal), and (d) posteroinferior.

- *Anterosuperior border* is curved; forms parts of the inferior and lateral orbital margins and separates lateral surface from the orbital surface.
- *Anteroinferior border* articulates with the zygomatic process of maxilla.
- *Posterosuperior border* extends from the frontozygomatic suture to the zygomaticotemporal suture; separates the lateral and temporal surfaces.
- *Posteroinferior border* forms the anterior part of the lower border of the zygomatic arch; extends from the zygomaticomaxillary suture to the zygomaticotemporal suture.

Temporal surface ends medially in a posteromedial border; articulates with the greater wing of sphenoid (in anterior wall temporal fossa) and inferiorly with the maxilla.

Ossification

It ossifies from three centers (one for malar; two for orbital portion); appear about eighth week and fuse at the fifth month of fetal life.

After birth, the zygomatic bone is divided by a horizontal suture into an upper larger and a lower smaller division.

> **QUESTIONNAIRE**
> - Hold the bone in anatomical position and identify the side it belongs.
> - Enumerate its parts.
> - Enumerate the articulations of zygomatic bone.
> - Name the foramina seen and the structures passing through them.
> - Comment on its ossification.

FRONTAL BONE

The frontal bone forms the wall of the cranial cavity in the region of the forehead. It ends in a median downward projection which constitutes its nasal part. On either side of the nasal part, the lower edge of the frontal bone forms the superior margin of the corresponding orbit. The right and left orbital plates constitute its orbital part. Passing backward from each orbital margin the orbital plate forms the greater part of the roof of the orbit. Lateral to the orbital margin there is a projection called the zygomatic process **(Figs. 8.19 and 8.20)**.

Features

Main part: The frontal bone has external and internal surfaces. The greater part of the external surface corresponds to the forehead. This part is bounded on each side by a prominent ridge that continues anteriorly with the upper border of the zygomatic process and posteriorly with

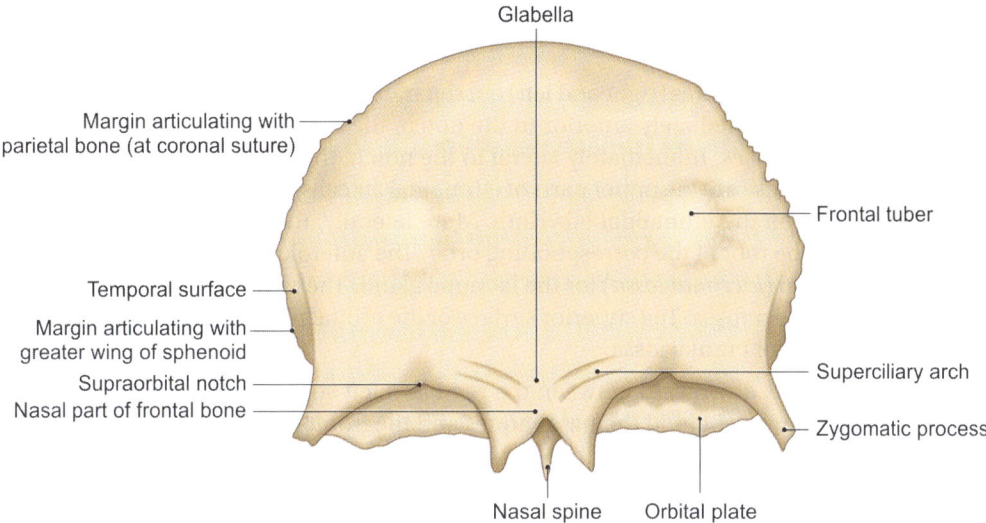

Fig. 8.19: Frontal bone from the front.

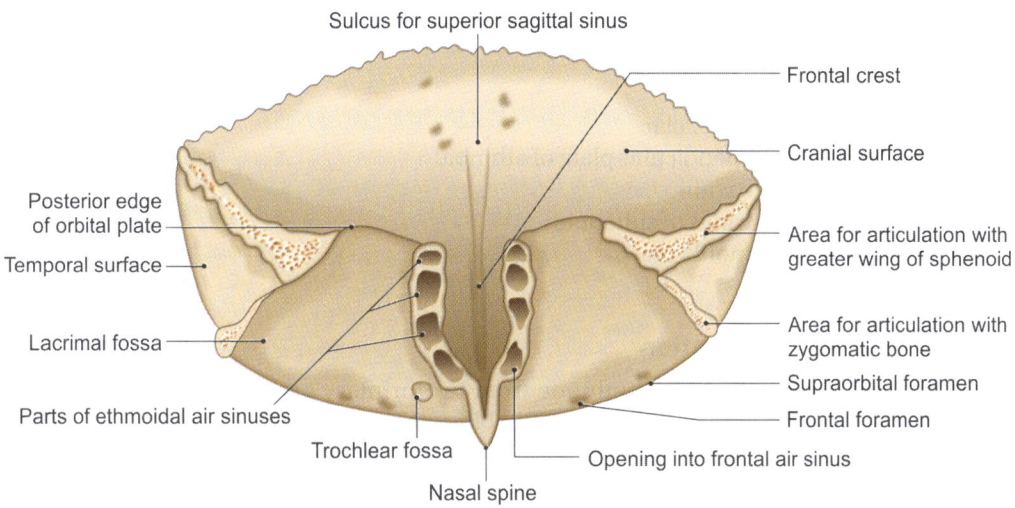

Fig. 8.20: Fontal bone from below.

the temporal lines. The part of the external surface behind this ridge and below the temporal lines forms part of the floor of the temporal fossa.

The features seen on the part of the external surface corresponding to the forehead are the frontal tuber (eminence), superciliary arches, glabella, supraorbital notch (*or foramen*), and frontal notch (*or foramen*). The internal surface is marked by a median sulcus for the superior sagittal sinus. The lips of this sulcus fuse to form a median ridge called the *frontal crest*. At the lower end of the crest the *foramen cecum* is seen.

Zygomatic process: It passes downward and laterally; joins the frontal process of the zygomatic bone.

Orbital part: The orbital plates (right and left) are separated by a wide notch; filled by ethmoid bone in intact skull. Immediately anterior to the notch, there are the openings into the right and left frontal air sinuses. Immediately lateral to the notch, the inferior aspect shows two or three depressions. These are the upper parts of ethmoidal air cells; completed in the intact skull by the depressions on the ethmoidal labyrinth. More laterally, the inferior surface forms the greater portion of the roof of the corresponding orbit. The anterolateral part of the roof shows a shallow depression (*lacrimal fossa*) for the lacrimal gland. The anteromedial part of the roof shows a small trochlear fossa. The superior surface of the orbital plate forms the greater part of the floor of the anterior cranial fossa.

Nasal part: It projects downward between the right and left supraorbital margins. The lower part of the projection lies behind the nasal bones and the frontal process of the maxillae. The nasal part bears the nasal spine; contributes to the nasal septum.

Articulations

- Posteriorly articulates with:
  - Right and left parietal bones (*at coronal suture*)
  - Greater wing of sphenoid
- Through zygomatic process it articulates with zygomatic bone
- Nasal part articulates with:
  - Nasal bones
  - Frontal processes of maxillae.
- Nasal spine meets: Perpendicular plate of ethmoid
- Orbital parts articulate with:
  - Greater and lesser wings of sphenoid
  - Orbital plate of ethmoid
  - Lacrimal bone.

Development and Ossification

The frontal bone is ossified in membrane from two primary centers (one for each half); appear at the end of the second month of fetal life, above each supraorbital margin. From each center ossification extends to form the corresponding half of the squamous part and the orbital plate.

The spine is ossified from two secondary centers, on either side of the middle line. Similar centers appear in the nasal part and zygomatic processes.

At birth the bone consists of two pieces separated by the frontal suture; usually obliterated by the eighth year (occasionally persists as *metopic suture*).

The frontal air sinuses are rudimentary at birth; develop fully after puberty.

Clinical Anatomy

Metopic suture: The lower part of the interfrontal suture (metopic suture) may persist in about 8% population. In a radiograph of the skull (AP view) it may be mistaken for a fracture (**Fig. 8.21**).

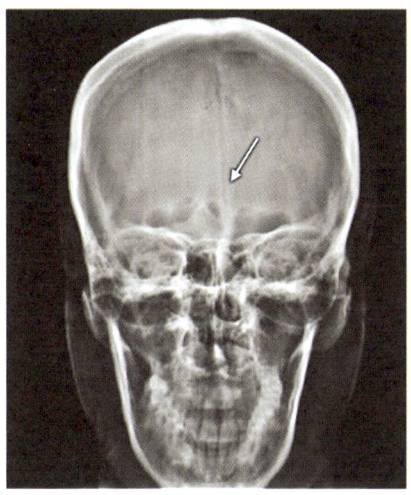 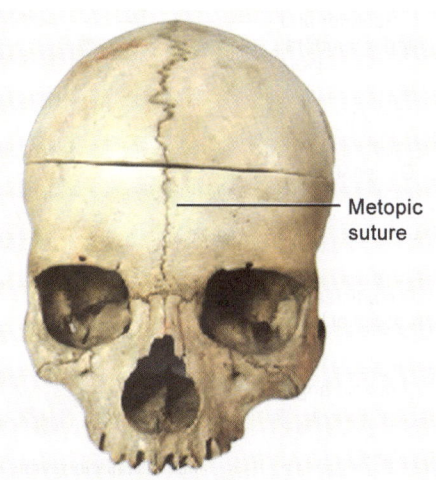

Fig. 8.21: Metopic suture.

Sinusitis: Inflammation of mucosal lining of paranasal sinuses is *sinusitis*. Frontal sinusitis causes heaviness and pain in the forehead. It may be a complication of upper respiratory infection or structural defect of nose.

Fracture of the frontal bone: In adults, localized injury to the bone causes a depressed comminuted fracture. The severity of the impact causing bleeding results in a black eye.

> **QUESTIONNAIRE**
> - Hold the bone in anatomical position and name its parts.
> - How would you classify this bone?
> - Enumerate the articulations of the frontal bone.
> - Mark the attachments of frontalis and orbicularis oculi.
> - What is metopic suture? What is its clinical relevance?
> - When does interfrontal suture close and in which direction?
> - Comment on its ossification.

PARIETAL BONE

The right and left parietal bones form the greater part of the roof and side walls of the cranial cavity. Each bone has an external surface and an internal surface **(Figs. 8.22 and 8.23)**.

Side Determination

- Superior (sagittal) border is straight; inferior border is irregular shaped
- Posteroinferior angle bears a groove for sigmoid sinus
- Medial surface is concave; lateral surface is convex.

Features

On the external surface it presents parietal tuber (eminence), superior and inferior temporal lines, and the parietal foramen.

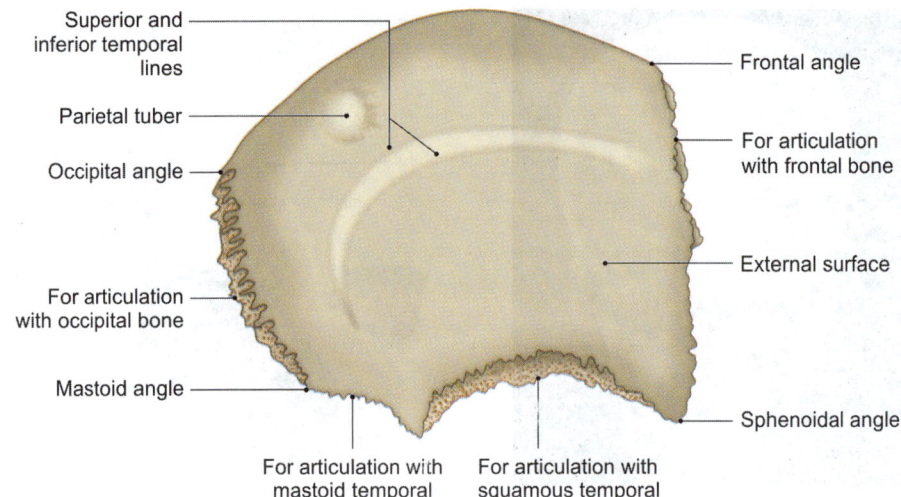

Fig. 8.22: Right parietal bone: Lateral aspect.

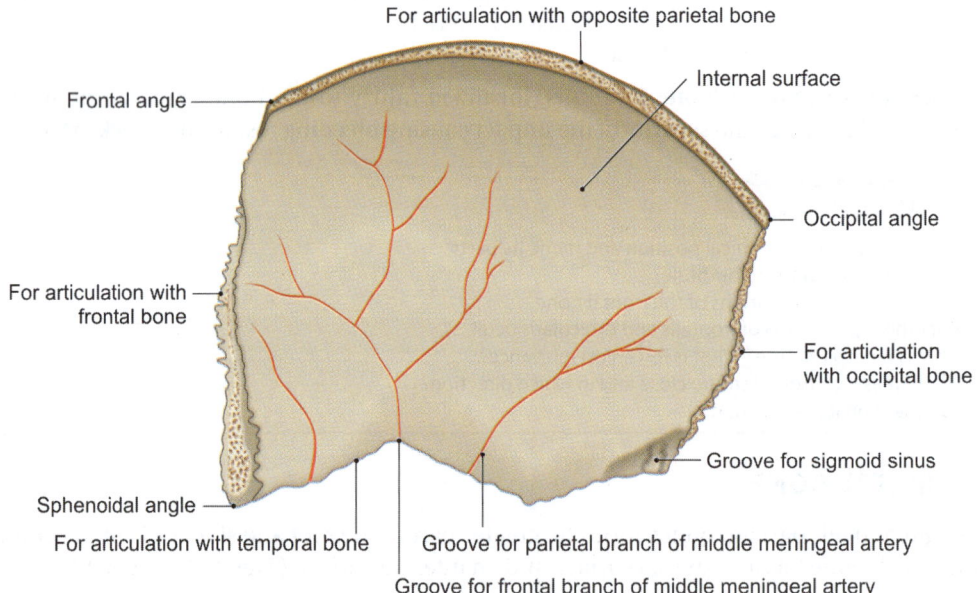

Fig. 8.23: Right parietal bone: Medial aspect.

The internal surface bears grooves for the frontal and parietal branches of the middle meningeal vessels. The posteroinferior angle presents a groove for part of the sigmoid sinus. There is a groove for the superior sagittal sinus along the upper border.

Articulations

- Right and left parietal bones articulate with each other at the sagittal suture.
- Anteriorly, each parietal bone articulates with the frontal bone at the coronal suture.

- Anteroinferior angle articulates with the greater wing of sphenoid.
- Inferior border articulates with the temporal bone (squamous and mastoid).
- Posterior border articulates with the occipital bone (at lambdoid suture).

Ossification

It ossifies in membrane from a single center; appears at the parietal eminence about eighth week of fetal life. Ossification extends in a radial manner from the center toward the bone margins; the angles form last. Occasionally, it is divided into two parts (upper and lower) by an anteroposterior suture.

Clinical Anatomy

Fig. 8.24: Parietal emissary foramen.

Parietal emissary foramen: This foramen (one in each bone close to sagittal suture) transmits emissary vein that connects superior sagittal sinus with scalp vein **(Fig. 8.24)**. These channels are valveless and blood can flow in either direction. Thus, an infection of scalp may pass through emissary veins to superior sagittal sinus resulting in sinus thrombosis or meningitis.

Pterion: At this bony landmark four bones meet namely: anteroinferior angle of parietal, squamous temporal, greater wing of sphenoid, and frontal bone **(Fig. 8.25)**. It is two fingers breadth above zygomatic arch and two-finger breadth behind orbital margin. Deep to it, anterior branch of middle meningeal vessels are related. This site is preferred for cerebral decompression by making a trephine hole.

Fractures of parietal bone: This involves maximum convexity—parietal eminence. This may be due to direct blow or in road traffic accidents.

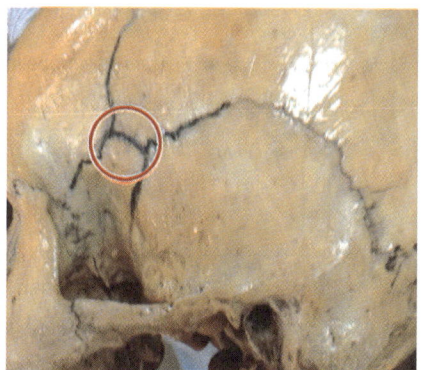 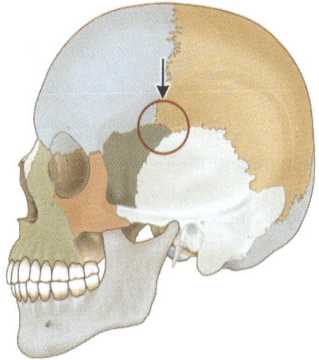

Fig. 8.25: Pterion.

> **QUESTIONNAIRE**
>
> - Anatomical position side determination.
> - How would you classify this bone?
> - Enumerate its articulations.
> - Identify parietal emissary foramen. Name the structures passing through it.
> - What is parietal eminence? What is its clinical relevance?
> - Comment on its ossification.

OCCIPITAL BONE

This unpaired bone lies in the posterior part of the skull. It is pierced by the *foramen magnum*. The part behind the foramen magnum is the *squamous part*; the part anterior to the foramen magnum is the *basilar part*; and the parts on either side of the foramen are the *condylar* (lateral) *parts*.

Features

Squamous part: It contributes to the posterior wall of the vault of the skull. It has external and internal surfaces. The features on the external surface include external occipital protuberance; external occipital crest and the nuchal lines (*highest, superior and inferior*). The internal surface is marked by four deep fossae. The area where the fossae meet is raised to form the *internal occipital protuberance*. Above the protuberance there is a wide median groove for the *superior sagittal sinus*; and on either side of the protuberance there is an equally wide groove for the *transverse sinus*. These grooves have prominent lips. Inferior to the protuberance, the internal surface presents a median ridge called the *internal occipital crest* (**Figs. 8.26 and 8.27**).

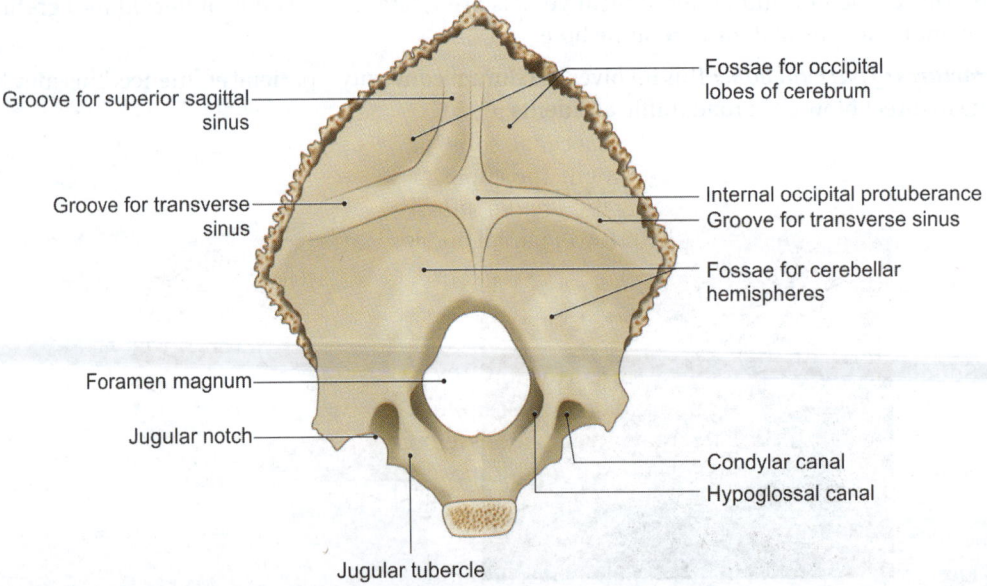

Fig. 8.26: Occipital bone: Anterosuperior view.

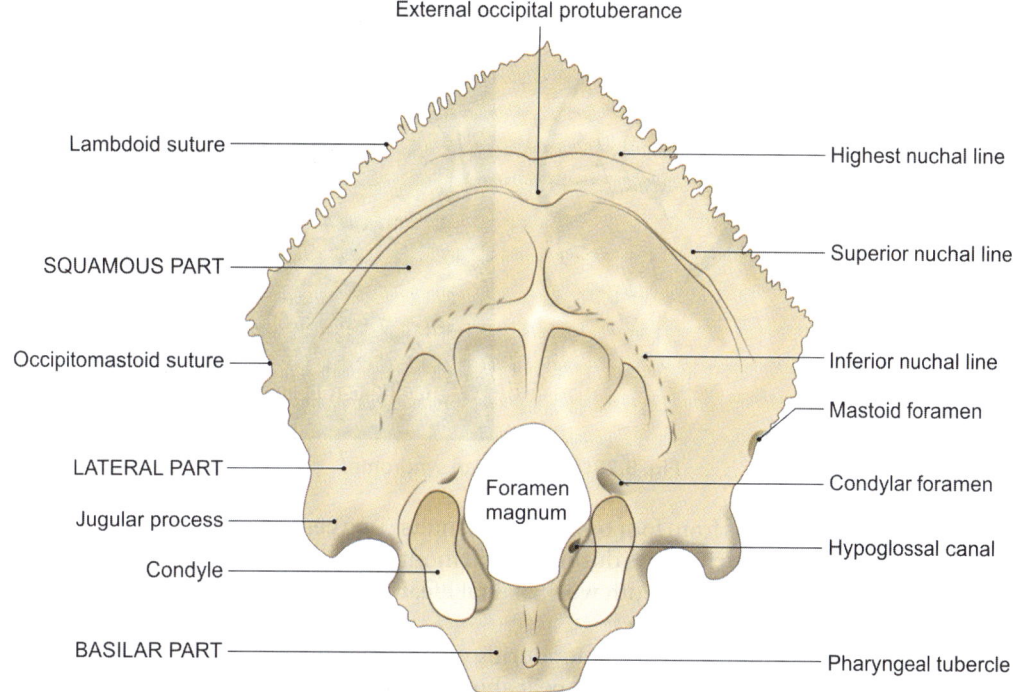

Fig. 8.27: Occipital bone: Posteroinferior view.

Basilar part: It lies in front of the foramen magnum. In adults, it directly continues with the body of the sphenoid; in the young, they are separated by a plate of cartilage. The inferior surface shows the *pharyngeal tubercle*. The superior surface forms the sloping median portion of the anterior wall of the posterior cranial fossa (*clivus*).

Lateral part: It shows superior and inferior surfaces. The features seen on the inferior surface include occipital condyles, hypoglossal canal, condylar fossa, condylar canal, jugular process, jugular fossa, and the jugular foramen. The superior surface forms part of the floor of the posterior cranial fossa. It presents the *jugular tubercle*. The superior aspect of the jugular process shows a deep groove for the lower part of the sigmoid sinus. The groove continues with the jugular foramen.

Articulations

- Squamous part articulates with corresponding parietal bone at lambdoid suture and corresponding mastoid temporal bone at occipitomastoid suture.
- Anterior margin of the lateral part meets petrous temporal; partially separated by jugular fossa.
- Anteriorly, basilar part is separated from the apex of petrous temporal by foramen lacerum.

Development and Ossification

- Occipital bone above highest nuchal lines develops in the membrane; rest part develops in the cartilage.

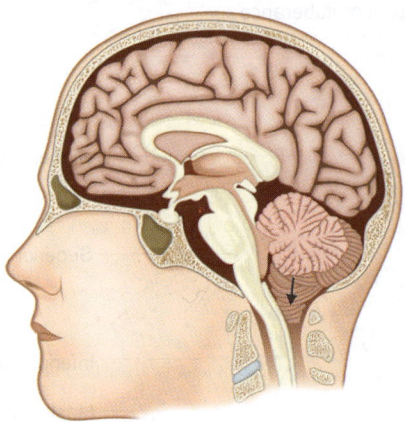
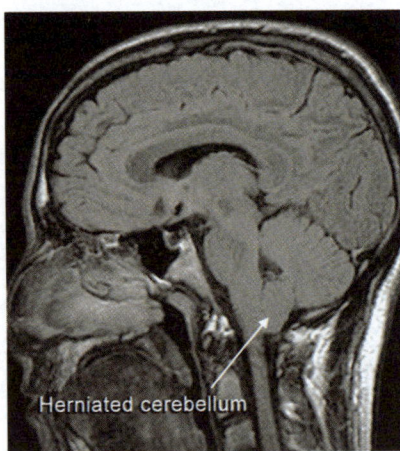

Fig. 8.28: Arnold-Chiari syndrome.

- *Squamous part* develops from four ossification centers. Two centers appear near the middle line above the highest nuchal lines during second month and two centers some little distance from the middle line about seventh week of fetal life. Union of upper and lower parts takes place in the third postnatal life.
- *Lateral part* ossifies from a single center during eighth week of fetal life.
- *Basilar part* ossifies from two centers; appear about sixth week of fetal life which soon coalesce.
- At fourth year squamous and two lateral parts unite; about sixth year the bone consists of a single piece.
- Between 18 years and 25 years, occipital, and sphenoid bones unite.

Clinical Anatomy

Arnold–Chiari syndrome: It is the most common congenital anomaly that involves cerebellum. The cerebellar vermis herniates into vertebral canal through the foramen magnum **(Fig. 8.28)**. This anomaly results in *communicating hydrocephalus*. The interference in the absorption of the CSF results in the dilatation of ventricular system. The anomaly is frequently associated with spina bifida with meningomyelocele.

> **QUESTIONNAIRE**
> - Hold the bone in anatomical position and name its parts.
> - How would you classify this bone?
> - Enumerate the articulations of this bone.
> - Identify foramen magnum. Enumerate the structures passing through it.
> - Show anterior and posterior condylar canals. Name the structures passing through them.
> - Mark the muscles attached on the nuchal lines and the intervening area between them.
> - Comment on its ossification.

TEMPORAL BONE

Each temporal bone is made up of squamous, petrous, mastoid, tympanic, and styloid parts. Its lateral aspect is marked by a prominent zygomatic process and by the external acoustic meatus.

Side Determination

❖ Zygomatic process is on the lateral side; directed forward
❖ Mastoid and styloid processes point downward.

Features

Squamous part: It contributes to lateral wall of skull, part of the base of skull and the part of the floor of the middle cranial fossa.

It has external (*temporal*) and internal (*cerebral*) surfaces. Zygomatic process arises from its external aspect. It joins the temporal process of the zygomatic bone to form the zygomatic arch (*zygoma*). Inferiorly, squamous part presents the mandibular fossa for articulation with the head of the mandible.

Features on the lateral aspect of the squamous temporal bone include temporal lines, supramastoid crest, anterior and posterior roots of the zygomatic process, tubercle of the root of zygoma, postglenoid tubercle, and suprameatal triangle. The inferior aspect of the squamous temporal bone presents mandibular fossa and the articular tubercle **(Figs. 8.29 to 8.31)**.

The cerebral surface of the squamous part forms the lateral portion of the floor and the lateral wall of the middle cranial fossa.

Mastoid part: It lies behind the external acoustic meatus. It presents a large downward projection called the *mastoid process*. Medial to the mastoid process, there is a deep mastoid

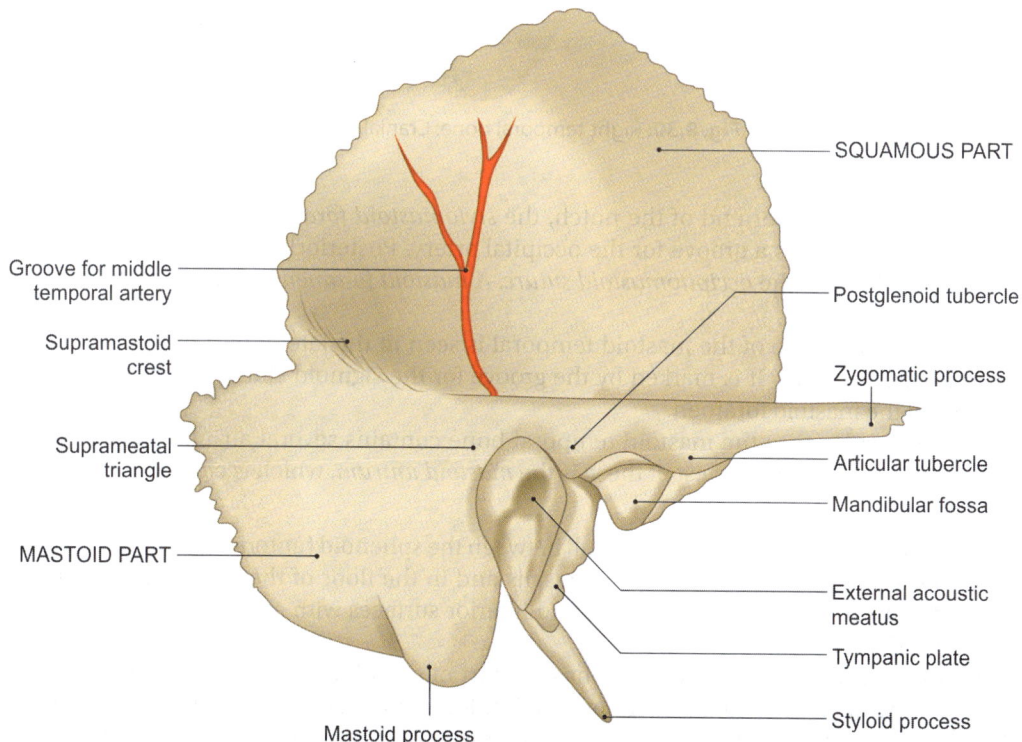

Fig. 8.29: Right temporal bone: Lateral aspect.

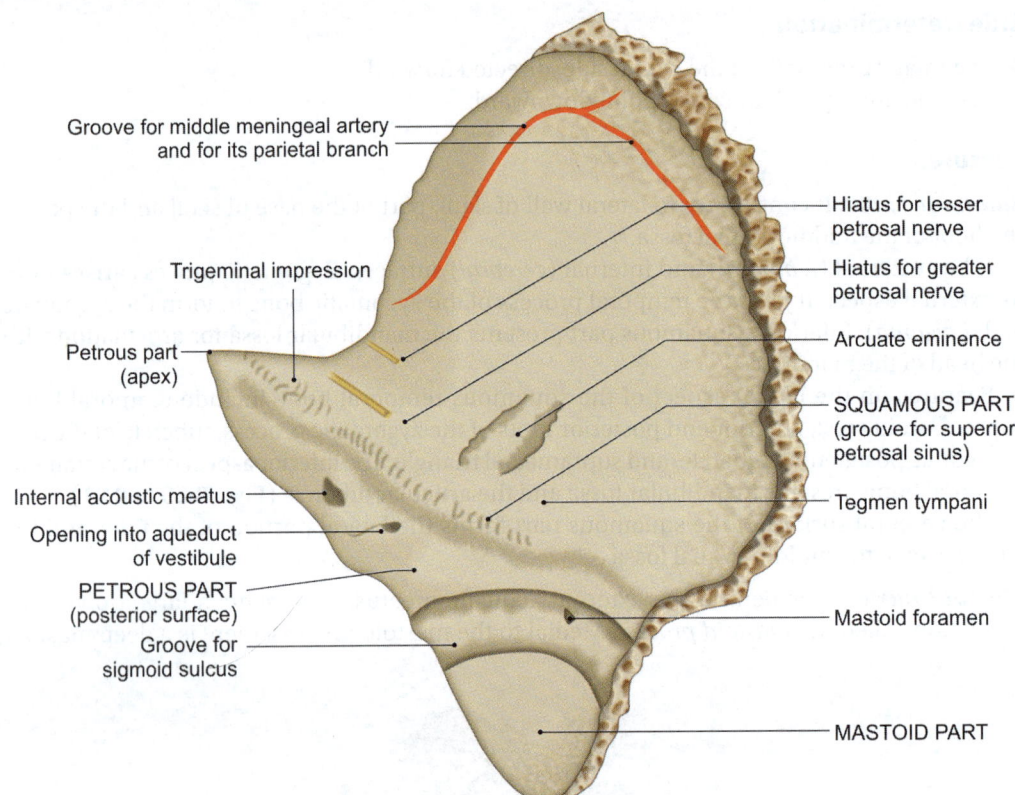

Fig. 8.30: Right temporal bone: Cranial aspect.

notch. Near the anterior end of the notch, the *stylomastoid foramen* is seen. Medial to the mastoid notch there is a groove for the occipital artery. Posteriorly, the mastoid part meets the occipital bone at the *occipitomastoid suture*. A *mastoid foramen* is present on or near this suture.

The internal surface of the mastoid temporal is seen in the lateral part of the floor of the posterior cranial fossa. It is marked by the groove for the sigmoid sinus, and by the internal opening of the mastoid foramen.

Within its substance the mastoid temporal bone contains several air-filled spaces called the *mastoid air cells*. The largest of these is the *mastoid antrum*, which is closely related to the middle ear.

Petrous part: It lies in the base of the skull between the sphenoid (anteriorly) and the occipital bone (posteriorly). It is seen in norma basalis and in the floor of the middle and posterior cranial fossae. It has anterior, posterior, and inferior surfaces with an apex which is directed forward and medially.

Apex lies in the angle between the basilar part of occipital bone (posteromedially) and the greater wing of sphenoid (anterolaterally). It forms the posterior margin of the foramen lacerum. This foramen separates the apex from the body of the sphenoid bone and from the basilar part of the occipital bone.

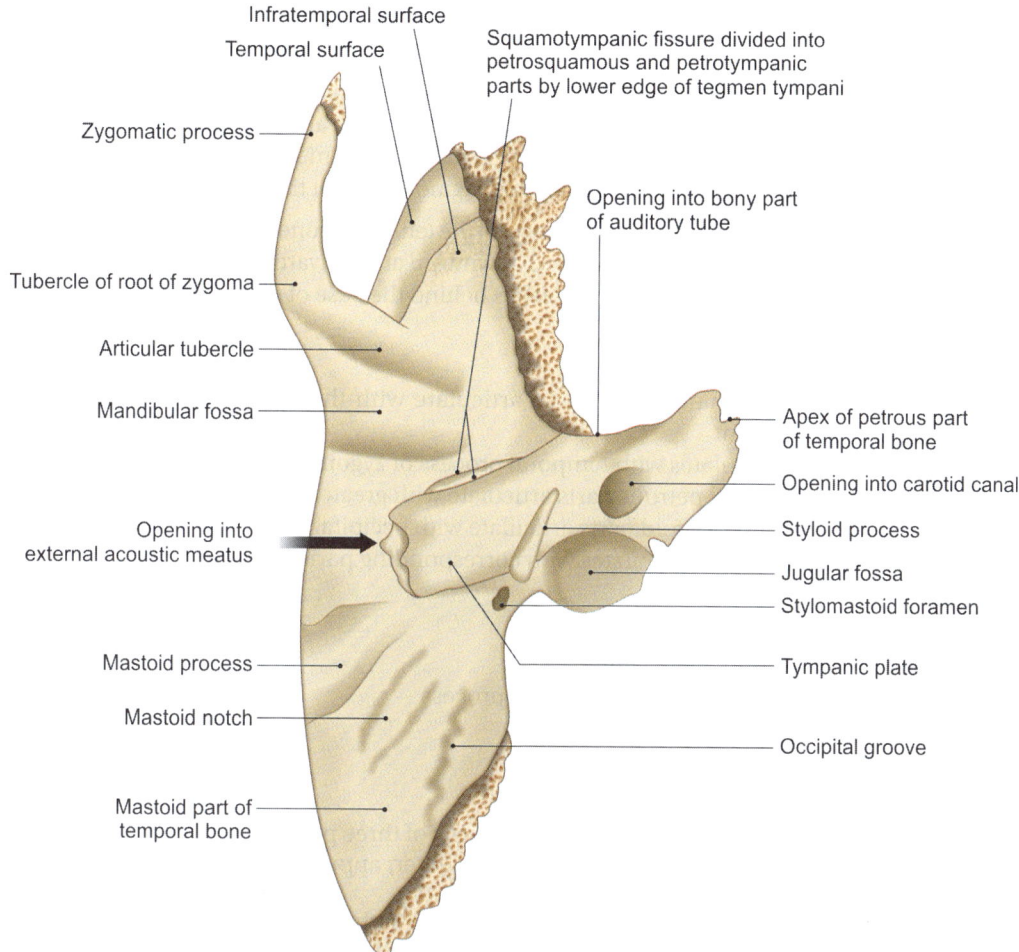

Fig. 8.31: Right temporal bone from below.

Anterior surface forms the sloping posterior part of the floor of the middle cranial fossa. The features include trigeminal impression, hiatus for greater petrosal nerve, hiatus for lesser petrosal nerve, arcuate eminence, and the tegmen tympani.

Posterior surface forms the lateral part of the sloping anterior wall of the posterior cranial fossa. It presents the opening of the *internal acoustic meatus*. Posterolateral to this opening a slit in the bone leads into a canal called the *aqueduct of the vestibule*.

The anterior and posterior surfaces are separated by a sharp superior border; separates middle and posterior cranial fossae. The border is grooved by the superior petrosal sinus.

Inferior surface presents the lower opening of the *carotid canal*. The canal passes through the petrous temporal bone to open into the posterior wall of the foramen lacerum. Behind the opening of the carotid canal, petrous temporal forms the anterior walls of the jugular fossa and jugular foramen. On the ridge between the opening of the carotid canal and the jugular fossa, a small opening is seen that leads into the canaliculus for the tympanic nerve. On the lateral wall of the jugular fossa there is the opening of the *mastoid canaliculus*.

The middle ear and the internal ear lie within the petrous temporal bone. The bony part of the auditory tube and the canal for the tensor tympani are associated with the middle ear.

Tympanic part: It is in the form of a bony plate called the *tympanic plate*. It lies between the mandibular fossa and the external acoustic meatus. It forms the anterior and the inferior walls and the lower part of the posterior wall of the external acoustic meatus. The plate has a rough lateral margin which gives attachment to the cartilaginous part of the meatus.

Styloid process: It is attached to the inferior aspect of the temporal bone. It is thin and pointed, and variable in length (usually 2.5 cm). It is directed downward and forward. Its base is ensheathed by the tympanic plate. The stylomastoid foramen lies behind the base of the styloid process.

Articulations

- Articular tubercle and mandibular fossa articulate with the head of mandible to form temporomandibular joint
- Zygomatic process articulates with temporal process of zygomatic bone
- *Anteriorly*: Squamous and petrous parts articulate with greater wing of sphenoid
- *Posteriorly:* Petrous and mastoid parts articulate with occipital bone
- *Superiorly*: Squamous part articulates with corresponding parietal bone.

Ossification and Development

Temporal bone ossifies from eight centers:
- One for squamous part including zygomatic process
- One for tympanic part
- Four for petrous and mastoid parts
- Two for styloid process

Just before the end of fetal life, temporal bone consists of three parts:
1. *Squamous part* ossifies in membrane from one center; appears near the root of zygomatic process about the second month.
2. *Petromastoid part* develops from four centers; appear in the cartilaginous ear capsule about the sixth month.
3. *Tympanic ring* (incomplete circle for the attachment of the circumference of tympanic membrane) expands to form the tympanic part; ossifies (in membrane) from one center that appears about the third month.

Styloid *process* develops from the proximal part of the cartilage of second branchial (hyoid) arch by two centers: one for proximal part (*tympanohyal*) appears before birth; other, comprising the rest (*stylohyal*) does not appear until after birth.

Tympanic ring unites with the squamous part shortly before birth; petromastoid and squamous parts join during first year and tympanohyal part of styloid process about the same time. Stylohyal does not unite with the rest of the bone until after puberty.

Clinical Anatomy

Bell's palsy: The course of facial nerve prior to its entry into the parotid gland from stylomastoid foramen remains unprotected especially in infants where mastoid process is not well developed. Thus, this part of nerve gets edematous in exposure to cold leading to weakness of ipsilateral facial muscles. This is a lower motor neuron (LMN) paralysis. Its features include facial asymmetry, epiphora, loss of nasolabial furrow, and the dribbling of saliva.

When patient is asked to perform specific actions of facial muscles, following features are observed on the affected side (**Fig. 8.32**):
- Loss of horizontal wrinkles
- Inability to shut the eye
- Inability to move angle of mouth
- Inability to whistle.

McEvan's triangle: This suprameatal triangle demarcates tympanic antrum, which is medial to it. It is about half inch deep to the triangle (**Fig. 8.33**). To drain pus from tympanic antrum an opening is made in the suprameatal triangle.

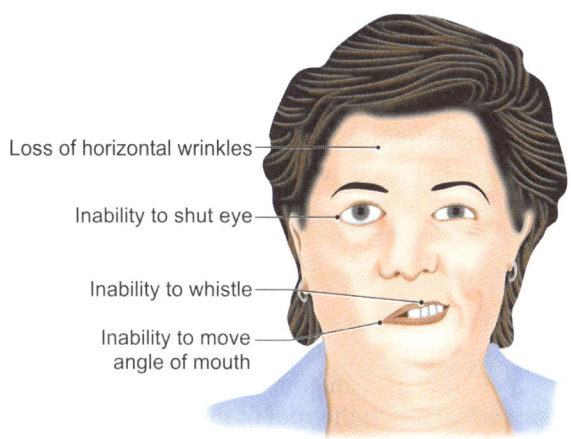

Fig. 8.32: Bell's palsy.

QUESTIONNAIRE

- Hold the bone in anatomical position to the side it belongs.
- Identify the parts of this bone.
- Mark the structures to the styloid process.
- Identify the suprameatal triangle. What are its boundaries and clinical importance?
- Show petrotympanic fissure. Name the structures passing through it.
- Identify internal acoustic meatus. Name the structures passing through it.
- Show arcuate eminence. What structure produces it?
- Identify trigeminal impression. Name the structure located there.
- Mark the nerve and vessels related to temporal bone.
- Mark the attachments of:

Ligaments	Muscles
Stylohyoid ligament	Sternocleidomastoid
Stylomandibular ligament	Posterior belly of digastric
	On the zygomatic process

- Comment on its ossification.

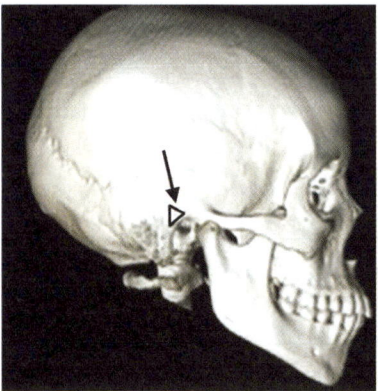 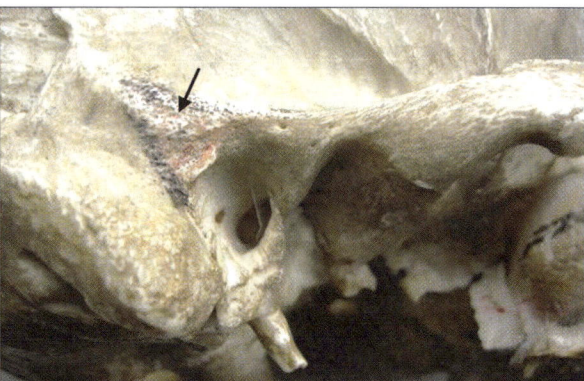

Fig. 8.33: McEvan's triangle.

SPHENOID BONE

This unpaired bone forms the middle part of the base of the skull. Parts of it extend into the lateral wall of the vault and into the orbit. The sphenoid consists of:
- Median part (body)
- Right and left greater wings
- Right and left lesser wings
- Right and left pterygoid processes.

Features

Body

It has superior, inferior, anterior, posterior, and right and left lateral surfaces **(Figs. 8.34 and 8.35)**. *Inferior surface* lies in the roof of the posterior part of the nasal cavity and in the roof of the

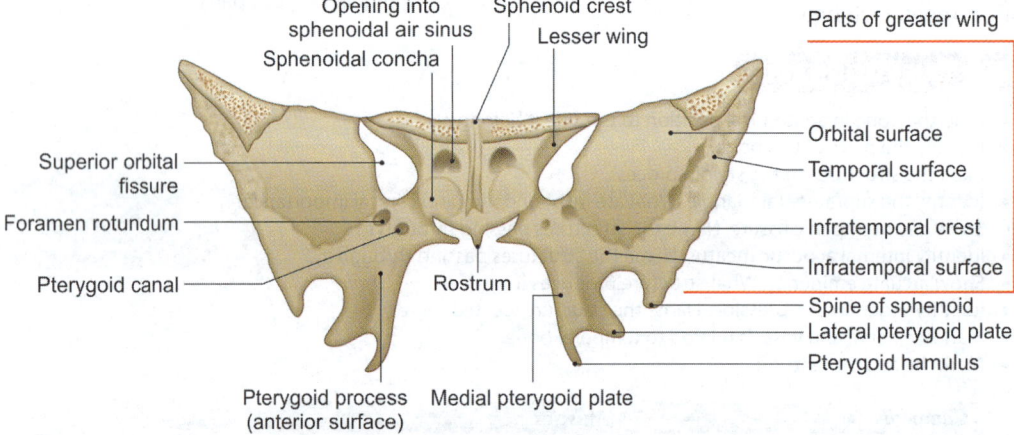

Fig. 8.34: Sphenoid bone: Anterior aspect.

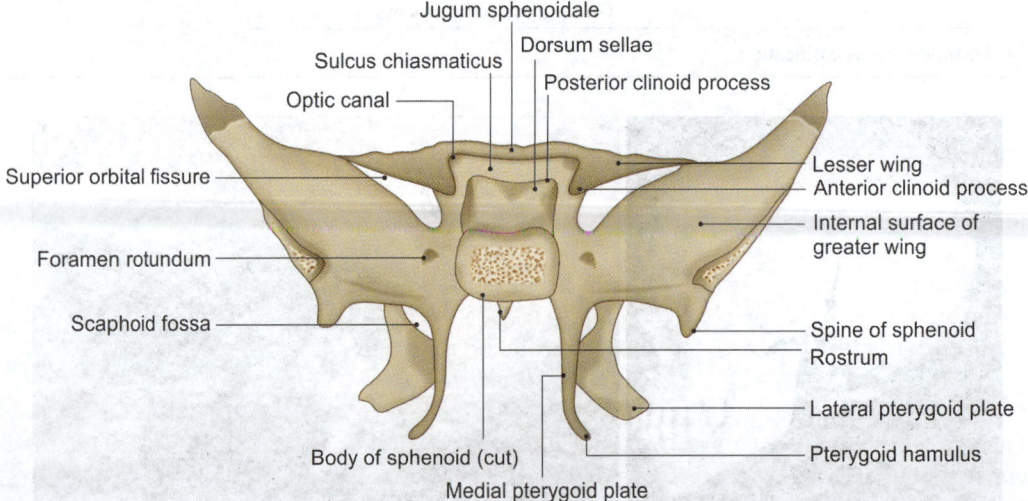

Fig. 8.35: Sphenoid bone: Posterior aspect.

nasopharynx. A median ridge (*rostrum*) projects downward from the body which fits into the gap between the alae of the vomer.

Superior surface forms the median part of the floor of the anterior cranial fossa (posteriorly) and median part of the middle cranial fossa. The features include jugum sphenoidale, sulcus chiasmaticus, tuberculum sellae, hypophyseal fossa, dorsum sellae, and the posterior clinoid processes.

Lateral surfaces are also seen in the floor of the middle cranial fossa. Each lateral surface is marked by the carotid groove.

Anterior surface takes part in forming the roof of the nasal cavity. It presents a median *sphenoidal crest* on either side of which there is the opening of the *sphenoidal air sinuses*. The lower margin of each opening is formed by a thin plate of bone called the *sphenoidal concha*. Sphenoidal air sinuses are within the body of the sphenoid.

Posteroinferiorly, the body of the sphenoid continues with the basilar part of the occipital bone. Both bones form the median part of the sloping anterior wall (*clivus*) of the posterior cranial fossa.

Greater Wings

These extend laterally and upward from each side of the body. Each wing presents cerebral, lateral, and orbital surfaces.

Cerebral surface is concave. It forms part of the floor of the middle cranial fossa. Anteriorly and medially, this surface has a sharp edge which is separated from the lesser wing by the *superior orbital fissure*. Just below the medial end of the fissure the foramen rotundum is seen. Posteromedially, the greater wing is separated from the apex of the petrous temporal bone by the foramen lacerum. Near the posterior margin of the cerebral surface foramina seen are the *foramen ovale, foramen spinosum, emissary sphenoidal foramen,* and sometimes the *canaliculus innominatus*.

Lateral surface is convex. It is divided into an upper part (*temporal surface*) and a lower part (*infratemporal surface*) by the infratemporal crest. The features on the infratemporal surface include foramen ovale, foramen spinosum, emissary sphenoid foramen, canaliculus innominatus, spine of sphenoid, and the groove for auditory tube.

Orbital surface forms the posterior part of the lateral wall of the orbit. Medially, it has a free edge that forms inferolateral margin of the superior orbital fissure. Inferiorly, it forms the upper boundary of the inferior orbital fissure.

Lesser Wings

They pass laterally from the anterior and upper part of the body. Each wing is attached to the body of sphenoid by anterior and posterior roots. The *optic canal* lies between these roots and the body of sphenoid. The medial part of the lesser wing shows a backward projection called the *anterior clinoid process*.

The lesser wing has superior and inferior surfaces. *Superior surface* forms part of the floor of the anterior cranial fossa. *Inferior surface* forms the posterior part of the roof of the orbit. It forms the upper boundary of the superior orbital fissure.

Pterygoid Processes

Each process projects downward from the junction of the body and greater wing of sphenoid. It consists of medial and lateral pterygoid plates. The upper part of the pterygoid process has an anterior surface which forms the posterior wall of the pterygopalatine fossa. On this surface the anterior opening of the pterygoid canal is seen. Posterior opening of pterygoid canal is located just above the scaphoid fossa, in the anterior wall of the foramen lacerum. A little above and lateral to this opening, the anterior opening of the foramen rotundum is seen.

Articulations

- Body of sphenoid:
  - Posteroinferiorly joins basilar part of occipital bone
  - Anteriorly, articulates with ethmoid bone
- Sphenoidal crest articulates with perpendicular plate of the ethmoid.
- Greater wing articulates with:
  - Posteriorly: Petrous temporal
  - Posterolaterally: Squamous temporal
  - Anteromedially: Frontal bone
  - Anteriorly and laterally: Zygomatic bone
  - Superiorly: Anteroinferior angle of the parietal bone
- Lesser wing articulates anteriorly with the orbital plate of frontal bone.
- Lower part of pterygoid process articulates anteriorly with maxilla.
- Anterior margin of medial pterygoid plate articulates with perpendicular plate of palatine bone.
- Pyramidal process of palatine bone fits into the interval between lower ends of medial and lateral pterygoid plates.
- Vaginal plate (*arises from medial side of pterygoid process*) articulates with:
  - Anteriorly: Sphenoidal process of palatine bone
  - Medially: Ala of vomer.

Development and Ossification

Till eighth month of fetal life, body of the sphenoid consists of two parts:
- One in front of tuberculum sellae (*presphenoid*) with which lesser wings continue.
- Sella turcica and dorsum sellae (*postsphenoid*) with great wings and pterygoid processes.

Greater part of the bone ossifies in cartilage. There are fourteen ossification centers: Six for presphenoid part, eight for postsphenoid part.

Presphenoid

About ninth week of fetal life, ossification center appears for each lesser wing lateral to optic foramen; two centers in the presphenoid part of body. Sphenoidal conchae develop from two centers; appear at fifth month. At about fourth year they fuse with ethmoidal labyrinths; between ninth and twelfth years they unite with the sphenoid.

Postsphenoid

Two ossification centers appear for the great wings about eighth week (between foramen rotundum and ovale).

Orbital plate, part of sphenoid in the temporal fossa and lateral pterygoid plate ossify in membrane. Soon centers for postsphenoid part of the body appear (one on either side of sella turcica); blend together about the middle of fetal life.

Medial pterygoid plate (except hamulus) ossifies in membrane; center appears about tenth week. Medial plate joins lateral pterygoid plate about sixth month. About fourth month, one center appears for lingula and joins the rest of the bone.

Presphenoid is united to postsphenoid part about eighth month. At birth, bone is in three parts:
- *Central part*: Consisting of body and lesser wings
- *Two lateral parts*: Comprising greater wing and pterygoid process.

In the first year after birth, greater wings and body unite. Lesser wings extend inward and meet with each other in the middle line to form *jugum sphenoidale*.

Sphenoid and occipital bone are fused by 25th year.

Sphenoidal air sinuses are small at birth; attain full size after puberty.

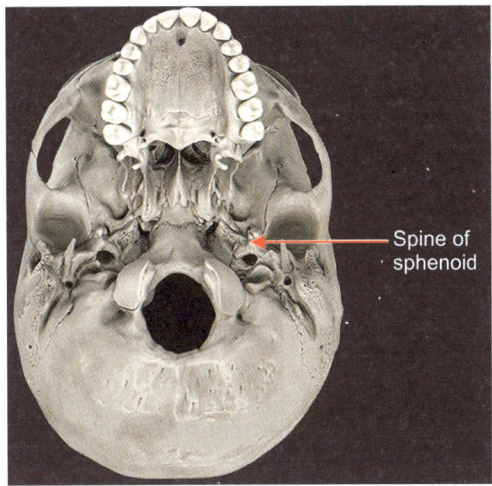

Fig. 8.36: Spine of sphenoid.

Clinical Anatomy

Fracture of spine of sphenoid (Fig. 8.36): Spine of sphenoid is related to auriculotemporal nerve and chorda tympani. Damage to auriculotemporal nerve would result in dry mouth (postganglionic parasympathetic pathway to parotid gland will be interrupted). Involvement of chorda tympani causes loss of taste sensations from anterior two-thirds of tongue (*gustatory to tongue*).

QUESTIONNAIRE

- Hold the bone in anatomical position and name its parts.
- Enumerate the articulations of this bone.
- Identify the foramina associated with this bone. Enumerate the structures passing through them.
- Identify clinoid processes. What is attached to them?
- Show sella turcica. What structure is located there?
- Where is sphenoidal air sinus located? Where does it opens?
- Comment on its ossification.

PALATINE BONE

Each palatine bone is consists of two parts: (a) perpendicular plate and (b) horizontal plate. The horizontal plate forms the posterior part of the bony (hard) palate. Its lateral margin joins the lower end of the perpendicular plate. The perpendicular plate lies in the posterior part of the lateral wall of the nasal cavity.

Features

It presents three processes: (a) Pyramidal, (b) orbital, and (c) sphenoidal.

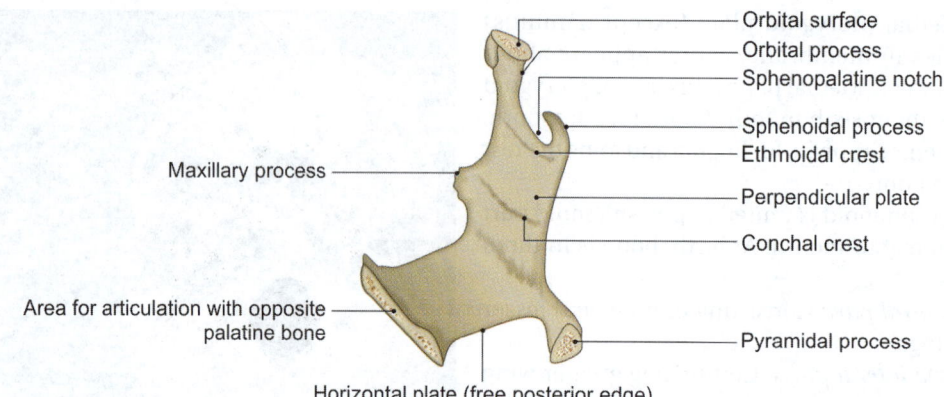

Fig. 8.37: Right palatine bone: Posteromedial aspect.

Horizontal Plate

It has superior and inferior surfaces. Each horizontal plate meets the opposite side plate at the *interpalatine suture*. Anteriorly, it meets palatine process of maxilla. The posterior edge of the plate is free; provides attachment to the soft palate. In the midline, the posterior edges of the right and left horizontal plates project backward to form the *posterior nasal spine*. A little in front of the posterior margin the inferior surface of the horizontal plate shows a raised *palatine crest*.

The superior surface forms the floor of the posterior part of the nasal cavity. In the midline (where two horizontal plates meet) there is an elevation called the *nasal crest*. It articulates with the vomer; contributes to the nasal septum **(Fig. 8.37)**.

Perpendicular Plate

It lies in the lateral wall of the nasal cavity. Anteriorly, it articulates with the maxilla and posteriorly with the medial pterygoid plate. It has medial and lateral surfaces. The lateral surface articulates with the maxilla converting the greater palatine groove on the maxilla into the *greater palatine canal*. This plate overlaps the posterior part of the maxillary hiatus. Superiorly, it forms the medial wall of the pterygopalatine fossa.

The medial surface forms part of the lateral wall of the nasal cavity. Inferiorly, this surface presents *conchal crest*; provides attachment to the inferior nasal concha. Superiorly, it has ethmoidal crest to which the middle nasal concha is attached.

The upper border of the plate has a notch which forms the lower part of the *sphenopalatine foramen (foramen is bounded above by the body of sphenoid)*.

Pyramidal Process

It passes backward and laterally from the posterolateral angle of the horizontal plate. It is wedged between the maxillary tuberosity (anteriorly) and the pterygoid process (posteriorly). It occupies the interval between the lower ends of the medial and lateral pterygoid plates. The *lesser palatine foramina* are on the inferior aspect of the pyramidal process.

Orbital Process

It arises from the anterosuperior angle of the perpendicular plate; forms a small part of the orbital floor.

Sphenoidal Process

It arises from the posterosuperior angle of the perpendicular plate. It meets the vaginal plate of the sphenoid; helps to form the *palatovaginal canal*.

Development and Ossification

It ossifies in membrane from a single center; appears during eighth week of fetal life at the junction of the two parts. From here, ossification spreads medially to horizontal part, downward into pyramidal process, and upward into the vertical part.
- *At birth*: Height of perpendicular plate is equal to the width of horizontal part.
- *In adult*: Perpendicular plate becomes twice the transverse width of horizontal part.

ETHMOID BONE

The ethmoid bone consists of a median vertical plate and right and left labyrinths. The median plate is subdivided into:
- Crista galli: Seen in the floor of anterior cranial fossa
- Perpendicular plate: Forms part of nasal septum

The labyrinth consists of a number of ethmoidal air sinuses. Labyrinth is bounded by:
- Laterally: Orbital plate (forms significant part of the medial wall of orbit)
- Medially: Medial plate (lies in the lateral wall of nasal cavity).

Two curved plates of bone form the *superior and middle nasal conchae* pass medially into the nasal cavity from the medial plate.

Each labyrinth is connected to the median plate by a narrow horizontal plate that passes laterally from the junction of the crista galli with the perpendicular plate. This horizontal plate has numerous perforations called the *cribriform* (= sieve like) *plate*. This plate forms part of the floor of the anterior cranial fossa and part of the roof of the nasal cavity.

Walls of many ethmoidal air cells are incomplete. In intact skull they are completed by parts of maxilla, frontal and lacrimal and sphenoid and palatine bones.

Articulations

Perpendicular plate articulates with:
- *Anteroinferiorly*: Nasal septal cartilage
- *Posteroinferiorly*: Vomer
- *Anteriorly*: Frontal and nasal bones
- *Posteriorly*: Sphenoid.

Cribriform plate articulates with:
- *Laterally*: Orbital plate of frontal bone
- *Posteriorly*: Sphenoid.

Labyrinth articulates with:
- *Above*: Frontal bone
- *Posteriorly*: Sphenoid
- *Laterally*: Maxilla, palatine bone and lacrimal bone.

Medial aspect of the labyrinth gives attachment to part of the inferior nasal concha.

Ossification

It ossifies in the cartilage of the nasal capsule from three centers:
- One for perpendicular plate
- One for each labyrinth.

Labyrinths develop (in the region of orbital plates) between fourth and fifth months of fetal life and extend into the conchae. At birth, ethmoid consists of the two small and poorly developed labyrinths.

During first year, perpendicular plate and crista galli ossify from one center; join labyrinths about the beginning of second year.

Cribriform plate ossifies partly from perpendicular plate and partly from labyrinths. Development of the ethmoidal cells begins during fetal life.

> **QUESTIONNAIRE**
> - Hold the bone in anatomical position and identify its parts.
> - Classify ethmoid bone.
> - Enumerate the articulations of this bone.
> - Identify crista galli. Why it is so named? What is attached to it?
> - Identify cribriform plate. What are the structures passes through it?
> - Identify perpendicular plate. What part of nasal septum does it form?
> - How many ethmoidal air sinuses are present? Where are their openings in the lateral wall of the nose?
> - What are the functions of the paranasal air sinuses?
> - Comment on its ossification.

LACRIMAL BONE

It is a small thin bony plate seen in the anterior part of the medial wall of the orbit. It has a lateral surface (seen in orbit) and a medial surface that helps to form the lateral wall of the nose.

The lateral surface is marked by a vertical lacrimal crest in front of which there is a vertical groove. This groove meets a similar groove on the frontal process of the maxilla to form the groove for the lacrimal sac.

Inferiorly, the lacrimal groove continues with the nasolacrimal canal. A descending process from the lacrimal bone helps to complete the medial wall of the canal (along with lacrimal process of inferior nasal concha). A curved spicule of bone called the *lacrimal hamulus* lies in the lateral wall of the upper end of the nasolacrimal canal.

Articulations

Lacrimal bone articulates with:
- *Anteriorly*: Frontal process of maxilla
- *Posteriorly*: Ethmoid
- *Superiorly*: Frontal bone
- *Inferiorly*: Maxilla

Ossification

It ossifies from one ossification center that appears about twelfth week of fetal life in the mesenchyme around the nasal capsule.

NASAL BONE

The right and left nasal bones form the bridge of the nose.

Articulations

Each nasal bone articulates with:
- *Medially*: Opposite nasal bone
- *Laterally*: Frontal process of maxilla
- *Superiorly (and by its posterior surface)*: Nasal part of frontal bone.

Inferior margin of the bone gives attachment to the lateral nasal cartilage.

Posterior surface of the bone is grooved and takes part in forming the anterior part of the roof of the nasal cavity.

The medial margins of the two nasal bones are thickened (on this aspect) and project into the nasal cavity as a crest which contributes to the nasal septum.

Ossification

It ossifies from one center that appears during third month in the mesenchyme over the cartilaginous anterior part of the nasal capsule.

THE VOMER

The vomer (*flat plate of bone*) forms the posteroinferior part of the nasal septum.

Articulations

Vomer articulates with:
- *Anterosuperiorly*: Perpendicular plate of ethmoid
- *Posterosuperiorly*: Body of sphenoid

Vomer has two alae; rostrum of the sphenoid fits into the interval between the alae. Inferiorly, vomer is attached to:
- Palatine processes of maxillae
- Horizontal plates of palatine bones.

Anteriorly, the vomer gives attachment to the septal cartilage of the nasal septum.

Development and Ossification

During development, the nasal septum consists of a cartilage plate called *ethmovomerine cartilage*. The posterosuperior part of this cartilage forms perpendicular plate of ethmoid and its anteroinferior part persists as the septal cartilage.

Vomer ossifies in the connective tissue covering its posteroinferior part.

Two ossification centers (one on either side of middle line) appear during eighth week of fetal life in this membrane; about third month these unite from below.

The union of the lamellae extends upward. By puberty, the lamellae are united to form a median plate.

INFERIOR NASAL CONCHA

This (*thin curved plate of bone*) lies in relation to the lateral wall of the nasal cavity. The plate is free inferiorly.

Articulations
- *Anteriorly*: Its superior margin is attached to the maxilla (*conchal crest*)
- *Posteriorly*: Conchal crest on the perpendicular plate of palatine bone
- Attached to lacrimal bone (*through lacrimal process*).
  Along with lacrimal bone it forms the medial boundary of the nasolacrimal groove.

Ossification
It ossifies from one ossification center that appears during fifth month of fetal life.

HYOID BONE

The hyoid bone is not a part of the skull; considered here for convenience. It is situated in the front of the upper part of the neck. It is not attached to any bone directly. It is held in place by muscles and ligaments attached to it. The most important ligaments are *stylohyoid ligaments* by which it is suspended from the base of the skull. It consists of central part (body) and two cornua (*greater and lesser*) on either side.

Features
Body: It is roughly quadrilateral. It presents two surfaces. The anterior surface is directed forward and upward; while posterior surface backward and downward. The anterior surface is divided into upper and lower parts by a transverse ridge and into right and left halves by a median vertical ridge. The posterior surface is smooth **(Figs. 8.38 to 8.40)**.

Greater cornua: These are attached to the lateral part of the body from which they project backward and laterally. They present upper and lower surfaces and medial and lateral borders. The posterior end of each cornu is enlarged to form a tubercle.

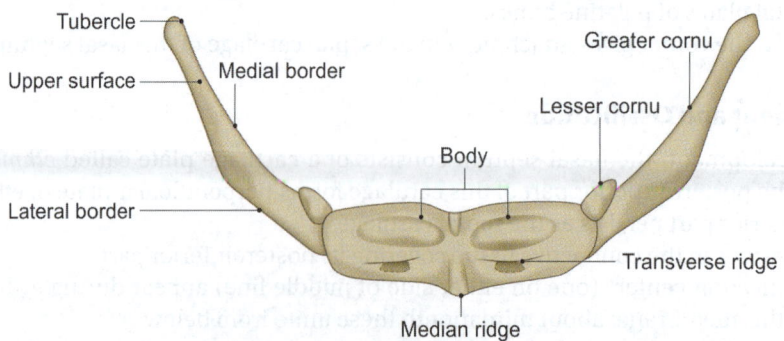

Fig. 8.38: Hyoid bone: From the front.

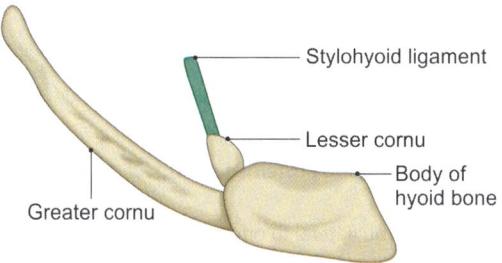

Fig. 8.39: Hyoid bone: From the lateral side.

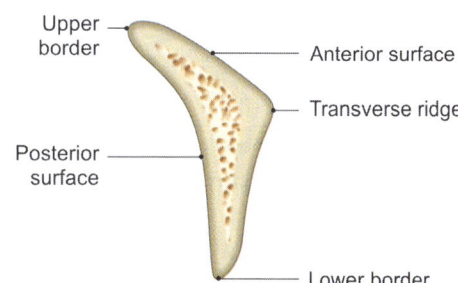

Fig. 8.40: Hyoid bone: Median section.

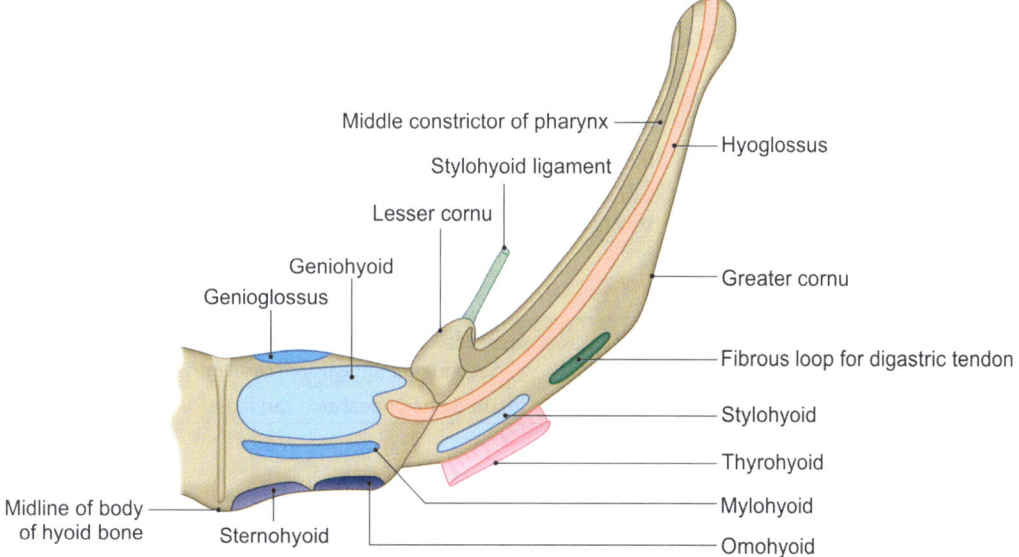

Fig. 8.41: Hyoid bone. Anterosuperior aspect: Attachments.

Lesser cornua: These (small and conical) project upward and laterally from the junction of the body and the greater cornua.

In the young, the union between the body and greater cornua is cartilaginous; but fuse in later life. The lesser cornua are attached by fibrous tissue; may be synovial joints between them and the greater cornua.

Attachments (Fig. 8.41)

Muscles

Muscle	Attachment
Genioglossus (lowest fibers)	Upper border of the body (*insertion*)
Geniohyoid	Anterior surface of the body (*insertion*)
Mylohyoid	Anterior surface of the body below insertion of geniohyoid (*insertion*)

(Contd...)

(Contd...)

Muscle	Attachment
Sternohyoid	Medial part of the inferior border of the body (*insertion*)
Omohyoid (superior belly)	Lateral part of the inferior border of the body (*origin*)
Middle constrictor of pharynx	Upper surface of the greater cornu and posterolateral aspect of the lesser cornu (*origin*)
Hyoglossus	Upper surface of the greater cornu (lateral to origin of middle constrictor) and lateral part of the body (*origin*)
Stylohyoid	Upper surface of greater cornu near its junction with body (*insertion*)
Thyrohyoid	Anterior part of lateral border of the greater cornu (*insertion*)

Other Attachments (Figs. 8.42 and 8.43)

Structure	Attachment
Stylohyoid ligament	Apex of the lesser cornu
Thyrohyoid membrane	Medial border of the greater cornu and upper border of body
Fibrous loop for the tendon of digastric	Lateral part of the upper surface of greater cornu (behind insertion of stylohyoid muscle)

Development

Part of bone	Developmental component
Upper half of the body and lesser cornu	Second pharyngeal arch cartilages
Lower half of the body and greater cornu	Third pharyngeal arch cartilages

Ossification

Hyoid ossifies from six centers:
- One center appears in each greater cornu at the end of fetal life.
- Two centers appear in the body at about the time of birth.
- Two centers appear in the lesser cornu at the age of puberty.

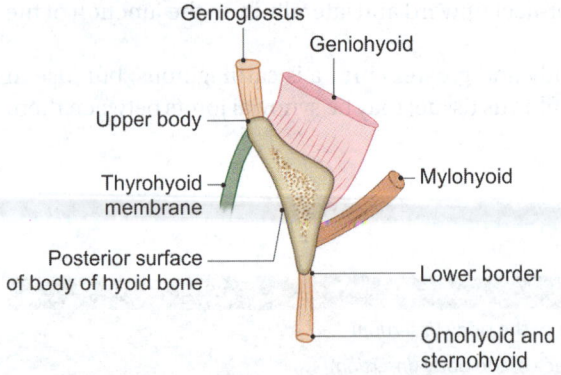

Fig. 8.42: Schematic parasagittal section through the body of hyoid: Arrangement of attached structures.

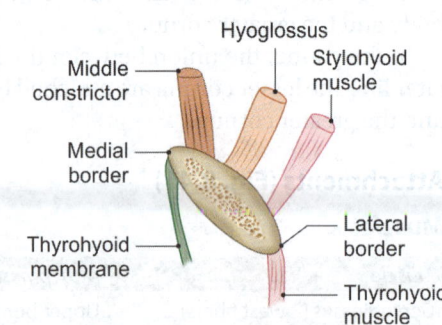

Fig. 8.43: Schematic vertical section through greater cornu of hyoid bone: Arrangement of structures attached.

CHAPTER 8 ✦ Individual Bones of Skull

QUESTIONNAIRE

- Hold the bone in anatomical position and identify its parts.
- How the hyoid bone is suspended in the body?
- Mark the attachments of:

Ligaments and structures	Muscles
Stylohyoid ligament	Strap muscles of the neck
Thyrohyoid membrane	On the greater cornu
	On the lesser cornu

- Comment on its ossification.

ATLAS OF MUSCLE ATTACHMENTS: HEAD AND NECK

Plate 1
Buccinator

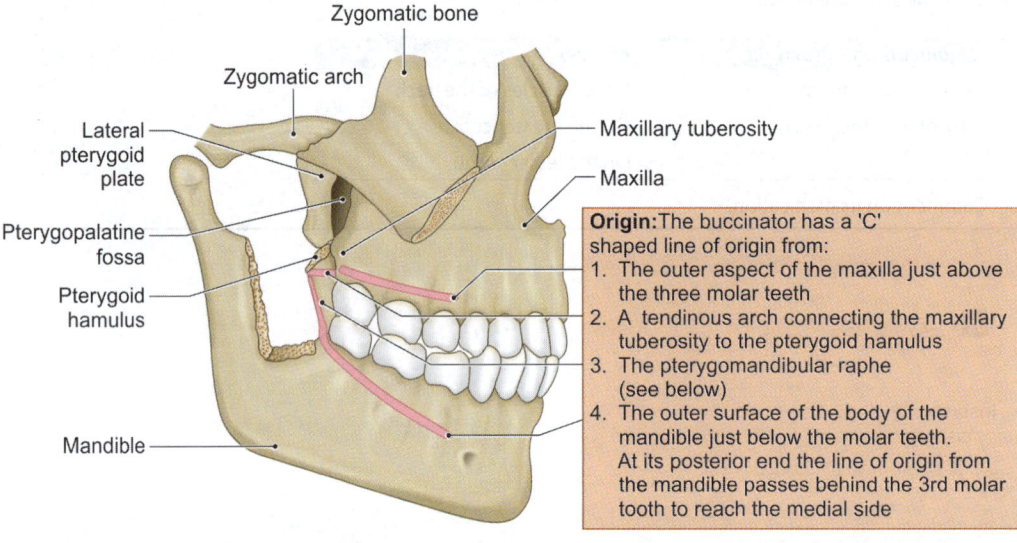

Origin: The buccinator has a 'C' shaped line of origin from:
1. The outer aspect of the maxilla just above the three molar teeth
2. A tendinous arch connecting the maxillary tuberosity to the pterygoid hamulus
3. The pterygomandibular raphe (see below)
4. The outer surface of the body of the mandible just below the molar teeth. At its posterior end the line of origin from the mandible passes behind the 3rd molar tooth to reach the medial side

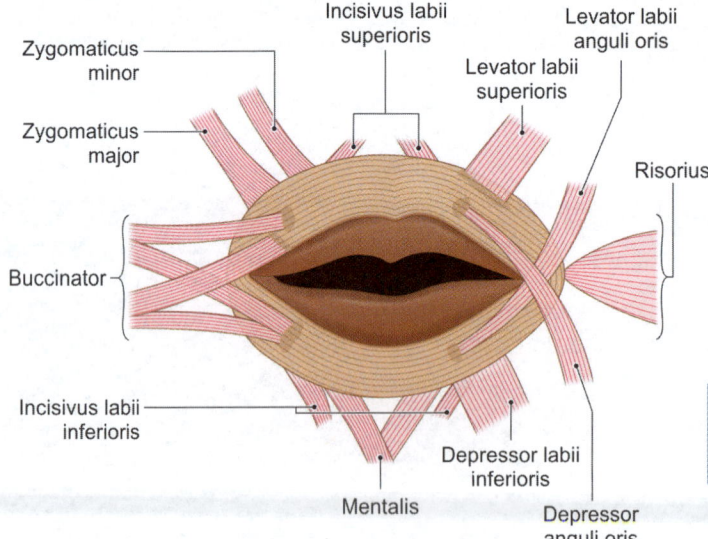

The pterygomandibular raphe is made up of interlacing tendinous fibers. It is attached above to the pterygoid hamulus (at the lower end of the medial pterygoid plate), and below to the posterior end of the mylohyoid line of the mandible.
The raphe gives attachment anteriorly to fibers of the buccinator, and posteriorly to fibers of the superior constrictor of the pharynx.

Insertion: The fibers of the buccinator run forward where they are continuous with the orbicularis oris.

Nerve supply: The muscle is supplied by the lower buccal branches of the facial nerve.

Actions: The buccinator aids mastication by pushing food between the teeth. The muscle increases air pressure within the mouth as in blowing (Laterally, the word buccinator means one who blows a trumpet).

Important relations: The muscle is lined on the inside by the mucous membrane of the mouth. It is related on its outer aspect to the parotid duct which pierces it opposite the third upper molar tooth; to the superficial muscles inserted into the angle of the mouth; to the facial artery and vein; and to branches of the facial and buccal nerves.

Atlas of Muscle Attachments: Head and Neck

Plate 2
Temporalis

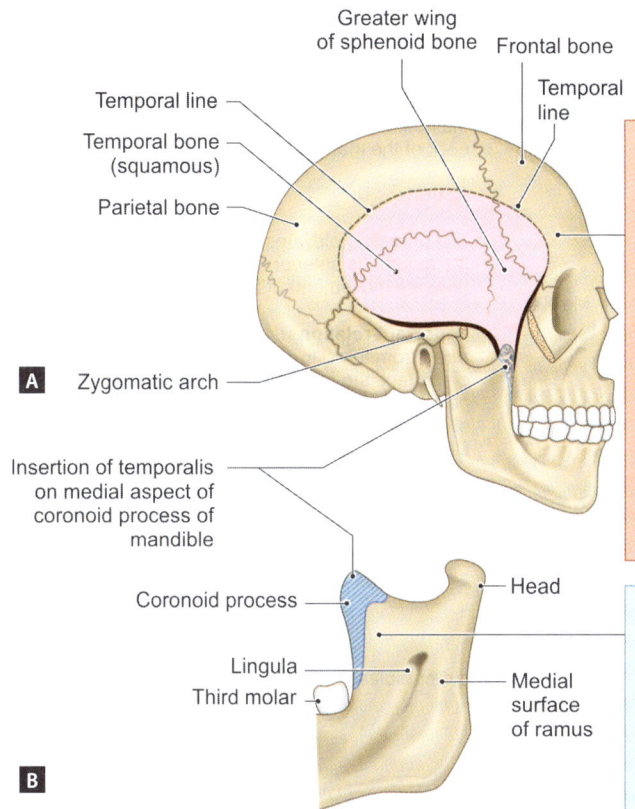

Origin:
The temporalis arises from the temporal fossa on the lateral aspect of the skull. The area is bounded above by the temporal line, and below by the zygomatic arch. It includes parts of the frontal, parietal, and squamous temporal and of the greater wing of the sphenoid bone.
The anterior fibers of the muscle run vertically downward; the posterior fibers run horizontally forward; while the intermediate fibers run obliquely to converge in a tendon. The tendon passes deep to the zygomatic arch.

Insertion:
The muscle is inserted into the coronoid process of the mandible. The region of insertion covers the entire medial aspect of the coronoid process (including its apex, anterior and posterior borders). Some fibers are inserted into the anterior border of the ramus.

Nerve supply:
The temporalis is supplied by the deep temporal branches of the mandibular nerve.

Actions:
The temporalis helps to close the mouth by elevating the mandible.
The movements of elevation and depression of the mandible have two components. Firstly, there is a hinge like movement between the condyle of the mandible and the inferior surface of the articular disc of the temporomandibular joint. The second component is a gliding movement of the disc (along with the head of the mandible). In wide opening of the mouth the disc glides forward so that the head of the mandible comes to lie below the articular eminence.
In closing the mouth the posterior horizontal fibers of the temporalis pull the mandible backward (along with the intra-articular disc), whereas the anterior vertical fibers produce the angular hinge like movement.

Temporal fascia:
The temporalis is covered by a thick temporal fascia. The fascia is attached above to the (superior) temporal line, and below to the zygomatic arch.

Plate 3

Masseter

Origin of masseter from: Zygomatic arch formed by
- Zygomatic process of temporal bone
- Temporal process of zygomatic bone

Maxilla

Mandible

Insertion of masseter into: Lateral surface of ramus and angle of mandible

Nerve supply:
The masseter is supplied by a branch of the anterior division of the mandibular nerve. The nerve reaches the muscle by passing through the notch between the coronoid process and neck of the mandible.

Actions:
The masseter elevates the mandible to close the mouth. Its anterior fibers help in protraction (forward movement) of the jaw.

Important relations:
Apart from the skin and some superficial muscles of the face the masseter is overlapped by the anterior part of the parotid gland, the parotid duct, the branches of the facial nerve and the transverse facial vessels. Deep to the masseter there are the ramus of the mandible, the lower part of the temporalis and the posterior part of the buccinator.

Origin of Pterygoid Muscles

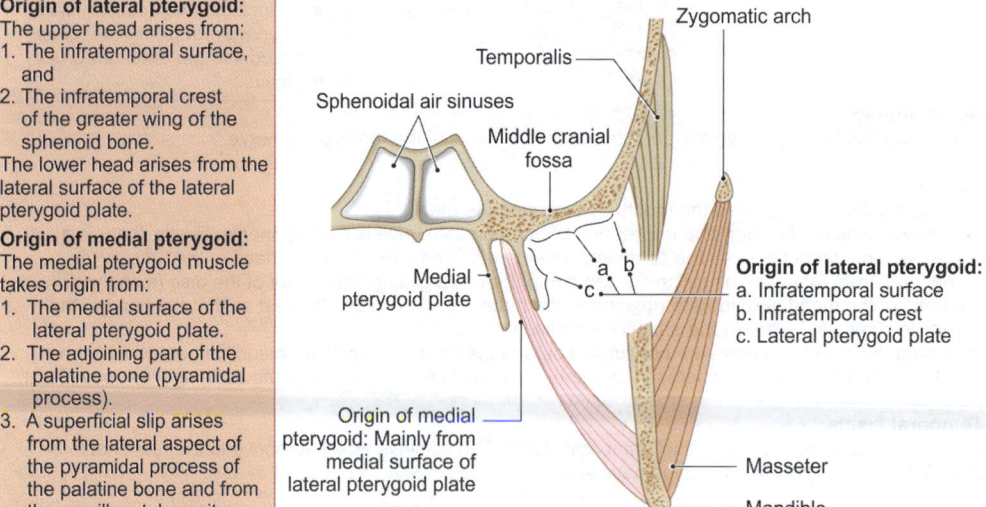

Zygomatic arch
Temporalis
Sphenoidal air sinuses
Middle cranial fossa
Medial pterygoid plate

Origin of lateral pterygoid:
a. Infratemporal surface
b. Infratemporal crest
c. Lateral pterygoid plate

Masseter
Mandible

Origin of medial pterygoid: Mainly from medial surface of lateral pterygoid plate

Origin of lateral pterygoid:
The upper head arises from:
1. The infratemporal surface, and
2. The infratemporal crest of the greater wing of the sphenoid bone.

The lower head arises from the lateral surface of the lateral pterygoid plate.

Origin of medial pterygoid:
The medial pterygoid muscle takes origin from:
1. The medial surface of the lateral pterygoid plate.
2. The adjoining part of the palatine bone (pyramidal process).
3. A superficial slip arises from the lateral aspect of the pyramidal process of the palatine bone and from the maxillary tuberosity (See next page also)

Plate 4

Medial and Lateral Pterygoid

(First see description of origins on previous page)

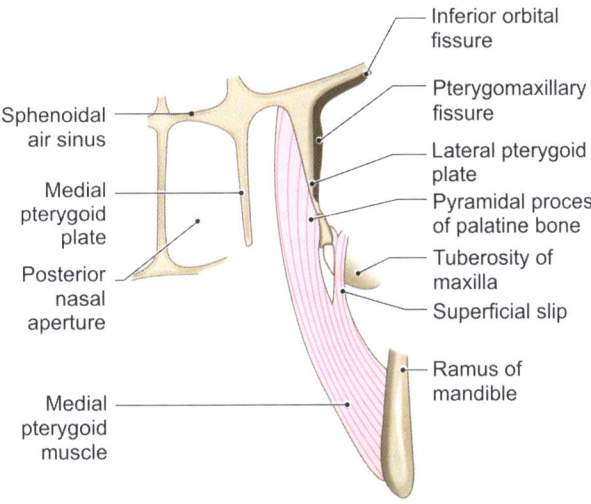

Actions of pterygoid muscles:
1. The medial and lateral pterygoids of both sides acting together protract the mandible.
2. The medial and lateral pterygoids of one side acting together pull the mandibular condyle of that side forward (and medially). As a result the chin moves forward and to the opposite side. Alternate action of the muscles of the two sides results in side-to-side chewing movements.
3. The two pterygoid muscles have opposite actions as far as opening and closing of the mouth is concerned. The medial pterygoid elevates the jaw. The lateral pterygoid helps in opening the mouth by pulling the head of the mandible forward along with the intra-articular disc.

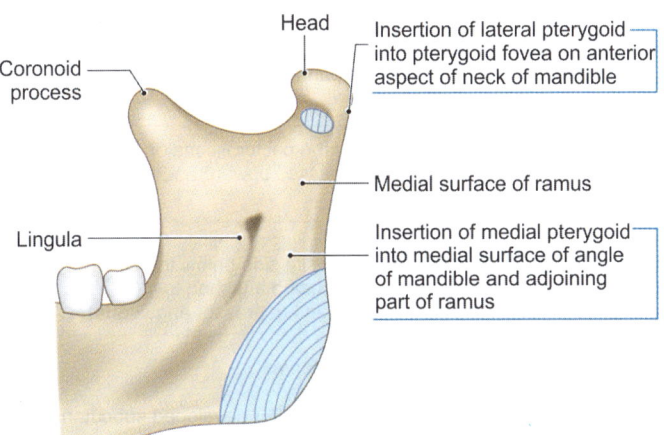

Insertion of lateral pterygoid:
The fibers of both heads run backward and laterally to be inserted into a depression (pterygoid fovea) on the anterior aspect of the neck of the mandible. Some fibers are inserted into the intra-articular disc and some into the capsule of the temporomandibular joint.

Insertion of medial pterygoid:
The fibers of the muscle pass downward, backward and laterally to be inserted into the medial surface of the angle of the mandible and the adjoining part of its ramus.

Nerve supply of medial and lateral pterygoid muscles:
Mandibular nerve.

Plate 5
Platysma

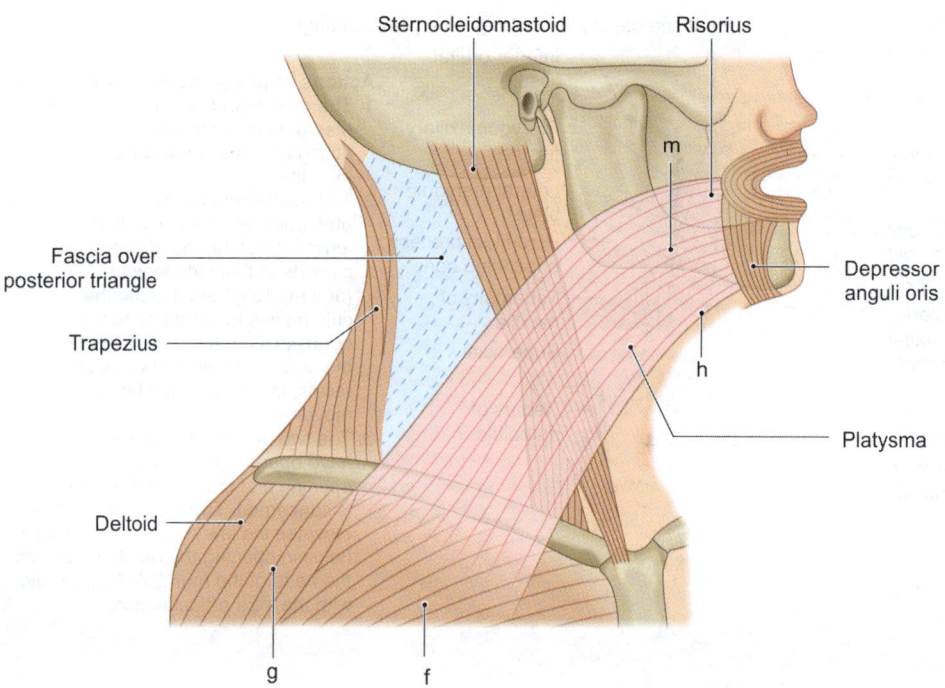

This is the most superficial muscle in the neck. Like the muscles of the face it lies in the superficial fascia. It is a remnant of an extensive sheet of subcutaneous muscle (called the pannulus carnosus) to be seen in some animals.

Origin: The muscle arises from the deep fascia covering the upper part of the pectoralis major (f in figure) and the anterior part of the deltoid (g). The fibers form a broad thin sheet that passes upward and forward across the clavicle, and then across the sternocleidomastoid.

Insertion: The most anterior fibers end by interlacing with those of the opposite side below the chin (h). The remaining fibers cross the lower border of the mandible, some of them being attached to it (m). The fibers end by merging with muscles at the angle of the mouth (especially risorius and depressor anguli oris).

Nerve supply: The muscles is supplied by the cervical branch of the facial nerve.

Action: The platysma produces wrinkles over the skin of the neck (the much better developed subcutaneous sheet of muscle present in some animals, e.g. the horse, enables them to move their skin over underlying structures).

Plate 6
Sternocleidomastoid

Insertion:
The muscle is inserted into the:
1. Lateral half of the superior nuchal line (d);
2. The lateral surface of the mastoid process from its apex to the upper border (e).

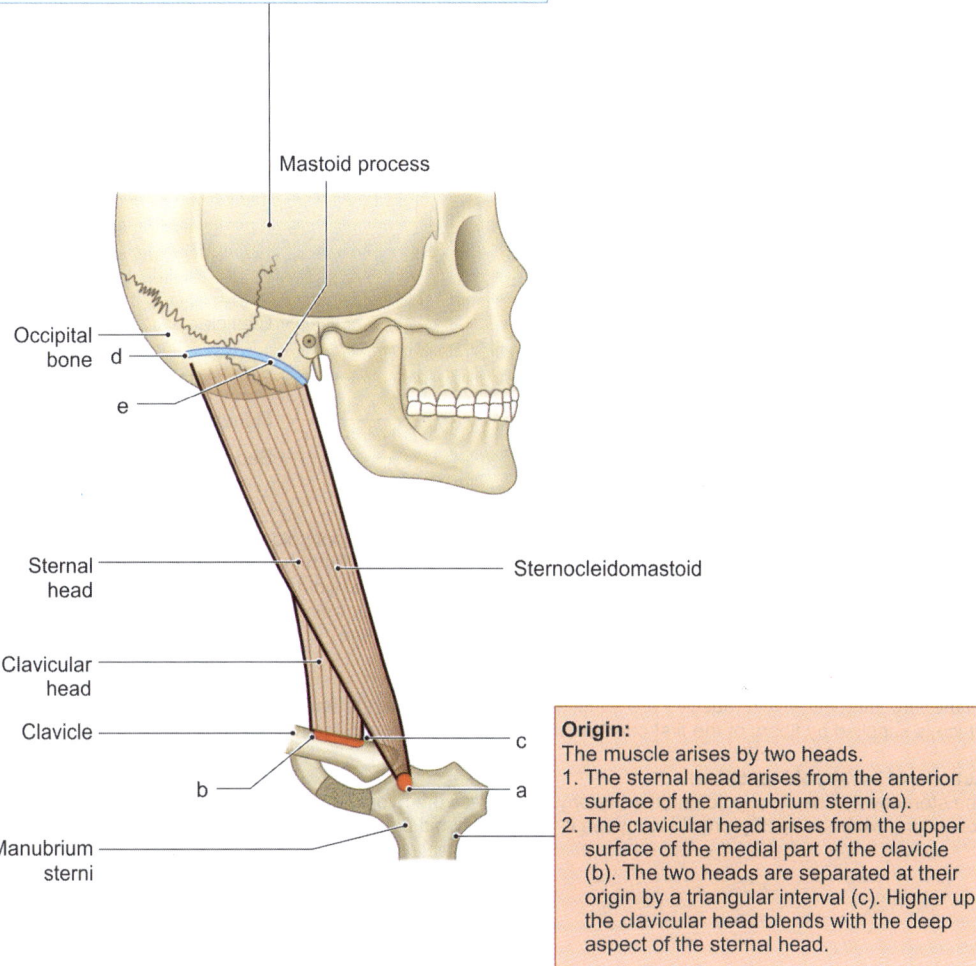

Origin:
The muscle arises by two heads.
1. The sternal head arises from the anterior surface of the manubrium sterni (a).
2. The clavicular head arises from the upper surface of the medial part of the clavicle (b). The two heads are separated at their origin by a triangular interval (c). Higher up the clavicular head blends with the deep aspect of the sternal head.

Relations:
The sternocleidomastoid forms an important landmark in the neck, and divides it into anterior and posterior triangles.

Plate 7
Infrahyoid Muscles

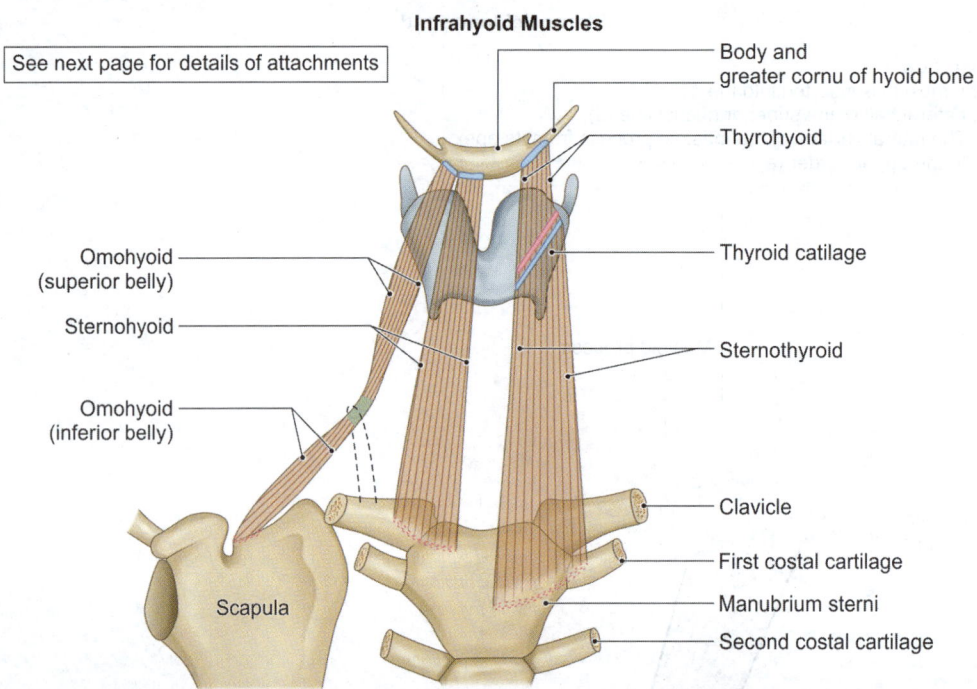

These are the sternohyoid, the sternothyroid, the thyrohyoid and the omohyoid muscles. The sternohyoid passes from the sternum to the hyoid bone. The sternothyroid passes from the sternum to the thyroid cartilage (of the larynx). The thyrohyoid passes from the thyroid cartilage to the hyoid bone. The omohyoid is made up of upper and lower bellies united by an intermediate tendon. The lower belly is attached to the scapula, and the upper belly to the hyoid bone. For details of attachments see next page.

Nerve supply of infrahyoid muscles:
All the foregoing infrahyoid muscles are supplied by branches from the ansa cervicalis except the thyrohyoid which is supplied by fibers of the first cervical nerve that travel through the hypoglossal nerve.

Actions of infrahyoid muscles:
The sternohyoid, the omohyoid and the thyrohyoid depress the hyoid bone. The sternothyroid pulls the larynx downward, whereas the thyrohyoid can raise it when the hyoid bone is fixed.

INFRAHYOID MUSCLES (DETAILS OF ATTACHMENTS)

Sternohyoid

Sternohyoid takes origin from:
- Posterior aspect of the manubrium sterni (upper part)
- Medial end of the clavicle (posterior aspect)
- Capsule of the sternoclavicular joint.

The fibers pass upward and medially; inserted into the body of the hyoid bone (lower border).

Thyrohyoid

- Arises from the oblique line on the lamina of the thyroid cartilage.
- Inserted into the lower border of the greater cornu of the hyoid bone.

Sternothyroid

- Arises from the posterior surface of the manubrium sterni below sternohyoid and from the medial end of the first costal cartilage.
- Inserted into the oblique line on the lamina of the thyroid cartilage just below the origin of the thyrohyoid.

Insertion of the sternothyroid corresponds to the origin of the thyrohyoid.

Omohyoid

Omohyoid has two bellies (superior and inferior); joined by an intermediate tendon.

Interior belly arises from a small area on the upper border of the scapula (near scapular notch). From here the inferior belly passes forward, upward, and medially across the floor of the posterior triangle. It ends deep to the sternocleidomastoid by joining the intermediate tendon.

Superior belly arises from the intermediate tendon and passes upward and medially to reach the hyoid bone.

It is inserted on the hyoid bone (lower border of the body, lateral to sternohyoid).

Intermediate tendon is kept in place by a band of deep fascia which stretches from the tendon to the clavicle.

Plate 8

Lateral Vertebral Muscles

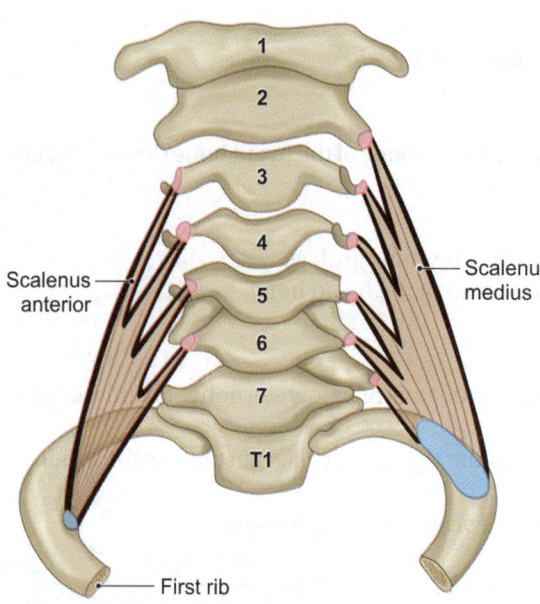

Scalenus Anterior

The scalenus anterior arises from the anterior tubercles of the transverse processes of vertebrae C3 to C6. It passes downward and laterally to be inserted into the inner border of the first rib (scalene tubercle) and to a ridge on its upper surface.

Nerve supply and action:

It is supplied by the ventral rami of spinal nerves C4, C5, and C6. It bends the neck forward and laterally and rotates it so that the face turns to the opposite side.

Scalenus Medius

The scalenus medius takes origin from the transverse process of the axis, and from the transverse processes (posterior tubercles) of vertebrae C3 to C7.
The muscle passes downward and laterally to be inserted into the upper surface of the first rib between its tubercle and the groove for the subclavian artery.

Nerve supply:

The scalenus medius is supplied by ventral rami of spinal nerves C3 to C8.

Action:

The muscle bends the cervical spine to its own side. It can raise the rib during forced inspiration.

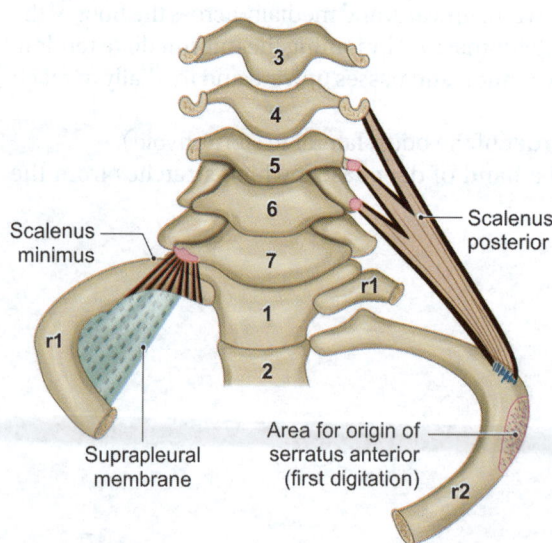

Scalenus Posterior

The scalenus posterior takes origin from the posterior tubercles of the transverse processes of vertebrae C4, C5, C6. Its fibers pass downward and laterally to be inserted into the outer surface of the second rib (behind the attachment of the serratus anterior).

Nerve supply and action:

The scalenus posterior is supplied by the ventral rami of spinal nerves C6, C7, C8. It bends the cervical spine to the same side. It can elevate the second rib.

Scalenus Minimus

The scalenus minimus is a small muscle arising from the transverse process of the seventh cervical vertebra. The fibers of the muscle spread out to be inserted into the inner border of the first rib in its posterior part. Some of its fibers are continuous with the suprapleural membrane, which is sometimes considered to be an expansion of the muscle.

Plate 9

Anterior Vertebral Muscles

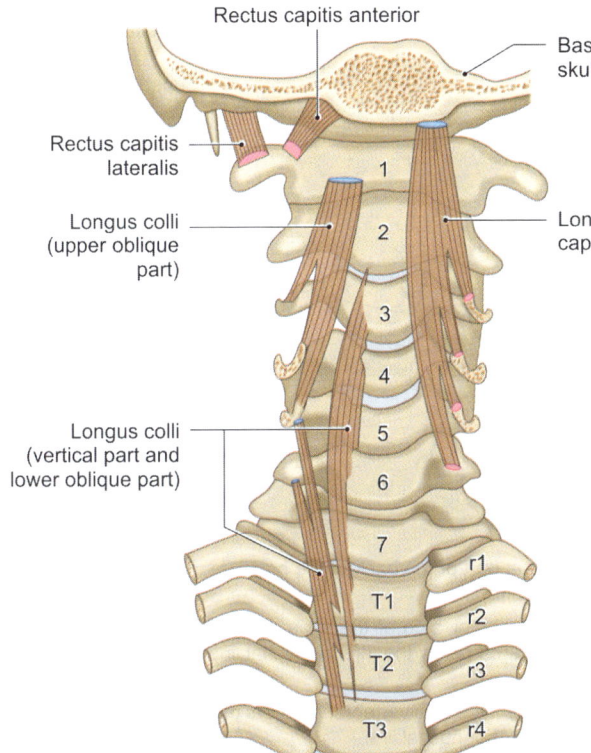

Rectus Capitis Anterior

The rectus capitis anterior arises from the atlas vertebra (lateral mass and root of transverse process).

It runs upward to gain insertion into the basilar part of the occipital bone.

The rectus capitis anterior is supplied by the ventral rami of spinal nerves C1 and C2. It is a flexor of the head.

Rectus Capitis Lateralis

The rectus capitis lateralis arises from the transverse process of the atlas.

It runs upward to the base of the skull where it is inserted into the jugular process of the occipital bone (just behind jugular fossa).

It is supplied by the ventral rami of spinal nerves C1 and C2. It bends the head to its own side.

Longus Colli

The longus colli is placed in front of the vertebral column. It extends vertically from the atlas above, to the third thoracic vertebra below. It consists of an upper oblique part, a middle vertical part, and a lower oblique part.

The upper oblique part runs upward and medially from the transverse processes (anterior tubercles) of vertebrae C3, C4, and C5 to the anterior arch of the atlas.

The vertical part arises from the bodies of vertebrae C5, C6, C7 and T1, T2, T3. It runs upward to be inserted into the bodies of vertebrae C2, C3, C4.

The inferior oblique part arises from the bodies of upper thoracic vertebrae and passes upward and laterally to the transverse processes (anterior tubercles) of vertebrae C5 and C6.

The longus colli is supplied by the ventral rami of cervical nerves C2 to C6. It is a flexor of the neck. It can help in lateral flexion and in rotation of the neck.

Longus Capitis

The longus capitis arises from the transverse processes (anterior tubercles) of cervical vertebrae (C3 to C6) and runs upward and medially to be inserted into the base of the skull, on the basilar part of the occipital bone.

Nerve supply and action:

The longus capitis is supplied by the ventral rami of spinal nerves C1, C2 and C3. It is a flexor of the head.

Plate 10

Suboccipital Muscles

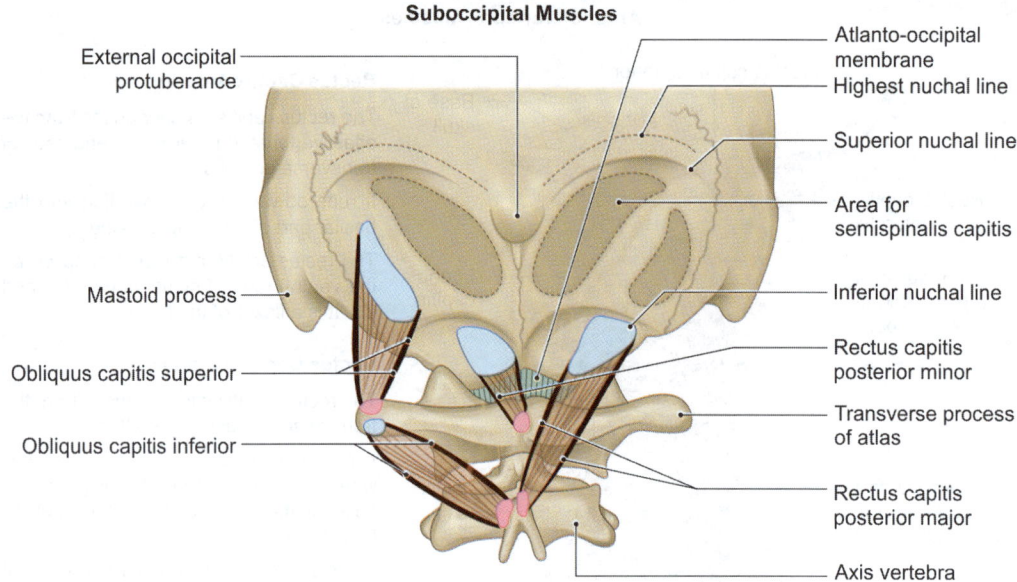

This is a group of small muscles placed in the uppermost part of the back of the neck, deep to the semispinalis capitis. They form the boundaries of the suboccipital triangle.

The **rectus capitis posterior minor** arises from the posterior arch of the atlas. Its fibers pass upward to be inserted into the occipital bone in the medial part of the area below the inferior nuchal line (i.e. between the line and the foramen magnum).

The **rectus capitis posterior major** arises from the spine of the axis vertebra. Its fibers pass upward and laterally to be inserted into the lateral part of the area below the inferior nuchal line.

The **obliquus capitis inferior** arises from the spine of the axis vertebra. Its fibers pass laterally and somewhat upward to be inserted into the transverse process of the atlas vertebra.

The **obliquus capitis superior** arises from the transverse process of the atlas. Its fibers pass upward (and somewhat medially) to be inserted into the lateral part of the area between the superior and inferior nuchal lines.

Nerve supply and actions:

The suboccipital muscles are supplied by the dorsal ramus of the first cervical nerve. The main action of the suboccipital muscles is to maintain the posture of the head. Note that the head tends to fall forward due to gravity. This is resisted by the two recti and the superior oblique which extend it. The obliquus capitis inferior rotates the head at the atlantoaxial joint turning the face to its own side. The rectus capitis posterior major can also produce slight rotation of the face to its own side. The superior oblique tilts the head laterally to its own side.

Plate 11

Erector Spinae

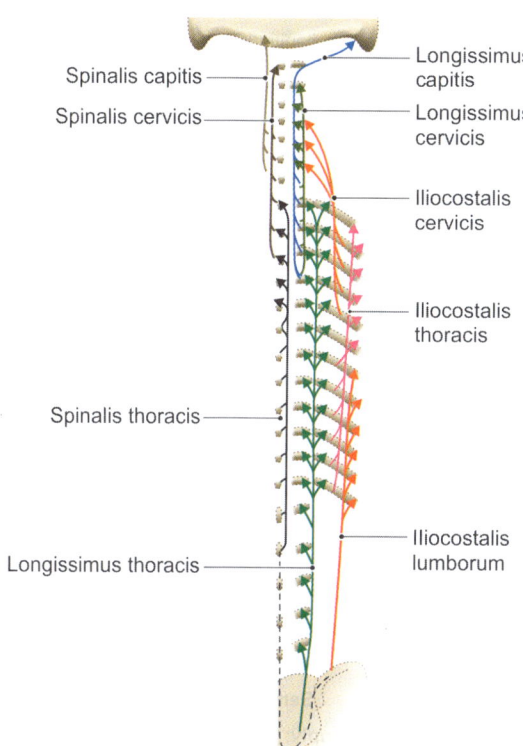

The erector spinae is deep to the splenius group and superficial to the semispinalis group. It consists of a lateral part, the iliocostocervicalis; an intermediate part called the longissimus; and a small medial part, the spinalis.

Origin:

The main origin of the muscle is from the back of the sacrum through a U-shaped tendon attached to the median and lateral sacral crests. The medial limb of the 'U' extends upward to the lumbar and lower thoracic spines. The lateral limb extends on to the dorsal part of the iliac crest and the sacrotuberous and sacroiliac ligaments (The origin is indicated by thick interrupted line in the lower part of figure).

The muscle mass passes upward and divides into three main parts.

The **spinalis** part is most medial and least developed. Its fibers pass from spines to spines. It is subdivided into the following:
1. The spinalis thoracis
2. The spinalis cervicis
3. The spinalis capitis.

The **longissimus** is the largest division of the erector spinae. It is subdivided into the following:
1. The longissimus thoracis
2. The longissimus cervicis
3. The longissimus capitis.

The **iliocostocervicalis** lies lateral to the longissimus and consists of:
1. The iliocostalis lumborum
2. The iliocostalis thoracis
3. The iliocostalis cervicis.

Note that out of the large muscle mass of the erector spinae only three slender slips (namely the iliocostalis cervicis, longissimus cervicis and longissimus capitis) reach the neck.

Nerve supply and actions of erector spinae:

The erector spinae is supplied by dorsal primary rami of spinal nerves.
As a whole the erector spinae is an extensor and lateral flexor of the vertebral column. The longissimus capitis turns the face to its own side.
The erector spinae is a very important postural muscle. In persons who lead a sedentary life, and with old age, the muscle becomes weak. The vertebral column then tends to bend forward. This puts excessive strain on ligaments of the vertebral column and also predisposes to prolapse of intervertebral discs. These are common causes of backache. Tone in the erector spinae can be maintained by exercises and also by brisk walking.

Atlas of Muscle Attachments: Head and Neck

Plate 12

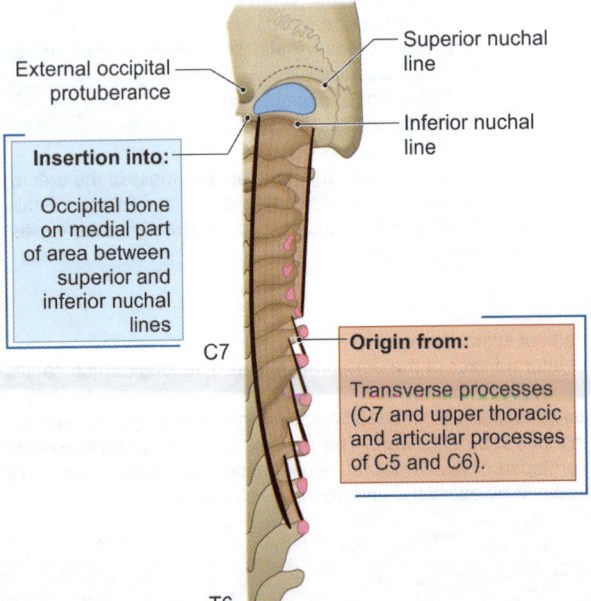

Splenius Capitis

Origin from:
Lower half of ligamentum nuchae
and
Vertebral spines C7 to T3

Insertion into:
Back of mastoid process (a)
and
Occipital bone below lateral one-third of superior nuchal line (b)

Splenius Capitis

Nerve supply:
The splenius capitis is supplied by dorsal rami of cervical nerves.

Action:
When the splenius capitis (and cervicis) of both sides contract the head is pulled backwards. When the muscles of one side contract the face is rotated to the same side.

The splenius capitis forms the (upper and posterior) part of the floor of the posterior triangle of the neck.

Semispinalis Capitis

Insertion into:
Occipital bone on medial part of area between superior and inferior nuchal lines

Origin from:
Transverse processes (C7 and upper thoracic and articular processes of C5 and C6).

Semispinalis Capitis

Nerve supply:
The semispinalis capitis is supplied by dorsal rami of cervical and thoracic spinal nerves.

Action:
The main action of the semispinalis capitis is to extend the head. It also has a slight rotatory action turning the face to the opposite side.

The muscle forms the roof of the suboccipital triangle.

Index

Page numbers followed by *f* refer to figure

A

Abdomen 225
　anterolateral muscles of 230
　external oblique muscle of 215, 228
　internal oblique muscle of 229
Abduction 2, 12, 67*f*, 68*f*
Abductor digiti minimi 62, 157
Abductor hallucis 154
Abductor pollicis
　brevis 61
　longus 41, 61, 102
Acanthion 273
Accessory meningeal artery 307
Accessory nerve 309
　spinal part of 244, 309
Acetabular notch 110
Acetabulum 17, 105, 110
Acromioclavicular joint 22
　articular capsules of 20
　capsule of 27
　dislocation of 22
Acromion process 23, 26
Adduction 2, 12, 67*f*, 68*f*
Adductor brevis 112, 119, 172
Adductor canal 171
Adductor hallucis 157, 205
Adductor longus 111, 119, 170
Adductor magnus 112, 119, 173
Adductor pollicis 62
Alaeque nasi 281
Alveolar index 327
Alveolar process 279, 322
Amphiarthroses 10
Ankle
　joint 132, 133, 162, 162*f*
　　articular capsules of 131
　　lateral ligament of 160
　　nerve supply of 132
　　superior extensor retinaculum of 131, 138
Annular ligament 39*f*, 43
Annulus fibrosus 239
Anterior atlanto-occipital membranes 300
Anterior cranial fossa 272, 300
　parts of 302*f*
Anterior cruciate ligament 121, 131

Anterior ethmoidal
　canal 306, 310
　foramina 283
　nerves 306
　sinus 314
　vessels 306
Anterior fontanel 276, 318, 320, 320*f*
Anterior gluteal line 108
Anterior inferior iliac spine 107
Anterior lacrimal crest 278
Anterior longitudinal ligament 240
Anterior nasal
　aperture 279, 311
　spine 279, 331
Anterior sacral foramina 255
Anterior superior iliac spine 106
Anteroinferior border 334
Anterolateral fontanel 318
Anthropoid 264
Appendicular skeleton 13
Arch, anterior 243
Arcuate eminence 303
Arm
　bone 30
　mechanism of abduction of 75
Arnold-Chiari syndrome 342, 342*f*
Artery 326
　articular 6
　epiphyseal 6
　medullary 6
　metaphyseal 6
Articular facets, direction of 238
Articularis genu 121
Articulations 7, 277, 284, 333, 336, 341, 346, 350, 353-356
Ascending pharyngeal artery, meningeal branch of 308, 309
Asterion 274, 287
Atavistic epiphysis 5
Atlantoaxial joints 246
Atlanto-occipital joint 243, 246, 299
Atypical cervical vertebrae 243
　features of 243
Atypical thoracic vertebrae 249, 250*f*
Auricular point 274
Auscultation, triangle of 28
Avascular necrosis 51
Axial skeleton 13

B

Ball and socket joints 12
Baseball finger 65
Bell's palsy 346, 347*f*
Biceps
　brachii 40, 43, 79
　femoris 112, 121, 137, 183
Bifid sternum 211, 212*f*
Bifurcate ligament 158
Biparietal diameter 319, 320*f*
Black eye 283, 283*f*
Body 109, 207, 209, 234, 252, 330, 333, 348, 350, 352, 356, 358*f*
　positions 1
Bone 4, 18, 105, 248
　cells 4
　flat plate of 355
　fusion 8
　general features of 4
　graft 115, 134, 140
　marrow 4
　　aspiration 115
　matrix 4
　temporal 13, 275, 285, 296, 318, 342
Bony orbit 281
Bony pelvis 17, 105, 261, 262
　types of 265
Brachialis 34, 37
Brachioradialis 34, 40, 43, 94
Breadth 274
Bregma 273, 276
Buccinator 360
Bucket
　handle movement 214*f*, 215
　handle tear 134, 134*f*
Bulla ethmoidale 311
Bunion 160

C

Calcaneocuboid joints 147
Calcaneofibular ligament 157
Calcaneus 17, 141, 158
Caldwell-Luc operation 332
Calvaria 272
Canaliculus, anterior 311
Canalis innominatus 307, 307*f*
Canine
　eminence 279
　fossa 279

Index

Capitulum 32
Carotid
　canal 298, 307, 308f, 345
　cavernous aneurysm 284
　groove 302
Carpal bones 15, 50
Carpal fractures 51
Carpal tunnel syndrome 56
Carpometacarpal joint 16, 60
Carrying angle 48, 49f
Cartilage 6, 7f
　epiphyseal plate of 5
　types of 6
　Y-shaped 114
Cartilaginous joint
　primary 10
　secondary 10
Cavernous sinus 307
Cavum trigeminale 303
Centrum 242
Cephalic index 274
Cerebellum, tonsil of 309
Cerebral surface 349
Cerebrospinal fluid 275
Cervical ligament 157
Cervical rib 218
　bilateral 218f
Cervical spondylosis 248
Cervical vertebra 235, 236, 243, 247
　articular facets of 239f
　fracture of 248
　second 245
　typical 236f
Cervicothoracic ganglion 218
Chin, prominence of 326
Chondrocytes 6
Circulus vasculosus 6
Circumduction 2
Clavicle 15, 18, 19
　fracture of 21
　medial end of 20f
　ossification 21f
　peculiarities of 18
Clavicular notches 207
Clavipectoral fascia 20
Claw foot 159, 159f
Cleft lip 332, 332f
Clergyman's knee 125, 125f
Club foot 159, 159f
Coccygeus 112
Coccyx 258
　dorsal aspect of 259f
　pelvic aspect of 259f
Cold abscess 250
Collar bone 18
Colles' fracture 42

Common peroneal nerve, palpation of 140
Complete tear 134f
Condylar joints 11
Conjoint ischiopubic ramus 109
Conjoint tendon 112
Conjunctiva 275
Conoid tubercle 18
Coracoacromial ligament 27
Coracobrachialis 34, 37, 80
Coracoclavicular ligament 27
　conoid part of 20
　parts of 22
　trapezoid part of 20
Coracoid process 23, 27
Cornua
　greater 356
　lesser 357
Corona sutures 9
Coronal suture 269, 285
Coronoid
　fossa 32
　process 44, 322
Corrugator supercilii 280
Costal cartilages 15, 213, 223, 224
Costal facets 235
Costochondral joints 216
Costoclavicular ligament 20, 21
Costodiaphragmatic recess 222
Costotransverse joints 216
　movements of 216
Costovertebral joints 216
　movements of 216
Coxa valga 122, 122f
Coxa vara 123, 123f
Cranial capacity 319
Cranial cavity 13, 272
　floor of 273f
Cranial fossae 272, 300
　floor of 310
Craniocleido-dysostosis 22, 22f
Craniometry 319
Cranium bones 269
Cribriform plate 300, 310
Crista galli 300, 353
Cruciform ligament, superior band of 309
Cubital tunnel syndrome 36
Cubitus valgus 48
Cuboid 159
　bone 146
Cuneiform, lateral 149, 159
Curvatures, primary 242

D

Dacryon 274
Deep fibers 119

Deep petrosal nerve 308
Deltoid 34, 75
　ligament 133, 160
　tuberosity 32
Demifacet 236
Dens
　alar ligaments of 300, 309
　apical ligament of 309
Dentate suture 9
Deviated nasal septum 316, 317f
Diaphragm 227
　attachments of 227
Diaphysis 4, 5
Digastric fossa 323
Digits 50
Dinner fork deformity 42
Diplopia 276
Dorsal digital expansions 62f, 63f, 98
Dorsal interossei 63, 93, 157, 160, 206
　attachments of 63f, 158f
Dorsal sacroiliac ligament 258
Dorsal scoliosis 251f
Dorsal tubercle 39
Dorsiflexion 133
Dorsum sellae 302
Dupuytren's ischemic contracture 65
Dura mater, outer layer of 8
Dural venous sinus thrombosis 276

E

Ectopia cordis 211, 211f
Elastic cartilage 7
Elbow
　dislocation of 48
　joint 67, 67f
　　capsular ligament of 34
　　capsule of 37, 43
　　radial collateral ligament of 37, 43
　　ulnar collateral ligament of 37, 43
Eleventh rib 220
　features 220
Eleventh thoracic vertebrae 249
Ellipsoid joints 11
Emissary sphenoidal foramen 303, 307, 349
Emissary veins 276, 307-309
Endosteum 4
Epicondyles, lateral 32
Epiphysis 5
　aberrant 5
　types of 5f

Index

Erector spinae 110, 371
 actions of 371
 nerve supply of 371
 part of 215
Ethmoid 269, 270
 bone 275, 311, 353
 parts of 316*f*
 cribriform plate of 310
Ethmoidal air sinuses 314
Ethmoidal infundibulum 314
Ethmoidal sinus 314
Eversion 3, 145
Extensor carpi radialis
 brevis 61, 96
 longus 34, 61, 95
Extensor carpi ulnaris 47, 61, 100
 tendon of 47
Extensor digiti minimi 99
Extensor digitorum 61, 97
 brevis 154, 188
 longus 137, 154, 187
Extensor hallucis
 brevis 154
 longus 137, 154, 186
Extensor indicis 103
Extensor pollicis
 brevis 41, 61, 103
 longus 61, 102
Extensor retinaculum 41, 64, 104
External occipital
 crest 284, 299
 protuberance 284, 299
Eyeball 284

F

Fabella 6
Face, length of 274
Facial bones 269
 fracture of 284
Facial nerve 310, 311
Facial skeleton 268
Fascia lata 112
Fawcett's method 253*f*
Female pelvis 263
 variants of 264
Femoral head
 fracture of 122
 ligaments of 121
Femoral neck, fracture of 122, 266
Femoral shaft, fracture middle third of 122
Femur 17, 116
 condyles of 5
 ossification 122*f*
 shaft of 171
Fetal skull 316, 317*f*

Fibers 43
 anterior 112
 posterior 112
Fibrocartilage 7
Fibrous capsule 258
Fibrous flexor sheath 64, 87, 158
Fibrous sheath 4
Fibula 135, 139
 fracture neck of 140, 140*f*
 ossification 140*f*
Fifth lumbar vertebra 252
Fissure, pterygomaxillary 290, 295, 306
Flail chest 223
Flat bone 207, 213
Flat foot 159, 159*f*
Flexion 2, 12, 67*f*, 68*f*, 240
 lateral 2
 opposite of 2
Flexor carpi
 radialis 60, 83
 ulnaris 47, 60, 84
Flexor digiti minimi 62
 brevis 157, 204
Flexor digitorum
 accessorius 154, 203
 brevis 154, 200
 longus 130, 154, 157, 197
 profundus 47, 60, 86
 superficialis 41, 43, 47, 60, 85
Flexor hallucis
 brevis 154, 204
 longus 137, 154, 196
Flexor pollicis
 brevis 62
 longus 41, 43, 47, 60, 88
Flexor retinaculum 56, 64, 89, 131, 158, 199
Fontanel 318
 posterior 276, 318
Foot 184
 articulated 105
 deformities of 159, 159*f*
 dorsal interossei of 206
 drop 140
 phalanges of 154
 plantar aspect of 154
 skeleton of 141, 142*f*, 143*f*
Foramen
 cecum 276, 300, 310, 335
 lacerum 295, 298, 302, 307, 308*f*
 magnum 298, 303, 309, 310*f*, 340
 ovale 303, 307, 307*f*, 349
 rotundum 302, 310
 spinosum 303, 307, 349
 transversarium 235, 243
Foramina 279, 286, 296, 305

Forearm 34
 muscles of
  anterior compartment of 60
  posterior compartment of 61
Fossa
 sublingual 323
 submandibular 323
 temporal 287
 trochanteric 117
 trochlear 281
Fracture 133, 320
 cervical vertebra 248*f*
 clavicle 22*f*
 femoral neck 122*f*
 orbital plate 276*f*
Frankfort plane 268
Free limb 15, 16
Frontal air sinuses 314
Frontal bone 13, 275, 278, 284, 316, 334
 fracture of 337
 orbital plate of 275
Frontal crest 300, 335
Frontomaxillary suture 277
Frontonasal suture 277
Frontosphenoid suture 285
Frontozygomatic suture 277
Frozen shoulder 29
Funnel chest 212*f*

G

Gastrocnemius 121, 133, 154, 193
Gemellus, superior 112
Giant cells 4
Ginglymus joints 11
Glabella 273
Gland
 sublingual 326
 submandibular 326
Glenoid
 cavity 23, 25
 labrum 27
Glossopharyngeal nerve 309
Gluteal line, posterior 108
Gluteal tuberosity 118
Gluteus maximus 110, 119, 174, 175
Gluteus medius 110, 119, 176
 paralysis of 266
Gluteus minimus 110, 119
 paralysis of 266
Gnathic index 327
Gnathion 273
Golfer's elbow 36, 37*f*
Gomphosis 8, 9, 10*f*
Gonion 274
Gracilis 128, 168

Index

Greater palatine
  canal 352
  foramina 294, 307
  nerves 307
Greater sciatic
  foramen 113
  notch 108, 109
Greater wing 287, 296, 349
Growth 318, 319
  endochondral 318
  mechanism of 318

H

Hallux valgus 160, 160*f*
Hallux varus 160
Hamate 55
  fracture of 65
Hand
  phalanges of 60, 60*f*
  skeleton of 50, 50*f*, 60
Hard palate 294
Harelip 332
Haversian canals 6
Head 30, 38, 213, 322
  and neck 360
    bones of 268
  circumference 318
  skeleton of 13
Hemorrhage, subconjunctival 275, 276*f*
Hiatus 303
  semilunaris 311, 314
Hilton's law 12
Hinge joints 11
Hip bone 16, 105, 113, 115*f*
  external aspect of 110
  fracture of 115, 115*f*
  internal aspect of 112
Hip joint 12, 17, 160, 161*f*
  capsule of 112, 121
  dislocated 266
Housemaid's knee 125, 125*f*
Human skeleton 13
Humerus 15, 30
  attachments 33
  head of 5
  ossification 35*f*
  supracondylar fracture of 36, 36*f*
  surgical neck of 35
Hyaline cartilage 7, 223
  joint 10
Hydrocephalus 342
Hyoid
  body of 358*f*
  bone 356, 356*f*, 357*f*
    greater cornu of 358*f*
Hypoglossal canal 303, 309
Hypophyseal fossa 302
Hypothenar muscles 62

I

Iliac crest 105, 110, 115
  vertical section 108*f*
  tubercle of 107
Iliac fossa 108, 261
Iliac tuberosity 108
Iliocostalis cervicis 215
Iliocostocervicalis 371
Iliopubic eminence 109
Iliotibial tract 131
Ilium 16, 105, 106, 110
Incisive fossa 279, 294, 322
Inferior extensor retinaculum 158
  upper limb of 131
Inferior iliac spine, posterior 108
Inferior nasal concha 269, 279, 311, 312*f*, 356
Inferior oblique capitis 245
Inferior orbital fissure 305, 306*f*
Inferior radioulnar joint 11, 67
  articular disc of 41, 43
Inferior tibiofibular joint 132
  interosseous ligament of 138
Inferior tympanic canaliculus, opening of 309*f*
Infraorbital canal 305
Infraorbital foramen 279, 282
Infraspinatus 34, 77
Infraspinous fossae 23
Infratemporal crest 289
Infratemporal fossa 289, 290*f*
Inguinal ligament 112
Injury, mechanism of 42
Intercarpal joints 16, 50
Interchondral joints 216
Interclavicular ligament 20, 21
Intercondylar eminence 126
Intercondylar notch 118
Intercostal muscles 225, 226
  actions of 225
  attachments of 225
  external 215
Intercostalis intimus 215
Intermaxillary suture 277, 294
Intermediate cuneiform 149, 159
Internal acoustic meatus 304, 310, 345
Internal intercostal
  membrane 215
  muscle 215
Internal jugular vein 309
Internal oblique abdominis 110
Internal occipital
  crest 304, 340
  protuberance 304, 340

Internasal suture 277
Interossei 157
  attachments of 62
Interosseous membrane 41, 43, 131, 138
Interosseous sacroiliac ligament 112, 258
Interosseous talocalcaneal ligament 158
Interosseous tibiofibular ligament 131, 131*f*
Interpalatine suture 294, 352
Interphalangeal joints 16, 17, 68, 68*f*, 162
Interspinous ligaments 240
Intertarsal joints 17
Intertransverse ligaments 240
Intertubercular sulcus 30, 34
  lateral lip of 31
  medial lip of 31
Intervertebral discs 234
Intervertebral foramina 235
Intervertebral joints, movements of 241
Intramembranous ossification 21, 248, 275
Intrinsic muscles, attachments of 154
Inversion 3, 145
Ischial ramus 110
Ischial spine 106, 109
Ischial tuberosity 109
Ischium 16, 105, 109, 110
  ramus of 109

J

Joints 7
  cartilaginous 10, 10*f*
  classification of 7, 8
  fibrocartilaginous 10
  fibrous 8
  fusion 29
  general features of 4
  nerve supply of 12
  trochoid 11
Jugular foramen 298, 299, 308, 308*f*
Jugular fossa 298
Jugum sphenoidale 300

K

Klippel-Feil syndrome 29, 248
Knee
  cap 124
  joint 11, 17, 161, 161*f*
    capsule of 121, 131
    fibular collateral ligament of 138
    menisci of 7
Kyphosis 250, 251*f*

Index

L
Lacrimal bone 311, 312f, 354
Lacrimal fossa 281, 336
Lacrimal hamulus 354
Lacunar ligament 112
Lambdoid suture 9, 269, 285
Lamina 234, 237
Lateral incisive foramina 294, 307
Lateral meniscus
    anterior horn of 131
    posterior horn of 131
Lateral pterygoid 299, 363
    muscles, nerve supply of 363
    plate 296
Lateral vertebral muscles 368
Latissimus dorsi 34, 73, 110, 215
Left iliac fossa 113
Left winged scapula 29f
Leg 184
    tendons, insertion of 154
Lesser palatine
    foramina 294, 307, 352
    nerves 307
Lesser pelvis, cavity of 261
Lesser petrosal nerve 307, 310
    hiatus for 303
Lesser sciatic
    foramen 114
    notch 109
Levator anguli oris 281
Levator ani 112, 233
    nerve supply of 233
Levator costae 215
Levator labii superioris 281
Levator palati 299
Levator scapulae 74, 245
Ligamenta flava 240
Ligaments 21, 23, 27, 30, 43, 49, 116, 123, 126, 134, 141, 144, 157, 160, 244, 246, 258, 260, 325, 329, 347
    accessory 11
    true 11
Ligamentum
    nuchae 300
    patellae 126
Limbus suture 8
Linea
    aspera 171
    terminalis 261
Lingual nerve block 328
Lingula 322
Lithotomy position 1
Long bone 30
    blood supply of 6
    modified 18
    nerve supply of 4
    parts of 4, 5f
Long plantar ligament 158, 160
Longissimus 371
Longitudinal ligament, posterior 240
Longus
    capitis 299, 369
    colli 245, 369
Lordosis 251f
Lower limb 163
    bones of 105
    joints, major 160
    skeleton of 16
Lower motor neuron 346
Lumbar scoliosis 251f
Lumbar vertebra 235, 236, 243, 252
    articular facets of 239f
    atypical 252
    features of 252
    identification of 253f
    sacralization of 252
    typical 237f
Lumbrical muscles 89
Lunate 52
    articulates 53
    surface 110
Lungs 220

M
Male pelvis 262
Malleolar fossa 135, 136
Mallet finger 65, 66f
Mandible 269, 318, 322, 322f, 325, 326
    fracture of 328
    median part of 324f
    right half of 323f
Mandibular canal 322
Mandibular foramen 322
Mandibular fossa 296
Mandibular nerve
    block 329f
    meningeal branch of 307
Mandibular notch 322
Manubriosternal joint 207, 208, 211
    movements of 211
Manubrium 207
    sterni 16f
March fracture 159, 159f
Masses, lateral 243
Mastoid
    antrum 344
    canaliculus 299, 309, 309f, 345
    fontanel 318
    foramen 286, 307, 344
    notch 298
    process 287, 296, 343
Maxilla 269-271, 275, 278, 285, 329, 331
    medial aspect of 312f
Maxillary air sinus 314
Maxillary artery 306
Maxillary hiatus 311
Maxillary nerve 306
Maxillary sinusitis 332, 332f
Maxillary tuberosity 293
McEvan's triangle 347, 347f
Meatus, inferior 311
Medial cuneiform 148, 159
Medial epicondyle 32, 35
Medial intermuscular septa 34
Medial ligament 133
Medial malleolus 126
Medial meniscus
    anterior horn of 131
    posterior horn of 131
Medial patellar retinacula 126
Medial pterygoid 299, 363
    muscles, nerve supply of 363
    plate 295
Medial supracondylar ridges 32
Median atlantoaxial joint 11
Median atlanto-occipital joint 244, 245
Median sacral crest 256
Mediastinum
    anterior 209
    boundaries of 208
    inferior 209
    middle 209
    posterior 208, 209
    superior 209
Medulla, lower end of 309
Membrana tectoria 309
Meningeal artery, middle 307
Meninges 244, 309
Meningitis 276
Meniscal tears 134, 134f
Mental foramen 322
    direction of 326
Mental protuberance 323
Mental tubercle 322, 323
Metacarpals 15, 56, 59
    parts of 56
Metacarpophalangeal joint 16, 65, 68, 68f, 162
Metaphysis 5
Metatarsals 17, 150, 153
    bones, articulations of 151f
    identification of 152
Metatarsophalangeal joints 17
Metopic suture 275, 336, 337f

Middle cranial fossa 272, 290f, 301, 302
  anterior wall of 303f
  fracture of 276
Middle ethmoidal sinus 314
Miner's elbow 48
Movements 2, 3f, 65, 258, 326
  demonstration of 214, 215
  mechanism of 214, 215
  sequence of 148
Muscles 19, 23, 27, 30, 34, 37, 40, 41, 43, 47, 49, 60-62, 110, 112, 116, 119, 121, 126, 128, 130, 134, 141, 144, 154, 160, 208, 215, 219, 221, 224, 245, 246, 259, 291, 299, 323, 324, 329, 347, 357
  anterior vertebral 369
  attachments 110
    atlas of 69, 163, 225, 260
  infrahyoid 366, 367
  insertion 40, 45
  origin 41, 47
Musculus uvulae 299
Mylohyoid groove 323

N
Naegele's pelvis 266
Nasal
  apertures, posterior 294, 311
  bone 355
  cavity 311, 314, 315f
    communicates 314
    lateral wall of 313f, 315f
  conchae, middle 279
  crest 352
  index 316
  septum 313f
  spine, posterior 294, 352
Nasion 273, 278
Nasolacrimal canal 305, 314
Nasomaxillary suture 277
Nasopalatine nerve 306
Navicular bone 146
Neck 213
Nerve 326
Neurocentral joints 242
Norma basalis 271, 292, 293f, 299, 301f
Norma frontalis 269, 277, 280, 280f
  features of 268
Norma lateralis 270, 284, 288f, 291, 292f
Norma occipitalis 284
Norma verticalis 269, 276
Nose, lateral wall of 312f
Nuchal lines, superior 284

Nucleus pulposus 239
Nutrient artery 6

O
Oblique cord 41
Obturator externus 112, 119, 180
Obturator foramen 105, 110
Obturator groove 109
Obturator internus 112, 119, 178
Obturator membrane 110
Obturator surface 109
Occipital artery, meningeal branch of 309
Occipital bone 13, 275, 284, 285, 298, 318, 340, 340f, 341f
Occipital condyles 299
Occipital veins 309
Occipitomastoid suture 284, 287, 299, 344
Olecranon fossa 32
Omohyoid 367
Ophryon 274
Opisthion 274
Opisthocranion 273
Opponens
  digiti minimi 62
  pollicis 62
Optic canal 283, 283f, 302, 305, 306f, 349
Optic chiasma 301
Orbicularis oculi 280
Orbit 282, 282f, 305
  lateral wall of 306
  medial wall of 306
  walls of 306
Orbital index 283
Orbital margins 281
Orbital process 352
Orbital surface 334
Orbital walls 281
Osseous tissue 4
Ossification 21, 28, 28f, 35, 42, 48, 64, 115f, 121, 132, 139, 158, 210, 248, 258, 334, 339, 346, 354, 356, 358
  laws of 6
Osteoblasts 4
Osteoclasts 4
Osteocollagenous fibers 4
Osteocytes 4
Osteology 1
Osteomyelitis, acute 133
Osteoprogenitor cells 4

P
Painful arc syndrome 29
Palatine bone 311, 312f, 351
  overlapping maxilla 312f

Palatine crest 294, 352
Palatomaxillary suture 294, 331
Palatovaginal canal 295, 353
Palm 50
Palmar interossei 63, 92
  attachments of 62f, 158f
Paranasal sinuses 314
  openings of 315f
Parietal bone 13, 275, 285, 316, 337
  fracture of 339
Parietal emissary foramen 307, 339, 339f
Parietomastoid suture 284, 285, 287
Parietosphenoid suture 285
Parietosquamous sutures 285
Parotid gland 326
Patella 6, 17, 124
Patellar retinacula, lateral 126
Pectineus 111, 169
Pectoral girdle 15
Pectoralis major 34, 69
Pectoralis minor 70, 215
Pedicles 234, 236, 252
Pelvic
  aperture, inferior 261
  brim 261
  cavity, boundaries of 261
  girdle 16
  inlet 262
    boundaries of 261
    orientation of 263f
  outlet 262
    boundaries of 261
    orientation of 263f
  part 108
  surface 109
Pelvis 261f-263f
  contracted 266
  diameters 262
  false 262
  fracture of 266
  greater 261
  orientation 262
  sagittal section of 263f
  skeleton of 17f
  true 262
  types 265
Periosteum 4, 6
Peroneal retinacula 158
Peronei 160
Peroneus
  brevis 137, 154, 160, 192
  longus 137, 154, 160, 191
  tertius 137, 154, 160, 189
Pertrochanteric fracture 122
Pes cavus 159
Pes planus 159
Petromastoid element 275

Index

Petrosal nerve, greater 303, 308
Petrosal sinus, inferior 308
Petrosquamous fissure 297
Petrotympanic fissure 297, 311
Phalanges 15, 17
    parts of 56
Pharynx, superior constrictor of 300
Pigeon chest 212*f*
Piriformis 111, 119, 177
Pisiform 6, 53, 54
    peculiarities of 54
Pivot joint 11, 38, 39, 44, 45, 245
Plantar 142
    aponeurosis 202
    calcaneonavicular ligament 158
    interossei 160, 206
Plantaris 154
Platypelloid 264
Platysma 364
Pleural tap 222
Pond fracture 320, 320*f*
Popliteal surface 118
Posterior arch 243
Posterior atlanto-occipital
        membranes 300
Posterior auricular artery,
        stylomastoid branch of 310
Posterior condylar canal 299, 303, 310
Posterior cranial fossa 273, 303, 304*f*
    fracture of 276
    parts of 302*f*
Posterior cruciate ligament 121, 131
Posterior ethmoidal
    canal 306, 310
    foramina 283
    nerves 306
    sinus 314
    vessels 306
Postsphenoid 350
Pott's fracture 140, 140*f*
Pott's spine 250, 251*f*
Preauricular sulcus 108
Premaxilla 294
Prepatellar bursitis 125
Presphenoid 350
Pressure epiphysis 5
Prolapsed intervertebral disc 248, 248*f*
Pronation 3
Pronator
    quadratus 40, 43, 47
    teres 34, 40, 47, 82
Prosthion 273
Psoas
    abscess 250
    major 119, 163
    minor 112, 163

Pterion 274, 339, 339*f*
Pterygoid
    canal, nerve of 308
    fovea 322
    hamulus 296
    process 285, 295, 296*f*, 349
    venous plexus 307
Pterygomandibular ligament 300
Pterygopalatine fossa 290, 291*f*
Pterygospinous ligament 300
Pubic
    arch 110
    crest 109
    symphysis 17, 105
    tubercle 106, 109, 114
Pubis 16, 105, 109, 110
    posterior surface of 113
    superior ramus of 106
    symphyseal surface of body of 106
Pump handle movement 214, 214*f*
Pyramidal process 285, 294, 352
Pyramidalis 111

Q

Quadrate ligament 43
Quadratus
    femoris 112, 119, 167
    lumborum 110, 232
Quadriceps femoris 128, 166
    components 126
Quadrilateral sternal end 18

R

Rachitic flat pelvis 266
Radial collateral ligaments 34
Radial fossa 32
Radial groove 32, 35
Radial head 41
    subluxation of 42
Radial tuberosity 38
Radioulnar joints 67*f*
Radius 15, 37, 40
    lower end of 41
    ossification 42*f*
Ramus 109, 322
    inferior 109
    superior 106, 109
Rectus abdominis 111, 231
Rectus capitis
    anterior 245, 299, 369
    lateralis 245, 300, 369
    posterior
        major 300
        minor 245, 300
Rectus femoris 110
Reid's base line 268

Ribs 207, 216, 217*f*
    anterior end of 213
    atypical 216
    false 213
    fracture of 223
    movements of 214
    notching of 222, 223*f*
    ossification 216
    true 213
Rider's bone 115
Right calcaneus 144*f*
Right carpus 51*f*
Right clavicle 18*f*-20*f*
Right cuboid bone 147*f*
Right femur 117*f*-120*f*
    attachments 120*f*
Right fibula 135*f*, 136*f*
    attachments 138*f*, 139*f*
    transverse section shaft of 137*f*
Right foot, skeleton of 155*f*
Right hamate 55*f*
Right hand, skeleton of 61*f*, 64*f*
Right hip bone 106*f*, 107*f*
    attachments 111*f*, 113*f*
    medial part of 108*f*
Right humerus 33*f*
    upper end of 32*f*, 33*f*
Right iliac fossa 113
Right intermediate cuneiform bone 149*f*
Right ischial tuberosity 108*f*
Right lateral cuneiform bone 150*f*
Right lower limb 17*f*
Right lunate 52*f*
Right maxilla 330*f*
Right medial cuneiform bone 148*f*
Right navicular bone 146*f*
Right palatine bone 352*f*
Right parietal bone 338*f*
Right patella 124*f*
Right pisiform 53*f*
Right radius 38*f*, 40*f*
    lower end of 40*f*, 41*f*
Right scaphoid 52*f*
Right scapula 24*f*-26*f*
    upper part of 25*f*
Right talus 145*f*
Right temporal bone 343*f*-345*f*
Right tibia 127*f*, 129*f*-131*f*
    upper end of 128*f*
Right trapezium 54*f*
Right ulna 44*f*, 46*f*
    lower end of 47*f*
    upper end of 46*f*
Right zygomatic bone 333*f*
Road traffic accidents 115

Index

Root, anterior 237
Rostrum 295
Rudimentary spine 244

S

Sacral
  hiatus 256
  index 257
  promontory 255
  vertebra 252
Sacroiliac joint 257, 257f
  capsule of 112
  movements of 257
Sacropelvic surface 108
Sacrospinous ligament 112
Sacrotuberous ligament 112
Sacrum 255, 255f-257f, 260
  dorsal aspect of 259f
  pelvic aspect of 259f
Saddle joints 12
Safety valve hematoma 277
Sagittal suture 9, 285
Salivary glands 326
Sartorius 110, 128, 165
Scalenus
  anterior 368
  medius 368
  minimus 368
  posterior 368
Scaphoid 51
  fossa 295
  fracture 51, 52f
  scapula 29
Scapula 15, 23, 28
  coracoid process of 5
  head of 25
  inferior angle of 28
  ossification of 28f
  winging of 28
Schindylesis 8, 9, 10f
Scoliosis 250
Second rib 219, 219f
  superior aspect of 219f
Sellar joints 12
Semimembranosus 182
Semispinalis capitis 300, 372
Semitendinosus 112, 128, 181
Serrate suture 9
Serratus anterior 71, 215
Sesamoid bone 6, 17, 124
  largest 124
Seventh cervical vertebra 247
Short plantar ligament 158
Shoulder
  arthrodesis 29
  blade 23
  cuff muscles 37
  girdle 15
  bones of 15f
  joint 12, 65, 66f
    arthrodesis of 29f
    capsular ligament of 34
    capsule of 27, 37
    dislocation of 36, 36f
Sigmoid sinus 309
  lower end of 309
Sigmoid sulcus 304
Sinus tarsi 142
Sinusitis 337
Skeleton 13
Skull 14f, 268, 269f-272f, 276, 277, 284, 285f, 287f, 293
  anatomical position of 268
  bones 269
  classification 274
  foramina of 305
  functions 271
  growth of 318
  individual bones of 322
  lateral aspect of 286f
  measurements 274
  methods of study of 268
  ossification 275
  preliminary review of 13
Smith-Petersen fracture 42, 43f
Socket joint 9
Soleus 154
Spermatic cord 115
Sphenoid 270, 271, 295
  body of 350, 352
  bone 275, 296f, 297, 348, 348f
  greater wing of 287, 296
  spine of 351, 351f
Sphenoidal air sinuses 314, 349
Sphenoidal concha 349
Sphenoidal fontanel 318
Sphenomandibular ligament 300
Sphenopalatine foramen 306, 314, 352
Spheroidal joints 12
Sphincter urethrae 112
Spina bifida 252, 254f
  occulta 253
Spinal artery
  anterior 244, 309
  posterior 244, 309
Spinal cord 244
  compression of 251
Spinalis 371
Spine 234, 255, 289
  crest of 26
  deformities 251f
  root of 26
Spinoglenoid notch 23, 26
Spinous process 23, 26, 234, 237, 252
Splenius
  capitis 372
  cervicis 245
Spondylolisthesis 253
Spondylolysis 253
Sprengel's deformity 29, 29f
Spring ligament 158, 160
Squamomastoid suture 287
Squamotympanic fissure 289, 296, 297
Squamous suture 8
Squint 276
Stephanion 274
Sternal angle 207, 210
Sternal foramen 211
Sternal fracture 212
Sternal puncture 211
Sternebrae 207
Sternoclavicular joint 207, 208
  articular
    capsules of 20
    disc of 20, 21
  capsule of 21
Sternoclavicular ligaments
  anterior 21
  posterior 21
Sternocleidomastoid 365
Sternocostalis 226
Sternohyoid 367
Sternothyroid 367
Sternum 207, 208f, 209, 210f
  body of 209
  ossification 211f
  salient features of 207
Stress fracture 159
Student's elbow 48, 49f
Styloglossus muscle 293
Stylohyoid
  ligament 293, 356, 358, 359
  muscle 293
Styloid process 39, 44, 58, 135, 293, 296, 346
Stylomandibular ligament 293
Stylomastoid foramen 298, 310, 344
Stylopharyngeus muscle 293
Subcostales 226
Subcutaneous infrapatellar bursitis 125
Suboccipital muscle 370
Subscapularis 34
Subtalar joints 145, 162, 162f
Sulcus
  calcanei 142
  chiasmaticus 301
  tali 142

Index

Superciliary arch 278
Superficial flexors 34
Superficial inguinal ring 115
Superficial transversus perinei 112
Superior iliac spine, posterior 106
Superior oblique capitis 245, 300
Superior orbital fissure 282, 283f, 302, 305, 306, 349
Superior peroneal retinaculum 138
Superior radioulnar joints 11, 67
Superior sagittal sinus 340
Superior tibiofibular joint 132, 135
   capsule of 131, 138
Supinator 43, 101
   crest 44
Supine position 1
Supraglenoid tubercle 25
Supramastoid crest 286
Suprameatal triangle 289
Supraorbital nerve, compression of 284
Suprascapular ligament 27
Supraspinatus 34, 76
   syndrome 29
Supraspinous fossae 23
Supraspinous ligaments 240
Surgical neck 31, 35
Sutural bones 284
Sutural growth 318
Sutural ligament 8
Sutures 8, 9f, 284
   closure of 319
Symphysis 10, 207
   menti 323, 325f, 328
Synarthrosis 8
Synchondrosis 10, 207
Syndesmosis 8, 9, 10f
Synostosis 10
Synovial joints 11, 11f, 207, 224, 239, 246
   morphological classification of 11
   types of 12f
Synovial membrane 132
Synovial sheaths 87

T

Talipes
   calcaneus 159
   equinovarus 159
   equinus 159
   valgus 159
   varus 159
Talocrural joint 133
Talofibular ligaments
   anterior 157
   posterior 138, 157

Talonavicular joints 147
Talus 159
Tarsal bones 17
Tarsometatarsal joints 17
Tear, incomplete 134f
Teeth eruption 327
Tegmen tympani 297, 303
Temporalis 361
Temporomandibular joint 11, 268, 326, 327f
   dislocation of 328, 328f
Tendocalcaneus 133
Tendon 47, 154
Tennis elbow 36, 37f
Tensor
   fasciae latae 110, 164
   palati 299
   tympani 299
Tenth thoracic vertebrae 249
Teres
   major 34, 78
   minor 34
Thenar muscles 61
Thigh, deep fascia of 112
Thoracic cage, movements of 214, 214f
Thoracic inlet syndrome 209, 218
Thoracic vertebrae 235, 236, 237f, 249, 249f, 250
   articular facets of 239f
Thorax 225
   skeleton of 14, 15f
Thumb joint 60
Thyrohyoid 367
   membrane 358, 359
Tibia 17, 126, 131, 134
   ossification 132f
   upper end of 121
Tibial collateral ligament 131
Tibial fracture 133f
Tibial tuberosity 126
Tibialis
   anterior 130, 154, 185
   posterior 130, 137, 154, 160, 198
Tibiocalcaneal ligaments 133
Tibiofibular joint 17, 132
   middle 132
Tibiofibular ligaments, posterior 138
Tibionavicular ligaments 133
Tibiotalar ligament
   anterior 133, 157
   posterior 133, 157
Traction epiphysis 5
Transpyloric plane 242
Transverse
   axis 11, 133
   ligament 243

   patellar fracture 125
   plane 2
   process 235, 237, 249, 252
   sinus 340
   sulcus 304
   tarsal joints 147
Transversus abdominis 110, 230
Trapezius 72, 300
Trapezoid 8, 54
Trendelenburg's sign, positive 266
Triceps 34, 37, 81
Trigeminal nerve, mandibular division of 307
Trochanter
   greater 117
   lesser 117
Trochlea 32
Trochlear articular surface 144
Trochlear notch 32, 44
Tubercle 107, 213, 296
   anterior 237, 244
   articular 296
   genial 323
   greater 30
   infraglenoid 25
   jugular 303, 341
   lesser 30
   pharyngeal 299, 341
   posterior 237, 244
   postglenoid 288, 296
Tuberculum sellae 302
Tuberosity 146
Twelfth thoracic vertebrae 249
Tympanic canaliculus 299, 309
Tympanic plate 289, 296, 297, 346
Tympanomastoid fissure 309
Typical ribs 213, 215
   salient features of 213
Typical vertebra 234, 242
   salient features of 234

U

Ulna 43
   attachments 45
   ossification 48f
   transverse section middle of shaft of 45f
Ulnar collateral ligaments 34, 37, 43
Ulnar head 47
Ulnar nerve, palpation of 35
Ulnar notch 39
Upper limb 69, 131
   bones of 18
   joints, major 65
   measurement of 22
   skeleton of 15, 16f

Urogenital diaphragm
   inferior fasciae of 112
   superior fasciae of 112

V

Vagus nerve 309
Vastus
   intermedius 121
   lateralis 121
   medialis 121
Ventral sacroiliac ligament 258
Vertebrae 235, 239
   fracture of 251
Vertebral arch 234
Vertebral artery 244, 309
Vertebral bodies 236
Vertebral canal 234
Vertebral column 14, 14f, 234
   curvatures 241, 241f
   development 242
   intervertebral movements 241
   movements 240, 241f
   ossification 242

Vertebral foramen 234, 236
Vertebrochondral ribs 15
Vertebropelvic ligaments 258
Vertebrosternal ribs 15
Vertical index 274
Vessels 306
Vestibule, aqueduct of 304, 345
Volkmann's ischemic contracture 36
Vomer 269, 294, 355
Vomerovaginal canal 295

W

Whitnall tubercle 281
Wings, lesser 349
Wormian bones 284
Wrist 50
   joint 67, 67f
      articular capsules of 41

X

Xiphisternal joint 207, 211
   movements of 211
Xiphoid process 207, 209

Z

Zygoma, tubercle of root of 296
Zygomatic
   arch 270, 288, 289f
      formation of 288
   bone 285, 333
   process 290f, 296, 330, 331, 336, 343
Zygomaticofacial
   foramen 279, 283, 306
   nerves 306
   vessels 306
Zygomaticomaxillary suture 277
Zygomaticotemporal
   foramen 283, 286, 306
   nerves 306
   vessels 306
Zygomaticus
   major 280
   minor 280